THE FEEDING WEB:

ISSUES IN
NUTRITIONAL ECOLOGY

THE FEEDING WEB:
ISSUES IN
NUTRITIONAL ECOLOGY

Joan Dye Gussow, Ed.D.

BULL PUBLISHING CO.

BERKELEY SERIES IN NUTRITION

Food for Sport, Nathan J. Smith, M.D. (1976)

Realities of Nutrition, Ronald M. Deutsch (1976)

The Feeding Web, Joan Dye Gussow (1978)

The Berkeley Series in Nutrition is a series of significant books about foods and nutrition, as they relate to the health and well being of people. It is our intent that all publications in this series will be carefully reviewed and evaluated before publication, to insure that the information is consistent with the current understanding of scientific research studies and practices in nutrition as it relates to the needs of humans.

Some books will provide an overview of the subject for the reader wanting reliable non-technical information. Others will be useful as college text books in non-major and major courses in nutrition. Still other books in the series are expected to contain specialized, technical information, for the professional in food and nutrition and related fields.

George M. Briggs, Ph.D.
Professor of Nutrition
Biochemist, Agriculture Experiment Station
University of California, Berkeley

Helen D. Ullrich, M.A., R.D.
Editor, Journal of *Nutrition Education*
Lecturer in Nutrition
University of California, Berkeley
Editors

Cover design: Joseph del Gaudio
Interior design: Anita Walker Scott
Composition: The Bookmakers, Inc.
Printing: Delta Lithograph Company

Printed in the United States of America

© Copyright 1978
Bull Publishing Co.
P.O. Box 208
Palo Alto, California 94302

ISBN 0-915950-15-4 paper
ISBN 0-915950-14-6 cloth
Library of Congress Catalog No. 78-8579

Trade distribution in U.S. by Hawthorn Books, Inc.
In Canada by Prentice-Hall of Canada

To my mother and father who taught me not to be afraid of hard work—or controversy; to my husband who gave me the confidence to try to save the world; and to my sons, Adam and Seth, for whose sake, among others, I am trying to save it.

Other Nutrition Books by BULL

Ronald M. Deutsch, *The Fat Counter Guide*

Ronald M. Deutsch, *The New Nuts Among the Berries*

Ronald M. Deutsch, *Realities of Nutrition*

James M. Ferguson, M.D. and C. Barr Taylor, M.D., *A Change for Heart*

James M. Ferguson, M.D., *Habits, Not Diets*

James M. Ferguson, M.D., *Learning to Eat*

James L. Free, *Just One More*

Bob Gaillard, William Haskell, Ph.D., Nathan J. Smith, M.D., Bruce Ogilvie, Ph.D., *Handbook for the Young Athlete*

Joyce Nash, Ph.D. and Linda Ormiston, Ph.D., *Taking Charge of Your Weight and Well-Being*

Jean Pennington, Ph.D., *Nutritional Diet Therapy*

Barbara Shannon, Ph.D., *Student Supplement for Realities of Nutrition*

Nathan J. Smith, M.D., *Food for Sport*

Albert J. Stunkard, M.D., *I Almost Feel Thin*

Albert J. Stunkard, M.D., *The Pain of Obesity*

Acknowledgements

The "author" of any book made up in large part of the words of other people must first acknowledge her debt to those who have put their thoughts to paper. My thanks to all those whose words are here reproduced; thanks for writing them, thanks for letting them be here incorporated— frequently at less than their originally intended length. All of you together—including (perhaps especially) those of you with whom I disagree—have shaped my own thinking and I am grateful for your permission to send your words out in this volume where they may, perhaps, shape the thinking of others.

My second debt is to all those writers whose work does *not* appear in these pages though it has frequently appeared in the course from which this book derives. Books are shorter than courses as it turns out. And they are also different. It is possible—and perhaps even desirable—to make students wade through impenetrable thickets of prose to find the tree of knowledge. Readers are, alas, seldom so inclined. In the end, I also had to cut, for a variety of reasons not interesting enough to report on, a number of pieces which were both well written and in their own way important. Some of those authors wrote such nice permission letters that I found the final choices painfully hard.

Colleagues and friends have sometimes looked at the reading lists for my nutritional ecology course and asked, "How did you find all these things?" The answer is, "I didn't." Over the years friends and acquaintances (among them students, ex-students, colleagues, and other friends—and even adversaries) have sent me copies of articles that they thought would interest me. It has occurred to me that I might transform this acknowledgment into a kind of provenance for the book—"This article, originally out of the collection of Countess X, has come to us by way of a poor photo copy from the hand of Dr. Y in whose collection it has resided for three years...The torn edge suggests it was originally ripped from a journal, not, presumably, from a library copy..." With some effort it would probably be possible to recall from whose hand each of the inclusions reached mine but it would be unfair; for all those other articles, often equally important and equally influential in the development of my thinking (though not just right for this book), would go unacknowledged.

I must, however, acknowledge at least one of the sources of the material herein, for she provided me not only with readings but with a model of openness and excitement in teaching. The very first version of this course was a joint venture between Eleanor Williams and myself. She is the source of (at least) the wonderful Philip Wylie assault on contemporary food (page 163), of the equally wonderful Magnus Pyke article on the social effects of food technology (page 186), and of the Richard Koff article on the end of the world (page 6) which first ran in *Playboy*. (*Playboy*, Eleanor?!)

Articles and reprints aside I would like to thank my students for raising questions I had to scramble to find the answers for, for making it clear to me that I could not arouse their concern without helping them figure out what to do with it, for being loving and enthusiastic and stimulating, and for caring enough to want to change the world, too.

And because this book is, for better or worse, what I am at the moment, I would like to end with a slightly eccentric list of some of the people (beyond those to whom I have dedicated the volume) who have *brought* me to where I am. Thanks to: Nelson Smith who showed me that good teaching could make even chemistry fun; Nadine Dutcher who taught me that friendship really can last a lifetime; the late Julia Hammer who taught me the difference between wisdom and knowledge; the late Herbert Birch, my severest critic, who taught me clear thinking (and should not be held accountable for any lapses therefrom); Ruthe Eshleman whose friendship supported me through graduate school among other crises; Orrea Pye who always let me teach what I believed even though my ideas sometimes alarmed her; Robert Choate who forced my ideas into public early, thus overcoming my fear of getting shot at; Mary Alice White who, believing in positive reinforcement, always knew when to give it; Tess Nakamura for joining with wisdom, compassion, *and* patience; and finally to Janice Dodds who never fails to be a model for me of what the citizens of a better world might be like. If you all didn't mean to play such a significant role in my life, you should have been more careful.

I cannot close without thanking two people without whom this volume would never have seen print. Thanks to David Bull for his insistent patience, for his commitment to quality, and for his conviction that *"everything* can be improved by cutting"; and to Diane Winkleby for the unfailingly cheerful impatience with which she has brought this physical book to birth.

Contents

4 SELLING IT! 205

5 ENERGY AND FOOD—THE INTERLOCKING CRISES 271

6 EARTH, AIR, FIRE AND WATER: SOLUTIONS AND THEIR PROBLEMS 335

7 EPILOGUE: WHAT CAN I HOPE FOR? 431

Prologue

Once in junior high school, in what I remember to be a "geography" class, I was assigned to do a term report on South America. A week or so after I began the project, I went to the teacher and asked if I couldn't just do the *history* of South America. And the week after that—deep into my family's *Encyclopedia Britannica* (which always told you more about everything than you really wanted to know)— I went back to the teacher and asked if it would be all right if I did just the history of *Peru*. My final hour-long report, which seemed to me to be frustratingly general, was on Pizarro's conquest of Peru.

I tell this story because it relates to this book. This book will probably strike some of the people who look through it as the intellectual equivalent of attempting to do a one-hour report on South America. It has struck me that way often, but I have as often fought down the impulse to ask myself for a reduction in my assignment. For I have grown up some in the three-plus decades since that geography class, and I have discovered that generalists, too, have their place. Without them, those engaged in the pursuit of knowledge run the risk of strolling through the woods, eyes down, examining each fascinating detail directly underfoot while failing to notice that just ahead the earth has turned sere.

This is a book of readings—and of interpretations of those readings—based on a good deal of exploration, on incessant thought, and on an ongoing attempt to come to terms with what the facts about the present state of the world seem to imply for living human organisms who are totally dependent on complex foodstuffs for their survival. The book grows out of a class which I have now taught for some seven years. Seven years ago, when I put the first version of the course together, my husband (a supporter in all things) took a look at the topics and readings and announced, "It sounds like a terrific course, but you don't know enough to teach it." "I know," I said, "but if I don't teach it, no one will."

While I have learned a bit more in the intervening years, I still begin the first session of each year's class with a disclaimer about expertise. I do this partly for myself and partly for the students. One year, three or four sessions into the semester, one of the students reacted to a series of readings on the disappearance of the American farmer by saying that she had no opinions on the subject because—although she had done the readings and found them convincing—she wasn't really an expert in agriculture and never would be.

Nowadays one is usually forced to choose between going deeper and deeper into a narrower and narrower hole—which is both very confining and, for some purposes, very necessary—and standing back away from the details in order to comprehend how things fit together. Where nutrition and food are concerned, there has been far too little of the latter activity, especially among nutritionists.

The course from which this book derives is called "nutritional ecology," and it describes itself immodestly in the catalogue as "an examination of the biological, technical, social, scientific, and commercial matrices in which the production, purchasing, and consumption of food are embedded." It seemed to me when I designed the course—as it seems to me when I think about this book—that there are here pulled together a good many topics that impinge on food and nutrition but which have seldom been seriously dealt with in any kind of organized context by majors in these fields.

The readings themselves are—as in any selection of this sort—arbitrarily chosen because they seem to the chooser to present, in a relatively concise manner, a piece of an issue that needs covering. Obviously there are biases operating in the selection. The initial bias is intentional. I am unabashedly partisan toward logical thought—and its usual companion, good writing. I am sure it is possible to think clearly and write turgidly—but it is probably not the best way to get ideas understood. And a good idea which is not understood is unlikely to extend its influence much beyond the small circle of the author's friends (or enemies) who will go to great lengths to understand it.

Which is not to say that all the writing herein presented is superb. Rather it is to say that where two articles have otherwise equal informational content, and one "says it" well, I am very likely to have chosen what is well said—whatever the relative credentials or fame of the authors. Thus it happens that even though I think this book is about food and nutrition, many of the authors are not nutritionists and many of the publications from which the articles are drawn are not food and nutrition journals. The reader is free to draw such conclusions from that as he/she will.

The second bias is unintentional, but probably unavoidable. It is that I am unable to present all points of view with equal conviction. I have always tried, in my class as in this volume, to present both sides of every issue I deal with. But I am certain I am not wholly successful in this effort.[1] The problem does not arise solely out of the difficulty of being fair to the side one has found less convincing. It is a much more fundamental problem, having to do even with how one defines "the sides."

This was not really clear to me until I recently looked through another book of readings in the field of nutrition. The author of that collection indicated in his introduction that he had tried to give both sides of each issue; yet when I finished reading the book, it was clear to me that *his* two sides and *my* two sides were very different from each other. We did not even share a common definition of *his* issues. He, for example, might wonder whether or not the evidence concerning fiber and health was sufficiently convincing as to warrant fiber replacement in processed foods. My question would be whether, in the light of resource constraints (and limitations on our knowledge), the fiber ought to have been processed out in the first place—whatever the evidence about its relationship to health.

How does this sort of bias arise? Theoretically, if one is attempting to be intellectually honest, one arrives at certain conclusions only after examining all the relevant evidence—at least all the relevant evidence that time permits one to examine. In real life, of course, the temporal constraint is a critical one, for none of us can read everything—not even everything we define as relevant. And it is clear that one's conclusions about the nature of the important issues in the world (and in one's profession) will differ markedly depending on where along the literature continuum one stops to browse—down near the glossy-paged stacks of *Food Technology* and *Food Product Development*, or philosophical light-years away amid the homely piles of the *Co-Evolution Quarterly* and *Mother Earth News.*

Once he/she has picked a spot and settled down for a good read, even the most diligent truthseeker will find it difficult, later, to remember which came first, the point of view or the choice of material—*especially when the material is outside the immediate area of his/her "expertise."* Why select *that* journal to scan and ignore *that* one? Why select *this* article to read thoroughly and skip the one adjacent? Why underline that paragraph—or that phrase—rather than another?

We are all—eventually if not initially—prejudiced in the original sense of that word. We all do make—indeed, must make if we are to function at all—prejudgements. We all develop some kind of

---

[1] It should be noted here that the volume is probably somewhat less balanced than the class simply because we were not given permission to use several articles presenting what for me is "the other side."

"cognitive frame"—sets of pigeon-holes into which we slip new pieces of data. And since we really cannot check personally on the accuracy of each new data bit, we learn as we proceed through life to trust some people and distrust others, to discount certain new information as questionable and to accept other new information as "fitting the scheme." At what point does our prejudgement based on accumulated prior knowledge become closed-mindedness—prejudice in the Archie Bunker sense? When do we stop being willing to examine openly new data that might require extensive remodeling of the entire carefully-crafted framework we carry around in our heads? Never—so we hope. But since we know that we cannot maintain objectivity, the most we can really hope for is a perpetual caution in our subjectivity—what Eric Sevaried recently referred to as having the "courage of one's doubts."[2]

What all this adds up to, of course, is that no one has *the* truth, especially about large important issues. All of us have only present approximations. My present approximations—presented in these pages—are hung on a cognitive framework which says that our determination to continue our profligate ways with the biosphere is suicidal, and that some radically different attitudes and behaviors may be required of us if we are to survive as a species into the twenty-first century. That is my bias. To the extent possible, I live in keeping with its implications, since I find living what I perceive as a responsible life-style to be intrinsically rewarding.

My third bias is perhaps surprising—even to me—in a book which has a great deal to do with the future. It is a bias against "up-to-dateness." In teaching the course on which this book is based, I change at least some of the readings every year to reflect my own changing understanding of the issues. None of my former students will be familiar with all the pieces included here, but probably all of them will find some old friends. My yearly changes are not always in the direction of recency. Pieces come in, drop out, are retrieved—are dropped again, and so on. In some cases articles have stayed in the course since the very beginning—Koff's article, "An End to All This," goes way back; so does the Hadsell piece on food processing (page 131).

Thus, in putting together this book I have had to ask myself several times why I was hanging on to certain selections—and whether there wasn't something "more recent" I could use to say the same thing. Is newer really better? Students tend to be contemptuous of a teacher in a "scientific" field who gives citations to anything more than two years old (in some fields more than two months old). It is necessary sometimes to remind ourselves that for all our assiduous piling up of data in science, we are not making that many important breakthroughs in the realm of "major ideas."

Of course, things are changing fast—but there is no need to throw away basic understandings just so we can recapture them years later. I have, for example, a very beautiful poster on the wall of my dining room. It shows a group of fish swimming through what appears to be rockweed and it says "Save the products of the land. Eat more fish—they feed themselves." The poster was published during World War I, but I first saw it in the midst of the furor over feeding grain to beef when high beef prices led our president to suggest that we eat more fish.

In 1916, Henry T. Sherman of my university wrote a pamphlet entitled "Food Gains from the War Conservation Movement," in which he urged that we stop feeding grain to beef and that we start growing our own vegetables to save the energy required for transport and preservation of fresh produce. Remember Henry T. Sherman when you read the chapter on energy and food. Old truths may actually be truer than new truths, since they have less of a tendency to get tricked out with irrelevant data and impenetrable jargon.

It is, therefore, not a lust for the new that leads me to a bias in favor of newspaper research. Nor is it a search for the newsy fact. As an ex-journalist, I consider it positively foolhardy to mine the

2 *The New York Times*, p. C21 (21 December 1977).

daily papers (even the Good Gray *New York Times*) for "facts." Yet I rely heavily on an elaborate file of newspaper clippings; for it is my fourth bias that if you care about predicting the future, you must count on newspapers to warn you of the large incoming truths, even if you cannot count on them to give you the details.

Let me give an example of what I mean. Several years ago I paid little attention as the Toxic Substances Control Bill wended its slow way through various committees of Congress. I did not see its relevance to my field. Substances deliberately *added* to foods were already controlled by the Food and Drug Administration, while substances used on or near food plants—herbicides, fungicides and so on—were already controlled by the Department of Agriculture. Then, in a tiny trickle, the news stories began. At first they were little filler items—about chicken feed accidentally contaminated with a highly toxic lubricant from a leaking machine, of fish found to be burdened with dangerously high levels of poisons never intended for use in, on, or near food. Then came full-page stories about the animal-feed PBB disaster in Michigan. As those stories accumulated, and as I had to figure out where to file them, it became clear that a new truth was emerging. Out of these bits of information—each of them more or less true, each of them more or less alarming, each of them later discounted, perhaps, or later confirmed—a much less discountable truth was emerging: in an environment saturated with toxic chemicals you cannot for long hope to produce safe food.

Such larger truths are what I have aimed for in this book. It has been my goal in writing it to do only one thing. I should like to encourage other people, who don't yet know enough to think about how the world might be made to survive (yet have a feeling such things ought to be thought about), to cut through the barbed wire isolating one discipline from another, and begin to work together to figure out how the world their children will inherit really works.[3]

[3] Some of the articles in this book have been abridged because of space limitations. References following them are complete to provide additional sources of information for the reader. As a result, reference numbers within these articles may not be consecutive.

CHAPTER 1

Limiting Growth in a Finite World

Advertisement

Progress
has become a matter
of doing what nature never intended.

Doing it with materials nature never dreamed of.

Man wants to touch the moon and farm the sea.

Man
wants a world of highers and deepers,
hotters and colders,
strongers, lighters,
fasters.

And Nature hands him some wood, some rock, and some ores.

But tomorrow is beyond the limits of these.

From here on,
what you need new
must be custom made.

Carborundum will help.

By making materials never found in nature.
Materials to stand the heats, the speeds, the pressures
that progress generates.

"CARBORUNDUM" has progressed.

From
the name
of a sharpening stone,
to that of
an international
materials systems company.

From
the very first
manmade mineral abrasive,
to what you'll need
for tomorrow.

This
special magazine
shows some of the ways
you'll get
where you're going.

Some
of the new routes
being cleared by
The Carborundum Company.

Reprinted with permission from Carborundum Company, Niagara Falls NY.

Peoplepeoplepeople

LINDA STEWART

Is our society growing too fast? Do we have to stop? Is it too late? "Peoplepeoplepeople" written in mid-1972 by a former advertising copywriter named Linda Stewart, brings a writer's wit and a human's pain to confronting the possibility of apocalypse. "People. . ." was the lead article in a population issue of a now-defunct newsletter briefly published by a still-lively consumer group, Consumer Action Now.

The end of the world is a highly resistible idea. It's a paranoid's dream, a New Yorker cartoon (the wild-eyed prophet with the cardboard sign, "Repent, for the End of the World is at hand"). It just won't wash in our empirical scheme (the world has never ended *before*) and besides, how can we believe the apocalypse when we still don't really believe in death? (Oh, maybe once we had a moment... when the fever bolted, when the car seemed to have a mind of its own ... but the moment was defied, deliciously vanquished, and then mythologized to be dined-out on ("For a moment there, I really thought I was a goner . . .").

We do not believe in our own certain death. The fact that we don't is a minor embarrassment. We don't talk about it to each other any more than we mention the disquieting conviction that we could fly, if we really *had* to. So we pay the upkeep on family plots, and make out wills, and buy insurance, pretending to believe the superstition, humoring Death as we would a madman. (Yes, of course. You're going to kill us. Now how about a nice warm glass of milk?)

So how can we believe the end of the world? Most of us can't. Even when presented with convincing evidence.

For instance, The Club of Rome report—an elaborate, expensive study, carried out by a team of scientists and a pessimistic computer, which seemed to prove incontrovertibly that The End was in sight. The widely publicized report, published under the title "The Limits to Growth" stated rather flatly that unless we make radical changes in the growth-rate of population and, most especially, of industrialization, our planet's limits will be reached within 100 years. After which, no efforts to save us can succeed. We must act, they say, before those limits are reached.

According to the computer, there's no way out. Even if pollution were controlled, the birth rate halved, food production doubled, new resources discovered, still the results of geometric growth all and always end in disaster. (For instance, if new resources were discovered, industrialization would increase, as would the pollution it causes, with the result: We'd poison ourselves to death. On the other hand if we controlled pollution, more people would survive and produce more people, and the population would surpass the food supply and the available land space.) And so on.

The report itself was highly controversial. There were those who denied its validity on the grounds that the projections were the mechanical whims of a computer, "an intellectual Rube Goldberg device" fed with "arbitrary assumptions" and spewing out "arbitrary conclusions."

(And after all, how can you believe a computer when its cousins can't even get your Macy's bill straight?)

Others disregarded the conclusions on the grounds of insufficient input. The machine, they argue, was fed with facts as we know them *today*—and as a British editor pointed out "an extrapolation of the trends of the 1880's would show today's cities buried under horse manure."

On the other hand, 33 of Britain's most eminent scientists and philosophers, engaged in global environmental studies, published a report whose conclusions are unhappily similar to the Club of Rome's computerized Doom—a prophesy of "inevitable breakdown within the lifetimes of our children." Their "Blueprint for Survival" advised that Britain halve her population, tax raw materials, and put a tax penalty on non-recyclable goods. A blueprint not unlike the Club of Rome's, which urges a vigilant slowdown in industrialization to a state of "Equilibrium." In the present scheme of things such advice seems synonymous with a slowdown of "progress"—at least, progress defined as a Ford in your future, a new factory in your town, and disposable bottles in your garbage can.

But progress isn't that one-sided and the economics of Utopia aren't simple. It is all well and good to lecture on the fundamental things of life vs. the triviality of plastic, General Motors, pop-tops and all the other paraphernalia of the Trevira Era. But how do we dislodge the progress we like from the "progress" we don't? And at the moment, like it or not, it's all tied up with GNP. What do we do with that whole big machine? And the people who run it? The mechanics of Utopia aren't simple.

It could be done, of course. And the Commission on Population and the American Future indicated a slowdown would increase rather than decrease per-capita income. But the change-over requires a change of values. A change from a materialistic to a humanistic ideology. An aspiration for services (including art, education, travel, recreation) rather than

goods (color TV's, cars—products that encourage industrial growth and pollution); a search for quality rather than quantity. Accordingly, The Club of Rome stresses that a *limit* to growth does not have to mean a no-growth economy, but merely a redirection and redefinition of growth into non-industrial areas.

But the philosophy of Utopia isn't simple either. That old dogs can't learn new tricks is a wisdom shared by all revolutionaries. Phoenixes seem only to rise from ashes. Writing has appeared on walls before. The British who wrote the Stamp Act must have seen it. And Nicholas and Alexandra. And Marie and Louis. It has always been easier to die than to change.

Will it be different this time? The stakes are higher, but can it be different?

It's easier not to believe the Club of Rome report, to leave things as they are, and please pass the pie.

I believe the report. If not in all its details, at least in essence. I believe in the sheer logic of the population chart and the pollution statistics and in the sheer stupidity of Man which includes Women which includes me, who still smokes.

And I believe what's required of me is a foresight, a generosity, an adaptability, a sense of proportion and justice, commitment and co-operation, sacrifice and responsibility I'm not always sure I'm capable of. And if the whole world is in hands such as mine, I have the sense to pause and tremble for the planet.

But there are moments when I believe I could do whatever's called for. And that you can too. There are moments when I believe that Truth outs, and Good triumphs, and that human beings are capable of heroism and humanity, not to mention common sense and a million other miracles. But then, I must confess, I also believe—though I don't usually mention this in public—but I also believe that, if we really *have* to, we can fly.

Reprinted with permission from *Consumer Action Now*, p. 1 (May 1972).

An End to All This

RICHARD M. KOFF

Richard Koff's article, originally published in *Playboy*, and later reprinted for what one assumes was a different audience in the *Sierra Club Bulletin*, supplies some of the details about the employment and subsequent activities of the pessimistic computer, about which Linda Stewart warned us.

With the careful disregard of their respective governments, two dozen eminent men were gathered last June in one of the great old *grande luxe* Swiss hotels. They strode familiarly down wide, carpeted halls—an Italian industrialist, a Belgian banker, two university presidents, a professor at MIT, the director of a major Swiss research institute, a Japanese nuclear physicist, a science advisor to an international economics organization, several economists whose pessimism, if quoted in the press, could cause a stock-market crash.

They moved purposefully toward a conference room. They did not drift, though side conversations delayed several members of the executive committee. Their one common characteristic was a certain firmness about the lips and jaw indicating an intention to get things done. They were activists in the most responsible meaning of the term. Each had been invited to join the group, called the Club of Rome, by its founder, Aurelio Peccei, himself a member of the management committee of Fiat, vice-president of Olivetti and managing director of Italconsult. Each served quietly, without compensation nor even paid expenses, as a full-fledged member.

They represented the best analytical minds of the world, with considerable influence to make funds available if a promising approach could be found to stop the suicidal roller coaster man

now rides. Their concern during the two days in Bern was formidably titled A Project on the Predicament of Mankind. The predicament is simply stated: World population is growing by 70,000,000 people every year. This is the fastest growth in man's history, and the rate is still accelerating. We will number four billion in 1975 and, if current trends continue, we can expect to reach eight billion well before the year 2000. This population is making more and more demands on its environment. We are taking fresh water out of the ground roughly twice as fast as natural processes replace it. The demand for electric power in the U.S. is doubling every ten years, and most power comes from the heavily polluting combustion of coal. We are building 10,000,000 cars a year—twice as many as we made only 17 years ago, and cars burn gasoline, grind rubber tires to dust, wear asbestos brakes into an acrid powder.

Until 1970, these figures were considered proud evidence of progress. After all, it was reasoned, if power demands, automobile production and water consumption are increasing even faster than population, then the standard of living of each individual must be improving; and for the advanced countries, this is certainly true. Edward C. Banfield, professor of urban government at Harvard, wrote a few years ago: "The plain fact is that the overwhelming majority of city dwellers live more comfortably and more conveniently than ever before. They have more and better housing, more and better schools, more and better transportation, and so on. By any conceivable measure of material welfare, the present generation of urban Americans is, on the whole, better off than any other large group of people has ever been anywhere."

It's not surprising, then, that the industrialized nations consider progress synonymous with economic growth and that the underdeveloped nations share that article of faith. The world wants and expects more people, more and faster jet planes, more television sets, more dishwashers. If one car in the garage is good, two must be better.

But consider the price of this plenty: Death due to lung cancer and bronchitis is doubling every ten years. The U. S. incidence of emphysema has doubled in the past five years. Crime in large cities has also doubled in the past five years.

Population biologist Paul Ehrlich describes an experiment in which a pair of fruit flies is put into a milk bottle with a small amount of food. In a matter of days, the population of fruit flies has multiplied to the point where the bottle is black with them. Then the limited food and their own effluvia raise the death rate, and the population drops suddenly down to zero. After 10,000 years of uninhibited propagation, mankind is beginning to sense the confines of its bottle. Man is beginning to realize that he's going to have to stop multiplying his numbers and gobbling up his world—and do it soon—because if the decision isn't made by him, it will be made *for* him by the laws of mathematics and nature.

The trouble is that man has never been very successful in controlling the destruction of community property. We have laws that keep a man from raping his neighbor's daughter, but we have few that keep him from despoiling his air. We have tried governmental action to remedy social ills before, but, as Banfield writes, "Insofar as they have any effect on the serious problems, it is, on the whole, to aggravate them."

This was the "predicament" facing the Club of Rome that June day. MIT professor Jay W. Forrester was a relatively new member of the club. He was lean, graying and spoke with the dry, didactic factuality of the trained lecturer. His theory was startling in its directness—that governmental inadequacy is an example of predictable and consistently self-defeating human behavior. His studies had suggested that the human mind is not adapted to interpreting the behavior of social systems, that human judgment and intuition were created, trained and naturally selected to look only in the immediate past for the cause of a problem. The hot stove burns the finger, not the curiosity that made one reach out to touch it.

All human solutions tend to be that simplistic. We see thousands of people in rat-infested, leaky-roofed tenements. Our traditional answer has been to tear down the tenements and put up large, low-income housing projects. The Pruitt-Igoe project in St. Louis was built to solve this problem and now 26 11-story glass and-concrete apartment buildings are being boarded up a scant 15 years after they were built—and long before they were paid for. Vandalism, physical deterioration and an impossible job of maintaining essential services made the project a social, architectural and financial disaster. Elevators stalled, windows were broken faster than they could be replaced, residents were assaulted in the halls, apartments were broken into and doors never repaired. The poorest of the poor refused to live there and vacancies climbed even as surrounding housing became more scarce. The buildings now stand vacant as monuments to governmental waste.

Our streets and highways are bumper to bumper with cars, so our answer has been wider and longer highways. But more highways attract more traffic, until the density is the same as—if not worse than—before. No highway system has ever caught up with the traffic it carries. When a rapid-transit system is in financial trouble, fares are raised to produce more income. But this only persuades more people to use cars, which clog the roads even more and provide less net income to the transit system. And it takes longer to drive through a modern city in a 300-horsepower automobile than it did in a one-horsepower buggy 100 years ago.

Forrester had his first hint of this social near-sightedness while analyzing corporate problems. "Time after time, we have gone into a corporation which is having severe and well-known difficulties—such as a falling market share, low profitability or instability of employment," he says. "We find that people perceive correctly what they are trying to accomplish. People can give rational reasons for their actions. They are usually trying in good conscience to solve the major difficulties. Policies are being followed on the presumption that they will alleviate the difficulties. In many instances, it then emerges that the known policies describe a system which actually *causes* the troubles. The known and intended practices of the organization are fully sufficient to create the difficulty, regardless of what happens outside the company. A downward spiral develops in which the presumed solution makes the difficulty worse and thereby causes redoubling of the presumed solution."

The same destructive behavior appeared when Forrester studied the solutions to urban problems. Actions taken to improve conditions in a city actually make matters worse. The construction of low-cost housing such as the Pruitt-Igoe project eventually produces more depressed areas and tenements, because it permits higher population densities and acommodates more low-income population than can find jobs. A social trap is created in which excess low-cost housing attracts low-income people to places where even their low incomes cannot be maintained. "If we were malicious and wanted to create urban slums, trap low-income people in ghetto areas and increase the number of people on welfare, we could do little better than follow the present policies," says Forrester. And, further, "The belief that more money will solve urban problems has taken attention away from correcting the underlying causes and has instead allowed the problems to grow to the limit of the available money, whatever that

amount might be."

Forrester's approach differs from that of ecologists, economists or demographers, because he does not narrow his attention to a single, specific cause-and-effect relationship. In his study, he was trying to make an all-encompassing, quantitative measure of the city as a social and biological system. It is a macrocosmic view that weaves the statistics of birth and death with the economics of mass production, variations in the job market with the realities of real-estate-investment returns. It is a complex, highly interrelated system of analysis that recognizes that you cannot break a city down into its component parts without distortion so extreme as to make the effort useless.

He had never tried to analyze the entire world, but his studies of the dynamics of corporations and of cities showed why programs begun in good faith worked out as badly as they often did. Why shouldn't the method be expanded to deal with the dynamics of the whole world system?

When men of action agree, obstacles disappear. A European foundation was happy to make a sizable grant to support the project. Two months later, under the direction of Professor Dennis Meadows, a team of nine researchers at MIT was being recruited to examine Forrester's theories in detail, expand the analysis and see what mankind could do to avoid the seemingly inevitable. As this article is written, almost a year into the project, it is confirming everything Forrester predicted.

Starting with cause-and-effect relationships he was sure of, Meadows went to the specialists for evaluations of exact, quantitative influences. We know that the death rate is directly affected by food availability, pollution levels and crowding. Experts can even reach consensus on how the material standard of living—meaning health services and housing, as well as the other fruits of technology—sharply reduces the death rate as it climbs above some minimum level necessary to sustain life. But further improvement in the standard of living doesn't do much to reduce the death rate, no matter how high it goes. Similarly, deaths caused by 1970 pollution levels are almost negligible when compared with the effects of the other factors. But if pollution levels climb ten or a hundred times higher than they have reached already—and pollution *will* reach such levels if current trends continue—we can anticipate a death rate high enough to make the worst plagues in history seem like mild outbreaks of flu.

Crowding also has its effect on the death rate. In the extreme case, people will kill one another for room to stand, but long before that limit is reached, the psychological effects and social stresses of crime, war and disease will do their damage. Garrett Hardin of the University of California writes of a more subtle effect of crowding. The cyclone that struck East Pakistan in November 1970 was reported to have killed 500,000 people. The newspapers said it was the cyclone that killed them. Hardin says crowding was the cause. "The Gangetic delta is barely above sea level," he says. "Every year, several thousand people are killed in quite ordinary storms. If Pakistan were not overcrowded, no sane man would bring his family to such a place.... A delta belongs to the river and the sea; man obtrudes there at his peril."

Birth rate is calculated in a similar way. Food production, pollution levels, crowding and material standard of living have their separate and predictable influences on the rate of growth. The difference between births and deaths establishes net population gain; and, given the current figures for standards of living, food availability, pollution and crowding, total population can be recalculated at annual intervals as far into the future as you like.

It isn't necessary to go into all the details of Forrester's method: The analysis includes all the effects mentioned here, plus such factors as natural-resource usage (dependent on population and capital investment) and capital investment (dependent on population, material standard of living, and discard or wear-out time of capital equipment). Forrester also calculates something he calls quality of life. This goes up when there are adequate food, medical service, housing and consumer goods, and low levels of crowding and pollution.

The amount of calculation necessary overloads the human brain. It would take 1000 men at 1000 calculators to work out the numbers year by year, following the labyrinthine relationships of the system. But it takes only a few seconds to run the projection on a computer. With the relationships agreed to up front by agricultural and industrial experts, census takers and financial and economic advisors, Forrester pushes the start button and lets the computer plot out curves that start with the year 1900 and go to 2100. The results offer some object lessons in how close man is to committing suicide.

The first thing we learn is that the enemy is our love of growth. Enormous pressures are now appearing on all sides that will act to suppress growth. Natural resources are being depleted; pollution levels, crowding and adequate food supplies, either separately or in concert, are going to arrest and reverse population growth forcibly and disastrously. Exactly which will deliver the *coup de grâce* is unclear, but the curves show the possible alternatives. It is for man to decide which he prefers.

In this first projection (below), Forrester showed mankind running out of natural resources. He assumed that irreplaceable coal, oil, gas and metal ores will require more and more effort to tear out of the earth and that technology will not find quick substitutes for them. Compared with some of the others, these curves look almost tolerable. This projection shows population rising steadily until about 2020, when natural resources start falling sharply. The world is already running out of easily mined ores and fuel for power that drives mass-production machinery and raises agricultural yields. But a growing population needs more resources—at first just for the amenities of life, later for survival. The industrialized nations are growing rapidly and are placing ever-increasing demands on the resources that often come from underdeveloped countries. What will happen when the resource-supplying nations start to hold back because they see the day when their own demands will require available supplies?

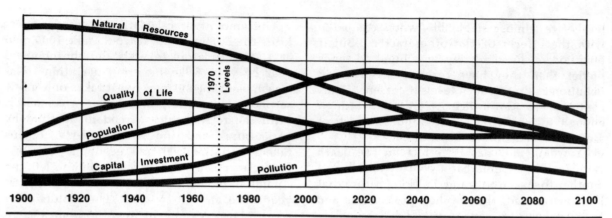

In this projection, the material standard of living (not graphed) will climb until about the year 2000; capital investment per person will continue to increase until then—before the depletion of natural resources has had a chance to make itself felt. Then, in about 2050, industrialization will turn down as resource shortages become grave. Pollution will rise to approximately six times 1970 levels, but this won't be high enough to create a runaway pollution catastrophe. There will, however, be widespread dissatisfaction because the quality of life will drop slowly as pollution grows and as crowding adds its irritations.

For his second projection, Forrester assumed we wouldn't be so lucky as to run out of natural resources. Suppose science finds plastic or glass substitutes for metals, and new power sources make it possible for us to reduce demands on coal, gas and oil reserves. He went back to the computer with the natural-resources-depletion rate after 1970 reduced to 25 percent of its former value (below).

In this case, capital investment and population grow until pollution levels get so high that death rate, birth rate and food production are drastically and dangerously affected. Population goes to almost six billion by 2030 and then, in a scant 30 years, drops to one billion. This is a world-wide catastrophe of mind-boggling proportions. War, pestilence, starvation and infant mortality turn the world into a morgue. The highly industrialized countries probably suffer most, because they are least able to survive the disruption to the environment and to the food supply.

Some writers have suggested that before we experience a catastrophe of this magnitude, mankind will stop the pollution-generating process by legislation or even revolution; but this is not very likely. The most important generator of pollutants is industrialization, which is also the major contributor to a higher standard of living. It is difficult to imagine underdeveloped

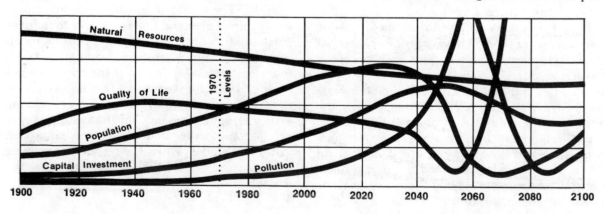

nations agreeing to a curtailment of their industrial growth. The rich nations cannot say to the poor ones, "OK, we've gone as far as we can go. Let's hold still right here." It is just as impossible to say to the poor of our own country, "We've really got to stop. Sorry, you can't have shoes for the children, an indoor toilet, a gas stove, a hearing aid for grandma." Yet, if the poor of all nations were to move up to the standard of living now enjoyed by a majority of Americans, we would have a pollution load on the environment ten times today's level.

The conclusion is inescapable. If the world is to achieve equilibrium at a material standard of living at or close to the level now enjoyed by the developed nations, world population and industrialization must be considerably lower than the current averages. And that is political dynamite.

This projection demonstrates a vitally important characteristic of the world system: It is going to reach equilibrium one way or another. We are entering a turbulent time, a time when the dedication to growth in the advanced nations will have to give way. It is impossible for every citizen of the world alive today to enjoy the standard of living that has been taken for granted in the West. The goals of our civilization will have to change, and when goals change, traditions no longer serve. We can predict a period of great unrest and uncertainty, with a frighteningly greater possibility of world war, unless enough people see that the true enemy is the system, not one another.

A second discouraging characteristic of the system is that major scientific achievement in the form of reduced depletion of natural resources has the effect only of postponing the date of catastrophe. It permits greater overshoot of industrialization and population and will actually magnify the catastrophe when it finally comes.

With this firmly in mind, it is relatively easy to predict what will happen if the next solution is attempted. Suppose we agree with the underdeveloped nations that their material needs should be met, and they agree to join us in trying to curb population growth. That means we increase capital investment (to give them a better standard of living) but apply extreme moral and economic pressure to hold down the birth rate. In the projection (below), Forrester assumed we cut the birth rate in half in 1970 and increase capital investment by 20 percent. For the first few years, things look good. Food per person increases, material standard of living rises and crowding is held close to present levels. But the more affluent world population ends up using natural resources too fast. Capital investment zooms and the pollution load on the environment reaches the critical level even earlier than it did in the previous run.

The reduction in birth rate temporarily slows population growth, but lower death rate, greater food production and eased crowding conditions soon encourage the population to start up again, and it is now a richer and more polluting population. This shows the curious interrelationships of what systems analysts call negative feedback. By starting a promising birth-control program, we simultaneously re-

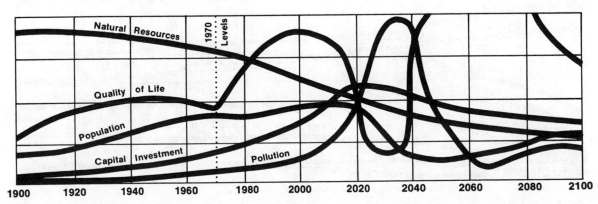

lease other natural pressures that help defeat the program. Here is the core of the nature of systems. When one pressure or combination of pressures is lightened, the result is likely to be the substitution of a new problem for the old. Often the new problem is more difficult to solve or less tolerable to live with than the old one. Advanced societies have come to expect technology to solve their problems. Technology works well when there are unlimited natural resources and geographical space to expand into; but in the real world, we reach limits. Ehrlich's milk bottle is close around us.

The projections also demonstrate the trade-off between short-term and long-term consequences of a decision. The developed nations all achieved their higher material standard of living by devoting a generation or two to building up a store of capital equipment. They used the productive capacity of labor to make machines and factories rather than food and other consumable goods. Robber barons did it for England during the Industrial Revolution and for the U. S. during the early expansion phase of its growth. The Soviet Union achieved the same result by arbitrarily denying its citizens the immediate fruits of their labor.

But there are few social mechanisms in the underdeveloped nations to defer short-run benefit for long-term return. The scarcity of such mechanisms may turn out to be a good thing, because it has the desirable effect of keeping average world capital investment under control. If we can simultaneously reduce capital investment, agree to hold the material standard of living at present levels, reduce the birth rate to half its current level, reduce pollution generation to half its current level (by a cutback in industrialization and by application of science to the problem), perhaps hold back on food production somewhat (if population is stabilized at or below the current level, we won't be needing much more food than is now produced), then, for the first time, we see the possibility of reaching equilibrium without catastrophic overshoot and population decline (below).

On the surface, it seems anti-humanitarian to reduce capital investment and stop the effort to raise food production. Such drastic measures couldn't possibly be accepted without years of study and discussion. But the alternatives are dire and inescapable. The population explosion and pollution are direct descendants of old gods—industrialization and science. Without drastically changing its priorities, world population will collapse in less than a century from the effects of pollution, food shortage, disease and war.

Forrester emphasizes that his analyses are not intended as literal year-by-year predictions; but he does insist that man's viewpoint must become world-wide and centuries deep if the species is to survive. Dennis Meadows and nine clean-cut young researchers, meanwhile, study dull books of statistics, scribble numbers on lined pads and occasionally push a few buttons on a computer console in what surely must be the least dramatic attempt ever made to save the world.

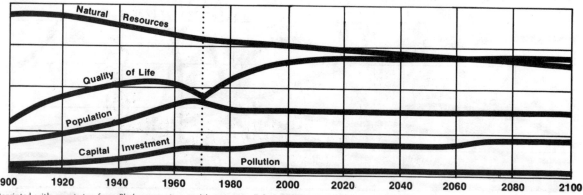

Reprinted with permission from *Playboy* magazine, 18 (7): 112–114+ (July 1971). Copyright 1971 by *Playboy*.

WE CAN'T GROW ON LIKE THIS.

We've always operated on the assumption that bigger is better. But is it?

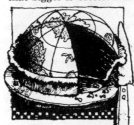

Like the dinosaurs, societies and economies can grow too big for their own good.

America is fast approaching that point. The natural resources we need to live – clean air, water, land fuels, metals – are getting scarcer. Some are on the verge of extinction. Others are becoming prohibitively expensive.

At the same time we're wasting tremendous amounts of these precious resources. And our wastes pollute our communities, our nation, our world.

We need to learn to use our resources efficiently and economically and to share them better so that everyone gets a piece of the pie.

We need to conserve the raw materials that jobs depend on, because if we deplete our resources now, things will be that much tougher later.

We need to put people to work *doing* things instead of just making things. The things we *do* make have to save resources instead of wasting them. We can build mass transit instead of freeways, rebuild our cities instead of spawning new suburban sprawl, put people to work cleaning up our environment instead of despoiling it. Harsh prescriptions? Maybe. But ones that will assure a more prosperous future.

For a better tomorrow, let's stop using resources like there's no tomorrow.

CENTER FOR
Growth Alternatives
1785 Massachusetts Avenue NW
Washington, D.C. 20036
202/387-6700

A television/radio public service advertising campaign is available on growth and resource consumption.
To order, write Public Media Center, 2751 Hyde Street, San Francisco, CA 94109, or call 415/885-0200.

Reprinted with permission from Public Media Center, San Francisco CA.

Growth is not a four-letter word.

Some people equate all our urban and environmental problems with economic growth. A few even advocate a no-growth economy.

Environmentalist Barry Commoner, however, points out that these problems "do not mean that any increase in economic activity automatically produces more pollution. What happens to the environment depends on how the growth is achieved."

Only growth offers hope for solving many of the problems mankind faces. Without strong, sound, responsible growth, progress falters and halts. All that is now wrong becomes worse, with even less hope for cure.

We think the Honorable Anthony Crosland, a Labor member of the British Parliament and Shadow Cabinet Minister for the Environment, offers a cogent argument for continued growth and its importance to all people. In a paper published recently by the Fabian Society, Mr. Crosland says, in part:

"We are concerned, here as in other fields, with the quality and composition of growth. We must continuously bring the environmental argument into the balance sheet; and we must devote part of the growth to combating its costs.

"This can be done. We know the technical answers to most forms of pollution. We can, in the long run, produce quieter aircraft, pollution-free cars, clean rivers, safe pesticides, effective waste disposal. Sensible planning can conserve the countryside even in the face of more people with cars and more leisure.

"Here we must beware of some of our friends. Their approach is hostile to growth in principle and indifferent to the needs of ordinary people. It has a manifest class bias, and reflects a set of middle and upper class value judgments. Its champions are often kindly and dedicated people. But they are affluent; and fundamentally, though of course not consciously, they want to kick the ladder down behind them. They are militant mainly about threats to rural peace and wildlife and well-loved beauty spots; but little concerned with the far more desperate problem of the urban environment in which 80 percent of our citizens live.

"We cannot accept a view of the environment which is essentially elitist, protectionist, and anti-growth. In fact, the anti-growth argument is not only unacceptable in terms of values; it is absurd in terms of the environment itself, however narrowly defined. For the greater part of the environmental problem stems not from present or future growth, but from past growth.

"Even if we stopped all further growth tomorrow, we should still need to spend huge additional sums on coping with pollution. We have no chance of finding these huge sums from near-static GNP, any more than we could find the extra sums we want for health or education or any of our other goals.

"Only rapid growth will give us any possibility."

Well said, Mr. Crosland.

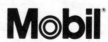

Reprinted with permission from Mobil Oil Corporation, New York NY. Copyright by Mobil Oil Corporation.

Debunking Madison Avenue

HERMAN E. DALY

The Mobil Oil Company got into the "public education" business early in the debate over whether there really were limits to growth, arguing in essence that there were not. This particular ad, published in August of 1972 in the *New York Times* and elsewhere is remarkable only because it triggered the response from economist Herman Daly reprinted on the next few pages. Daly's answer to Mobil, first published in *Environmental Action* in October of 1972, disagrees strongly with both the premises and the conclusions of the ad.

This meretricious ad is a slick sales job on a flimsy argument, selectively quoting "authorities" and pandering to the presumed interest of uninformed readers.

Mobil's first authority, Barry Commoner, can easily be quoted against the company, but before doing that it should be noted that there is considerably less to his quoted statement than meets the eye. No one argues that "any increase in economic activity automatically produces more pollution." Obviously pollution per unit of output can be cut by improved technology and thus allow for more units to be produced with the same aggregate pollution. But there are limits to how far pollution per unit of Gross National Product (GNP) can be reduced. The second law of thermodynamics[1] implies that a totally pollutionless product is impossible. Production and consumption always involve some conversion of useful matter and energy into useless waste. Thus growth in units of physical output cannot continue indefinitely because pollution per unit cannot be reduced indefinitely, and long before absolute physical limits are reached, extra output will cost more in terms of destruction of amenities, not to mention life support systems, than it is worth in terms of added services. When that point is reached, growth will make us *poorer*, not richer. Elementary economics teaches that marginal costs of output rise while marginal benefits fall. At some point the growth of anything, including GNP, becomes uneconomic. Technical progress can postpone that point, but not beyond thermodynamic limits. Furthermore, anyone who appeals to technological progress as the answer should begin by explaining why we should expect future technical change to be ecologically sound when recent post-war technical change has been, on balance, environmentally destructive (as Commoner himself has convincingly shown).

How do we know that the extra benefits of growth are at present greater than the extra costs? The answer is that we do not know, since we count true benefits imperfectly (leisure and many amenities are omitted), do not count costs at all (GNP is considered as measure of benefits and there is no comparable statistical series that purports to measure costs of growth), and even count many real costs as benefits (purely defensive expenditures such as extra medical bills occasioned by pollution-induced emphysema). Many reasonable people are beginning to suspect that the extra costs of growth now outweigh the extra benefits. If so, growth is making us poorer. As we experience a diminished

[1]For a more detailed discussion of the second law of thermodynamics, see Paul and Anne Ehrlich's *Population, Resources, Environment* (W.H. Freeman, 1970), pps. 54-55.

sense of total well-being we attribute it to traditional scarcity and call for still more growth, which makes us still worse off, etc.! This hypothesis is also debatable, but the important point is that the ad simply assumes that growth will make us richer, when that is the very question at issue! In other words, the whole ad is an expensive exercise in begging the question.

As for Barry Commoner, one can also "prove" the opposite from his writings. For example: "Environmental degradation represents a crucial, potentially fatal, *hidden* factor in the operation of the economic system. . . . A more theoretical basis for the incompatibility between the private enterprise system and the eco-system relates to the matter of growth." (*The Closing Circle*, pages 273-74, emphasis original.) I wonder why the ad hucksters did not choose the latter quotation? Although Barry Commoner might not be everyone's first choice for a reliable authority, he is certainly not the growth booster that Madison Avenue tries to make of him.

As for Mobil's other "authority," British Labor M.P. Anthony Crosland, the ad quotes him at sufficient length for him to hang himself in his own word rope. Consider first the by-now-familiar allegation that the environmental movement is elitist and cares not for the poor. By and large environmentalists have taken pains to emphasize the radical implications of stopping growth—it would mean that poverty must be cured by redistributing existing levels of wealth and income. There is just not enough environmental room to "grow our way out of poverty" even assuming that there exists a tendency for growth to reduce poverty, which is very doubtful. There is no alternative but to *share*. That is what *really* bothers the Mobil Moguls, who are joined in their crocodile tears on behalf of the poor by Yale economist Henry Wallich. Wallich states, much too bluntly for the Madison Avenue soft sell, that "Growth is a substitute for equality of income. So long as there is growth there is hope, and that makes large income differentials tolerable." (*Newsweek*, January 24, 1972, page 62) In short, the only

answer to poverty offered by these latter-day Marie Antoinettes is, "Let them eat growth." Better yet, let the poor merely hope to eat growth in the future, since as long as there is hope large differentials in wealth and income are "tolerable."

Mr. Crosland also makes a puzzling concession to growth critics when he says, "the greater part of the environmental problem stems not from present or future growth, but from past growth." Past growth causes present problems, but present and future growth do not. Therefore let us grow in the present and future so we will be rich enough to pay for past growth. Very well, Mr. Crosland, but how do you propose to keep benign present and future growth from eventually becoming pernicious past growth? And how do you know that growth is in fact making us richer rather than poorer? These questions are fundamental and they cannot be begged forever.

If this ad contains the heaviest artillery that Mobil and Madison Avenue have in their vast arsenal, then the environmental movement has cause for increased confidence. No, Mobil, "growth" is not a four-letter word—but your ad of that title is "pure bull," which is two four-letter words!

But what is the alternative to economic growth? What characterizes a non-growing or steady-state economy? The steady-state economy is basically a physical concept, but with important social and moral implications. It is defined as constant stocks of physical wealth and people, each maintained at some desirable, chosen level by a low rate of maintenance throughput—i.e., by physical production flows equal to physical depreciation flows, and births equal to deaths, at low rates, so that longevity of people and artifacts is high. The throughput is viewed as the cost of maintaining the stocks, which are steady-state open systems that maintain their organization by continually importing usable energy from, and exporting waste back to the environment. It is the stock that yields services that satisfy human wants. One cannot cross a river on the maintenance flow of a bridge, but only on an existing bridge which yields a service that satisfies a human want. Or, if we can maintain a desired, sufficient stock of cars with a lower throughput of iron, coal, petroleum, etc., we are better off, not worse off. Throughput is roughly equivalent to GNP, the annual flow of new production. Currently we attempt to maximize the growth of GNP, whereas the above reasoning suggests that we should follow Kenneth Boulding's advice, to relabel it GNC ("C" for cost), and minimize it, subject to the maintenance of a chosen level of stocks. To maximize GNP-throughput for its own sake is absurd. To maximize the input end of the throughput for the sake of building up a larger stock is a limited process. Physical and ecological limits to the volume of throughput imply the eventual *necessity* of a steady-state economy. Less recognizable, but probably more stringent, social and moral limits imply the desirability of a steady state long before it becomes a physical necessity. For example, the effective limit to breeder reactor usage will more likely be the social problem of safeguarding plutonium from theft and immoral uses, than, say, thermal pollution or low-level radiation.

Once we have attained a steady state at some level of stocks, we are not forever frozen at that level. Moral and technological evolution may make it both possible and desirable to grow (or decline) to a different level of stocks. But growth will then be seen as a temporary adjustment process necessary to move from one steady state to another, not as an economic norm. This requires a substantial paradigm shift in economic thought. Ecological conservatism breeds economic radicalism.

The major challenges facing us today are: for physical scientists to define more clearly the limits and interactions of the ecosystem which determine the feasible levels of the steady state, and to develop technologies more in conformity with those limits; for social scientists to design the institutions which will bring about the transition to the steady state, and permit its continuance once attained; for philosophers and theologians to stress the neglected traditions of stewardship and distributive justice which exist in our cultural and religious heritage. The latter is of paramount importance since the problem of sharing a fixed total is much greater than that of sharing a growing total. Indeed, as is apparent in the Mobil ad, this has been the major reason for giving top priority to growth—i.e., to economize on scarce moral resources. But as physical growth reaches limits it can no longer serve as a substitute for moral growth—assuming that it ever was an acceptable substitute. Progress must henceforth be made in terms of the things that really count rather than in terms of things that are merely countable.

Reprinted with permission from *Environmental Action* magazine (14 October 1972), the biweekly publication of Environmental Action Inc., 1346 Connecticut Ave., Washington DC 20036. A one-year subscription is $15.

Interview with Dr. Sicco Mansholt

VANYA WALKER-LEIGH

If the art of politics is the art of resource allocation, then it is the politicians of the world who will be forced to come to terms with resource limits. The question of whether they could, and would so respond is addressed by Dr. Sicco Mansholt, former Head of the European Common Market in this excerpt from an interview first published in the August/September 1974 issue of *The Ecologist*.

The Ecologist: First of all, would you say that MIT's "Limits to Growth" and The Ecologist's "A Blueprint for Survival" have had an impact on European politicians or businessmen?

Sicco Mansholt: Not very much, though they did have a big impact on the general public. They got a shock. They did make some impact on some business, more than on politicians, certainly. Businessmen directly concerned, like pesticide manufacturers in part agree with "Blueprint" and some research into non-persistent pesticides is underway. They do realise that the time will come when pesticides have to be strictly regulated, though they don't seem to show much interest in biological pest control. Certain industries running into shortages may have been impacted; oil companies certainly were. They pretended that they knew about the limits to growth all along, but they did not.

To my great regret, I must say that politicians in general have not been impressed in any way. Perhaps some of them do grasp the implications but they show no sign whatever of acting on them. Concorde is one of the politicians' virility symbols, a symbol that they are living in the past, and have not grasped the problem. . . . As for the EEC environment programme, it is obvious that my former colleagues don't understand the real problem either. The measures that have been adopted are just marginal nib-blings. No environmental measures taken in Europe so far have had any results . . . the waters of the Rhine will be much more polluted in 10 years than they are today. The Rhine is a test case. But take the development plans for power stations, industrial effluents pouring into the river. I am afraid it will be a test case, in a negative sense. No wonder the mass are disgusted with Europe. It's a Europe of Business only.

The Ecologist: What is the "real problem," you refer to?

Sicco Mansholt: Ever since 1968, I have been convinced we have to stop growth not only for ecological reasons but because of the enormous gap between developed and developing countries. The increasing gap is proof of our economic failure. Our politicians say that we must grow in order to help the third world grow: that is a lie, the opposite is true. There are not many resources left for the third world, and they are the biggest losers in our present economic system.

We in the rich countries, with our wealth, can buy at high prices the last scarce metals and oils. There may even be raw material wars soon. Already we should have a world energy board with broad powers, but there is nothing in the making. So the billions of poor in the world today will be faced with disaster. How can you increase their standard of living without cheap power? The Green Revolution has also failed....

The Ecologist: Do you expect the present "energy crisis" to modify attitudes?

Sicco Mansholt: Well, just look at the reactions of our politicians. It is to look for other types of power. No one is saying, couldn't we establish a kind of society that needs less energy? Personally, I welcome the crisis; in fact a year ago, I said I hoped the energy crisis would come soon, since it is one event which makes the mass of people realise the implications of limits to growth. Or should do....

The Ecologist: But do you see multi-national companies taking the lead towards ecological sanity?

Sicco Mansholt: Hardly, they are only interested in environmental problems, insofar as they can make a profit out of the whole mess. I have not much hope in business. Royal Dutch Shell, talking about economising on energy, other oil and chemical companies advertising what they are doing about the environment— it's demagogic eyewash.

The Ecologist: So it's up to governments to take the lead?

Sicco Mansholt: Definitely. Europe, US and Japan should undertake a billion dollar annual research programme as a minimum—a tiny fraction of research funds at present geared to economic growth and expansion. This world research should first develop non-pollutant and recycling processes, biological pest controls, "ecological" agricultural systems, energy-saving and conservation measures, while at the same time preparing the developed world for a no-growth economy....

The Ecologist: That brings us back to the politicians....

Sicco Mansholt: Exactly, that is why the ecological movements have to get into politics. The survival of mankind is not a political issue. It should be.

The Ecologist: Do you see any signs of a popular ecological movement in Europe?

Sicco Mansholt: Not yet. Only a tiny fraction of the population are really "Ecologically aware"

at the moment. The problem is that most measures that have to be taken are unpopular. In Holland, we have a little group of six people, studying the political consequences of ecological difficulties. We spent eight week-ends, brainstorming. Time and again, we saw that our conclusions meant "political suicide" on the present political scene. However, we have not given up. I am convinced that there are ways to unite socialists in Europe, around a modern radical European programme, a programme which doesn't just tinker with the symptoms.

We have to get to no-growth, de-materialise our society, have greater equality, abolish private cars. I will have to take a cut in my living standard myself. We must teach our children quite differently: at present, as I see with my five-year-old grandson, they are being programmed at school to take part in the economic rat race. People are defined by their occupation, not their talents or inclinations. We must have a society in which people say, when you ask them what they do, "I go fishing," "I play the piano," instead of "I am a banker" or "I am an unskilled worker."

But it is difficult, I realise. Young people feel things are wrong, they are willing to fight. Workers are another problem. At present they are as committed to growth as their bosses. As for the bourgeois, don't bother to convert them. They will have to be starved out, when the time comes.

The Ecologist: But can you foresee people supporting such changes? Or must some eco-disaster occur before they will face the facts?

Sicco Mansholt: What's happening in Africa right now is a disaster. So is the disappearance of plant and animal species in Europe, and so many other negative processes. I had hoped that man would use his reason, but he does not seem to. I had hoped that such a programme could be put into effect before a disaster. But when you ask me what I really feel, I don't think it is possible without a disaster. Only then will politicians and the people start to act as they should be doing now.

Reprinted with permission from *The Ecologist* (Wadebridge, Cornwall, U.K.), 4(7):259 (August/September 1974).

Marching backward into the future.

Even in the best of times, good news enjoys scant currency in the media. But now, there's much talk of everything simply winding down. A shambling toward doomsday.

We'd like to raise a voice of dissent. A "take heart" dissent rooted in man's historic cussedness and ingenuity in the face of adversity.

Today's doomsters, like yesterday's, suffer from tunnel vision. They are infatuated with projecting the gloomy absolutes of their own age upon future worlds they can't visualize. Worlds of fast-changing conditions and values which have repeatedly generated their own coping mechanisms.

In plotting their disaster charts, the doomsayers forget that both man's curse and salvation is his erratic behavior. Human events pursue a course predictable in only one respect: forever skirting the abyss.

History, happily, is strewn with the doomsayers' unfulfilled prophecies. Many early Christians abandoned all hope for the here and now. The philosopher, Oswald Spengler, saw World War I as the tragic epilogue to Western Civilization.

In the 1860's, the loss of whaling ships to Confederate cruisers threatened an energy crisis—whale oil. But America's lamps kept burning because petroleum was discovered in undreamed-of quantity. (Just as other fuels —though they're considered exotic today, or are as yet undreamed-of—will eventually turn oil into yesterday's fuel.)

Three years ago, members of a distinguished international group of academicians, the Club of Rome, produced a thick report called "The Limits of Growth." Drawing scientific authority from computer projections, this widely publicized doomsday forecast called for revolutionary changes in lifestyles so that mankind would not consume, pollute, and overpopulate civilization into total collapse within the century.

But a funny thing has happened on the way to the apocalypse. The same Club of Rome has issued a new report, "Mankind at The Turning Point," which may give us all a reprieve. Its authors could be the first alarmists to be frightened by their own visions of the future. In essence, they now say that with massive capital investment and global cooperation we can solve the world's shortages of goods and surfeit of people. We agree.

We agree, also, with the French poet, Paul Valery, that man too often marches backward into the future. But at least, being cussed and ingenious, he manages to get there.

Reprinted with permission from Mobil Oil Corporation, New York NY. Copyright 1975 by Mobil Oil Corporation.

Conditional Optimism about the World Situation

KENNETH E. BOULDING

Here is Mobil back again, announcing that the Club of Rome has recanted—that its newest study, *Mankind at the Turning Point,* has found growth acceptable after all. Once again Mobil's conclusions are brought into question on the succeeding pages by an economist giving an alternate reading of the same report. This time the economist is Kenneth Boulding, reviewing *Mankind at the Turning Point* for *Science* (March, 1975).

The first report to the Club of Rome, *The Limits to Growth* (D. H. Meadows *et al.,* Universe Books, 1972; reviewed by K. E. Boulding in *The New Republic,* 29 April 1972), had a remarkable resemblance to the Book of Jonah. Not only was a considerable part of it spewed out of the belly of the great fish of the computer, but its main message was that if Nineveh, that is, the great city of the developed world, did not repent it would be destroyed, though not so much by the wrath of an outraged God as by the sheer depletion of the resources on which it depended for its input and the depletion of sinks for its unwanted output of pollution. The Second Report to the Club of Rome[1] is almost the Second Book of Jonah, no doubt lost in the Biblical version, in which the prophet gives Nineveh fairly detailed instructions about how to repent, which the first book did not specify.

The first report was criticized on the grounds that it took a far too holistic view of an extremely diverse and complex planet, though one could perhaps defend this as a very first approximation. The second report seems to answer this criticism by breaking the world down into ten regions—North America, Latin America, Western Europe, the Eastern Socialist bloc, China, Japan, India, the Arab world, tropical Africa, and the Southern Hemisphere rich countries of Australasia and South Africa. Each of these has a model of its own, somewhat more detailed than the models of the first report but essentially similar, involving in different parts of the world inputs, outputs, and accumulations or decumulations of people and things. In addition, there are included the trade, investments, and aid relationships among the various regions, especially of course from the rich countries to the poor.

Scenarios are run off on the computer involving various degrees in timing of population control and "aid," that is, gifts of economic goods from the rich countries to the poor. The general message of all these scenarios is "the

[1]**Mankind at the Turning Point.** The Second Report to the Club of Rome. Mihajlo Mesarovic and Eduard Pestel. Dutton, New York, and Reader's Digest Press, New York, 1974. xiv, 210 pp., illus. $12.95.

earlier the better." If certain basic sets of decisions are made very soon the printouts give us some hope, but pretty soon it will be too late to avoid major catastrophes. As in all these computer models, there are assumptions of the constancy of certain parameters such as the efficiency of investment or aid or the success of population control, which are of course very risky assumptions. Nevertheless, provided we know what is going on and are not carried away by the esthetic delights of the "computer spaghetti," as it has been called, the plotting of these scenarios can be extremely useful, indicating at least the implications of the assumptions.

A particularly interesting scenario is one concerning the relations of the oil-rich countries to the food- and capital-rich countries, which turns out to be surprisingly optimistic, suggesting that a little monopoly squeeze in the oil market may not do the oil-importing rich countries very much harm and may end up doing the oil-rich countries a great deal of good by the time their oil is exhausted. One does worry, of course, about the cultural assumptions behind the parameters of these models. Again, however, one should be grateful for any gleam of hope.

In some ways, for all its modestly optimistic tone, this volume is even more depressing than the first report, perhaps because it is more specific. Its suggestions on what has to be done to repent (population control and large transfers *now*) are extremely plausible. Like Donne's great sonnet on the judgment, it points out that by the time the judgment has arrived it is too late to repent, and we have to repent now for repentance to do any good. What the report does not say is how we are to be persuaded to repent. If the only way to avoid catastrophe is immediate population control in the poor countries and an immediate vast outburst of generosity in the rich ones, the probability of catastrophe seems appallingly high. The failures of population control in India, for instance, are no accident, but are deeply involved with a social structure in the Indian village that seems

fantastically hard to change. In many countries, also, where there is fear of "outbreeding," that is, differential population growth in different groups, or even between different nations, even the will to population control can easily be destroyed, as we have seen in Romania and Ceylon. On this score the population conference of last summer in Bucharest was by no means reassuring. Repentance is extraordinarily difficult as long as the general view prevails that anything that is wrong with anybody is always somebody else's fault, and that is the official ideology of a large part of the world.

The theory of grants economics, furthermore suggests that generosity is a function of the image, especially in the mind of the donor, of the efficiency of grants. If by sacrificing a dollar I can benefit you ten dollars I am much more likely to do it than if I can only benefit you ten cents. The two items of repentance therefore feed back on each other. Without population control in the the poor countries the rich countries can argue that anything that is done for the poor countries will not benefit them in the long run and indeed will only lead to a larger eventual catastrophe. This is the "lifeboat principle" as enunciated by Garrett Hardin. The poor countries can argue, on the other hand, that without generosity on the part of the rich countries there is no point in their controlling their population as there is going to be a catastrophe anyway and they might as well have whatever fun is available while it lasts. How one can possibly link these two items of repentance in a reinforcing union is something the report does not suggest, and I must confess also I have no answer. Perhaps we simply have to look beyond catastrophe and to ask how one prepares the ground for learning from catastrophe. There have indeed been catastrophes in history which produced very fundamental learning, like the Irish famine of the 1840's and the Japanese catastrophe of World War II. Since these catastrophes the Irish have controlled their population and the Japanese have controlled their aggressiveness. I understand that a third report is on the way. Perhaps this one will deal with the question how we repent in time, before catastrophe, or, failing that, how we prepare for catastrophe by preparing the ground for repentance after it.

Like the first report, the second report does not reveal all its technical details, and there will no doubt be criticism of these when they are revealed. There is danger that computer modelers develop a "mystique" which makes the operation hard to criticize in detail. A dictionary of assumptions and parameters would be highly desirable. Nevertheless, the presentation is masterly. It consists of a general text interspersed with "briefs" which develop some, but not all, of the more technical details. It will be a rare person who is not moved as well as stimulated by this document. One hopes that these modern works will indeed have the same effect as Jonah's prophecies. It will be recalled that Nineveh did repent and was not destroyed even though this made Jonah furious. This is a slim thread on which to hang a hope for the future, but perhaps it is all the thread we have.

Reprinted with permission from *Science*, 187:1188+ (28 March 1975). Copyright 1975 by the American Association for the Advancement of Science.

Nature of Global Crises

MIHAJLO MESAROVIC and EDUARD PESTEL

What Boulding's review suggested about the "conditional optimism" of the second Club of Rome Report is confirmed by the excerpt from Mankind at the Turning Point *reprinted here. This overview suggests that the finiteness of the globe imposes some limits to business as usual.*

Crises are not new to human society. In fact, mankind has never been crisis-free for any substantial period of time. And history shows that sooner or later man has always been able to overcome the crises of his day. In retrospect it seems that all crises in modern times were solved soon enough to prevent a reversal of the triumphant march of progress.

Is there any reason to believe that the crises of our era will not be resolved as successfully as the crises of the past were resolved? Is there any reason why we should not go about our business as usual, confident that the precedents of the past will apply to the future, and that all our crises will be taken care of in due time?

The answer to these questions is yes, there is ample reason to believe that the problems of our time will *not* be solved in the routine course of events. For one thing, the numerous crises of the present exist simultaneously and with a strongly woven interrelationship between them. We do not have the luxury of dealing with one crisis at a time. Furthermore, the scale and global character of the present crises differ from the nature and scale of most past crises. The most important factor, however, that separates the current series of crises from the crises of the past is the character of their causes. In the past, major crises had *negative* origins; they were caused by the evil intentions of aggressive rulers or governments, or by natural disasters regarded as evil according to human values—plagues, floods, earthquakes, and so on. In contrast, many of the crises of the present have *positive* origins: they are consequences of actions that were, at their genesis, stimulated by man's best intentions. To reduce human labor by exploiting the non-human energy sources in Nature, for example, was a goal no one quarreled with but it led to the present energy crises. Strengthening of the group—be it the family, community, or nation—by having a large number of children was commendable; but it led to the population crises. To reduce human suffering and prolong human life by conquering disease was certainly a noble aim; but it led to a substantial increase in the population. Large construction projects, such as building roads, dams and canals, agriculture and forestry practices, hunting and breeding of animals, mining and industrial engineering, etc.— in other words the imposition of man's design on the natural environment for man's own good—was man's way of "taming" Nature; but it led to the environmental crises. Today it seems that the basic values, which are ingrained in human societies of all ideologies and religious persuasions, are ultimately responsible for many of our troubles. But if future crises are to be avoided, how then should these values be readjusted? Should traditional "good" become revisionist "bad"? Is it necessary to abandon the values which have, so far, served man so well, as evidenced by his continuous progress?

In the last three centuries, human progress can be measured in terms of man's triumphs over Nature. Our successes have been so great that man's supremacy over Nature has been taken for granted: Nature has not yet been defeated, but it certainly has appeared to be in irreversible retreat. Where Nature has still held out, man has considered his ultimate control simply a question of time. The "war on cancer," for example, was not really launched as war—for a war is a struggle that may be lost—but as an expedition to liquidate the remnants of an enemy who may hold out for a while, but whose ultimate defeat was assumed to be inevitable. In the new crises, however, there is evidence that the adversary is Nature once again, an adversary who is not at all beaten, and who is in some ways more elusive and more formidable than we ever imagined.

Consider, for example, our attitude toward natural resources. In an unrestrained pursuit of economic and material growth, we have put faith in the presumably inexhaustible supply of natural resources: food, energy, raw materials, etc. But now we have discovered that these essential resources are by no means infinitely available. Even if we accept as plausible that substitutions will be found as the supply of presently essential resources dwindles, we can by no means be certain that the substitutions will be found exactly when they are needed and in the precise quantity that is needed. Given this uncertainty, we cannot be sure that progress will continue uninterrupted. And considering the complexity of the systems that govern the course of human society, any interruption is bound to have serious, and perhaps disastrous, consequences.

Man's dependency on Nature goes very deep indeed; his use and misuse of resources is only part of the picture. As man has become the dominant force in the shaping of life-systems on the Earth, his ascent has been accompanied by a reduction of the biological diversity in Nature. Species not perceived to be in the service of man have been systematically reduced in number or eliminated. Should this trend continue, Earth will soon be inhabited by a diminished number of species. Today we understand much better than our ancestors that the existence of all life on Earth—our own included—depends on the stability of the ecological system. An Earth with less diverse inhabitants might not continue to possess the stability essential for adaptation and survival. And if our ecosystem breaks down—even if only temporarily—the effect on mankind will be calamitous. The ultimate irony confronting technological man may well reside in the fact that Nature's most potent threats to human welfare are not her destructive power—earthquakes, tornadoes and hurricanes—but the fragility of the web of life, the delicacy of those skeins which bind species to species and which comprise the dynamic bonds which relate the animate and inanimate realms so inextricably in the processes of life.

Brief on Man's Interference in Nature

Being "but a part of nature," man has always affected and has always been affected by his environment. However, due to the disproportionate increase in numbers and due to increased sophistication of man's intervention in natural processes, the interference of man is taking on a completely new dimension with unpredictable and potentially catastrophic consequences; this is beginning to cause concern from an unsuspected source: the scientists who originated and developed such techniques of intervention. A good example is the most recent appeal by a group of microbiologists to the world scientific community at large to refrain from conducting the experiments that involve inserting into bacteria the genes which are resistant to antibiotics or the genes of viruses. The potential danger to which the appeal specifically addresses itself is due to the fact that the bacteria often used in scientific experiments of this kind is a common inhabitant in the human intestine. A prospect of such a resistant bacteria escaping and infecting the population must be taken into account; it implies the possibility of loosing new plagues upon the world. The event was properly hailed by the scientists themselves as a historical landmark of restraint to conduct experiments purely for the sake of scientific curiosity. It represents a reversal of the cherished tradition that nothing should interfere with the sciences' search for truth. However, even if the experiments in which new, resistant bacteria are created are foolproof, there exists a real danger in: (1) the potential of using such a new technique for biological warfare; (2) the possibility of such experiments being conducted outside of a properly controlled laboratory. Although the use of this less-than-a-year-old technique is still in the hands of experts, it will be a "high school project within a few years."[1] The solemn high-level warnings against conducting such experiments whose consequences cannot be predicted could hardly be considered as a sufficient deterrent then. But there are many others, even if considered less spectacular, examples of unknown and potentially harmful consequences of man's intervention in nature.

When man imposes his own design on Nature, he interferes with the process of natural selection. The consequences of such interventions cannot be predicted. In his pursuit of short-term gains, man is introducing into the ecosystem a large number of inadequately tested new chemicals, which may have serious and widespread biological implications. Countless living organisms could be affected, including man himself. In the interest of his own comfort in the present, and in the name of progress, man may thus degrade the quality of his own species in the future.

The ever-widening gap between man and Nature—his physical isolation and his mental estrangement from Nature—is the logical consequence of the traditional concept of progress; for progress in world development has led increasingly to a process of undifferentiated growth, based on man's erroneous assumption that Nature's supporting system was inexhaustible in every respect. The modern crises are, in fact, man-made, and differ from many of their predecessors in that they *can* be dealt with. The choices are complicated, but they exist. Obviously, we cannot clean up the air by turning off all the machinery (since that would instantly create other sorts of crises), but the fact is that modern man at least has that option, and that know-how. Medieval people had no choice but to allow the plague to run its course; they could not "turn off" disease-carrying rats.

If we are to deal effectively with the crises of the present, we must understand their origin and nature, their linkages and interactions. It is our intention in this book to analyze the crises in the world development in concrete rather than abstract terms; otherwise our analyses will be just another academic exercise, of which there is no shortage. Specifically, we shall ask the following questions:

1. Are the crises—energy, food, raw materials, etc.—persistent, or are they aberrations due, possibly, to oversight or neglect?

2. Can the crises be solved within local, national, or regional boundaries, or must truly lasting solutions be effected within a global framework?

3. Can the crises be solved by traditional measures which have always been confined to an isolated aspect of social development, such as technology, economics, politics, etc.—or must the strategy for solution be more comprehensive, involving all aspects of social life simultaneously?

4. How urgent is the resolution of the crises? Will delay buy time and make the implementation of solutions less painful? Or are solutions made more elusive by delay?

5. Is there a way to solve the total crises by cooperation without undue sacrifice on the part of any of the constituents of the world system; or is there the danger that some could gain permanently by seeking confrontation with their partners in the global context?

Whenever one deals with the sort of problems and questions outlined above, a decision concerning the time-horizon of the study has to be made. Most of the so-called "long looks" into the future do not extend beyond the year 2000. If things seem manageable by then, everything

---

[1]Paul Berg et al., "Potential Biohazards of Recombinant DNA Molecules," *Science,* Vol. 5, No. 4148, July 1974.

is proclaimed satisfactory. Granted, the degree of uncertainty grows with each extension of time. But the dynamics of the world system require twenty years or more for the effects of change to be accurately measured and fully revealed. Moreover, the delays involved in the implementation of decisions can be formidable. To construct a power plant takes five to ten years from the decision to build a plant to its actual operation. And this length of time is merely the product of technological and administrative requirements; when basic human attitudes must change and social adjustments must be made, implementation takes much longer. Given these delays, a twenty-five-year period cannot accurately reveal the dynamics of the system: basic and important trends simply cannot be assessed within such a "short" time period. What appears to be a minor deviation in a twenty-year assessment can become a major upset after forty years—that is, after the evolution has been subjected fully to the momentum of change. An example of the dynamics at work will be found in Chapter 9, in the analysis of the supply and demand for food. By the year 2000 the demand for food in South Asia will be about 30 percent greater than the supply—an alarming but conceivably a manageable gap. With advanced planning, the gap could be reduced to as low as 10 percent. However, if the same projections are extended another twenty-five years, the deficit rises to over 100 percent—clearly a catastrophic disparity.

The analyses in this book extend over a period of fifty years. If, during this coming half-century, a viable world system emerges, an organic growth pattern will have been established for mankind to follow thereafter. If a viable system does not develop, projections for the decades thereafter may be academic.

Reprinted with permission from *Mankind at the Turning Point*, pp. 10-17, by Mihajlo Mesarovic and Eduard Pestel. Copyright 1974 by Mihajlo Mesarovic and Eduard Pestel. Reprinted by permission of the publishers, E. P. Dutton and Hutchinson Publishing Group Limited.

Homo Sapiens, the Manna Maker

F. M. ESFANDIARY

Among some observers, technological optimism has remained undaunted through the entire *Limits* debate. Dr. F. M. Esfandiary, who teaches long-range planning (and clearly believes in it), demonstrates his dauntless faith in technology in this article first printed on the Op Ed page of the *New York Times* on August 9, 1975.

The world is moving toward an age of limitless abundance—abundant energy, food, raw materials. Decades from now this late 20th century will be remembered as a period in which the world shifted from age-old scarcity to a new era of plenty.

Paradoxically in the United States today there is growing concern that we are depleting our "finite" resources. Books and articles appear every day with cataclysmic titles: "The Coming Dark Age," "Limits to Growth," "The End of Affluence," "The End of the Consumer Society."

Such doomsday exaggerations are by now a familiar pattern, particularly in the United States.

What are the new sources of energy, the new methods of food production, the new accessibility of limitless raw materials?

Energy

Solar power, nuclear fusion, geothermal energy, recycled energy, wind energy, hydrogen fuel—these sources will soon provide cheap, nonpolluting limitless energy, enough to last for millions of years.

Small-scale application of solar energy has already begun. Widespread solar electrification and commercial application of nuclear fusion are expected in the 1990's. Scientists are also excitedly projecting a bountiful "hydrogen economy."

New technologies are increasingly mobilized in the development of energy. Computers and lasers are helping develop solar energy and nuclear fusion. Earth-orbiting satellites have located geothermal sites in Arizona, Central America and East Asia.

Food

Agriculture is undergoing an epochal revolution. We are evolving from feudal and industrial agriculture to cybernated food production. Computers, remote control cultivators, television monitors, sensors, data banks can now automatically run thousands of acres of cultivated land. A couple of telefarm operators can feed a million people.

Computers are also helping create a second Green Revolution. Through selective breeding, new crops are developed that need little or no fertilizers, grow in marshes, respond to salt-water irrigation, resist drought and disease, yield richer proteins. Such revolutionary crop engineering will help open up millions of acres of land that for ages have been sterile.

Desalination units and sprawling greenhouses are already helping grow year-round vegetables and fruits in the hot arid deserts of the Arab emirates, Mexico and California. Earth resource satellites are daily transmitting billions of bits of information crucial to food production.

Raw Materials

We now have the capability to extract limitless raw materials from recycled wastes, rocks, the earth's interiors, the ocean floors, space.

Vladimir Shatalov, chief of Soviet astronaut training, envisions atomic power stations in space, fueled by raw materials from the planets. "Would you say this is fantasy?" he asks. "But all space exploits come from fantasies."

How absurd the American panic over scarcity when we are entering an age of abundance. How absurd to focus on "finiteness" at the period in evolution when our world is transcending finiteness, opening up the infinite resources of an infinite universe.

How outrageous that after centuries of privation and sacrifice leaders can come up with nothing more than yet more sacrifice. How short-sighted the exhortations to no-growth at precisely the time when we urgently need more and more growth—growth not *within* but *beyond* industrialism.

How retrospective the preachings to lower living standards of the relatively rich to raise conditions of the poor, at a time when we can raise *everyone's* living conditions by vigorously developing and spreading abundance, not sharing scarcity.

Let it be well understood that people around the world fester in scarcity not because we lack resources. But because we still squander billions of dollars on armaments. And because we fritter away more billions shoring up obsolete industrial technologies and resources.

For instance, why does the United States dissipate billions of dollars on offshore drilling for oil and on the Alaska pipeline yet invest only a piddling $50 million a year on solar energy and on nuclear fusion?

Why are most Communist countries bogged down in anachronistic agrarianism and manual labor when instead they could computerize their agriculture and economies to move ahead more vigorously?

Why do Asia, Africa and Latin America still squander billions of dollars importing automobile and truck factories, and building outdated schools, when instead they should rapidly shift to automated mass transit and satellite-linked teleducation to quickly spread information on birth control, new agricultural techniques and so on?

This very day we have the post-industrial technology, the resources, the capital, the knowledge to flow to a new era of undreamed-of-abundance.

Reprinted with permission from *The New York Times*, p. 17 (9 August 1975). Copyright 1975 by The New York Times Company.

Nicholas Georgescu-Roegen: Entropy the Measure of Economic Man

NICHOLAS WADE

Science editor, Nicholas Wade, a frequent commentator on food and resource problems, brings his usual lucid style to a survey of the life and thought of Nicholas Georgescu-Roegen. He manages to make it clear why Georgescu-Roegen's linking of two complex topics—entropy and economics—has reshaped much of the thinking about the true limitations on material growth. The article first appeared in *Science* in October of 1975.

ashville, Tennessee. Nashville styles itself the Athens of the South, and sports a perfect concrete replica of the Parthenon to establish the point. Another local temple, the Hall of Fame, attests to Nashville's position as the national focus of country music. Yet despite its 14 centers of higher learning, the city cannot even support a decent orchestra, grumbles Nicholas Georgescu-Roegen, a long-time resident who is professor of economics at Vanderbilt University.

Georgescu-Roegen, a Romanian by birth and a statistician by early training, is himself one of the ornaments of Nashville, though probably few of its citizens have ever heard of him. Only in the last few years has his name become known beyond the select fraternity of mathematical economists. There he has long been regarded as one of the specialty's pioneers. His colleagues consider his work to be Nobel prize material. Nobelist Paul Samuelson of the Massachusetts Institute of Technology, in the foreword to a collection of Georgescu-Roegen's essays, describes him as "a scholar's scholar, an economist's economist," a man whose ideas

"will interest minds when today's skyscrapers have crumbled back to sand."

In the last few years Georgescu-Roegen has left the ivory tower altitudes of the pure theory of consumer choice and begun to adumbrate a theory of Malthusian comprehensiveness and all-but-Malthusian gloom. It implies, in brief, that unless man can reorient his technology and economy toward the energy that comes directly from the sun, his life as a species will be sharply limited by his "terrestrial dowry" of low entropy materials.

The theory has received less attention than it almost certainly merits. For one thing, Georgescu-Roegen believes that economic activity must not merely cease to grow, as the Club of Rome suggested in its *Limits to Growth*, but will eventually decline. Neither sentiment is at the pinnacle of economic intellectual fashion. For another, the full implications of the thesis have become apparent only within the last year. Its theoretical basis was laid out in 1971 in *The Entropy Law and the Economic Process*, a stimulating but difficult book which is probably more often praised than read. The practical consequences are described in "Energy and economic myths," a paper published this January [1975] in the *Southern Economic Journal*. The thesis has received resounding accolades from Georgescu-Roegen's intellectual allies, but has so far been largely ignored by orthodox economists. "The behavior of the economic growth people has been like the Sherlock Holmes case of the dog that barked in the night—strangely silent," comments Herman Daly of Louisiana State University. The thesis' claim to public attention, in other words, rests at present on its merits and on its author's formidable scholarly reputation, rather than on the unanimous plaudits of the economic profession.

The starting point of Georgescu-Roegen's theory is the entropy law, or second law of thermodynamics. The law is a broad, almost philosophical, concept which has had many formulations in its 110-year history. Central to all of them is the notion of irreversibility, that certain processes go in one direction only and can never be repeated except at far greater cost on the whole. A given lump of coal, for example, can be burned only once. There is of course the same amount of energy in the heat, smoke, and ashes as there was in the lump of coal (that is stipulated by the first law of thermodynamics governing the conservation of matter-energy), but the energy bound up in the combustion products is so dissipated that it is unavailable for use, unlike the "free" energy in the coal, and the process cannot be reversed.

Entropy is a measure of this bound or dissipated energy. The entropy law says that the entropy of a closed system always increases, the change being from free energy to bound, not the other way about. Entropy is also a measure of disorderliness (dissipated energy represents a more chaotic situation than that before the lump of coal was burned). So the entropy law is also saying that the natural state of things is to pass always from order to disorder. Whence the notion of entropy as time's arrow.

The idea of entropy as an index of disorder underlies the description of certain materials as possessing low entropy. An ingot of copper has low entropy because its atoms are disposed in a more orderly state than they were in the original copper ore. Did the refiner create low entropy in making the ingot? No, because in the smelting he engendered far more high entropy by converting free energy to bound. All man's activities, says the entropy law, end in deficit; you cannot get anything except at a far greater cost in low entropy.

There is one more tentacle of the entropy law to examine before considering how Georgescu-Roegen deploys it against the foundations of conventional economics. For a deep law of physics, the entropy law's distinction between free and bound, available and unavailable energy may sound strangely anthropomorphic. And indeed it is anthropomorphic. A pure intellect would not comprehend the distinction: it would just see energy shifting about. The difference is important only to living organisms, because they exist on the slope between low entropy and high. They absorb low entropy by feeding, directly or indirectly, on sunlight, and they give out high entropy in the form of waste and heat.

All species depend on the sun as their ultimate source of low entropy except man, who has learned also to exploit the terrestrial stores of low entropy such as minerals and fossil fuels. Life feeds on low entropy; and so does economic life. Objects of economic value, such as fruit, cloth, china, lumber, and copper, are highly ordered, low entropy structures. For low entropy is the true taproot of economic scarcity.

What Georgescu-Roegen is saying is both profound and yet very simple. He asserts that the entropy law rules supreme over the economic process. The physics student who considers that an obvious truth should try looking for it in an economics textbook. He won't find it, because standard economists (says Georgescu-Roegen) assume a physical model of the world in which everything is perfectly reversible, in which after every disturbance the system comes back into equilibrium and all goes on as before. Standard economists teach that economics is a closed, circular process, an endless pendulum movement between production and consumption in which the exhaustibility of natural resources raises no problem, and the cure-all for pollution is simply to get prices right. Such conceptions are based on the mechanistic framework which economists borrowed long ago from physics, and which they have never revised to redress its basic omission, that of the law of entropy.

Once we recall that none of man's activities eludes the entropy law, the economic process appears in a very different light. For one thing, the process can now be recognized to be not circular and timeless, but irrevocable. It consists quintessentially of the continuous and irreversible transformation of low entropy into high. The basic inputs are drawn from the solar flow of low entropy and from the terrestrial stocks. The material output is high entropy in the form of pollution and dissipated matter and heat. The true—that is, the intended—output of the economic process is in fact an intangible: the enjoyment of life.

This is a radically different view of the economic process from that in the textbooks and, not surprisingly, it stresses different aspects. It places paramount emphasis on the inputs to the process (energy and natural resources) and on the output (pollution). Both are aspects which for long escaped serious attention, says Georgescu-Roegen, because of the propensity of standard economists (and of Marxists) to ignore the natural environment.

The economic process being by the entropy law irrevocable, Georgescu-Roegen is led also to stress its place in history, particularly the way in which the present pattern of economic activity will affect that of future generations. Because the terrestrial dowry of ordered material structures is finite, every Cadillac or every Zim we make today, let alone any instrument of war, "means fewer plowshares for future generations, and implicitly, fewer human beings too." Economic development, Georgescu-Roegen considers, "is definitely against the interest of the human species as a whole if its interest is to have a lifespan as long as is compatible with its dowry of low entropy."

Mechanized agriculture, including the Green Revolution, is also against the long-run interest of mankind, because of the vastly different abundances of solar and terrestrial low entropy. The earth's outstanding recoverable reserves of fossil fuel are estimated to be the equivalent of about 2 weeks' sunlight. Yet the modern method of agriculture replaces the water buffalo and its manure (both the product of solar energy, which is almost a free good) with the tractor and chemical fertilizer (both derived from terrestrial sources of low entropy). In doing so, it substitutes scarce elements for one that is abundant. This is why the Green Revolution, even though it is the only way to feed populations now, is in the long run such a bad deal for mankind.

Mechanized agriculture allows a larger population to survive now at the expense of a greater reduction in the amount of future life. What of the life-span of mankind as a species? If the worst befalls, when his terrestrial dowry is completely exhausted, could not man revert to the cave and survive as once he did by berry picking? The thought ignores that, evolution being irrevocable, steps cannot be retraced in history. Mankind, Georgescu-Roegen believes, has become addicted to his "exosomatic" instruments, those organs which are part of his evolution but not part of his biological constitution. Man's exosomatic instruments, which economists call capital equipment, and which are the ultimate cause of the social conflict that distinguishes the human species (the advantage derived from their improvement became the basis of inequality between individuals and groups), are comforts that man will never give up.

How are we to preserve their share of the terrestrial dowry for future generations? "Standard" economists might suggest that the price mechanism will offset scarcities. But, says Georgescu-Roegen, prices are only a parochial expression of value unless everyone concerned can bid—and future generations are excluded from today's market, which is why oil, for example, still sells for the merest fraction of its true value. The only way to protect future generations from the present spasmic squandering of our energy bonanza is "by reeducating ourselves so as to feel some sympathy for our future fellow humans."

The monopoly of the present over future generations would be substantially reduced in an economy based primarily on the flow of solar energy. Such an economy would still need to tap the terrestrial dowry, especially for materials, and the depletion of these critical resources must therefore be rendered as small as posible. How is this to be accomplished? Georgescu-Roegen has proposed a "minimal bioeconomic program" which, though admittedly utopian, points in what he considers the right directions:

—Production of all instruments of war should be prohibited completely.

—With the productive forces thereby released, industrial nations should help the underdeveloped nations to arrive as quickly as possible at a good (but not luxurious) life.

—Mankind should gradually lower its population to a level that could be adequately fed only through organic agriculture, a burden that will fall most heavily on the underdeveloped nations.

—Until direct use of solar energy becomes a general convenience or controlled fusion is achieved, all waste of energy—by overheating, overcooling, overspeeding, and so forth—should be avoided, if necessary by regulation.

—Consumption for the sake of fashion, such as getting a new car each year, should be regarded as a bioeconomic crime; manufacturers should focus on durability, designing their products for long life and ease of repair.

"Will mankind listen to any program that implies a constriction of its addition to exosomatic comfort? Perhaps the destiny of man is to have a short, but fiery, exciting and extravagant life rather than a long, uneventful and vegetative existence. Let other species—the amoebas, for example—which have no spiritual ambitions, inherit an earth still bathed in plenty of sunshine."...

In conversation, Georgescu-Roegen speaks animatedly of his new theory and of the failure of the would-be critics among his colleagues to come out and debate with him. Asked the reason for his critics' muteness, he replies with a Romanian proverb— "'Don't mention the cord in the house of the hanged.'" "I am very unpopular with economists," he says, comparing his attack on standard economics to the action of a man who confiscates marbles from children. "They will never forget that, but the next generation of economists will speak only my language."

Coming from a lesser man, the prediction might sound vainglorious. But Georgescu-Roegen inspires favorable reviews from independents and sky-high praise from those who agree with him. Economist Kenneth Boulding, in a review of *The Entropy Law and the Economic Process* (*Science*, 10 March 1972), wrote that the book had real defects but that "If...the right 500 people were to read it, science perhaps would never be quite the same again." Joseph J. Spengler of Duke University, a past president of the American Economic Association, believes that his and Georgescu-Roegen's earlier book "will come to be recognized as two of the greatest books we have had in the first three quarters of this century." According to Herman Daly, a proponent of the steady-state economy, Georgescu-Roegen's new thesis has not yet been fully digested but when it has been, "it will win him a place as one of the most important economists of our time. What he has done is to tie economics back to its biophysical foundations—it is that divorce that has led to many of our current problems such as pollution."

Alvin Weinberg, director of the Institute for Energy Analysis and a man whose outlook on energy might be expected to make him an opponent of Georgescu-Roegen's, describes him as a "highly original thinker" whose views people are now beginning to take more seriously. But Weinberg begs off detailed discussion of the thesis, saying he is not an economist. Similarly economist Paul Samuelson professes incompetence to judge Georgescu-Roegen's ideas on entropy, but adds that his tennis partner, a scientist, informs him they are essentially sound. Samuelson finds "everything he writes extremely stimulating, " but notes that, as with Malthus, "there is not much refutable about 'Just-you-wait' statements."

Georgescu-Roegen is willing to put more urgency into his "just-you-wait statements" in conversation than he is in print. He regards man's present place in history as being near the end of an unrepeatable bonanza of cheap fuel. "When the bonanza disappears, we may get into the kind of experience similar to that of species like fish which find they have to adapt to living in shallower waters. But in our case it would be a political and sociological change, not a biological modification. Evolution, even exosomatic evolution, is not reversible—man would rather die in the penthouse than live in the cave."

Pressed to say how and when the crisis may come, Georgescu-Roegen replies, "For the near future, I don't know. But in 50 or 60 years the world might find itself in a half anarchic state. I am not saying there will not be a government in the United States. But the tendency for the state to become more and more important in the individual's life will reverse. People will live in isolation from the state. These hippies may be an avant-garde pre-adaptation. People would have to educate their children at home because there would not be enough taxes for schools. The population might have to go down. I don't know how—it might be from the disorganization in the means of communication or of hospital care."

Whether or not this verbal presentiment turns out to be accurate, Georgescu-Roegen's general theory is a powerful and ambitious synthesis that would seem to deserve more attention than has yet been its lot. Though some of his general conclusions have been touched on by others (notably Kenneth Boulding in his 1966 essay "The economics of the coming spaceship earth"), Georgescu-Roegen has developed the scholarly underpinning of a broad theoretical framework. The theory offers potential support to many of the ideas of ecologists, environmentalists, advocates of zero population growth, opponents of economic growth, alternative technologists, and other critics of the established economic order. Here at least, if not also among "standard" economists, Georgescu-Roegen should find an increasing following.

Excerpted with permission from *Science*, 190: 447-450 (31 October 1975). Copyright 1975 by the American Association for the Advancement of Science.

8,000,000,000 People? We'll Never Get There

PAUL EHRLICH and JOHN P. HOLDREN

Paul Ehrlich of *Population Bomb* fame, and his frequent collaborator John P. Holdren, wrote the article reproduced here for the *Development Forum*, a monthly United Nations' newspaper. It is included to remind us early on that the limits on our urge to grow are not merely things, but processes. It is a theme to which we will return again.

One of the most frequently repeated imbecilities in the world today is that in 30 or so years' time, there will be twice as many people living on the earth. This statement is bandied about because *if* the population of the globe were to continue to multiply at approximately the same rate as it has been doing for the last few years, the population would indeed double in about 35 years. Unfortunately however, a long history of exponential population growth in no way implies a long future. Although it may be theoretically possible at some time in the future to support eight thousand million people temporarily, even the most casual examination of ecological constraints under which mankind must operate, and of the lamentable failure of human political and social systems to produce an equitable and efficacious distribution of the world's limited resources, make it clear that the probability of supporting eight million people by 2010 is vanishingly small.

Consider briefly just the ecological constraints. Humanity is utterly dependent for its existence upon the functioning of immense and complex ecological systems. The conditions that make earth hospitable to human life result from complex and perhaps fragile balances among the great chemical cycles—water, nitrogen, carbon, oxygen, phosphorus, sulphur—all powered by the energy of the sun. Deadly ultraviolet rays are filtered out of the sun's radiation by a minute trace of ozone in the atmosphere, and traces of carbon dioxide and water vapour keep the surface temperature of the planet within limits tolerated by present-day organisms. Some of those organisms, in turn, regulate the environmental concentrations of nitrites, ammonia and hydrogen sulphide—all poisonous to most forms of life. Over the long term, organisms also control the atmospheric concentrations of oxygen and nitrogen.

Today, four thousand million people depend on such free "service" functions of ecosystems for the preservation of the atmosphere, for the bulk of their waste disposal, for most of the nutrient cycling that is essential to the production of all their food, and for the maintenance of a great store of genetic information from which new crops, domestic animals, biological pest controls and antibiotics will come. Furthermore, almost all potential pests for our crops are controlled by nature, not by man, and almost all fish and shellfish—the source of perhaps 10 to 20 per cent of the animal protein consumed by mankind—are produced by natural ecosystems. Natural vegetation reduces floods, helps to prevent erosion, moderates local weather conditions and affects the albedo (and thus the global weather balance). Soils themselves are the product of the interaction of an enormous variety of living organisms with inorganic particles which the plants and animals help to fragment from rocks.

As incomplete as our knowledge may be concerning the vital operation of the natural systems that support human life, one cardinal principle seems clear: the ability of these systems to persist and perform their functions in the face of inevitable environmental change is related to the complexity of these systems. The more species of plants, animals and micro-organisms that have co-evolved to share the energy flowing through an ecosystem, the more stable the system is likely to be—in other words, the less likely it is that small changes in conditions will cause major disruptions.

Mankind has been a relentless enemy of co-evolved complexity in ecological systems—hence a destabilizing force—at least since the agricultural revolution (the hunting activities of human beings may have been a factor in the extinction of some large mammals even earlier). Agriculture itself is the practice of replacing co-evolved natural ecosystems with simple artificial ones based on a few strains of highly productive crops. These croplands ordinarily require constant vigilance and inputs of energy (in the form of cultivation, fertilizers, pesticides and so forth) to stave off the collapse to which their biological simplicity makes them prone. Even with prodigious effort, however, it is unlikely that mankind could maintain this perilous enterprise for long without support from natural systems.

Earth is now littered with the remains of other civilizations that failed to come to grips with the ecological constraints imposed upon society: the hydraulic civilization of the Tigris and Euphrates valleys, the classic Mayans, the ancient Khmers and the Roman Empire are only

a few examples. While history books sometimes tend to credit these collapses to mysterious life cycles within the civilizations themselves, the record of silted irrigation canals, salted and laterized soils, deforestation, erosion and the like is clear for those who know how to read it. Fortunately, the civilizations that fell victim to earlier ecocatastrophes were relatively localized. Today, so-called Western civilization embraces the entire planet.

Many ecologists believe that an essential accompaniment to the intensively exploitive activities of mankind on land and increasingly in the oceans must be preservation of extensive, lightly exploited natural communities to serve as ecological buffers and reservoirs of diversity. Failure to establish such preserves and to protect our agricultural resources as carefully as possible could spell the end of our civilization as surely as a full-scale nuclear war, though perhaps less quickly.

Today, one of the best measures of the assault humanity is mounting against the all-important natural systems that support it is the level of society's energy consumption. The simplifying processes of agriculture are increasingly powered by inanimate energy, and so is the destruction of farmlands through paving and "development." The processes that lead to the release of hundreds of thousands of new synthetic compounds into the environment are energy-intensive—and these compounds often have profound effects on the living organisms of earth, which have no prior evolutionary experience with them. One can also regard per capita energy consumption as an index of the physical activity of a society—its moving of materials and people, its transforming of materials, its changing of temperatures and so on. In virtually all circumstances, these activities exact a cost from natural environmental systems.

In the Massachusetts Institute of Technology's prestigious "Study of Critical Environmental Problems" (SCEP), a majority of the global problems considered were directly involved with energy use. The fundamentally intractable problem of thermal pollution is shared by both nuclear and fossil-fuelled power technologies (at present, nuclear power is somewhat worse in this regard). If the "historic growth" scenario of the Ford Foundation's Energy Report (3.4 percent energy growth per annum, the 1950-1970 US average) is applied to the world, the associated heat release alone would almost certainly disrupt global climate significantly within about a century, with serious ecosystemic consequences, while climatic disruptions by the carbon dioxide and particles from fossil fuel combustion could occur much sooner.

What if we could miraculously develop a source of cheap, abundant power that was nearly "pollution-free" (for example, solar or a much improved nuclear technology)? Some of the environmental problems considered in SCEP would be abated. Carbon dioxide concentrations in the atmosphere would drop, as would particulates from direct energy use, and the problems of oil pollution and containment of radioactive wastes would be reduced or eliminated. Under any reasonable scenario about the uses to which superabundant energy would be put, however, one would expect other problems (most of which are considered in SCEP) to be exacerbated: atmospheric particulates from farming marginal land, particulates from mining lower grade ores (including perhaps common rock), particulates from off-road vehicles, formation of aircraft contrails, injection of synthetic organic poisons into the biosphere, destruction of estuaries and so on. As the population grew from four thousand million towards eight, the attempt clearly would be made to pave, develop, industrialize and exploit every last bit of the planet—a trend that would inevitably lead to a collapse of the life-support systems upon which that growing population would depend.

Such a collapse could take many forms. One might be the complete loss of oceanic fisheries through a combination of overfishing, marine pollution and the destruction of estuaries. This, in turn, could lead to global famine developing as a key source of protein was removed from a world already on a nutritional knife-edge. On the other hand, the end of civilization might be triggered by weather changes induced by worldwide attempts at "development"—weather changes to which agricultural systems could no longer respond because the decay of genetic variability of crops (one of today's most serious environmental problems) had proceeded too far. Or the end might be heralded by the rapid destruction of the ozone shield, posing a direct threat to *homo sapiens* as well as to all the ecosystems of the planet. Or, as has often been predicted, the accumulation of poisonous wastes might simply swamp the natural disposal systems, making air unbreathable and water unpotable.

Most likely, of course, is a combination of such events, as mankind, largely ignorant of both the functioning of ecological systems and the nature of human attacks upon them, follows the growth maniacs and the pied pipers of technology all the way to destruction. Those who believe that science will pull a technological rabbit out of the hat to save us at the last minute simply suffer from an inability to learn. Technological rabbits tend to create more problems than they solve—they usually have large appetites and abundant noxious droppings. The green revolution, broadcast use of antibiotics and chlorinated hydrocarbon pesticides, dependence on the automobile for personal transportation, and today's primitive nuclear power systems are prime examples.

Therefore, when one talks about having eight thousand million people in the year 2010, one must ask what are the possibilities that a sequence of events leading to ecosystem collapse can be avoided. We think that such a world can be designed in *theory*, but the theory would have to neglect all the realities of human behaviour. One hardly needs special expertise to evaluate the likelihood that human society will reform to the point where the kind of "Faustian bargain" that was envisioned by Alvin Weinberg can be made—not just relative to those technological rabbits, but with Mother Nature herself.

In short, believing that there will be eight

thousand million people in the year 2010 is somewhat akin to believing in Santa Claus. We will indeed be fortunate if the world can support four thousand million in the year 2010, and the population size may well be much less than that—as a result of a continuing sequence of disasters and a general deterioration of the carrying capacity of the planet. If by some combination of unlikely events there are eight thousand million people alive in A.D. 2010, it will be a fairly sure bet that their very presence and the techniques used to support them will be mortgaging the future of all humanity—dramatically degrading the environment and reducing future carrying capacities. It is always important to remember that the question is not just "How many people can we support?" but "How many people can we support, with what standard of living, and *for how long?*" And of course there is always that ultimate question: "Why have more people?"

Reprinted with permission from *Development Forum,* (April 1976), a newspaper published monthly by the United Nations to promote knowledge and interest in many of the major causes in which the United Nations is committed.

Another Utopia Gone

SAMUEL C. FLORMAN

The Club of Rome is back again—this time observed by an engineer/philosopher/businessman named Samuel Florman, author of a much-praised book entitled *The Existential Pleasures of Engineering*. In this article, first published in the August, 1976 issue of *Harpers*, he does not come down on one side or the other of the growth debate. Rather he ponders, painfully, the very problem Linda Stewart began with: Is a fundamental change in humanity required? Is humanity capable of fundamental change?

The gentle sophistries of the Club of Rome

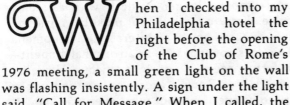hen I checked into my Philadelphia hotel the night before the opening of the Club of Rome's 1976 meeting, a small green light on the wall was flashing insistently. A sign under the light said, "Call for Message." When I called, the operator said, "There is no message." I asked why the light was flashing. She replied, "The system is broken; we're trying to fix it." During the next few days, I thought often of that light.

Clearly, the global system in which we live is malfunctioning. Warning lights blink wildly all over the world. So it is reassuring to know that the members of the Club of Rome are dedicated to finding out what is wrong, and to prescribing a solution. They are a remarkable body of scholars, industrialists, and civil servants who give fresh luster to that worn-out phrase "men of goodwill." Their three-day meeting in April was a beautiful demonstration of moral concern. At the same time, judged by the standard of intellectual content, much of it bordered on the absurd. I had come to Philadelphia looking for a message about the future. Like the telephone operator at the hotel, the Club of Rome

had no message, at least not one that I found intelligible. They filled the air with exhortations, inspiring visions, and noble proposals, hardly any of which came to grips with the problems of the world. At the close of the conference, I was left with a troublesome question: Can an intellectual disaster be a moral triumph?

A queer animal

The idea of holding the Club of Rome's meeting in Philadelphia is credited to Fulvio Oliveto, a member of the Philadelphia chapter of the Institute of Electrical and Electronics Engineers. Oliveto made his proposal to the club's chairman, the Italian industrialist Aurelio Peccei, who was enthusiastic. The idea was then taken to Philadelphia's prestigious Franklin Institute, and on to the First Pennsylvania Corporation, the city's leading financial institution, whose leaders had been looking for a suitable Bicentennial project. The corporation put up $240,000 to underwrite the cost of the conference, plus part of the cost of an exhibit on "futures" to be mounted at the institute. Surely the sponsors were not unmindful of the public-relations benefits to be reaped from such an enterprise, but compared to all the foolish, costumed stagings of Revolutionary War battles and other embarrassing Bicentennial manifestations, the decision to invite the Club of Rome to Philadelphia stood as a model of intelligence and good taste.

The Club of Rome had never before held one of its full-scale meetings in the United States. It was coming to these shores bathed in a mystique almost without parallel for an organization so young and lacking in wealth, power, or constituency. Part of the club's fame is, undoubtedly, attributable to its elegant name. The word *club* has a social flavor that cannot be duplicated by *organization, institute,* or even *society.* "Rome" connotes imperial majesty, ecclesiastical grandeur, and continental sophistication. Add to this fortuitous choice of name an arresting first report seeming to predict the imminent end of the world, and you have the beginnings of instant renown.

The club was founded in 1968 at the home of Aurelio Peccei, following a leisurely luncheon at the Accademia dei Lincei in Rome. As Peccei tells the tale, the weather was balmy, the view from the academy was lovely, and the wine flowed freely. Thirty concerned citizens from ten nations had gathered to discuss mankind's ominous prospects, and to consider what a small group like themselves might do to improve them. The urbane aura of that occasion characterizes the deliberations of the club leaders to this day, making their meetings seem a little dilettantish, but, at the same time, establishing a mood of cordial civility that inspires faith in the possibility of rational solutions.

The club is "a queer animal," in Peccei's words, with no organization or staff, keeping no formal minutes of its meetings, and having practically no budget. "When we first tried to get support," says Peccei with a smile, "we got much support. Moral support." However, the club has found a way around its lack of direct income. Its conferences, which take place almost every year, have been subsidized by the governments of Austria, Switzerland, and Canada, and by business groups in France, Japan, and now the United States. Its research projects are underwritten by governments, foundations,

and corporations. The power of persuasion is clearly not the least of its members' talents. Chartered in Switzerland as a nonprofit association, the club's membership is limited to 100, and is drawn from all parts of the world, with the notable exceptions to date of Russia and China. Peccei is at pains to make clear that he has no grandiose plans for bureaucratic growth. The club's purpose, he says, is to act as a catalyst, to point out the nature of world problems, to propose alternative solutions, to alarm and enlighten governments and entire populations.

The web of global crises—technical, social, economic, and political—is labeled by the club the *problematique humaine.* The most significant characteristic of the *problematique* is an all-encompassing, interrelated complexity. The club maintains that such problems as food, population, resources, pollution, poverty, et cetera can no longer be dealt with as identifiable, discrete matters, but must be considered as a dynamic maze of interacting phenomena. This does not appear to be an original thought—in fact, it seems downright obvious. However, the Club of Rome's great contribution was to try to be specific about what everyone knew to be generally true, to attempt to quantify and examine the forces at work. Seeking nothing less than a mathematical model for the whole world, it was inevitable that several club members should find their way in the summer of 1970 to MIT, where Prof. Jay Forrester and his group were performing pioneering work in the field of systems dynamics. With financial support from the Volkswagen Foundation, an international team of researchers was put to work under the directorship of Dennis Meadows, and a year later the first report to the Club of Rome was ready. A popularized version of this report was published in March 1972 under the title *The Limits to Growth.*

The essence of the report was that exponential growth trends in population, industrialization, pollution, food production, and resource depletion threaten to bring us to the limits of global capacity within 100 years;

resulting in catastrophe. No sooner had the ink dried (actually it never did dry, since the book has sold more than 2 million copies around the world and new editions are still being published) than the debate began between proponents of growth and no-growth. This issue, which made the Club of Rome world-famous overnight, has also proved to be something of an albatross. Peccei has tried vainly to explain that *Limits to Growth* was merely a first report *to* the club, and that it was not intended to be a statement of club policy. Club members have learned that it is easier to get your name into the newspapers than to get the story told to your satisfaction.

The argument about growth and no-growth seems to have generated much more heat than light. What Meadows said, after all, was that destructive growth is destructive, not exactly the sort of statement that should enrage reasonable men. Those who have attacked the report because it does not allow for the corrective actions people will take are coming very close to a tautology. People will indeed take action, not only because of automatic factors such as price changes (the effect of which perhaps the report has underestimated), but because of reasoned action resulting from forecasts such as the report itself. In your warning, say these critics, you have neglected to consider that we might listen to your warning. Adding to the confusion is a lack of agreement about what exactly is meant by "growth." *The Limits to Growth* does not advocate a cessation of constructive activity, as some critics have assumed. Continuing technological advance, according to the text, will be "both necessary and welcome," as will "higher productivity," which could be "translated into a higher standard of living or more leisure or more pleasant surroundings for everyone." In short, the public debate, while not entirely without substance, proved to be an emotional argument between worried advocates of planning on the one hand and mildly optimistic advocates of laissez-faire on the other.

Members of the Club of Rome, although professing dismay at all the confusion and tumult, could not have helped but feel that *The Limits to Growth* was a success beyond their wildest dreams. The controversy it sparked had inspired the very debate it was the club's aim to encourage.

Then, suddenly, the entire picture changed. This animated, essentially academic, colloquy was interrupted by an outraged clamor of protest from an unexpected source—the underdeveloped nations of the Third World. "How can you have the effrontery," they asked, "to talk about limiting growth while we are starving and impoverished, just planning to embark on some growth of our own?" *The Limits to Growth*, they maintained, could only be viewed as part of a conspiracy to further subdue the exploited peoples, and the Club of Rome, as its name implied, was obviously an elitist agent of the imperialistic West.

The good and gentle members of the club were shocked and abashed. Certainly they had not intended to slight any of their brothers on this planet. They resolved to make amends. In so reacting they were already expressing the moral compassion and intellectual chaos that were to mark the Philadelphia meeting of April 1976.

A sermon and a hymn

Computerized forecasting on a global scale has not been abandoned by the club. A new world model has been created by members Mihajlo Mesarovic and Edward Pestel, and stored in Mesarovic's computer at Case Western Reserve University. This model is more complex than the *Limits* model; it divides the world into ten distinct geographical regions, and has data on different "levels" (individual, group, demoeconomic, technology, and environment). It contains statistical information on about 100,000 relationships, such as birth rate to population growth, oil prices to fertilizer production, and capital stock to economic output. Scenarios can be played showing the probable impact of various alternative policies in the fields of agriculture, economy and finance, industrial investment, energy, and population control.

Work with this model formed the basis of the second report to the Club of Rome, published in 1974, entitled *Mankind at the Turning Point*. At the Philadelphia meeting, which was called "New Horizons for Mankind" (the titles begin to pall), one session was devoted to a report by Mesarovic and Pestel on current use of the model as an alternative policy tool. At Case, Mesarovic is studying how alternative U.S. policies might affect the global food crisis. Other projects are under way in Germany, Iran, Venezuela, and Egypt. The progress reports on these projects were, I thought, the most substantial and interesting part of the conference. I heard some knowledgeable people complain that the model contains assumptions that are unwarranted, but to all such criticism Mesarovic and Pestel respond that they are learning by doing, and keeping the model "open" for modification.

If the club had restricted itself to improving such policy tools, advocating their use, and publicizing the results obtained with them, one could only report that they were performing a valuable service. Of course, this would mean diminishing headlines, and a sense of frustration for Peccei and his colleagues, whose aim it is to prod the world continuously, vigorously, and in every conceivable fashion. It would also fail to satisfy the Third World critics of *The Limits to Growth*.

So the club embarked on two new ventures which were unveiled in Philadelphia: the RIO project (Reviewing the International Order), under the direction of the Nobel Prize-winning Dutch economist Jan Tinbergen, and *Goals for Global Societies*, directed by the philosopher Ervin Laszlo. These two works may stimulate enough controversy to satisfy the club's zest for perpetual agitation, but they are likely to damage, permanently, the club's reputation with clear-thinking people.

The RIO report, the full version of which is to be published some time this year, contains much solid information, and reflects devoted consideration of world economic problems, but it is, I believe, fatally flawed. In brief, it proposes that the rich nations make gifts to the poor nations, with the objective of reducing the 13-to-1 ratio that exists between average income in the richest 10 percent of nations and the poorest 10 percent. The word *gift* is not used, to be sure. Various euphemisms are adopted. There should be "transfers" of fertilizers, and "transfers" of funds for development (more than $30 billion by 1980), "compliance" by transnational enterprises "with host countries' plans," "subventioning" of the cost of technological knowhow, and so forth. In addition, the developed countries should assist the underdeveloped countries—or "developing," to use the preferred word—by reducing tariffs, easing immigration restrictions, and levying taxes to support a central world treasury. "Continuation of the study," says a document distributed by the club, "may well indicate that the very concept of nation-state is outdated."

It takes no great insight into human affairs to conclude that citizens of the wealthier nations may not be willing to make the sacrifices called for in the RIO report. The report maintains that redistribution of wealth is required in order to avert worldwide disaster. It seems to me that the opposite argument can be made more compellingly. Impoverished masses are much less likely to cause trouble for us than developing nations, which are just beginning to feel their oats. Angola-like controversies can arise, of course, but the superpowers have developed ways of handling such confrontations. The brutal truth is that the poorest nations do not pose a substantial threat to our well-being. Knowing, however, that the emerging nations will emerge eventually, whether we want them to or not, we are seeking their goodwill. We need their raw materials, we would like to have them as markets, and we want them to fall within our sphere of influence. Also, although we are terribly selfish, we want to do what is *right*.

What the average American considers to be right tends to be expressed in the form of what

American leaders consider to be politically feasible. The outer limit of such policy at this time is defined by present aid programs, augmented by the plan which Secretary of State Kissinger proposed to the U.N. Conference on Trade and Development in Nairobi last May 6. The main feature of this plan is the establishment of a billion-dollar International Resources Bank designed to stimulate private investment in the development of Third World resources, and to help stabilize the prices of such resources. There are other elements designed to ameliorate some of the problems faced by the poorer nations, but nothing vaguely resembling the extravagant demands of the RIO package. RIO is not a rational proposal. It calls for more charity than people are willing to give. In order to become effective, it requires nothing less than a change in human nature. It is a sermon masquerading as a study.

If we protest, however, the Club of Rome is ready for us. It quickly brings Ervin Laszlo on stage with *Goals for Global Societies*. Human nature *can* change, says Laszlo. "Our researches show that the inner dimension of all major nations and cultures is capable of creative and humanistic transformation." His staff members are studying polls and newspapers, conducting interviews, and in a variety of ways trying to capture the philosophical mood in different parts of the world. They claim to have evidence showing that there are humanistic goals which all people can accept, and which will enable mankind to survive in a spirit of harmony. The final report, like RIO, will be published later this year. At Philadelphia, Laszlo presented some preliminary findings: Americans believe that their level of consumption is immoral, and that their politicians are not as forthright as they ought to be; in Western Europe the young are flocking to the ideals of the counter-culture—utter honesty and self-limitation; in Eastern Europe there are socialist goals; in Japan there are indications that the aspirations of the average citizen are less materialistic than they were in 1973; in the Arab nations there is an urgency to catch up with the West, but a

desire for something other than a consumer society; in Africa people are essentially religious; and so forth. "What we need," Laszlo said, "is an evolution of a new ethical consciousness." The lights dimmed, and a slide was projected with the heading "The Required Transformation in Contemporary Values and Beliefs." At this point my notes become sketchy: "all religions . . . universal compassion . . . brotherhood . . . world solidarity." It was late in the day, and there was restless stirring in the hall as the third session of the conference drew to an end. Yet a sudden hush seemed to descend as Laszlo concluded. "We all have a moral obligation," he said, "to spur development of a sense of solidarity." If RIO was the sermon, then *Goals for Global Societies* was the closing hymn.

Romantic reformers

At the opening session Peccei had invoked the ethical and moral imperatives of the Declaration of Independence. Throughout the conference, speakers kept referring to the Bicentennial and the spirit of the American Revolution. Yet the single element most conspicuously absent from the conference was the very pragmatism that characterized the American Founding Fathers. Jefferson and Franklin had ideals, but it never occured to them to hang their hopes on anything as ephemeral as the "evolution of a new ethical consciousness." Their great achievement was to create a government for people who were imperfect, yet who wanted to live in freedom under a system of law. They were clearheaded, skeptical men of Enlightenment.

The Club of Rome meeting was imbued with a very different spirit, a romantic neoidealism akin to that which prevailed in nineteenth-century Europe. Also, for all the lip service paid to the achievements of the U.S., I sensed undercurrents of resentment and disapproval. The mood brought to mind not Philadelphia in 1776, but in 1876, when the Centennial Exhibition attracted large numbers of European visitors. They crowded into the glass-and-iron

Machine Hall to marvel at the many new mechanisms powered by the gigantic Corliss steam engine. American technology had come into its own, and astute observers could see that this portended significant changes for the human race. Europeans were impressed, but grudgingly so, patronizing the young nation as being technologically strong but woefully deficient in culture. A hundred years later this attitude persists. The 1976 Club of Rome meeting was, perhaps more than anything else, a genteel confrontation between the new world and the old, between American pragmatism and European intellectualism.

The principal speakers at the meeting were all Europeans. Two of them, Mesarovic and Laszlo, were nominally Americans, but European born and educated. As for the Latins, Africans, Asians, Arabs, and other non-Europeans, most of them, having been educated in the European tradition, shared the European mode of thought. The Americans were outnumbered about 10 to 1, and outtalked about 100 to 1. However, when the final oratory died away, they seemed to have acquitted themselves very well.

For a while, things did not look promising for the image of the host nation. The ugly American arrived in the person of Vice-President Nelson A. Rockefeller, who almost soured the affair beyond redemption. The opening banquet at the Franklin Institute was one of those festive occasions that impress even the jaded partygoer. The invited guests included not only the eighty-odd conference participants from all over the world, about half of them Club of Rome members, but also a select group of Philadelphia citizens who had been invited by the sponsors. Everyone had been checked, and then checked again, by the Secret Service. The many agents with walkie-talkies and troopers with rifles heightened the pleasant feeling of dramatic tension. Dr. Bowen C. Dees, director of the institute, walked serenely around the room, greeting as notable a collection of guests as his venerable building had seen in some time. All of a sudden the Vice-President was there, moving into the heart of the crowd, smiling, reaching out to shake hands. The feeling of power was electric.

Soon we were seated in the Benjamin Franklin Memorial Hall, under the huge white statue of Franklin by James Earl Fraser, dining on crown roast of lamb, and basking in the festive atmosphere. Then, after the coffee had been served, Nelson Rockefeller stood up and gave a harsh, crude, insulting speech that embarrassed everyone in the room almost beyond endurance. It was not a bad or uninteresting speech, as speeches go—a no-nonsense Moynihan-like rebuke to unrealistic demands of Third World nations. However, before this group of benevolent humanitarians and invited guests, the effect was shocking. It is to the credit of Nelson Rockefeller's reputation for responsibility that the almost universal assumption amongst the guests was that he had not seen the speech before he stood up to deliver it. Each of the three times he said that the most meaningful thing America can do to solve world problems is to increase its own well-being, so as to serve as an example for others, he appeared to wince. When he called the Club of Rome naive for the second time, I felt that some speechwriter would soon be out of a job. He concluded by berating doomsday prophets and expressing total faith in the American people. There was hardly any applause. He shook hands with Peccei, who was flushed but grinning, trying to pretend that he had not been insulted. John Bunting, chairman of the First Pennsylvania Corporation, and host for the evening, gamely assured the Club of Rome members that they would have "equal time" the next day. The *Evening Bulletin* reported the event in the hockey parlance of the season: "Vice-President Nelson A. Rockefeller checked First Pennsylvania Corp. chairman John R. Bunting, Jr., into the boards last night. Bunting came up fast, saying it didn't really hurt."

John Bunting is a slight, trim man with an imperturbable manner, a man who appears to know that the world is undergoing upheavals, and that in the future only those with foresight and a fine sense of balance will be able to keep their footing. In his speeches and reports, which took note of the Club of Rome long before 1976, he has spoken of the danger of uncontrolled growth, while at the same time pointing out the vital role that growth, and even inflation, have played in making political and social change possible. His writings portray an orderly mind that sees the purposes served by an element of disorder. This contrasts sharply with the many members of the club who crave order but do not see the complexities—or the dangers—involved in getting it. Most American businessmen might think that sponsoring a Club of Rome meeting was a waste of hard-earned stockholder money. Bunting, one imagines, aside from Bicentennial publicity considerations, was intrigued by the intellectual and social chemistry which might result when these notables from all over the world gathered together, not only to talk to each other and to the public, but, incidentally, to absorb something of the flavor of Philadelphia, and of the United States of America.

On the first day, during the RIO session, after Idriss Jazairy of Algeria had excoriated transnational enterprises, reciting a "litany of exploitation," and calling for their control by international "antitrust" legislation, G. William Miller, Chairman of Textron, Inc., was called upon to comment. "We must consider," said Miller softly, "the realities of human nature from the beginning of recorded time. The arguments we have heard will not convince the 'haves' to turn over their wealth to the 'have-nots.' This is not a negative comment. It is realistic. We must seek a confluence of self-interest." If there is a receptive climate, he continued, investment capital will flow from the rich nations to the poor. He suggested that we build with the institutions that we have, trying to make the transnational corporations a force for good in the world.

I wondered if this straightforward approach might not bring about a change in the tone of the meeting; but it was not to be. The next speaker, Enrique Iglesias of Chile, responded defensively, "Do we appear rhetorical and

literary? Well, we are building a new code of moral conduct."

The following morning Richard Gardner of Columbia Law School tried to turn the meeting's attention to the limitations imposed on all action by the imperfections of human beings. He spoke of the ineffectual ways in which our political leaders function even when goals are not a matter of dispute. His wry humor evoked little response.

On the final morning Arthur Stern, senior vice-president of Magnavox, addressed the meeting briefly. Referring to the RIO proposal to redistribute resources in the world, he said, "The populations of the wealthy countries will perceive such redistribution as a sacrifice. We cannot postulate it as a categorical imperative. It won't 'sell.' These are all wishes." It is not merely a question of what is just, he tried to explain, as if talking to a child. We must consider what is possible.

In love with ideals

It is maddening to hear what seems to be pure common sense, and to see that it is making no impression on the audience. What is there about the people at this conference that makes them immune to persuasion by evidence? "Everyone tries to discourage us," Mesarovic told me. "We do not get discouraged." Yes, but there is more to it than that.

One element was touched on the first day by the Indian journalist Romesh Thapar, when he said that "those of us who come to conferences are an elite who live luxuriously, copying your ways." The members of this elite group in no way represent the reality of life as it is lived by the masses in their countries. Nor, on the other hand, do they represent the real power establishment (a few maverick industrialists like Peccei notwithstanding). This point was made by another Indian, Prof. Bacigha Singh Minhas of New Delhi, who said, "The ideology that we formulate may be tolerated by the upper class. But this is hypocrisy."

Members of the Club of Rome represent

neither the proletariat nor the ruling classes, but that very thin layer of society which used to be called the intelligentsia. To a certain extent this disqualifies them from speaking with authority about the future, for they represent nobody, and in any political upheaval they would be likely to disappear without a trace. One might even postulate that their interest in a world order stems in part from their frustration over the lack of a just order within their own homelands. During the three days of the conference there was no mention of the oppressive conditions that exist within the nations of so many of the participants. Not a word about political imprisonments, torture, corruption, violation of basic human rights, misappropriation of aid funds, and the rest. This may be in keeping with the etiquette of an international gathering, but it also reflects the willful blindness of those who are in love with their ideals.

During the final session of the conference a woman handed me a reprint of an article by Peccei entitled "The Humanistic Revolution." When I saw what it was, I felt like saying to her, "Dear lady, I have already read this, and I beg you to take all the copies of it that you can find and burn them quickly. Dr. Peccei is a good and kindly man, with wonderful talents for organizing and inspiring people. Tell him not to waste his time spinning these wild fantasies." I picked up the article which I had struggled through a few days previously: *"Something fundamental must be done to change human society and man himself.... The challenge, in other words, is that of a quantum jump in human quality. Nothing less or different can suffice. And only a humane philosophy of life—a new humanism firmly established as the inspiration and guideline of society—can generate and sustain this qualitative change."*

All Club of Rome literature makes liberal use of italics to stress apocalyptic warnings and transcendental solutions. At this point I would like to italicize a sentence of my own. *We dare not trust the future of our children to any scheme that insists upon a change in human nature, particularly since the Club of Rome and others have shown convincingly that we cannot afford to wait for the millennium, but must plan*

and act promptly and continuously to meet the crises that confront us. As Messrs. Miller, Gardner, and Stern told the conference, our only hope is to work with the people and institutions that exist. It is all very well to strive for the evolution of a new ethical consciousness. Who would not endorse such an effort? It is true, as Laszlo has said, that our attitudes are constantly changing, and sometimes such efforts have amazing success. Yet one thing has never changed, through the coming and going of great faiths, through the rise and fall of chieftains, emperors, doges, protectors, popes, and commissars, and that one thing is the struggle for wealth and power.

Such empirical reality does not impress the European intellectual. An Austrian graduate student tried to explain it to me once in a wine cellar in Salzburg: "You do not understand. We simply must have our theories."

It is all too easy to make fun of the implausible ideas of Peccei and his colleagues, and of the ornate sentences that filled the auditorium like music as the Club of Rome meeting drew toward its close. Ideas are wispy and have no reality until that sudden, unpredictable moment when they catch fire and explode. Then no one, least of all the person whose idea it was, can predict what will happen. From the witty conversation of Parisian salons, and some half-baked ideas of Jean Jacques Rousseau, we can trace a line to the fall of the Bastille, Robespierre, and finally Napolean. Ideas can be laughable, but they can also be frightening, particularly grandiose political ideas.

The ultimate expression of political intellectualism is to be found in the People's Republic of China. During the *Goals for Global Societies* session, Paul Lin of McGill University spoke of this phenomenon. "Freedom and welfare," he said, "are abstractions that mean nothing to the oppressed."

Beyond RIO and *Goals for Global Societies*, beyond all the Club of Rome visions of a new order, lies the reality of Communist China. It is the one place in the world where moral improvement is public policy. In our travail it beckons like easeful death, but not yet. Time enough for that if we fail.

"Be a little naive"

At the end, the 1976 meeting of the Club of Rome seemed both ludicrous and frightening—and yet, as I said at the outset, inspiring. The same Arthur Stern who on the final day counseled the club members to return to the world of the possible was at the previous night's dinner comparing them to Diogenes and Jesus. "The deep faith in these men shines through," he said. "With all its shortcomings, the Club of Rome is unique."

At the press conference that followed the final session, Peccei and his executive committee members responded to questions that, while not hostile, were plainly skeptical. From the point of view of press coverage the event was already a success, having received respectful front-page coverage in the *New York Times*, which in turn had brought representatives scurrying from *Time* and *Newsweek*. But Peccei, an evangelist to the end, was trying to persuade all the reporters present to carry the club's message forth continually to the public. He looked around the room, wistfully, wrinkling his brow like an aging Marcello Mastroianni. "Be a little naive," he said, "as we have been accused of being. It can be a better world."

A reported asked, "Are you personally satisfied in your conscience that you are a model world citizen?" There was an embarrassed pause.

"We are not saints," answered Peccei. "But I will die with the belief that I did what I could."

Reprinted with permission from *Harper's Magazine,* 253: 29-32+ (August 1976). Copyright 1976 by *Harper's Magazine.* All rights reserved.

The Talk of the Town

There is much, and little, to be said for surveys, of course, especially surveys which simply poll people about what they think, as opposed to measuring what they actually do. Nevertheless, both the *New Yorker* and I found encouragement on the eve of the Bicentennial year in what appeared to be a new acceptance of the notion that Americans might well be willing to consider lowering both their voices and their expectations.

Notes and Comment

A few years ago, a national debate arose over what the Club of Rome, in one of its publications, called "the limits to growth." Some people believed that economic expansion could go on indefinitely. Among them was President Nixon, who remarked, in a speech to the Seafarers International Union toward the end of 1973, "There are only seven per cent [actually, the figure was then five and a half per cent] of the people of the world living in the United States, and we use thirty per cent [actually, thirty-three per cent] of all the energy. That isn't bad; that is good. That means we are the richest, strongest people in the world, and that we have the highest standard of living in the world. That is why we need so much energy, and may it always be that way." President Nixon, of course, wanted the United States to be "No. 1" in just about every statistic you could think of. On the other side of the argument were people who believed that economic expansion would run up against certain natural limits—limits on the earth's capacity for supporting population, limits on the biosphere's capacity for enduring industrial pollution, and limits on the earth's natural resources. A few days ago, the results of a recent Louis Harris poll indicated strongly that, at least as far as the general public was concerned, the debate was over. By sixty-one per cent to twenty-three per cent, the public agreed with the statement that it was "morally wrong" for Americans to consume forty per cent (a later figure) of the world's energy and raw materials. By fifty-five per cent to thirty per cent, the public agreed that the disparity between population and consumption "hurts the well-being of the rest of the world." By fifty per cent to thirty-one per cent, the public agreed with the statement that America's continued high consumption "will turn the rest of the people of the world against us." By eighty-one per cent to ten per cent, the public agreed that high consumption "causes us to pollute the air, the rivers, and the seas." And by ninety per cent to five per cent the public agreed that "we here in this country will have to find ways to cut back on the amount of things we consume and waste." These figures seem to indicate a revolution in the popular attitude. The figures in polls, of course, are extremely changeable, as anyone who has followed political campaigns well knows. However, when they rise above a certain level—reach sixty or sixty-five per cent—there can be no doubt that something significant is happening to public opinion. And on the very rare occasions when the figures rise into the eighties or the nineties one recognizes that one is dealing with political reality of the first order.

Many currents of opinion must have flowed together to produce the shift reflected in the Harris poll. One of the currents, certainly, was the anti-materialist revolt of the young in the nineteen-sixties. Probably another was the revival of fiscal conservatism among politicians of the right, which took the form of an attack on the programs of social spending set up in the years of President Lyndon Johnson. A third current was probably the environmental movement. The decisive events may have been the oil embargo of 1973 and the recession, which began at about the same time. The concurrence of the energy crisis and the recession apparently taught the public that the penalties for overconsumption could be basic and severe. The threat, the public learned, was not just to "the quality of life"—that luxurious preoccupation of the nineteen-sixties—but to people's livelihoods, to life itself.

The people in politics, not for the first time in recent years, have been slow to discover the public's mood, and slow to respond to it. Among politicians who are visible on the national scene, only Governor Jerry Brown of California seems to be closely attuned to it, in his politics of austerity, and a recent poll has shown that he enjoys an approval rating of seven to one among California voters. The Presidential candidates of both parties have drawn close to the new consensus and circled around it, but not one has laid claim to it. Many of the Democrats have apparently decided that the thing to do is to "run against Washington"—an empty, wholly negative program that catches the bare fact of the public's disillusionment but not its con-

tent. The Republicans seem to have rested their political hopes on a campaign against federal spending, but federal spending, although it may be unpopular, is not exactly what is bothering the public, either. The public is not fed up with government and at the same time enamored of private enterprise. What seems to have happened is that the public, in a striking reversal of the American mood in the prosperous post-war years, has turned against excess and waste in all its forms—public, private, and even personal. In addition, the passion to be No. 1 has apparently subsided, leaving the people willing to let the United States take its place in the world simply as a nation among nations. It will do now to be No. 2 or No. 3 in a few areas. (And if the public does not want the United States to give offense to other nations by excessive consumption, how much less must it want the government to overthrow the governments of other countries and kill their leaders.) Next year, the United States will recall its origins through Bicentennial celebrations and set the course for the immediate future through a Presidential election. As that year of reflection and decision approaches, Louis Harris is telling us that the public is hoping for a new modesty of national purpose and a new austerity of means. He may have given us an early glimpse of the spirit of 1976.

Reprinted with permission from *The New Yorker,* 51 (43): 33-34 (15 December 1975). Copyright 1975 by The New Yorker Magazine, Inc.

Limiting Growth in a Finite World

There is a familiar "chase" sequence from my childhood that still turns up regularly on TV's Saturday morning cartoon shows. In it the chasee somehow lures the chaser into running off a cliff; the pursuer's momentum carries him (never—oddly enough—her) off the edge of the cliff and—still running—out into mid-air. Suddenly he realizes where he is, looks down—and falls.

What if he did not look down? Could he simply continue running? Has this "harmless" violence perpetrated by Tom and Jerry, Woody Woodpecker, Bugs Bunny and their friends helped generations of Americans to internalize that very American lesson: keep moving at all costs? Have we learned to believe that if we do not look down, we can forever escape the abyss?

Some such belief appears to motivate the angriest critics of the ideas which have been explored in this chapter. That material growth cannot be indefinitely continued on a materially finite globe seems almost childishly self-evident. Yet in the less than half a decade since the "no-growth" movement was first given a name, much of what has been said and written about the "irrationality," "impracticality," and "immorality" of such an idea appears to be founded on optimistic extrapolation from Looney Tunes logic—that if we just keep running, new ground will miraculously appear under our flying feet.

Linda Stewart in her opening paper, manages to capture with wit and feeling the barrier—not intellectual but emotional—which impedes our thinking. The world has not ended before, she concedes, a fact which has mistakenly led us to infer the existence of a celestial contract assuring the survival—no matter what—of the fragile crust of life on earth. Part of our confusion no doubt arises from our habit of believing with the Carborundum Company that progress means "doing what nature never intended"; as a consequence we find it difficult to believe that nature's intentions may be more serious than ours.

Richard Koff's article on page 6, first published in 1971, provides a brief but informative introduction to the Club of Rome, to the concept of the "counter-intuitive" solution developed by MIT Professor Jay Forrester, and to the doomsday conclusions of a team of scientists and a computer—conclusions which were published in book form some months later under the title *Limits to Growth*.[1] Since then, in much the same way that Kleenex has come to represent all tissue handkerchiefs in the public mind, "limits to growth" has become the generic descriptor for a whole cluster of ideas centering around the single notion that "we can't grow on like this." Perhaps because its title *became* generic; perhaps because *Limits'* computer printouts of disaster appealed to the American infatuation with the trappings of science; or perhaps simply because we in the U. S. are so unregenerately ethnocentric, *Limits* had a much wider impact than did its British counterpart—the much more radical "Blueprint for Survival"[2] mentioned by Stewart as having preceded *Limits* into

---

[1]D.H. Meadows, D.L. Meadows, J. Randers, W. Behrens III, *The Limits to Growth* (New York: Universe Books, 1972).
[2]E. Goldsmith, *et al.*, "A Blueprint for Survival," *The Ecologist*, 2: 1-42 (January 1972).

print. *Blueprint* urged not merely the cessation of growth, but the reconstruction of the entire society, including an ultimate *reduction* in the population of the British Isles.

Between them, *Blueprint* and *Limits* set off the debate. The Mobil Oil Company ad and the answer to it by economist Herman Daly, both reprinted here, give the flavor of the argument that ensued. For the growth advocates, "no-growth" was elitist, a position taken by those of us who "had it made" and were now warning the "have-nots" against adding to the pollution our affluence was already producing. Continuous material growth, they argued, is the only hope the poor have of bettering their lot. Daly's answer—laid out briefly in the article from *Environmental Action*—was both angry and eloquent. Growth alone will *not* help the poor, he insisted, only economic justice will, and we had better get on with it. To urge continued growth as a solution merely permits us to justify our own greed and to "economize on scarce moral resources."

His point is further explicated in Vanya Walker Leigh's interview with former Common Market President Dr. Sicco Mansholt. Dr. Mansholt points out that for us to continue to grow is to use up the cheap and readily available resource stocks so that there will be less left for those countries just beginning to industrialize. Moreover, he argues, the issue is not so much moral as political, since to act on the belief that there are "limits to growth" would require from politicians measures equivalent to political suicide.

But morality and political feasibility aside, what of the substance of the argument? Is the world coming to an end? If so, when? Is there really an urgent and immediate need to limit growth? Or change its direction?

Much early criticism of *Limits* was directed at technical or conceptual flaws in the model and at the fact that the basic data on which the computer runs were based were not published. The most trivial of these criticisms were silenced by the Arab oil boycott. The abrupt cutting-off of Middle-East fuel sources, though politically motivated and (as it happened) temporary, began to raise serious public questions about the *ultimate* finiteness of fossil fuel and other material resources. Moreover, the sudden rash of seemingly unrelated shortages—of paper, glass, plastics, fertilizer, pharmaceuticals and so on—served to illustrate on a small scale the inter-relatedness of problems—an inter-relatedness which on a much grander scale was the "problematique" to which the Club of Rome had originally addressed itself.

The second Club of Rome sponsored analysis, *Mankind at the Turning Point*, was published in 1974, by which time the lifting of the Arab oil boycott, the greed of the oil companies, and the political short-sightedness Dr. Mansholt had warned against had conspired to obscure once again the underlying limits the boycott had revealed.[3] The new motto was "energy independence," interpreted in some circles as a "drain America first," or "Strength Through Exhaustion" policy.[4]

The headline in *The New York Times* reporting on a conference called to discuss the new Club of Rome study, reflected the swing back to optimism: "Scholars Rebut Computer View that Disaster Awaits Mankind."[5] Mobil leaped once more into the role of public informer, hailing the new book as a "reprieve." Criticizing the original *Limits'* analysis, the authors of *Mankind* claimed to have found that growth was acceptable as long as it was "organic," and that certain disaster did not await us all if growth continued.

On closer reading, however, the author's apparent optimism takes on a decidedly less sanguine cast. *Limits*, by treating the whole world as a single unit, failed to take into account both the uneven

---

[3]The willingness of the public to believe good news, even while they were standing in gas lines, was astonishing. Surveys taken by the National Opinion Research Center in December 1973 and January-February 1974 showed that the general public expectation was that there would be "an absence of energy shortages before 1980" and that future fuel shortages were "not inevitable."
[4]David Brower, "Nonnuclear Futures," *Not Man Apart* (mid-July, 1975).
[5]*The New York Times* (18 October 1974).

distribution of people and the uneven distribution of resources in various countries. The model was, to use the standard terminology, too aggregated. The new analysis divided the world up into regions—with the result that in some areas where population was large and resources limited, the computer showed disaster occurring even more rapidly than in the Meadows' model.

Boulding's brief review of *Mankind*, published originally in *Science*, brilliantly captures the "attempting to be hopeful" flavor of the new analysis. The chapter from Mesarovic and Pestel's book which follows the Boulding review suggests the nature of the crises they foresee if, unlike Nineveh, we do not repent. It is a very conditional optimism indeed.

But some optimists remained unconditional. Professor Esfandiary is clearly one of them, and his brief brief for technological solutions is an appropriate introduction to the ecstatic growth scenarios of Herman Kahn and his colleagues at the Hudson Institute. In a volume called *The Next 200 Years*,[6] published (not inadvertently one suspects) at the end of America's *first* 200 years, Kahn confidently predicts that while "200 years ago almost everywhere human beings were comparatively few, poor and at the mercy of the forces of nature . . . 200 years from now, we expect, almost everywhere they will be numerous, rich and in control of the forces of nature." Even without space colonies (whose existence he assumes), there is no reason why we could not have by 2176, 15 billion people, ". . . give or take a factor of two [that is a range of 7.5 to 30 billion] . . .," with per capita incomes of $20,000.

How is this miracle to come about? Kahn's underlying assumption is that the rate of population growth has now peaked, so that "the problem of exponential population growth appears almost to be solving itself." He illustrates his contention with several charts, two of which are shown below.

Figure 1, "Population Growth Rate in Long-Term Historical Perspective," appears to show that, just as Kahn asserts, we are at the precise peak of an historically unprecedented upsurge in population growth which is now about to decline as rapidly as it has increased—levelling off, as predicted, around 2176 (give or take a few years.) The illusion created by Figure 1 is that the sense of overcrowding we feel is temporary, an illusion that is dispelled by Figure 2—or would be dispelled by Figure 2 were it to be continued beyond the "present."

For "population growth rate" and "population" are two different things, and there is nowhere any indication that the line representing the size of the total population is going to take a reassuring tumble. If one thinks about the cause of the "population explosion" of the past decades, what is happening will become obvious. For the rapid increase in rate of population growth was not caused by any apparent increase in *birth rates* (indeed birth rates have actually declined slightly), but by a decrease in *death rates*, especially among infants and children. It is obvious that once death rates have been reduced to a relatively low level, the *rate* of population increase will inevitably level off. But even the most optimistic estimates do not see birth rates declining rapidly enough to cause a sharp declination in the curve in Figure 2 which describes population size. Were the lines in Figure 2 to be continued beyond the present, the lower line would level off and begin to drop. The upper line would not.

To be fair, Kahn does acknowledge continued population growth. It is merely that his charts tend to obscure that acknowledgement. And while it is commonly agreed that population growth rate has begun to fall, for the reasons just outlined, it is a good deal less obvious that it will continue to fall for the reasons Dr. Kahn suggests—namely a near universal increase in affluence. Population growth ends as well in the *Limits* and *Mankind* scenarios, not from increasing affluence and declining birth rates, but from rapidly increasing death rates as local population growth outstrips local food supplies.

⁶Herman Kahn, W. Brown, L. Martel, *et al.*, *The Next 200 Years* (New York: William Morrow & Company, Inc., 1976).

Figure 1. Population Growth Rate in Long-Term Historical Perspective*

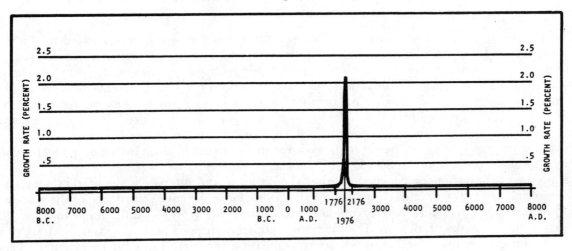

*Kahn, page 29.
Source: Adapted from Ronald Freeman and Bernard Berelson, "The Human Population," *Scientific American,* September 1974, pp. 36-37. Copyright 1974 by Scientific American, Inc. All rights reserved.

Figure 2. Population Growth—1750 to Present*

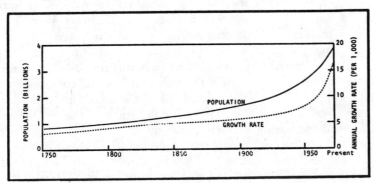

*Kahn, page 28.
Source: Adapted from Ansley J. Coale, "The History of the Human Population," *Scientific American,* September 1974, p.42. Copyright 1974 by Scientific American, Inc. All rights reserved.

The factors that *may* actually halt population growth—in time—will be discussed in the next chapter. Meanwhile, viewed closely, Kahn's optimism seems merely opportunistic. For it appears to be the burden of his argument that everything will be fine if Americans simply go on consuming even more than they presently consume. There are no serious resource problems, he asserts. Thus American businesses and multi-national corporations should go about their extractive activities as usual. And certainly none of us should feel guilty about our gluttony, since it is the enormous gap between us "haves" and those "have nots" which motivates them to try harder.

Such a cornucopian view of the future is, alas, not limited to the Hudson Institute. A recent report of the National Commission on Supplies and Shortages, *Government and the Nation's Resources,*[7] comes to an almost equally optimistic conclusion—that the nation's, and ultimately the world's supplies of raw materials are for all practical purposes inexhaustible, since the entire substance of the globe is at our disposal. (One wonders where we—like Atlas lifting the world—would stand to mine it!)

What is one to make of all this? The ultimate argument, stripped of its excesses, is straightforward. It centers on the question of what size population the earth can support at what level of living. Clearly the ultimate answer to that question does not lie in whether or not we have unlimited supplies of iron or copper in the ground (or in nodules on the ocean floor). Our ultimate survival depends on whether, in the face of rising demands for everything, we can maintain an environment fit to produce food and a supply of the inputs (including clean air and water) necessary to produce it.

A number of recent revelations regarding the extent of man's potential impact on the unseen systems that support him make the issue of whether we will run out of mercury, for example, comparatively trivial. These include: the long-term undetected "leakage" into the environment of persistent toxins like PCB's; the unexpected vulnerability of the protective ozone layer to everything from spray-can propellants to cow flatulence and fertilizers; the wide-scale land subsidence and salt-water incursions which have followed our mining and drilling activities. These are but a few of the surprises which have begun to suggest that mere access to the totality of crustal minerals—even if their extraction were economically feasible—would not provide for unlimited growth, since life is dependent upon the effective functioning of systems whose subtleties we have only begun to fathom.

Various aspects of this issue will be discussed at length in the sections which follow. Two of them seem worth mentioning here. One of the major constraints on material growth is energy—one of the topics to which a separate section will be devoted. Nicholas Wade's piece on economist Georgescu-Roegen was included in this chapter to suggest the extent to which the cornucopian notion is based—often apparently unwittingly—on an assumption of unlimited energy.

A second major constraint on the Kahnian vision of a bountiful 30-billion-person world is perhaps the most difficult of all to overcome—namely the vulnerability and complexity of the biological and social systems which support our civilization. Paul Ehrlich and John Holdren put it bluntly in "8,000,000,000 People. We'll Never Get There," pointing out the ecological strains which an increasing population and increasing affluence put on our life-support systems.

In this regard, even Kahn is less optimistic than he seems. In Table 1 below are listed what Kahn calls the "Eight Basically Solvable Issues" which he considers to be "at the center of current controversies." In Table 2 are what he calls "Eight Basically Uncertain Issues." Among the latter are "Effects of U.S. superindustrial economy on environment, society and culture of the U.S. and the world," and "Possible damage to earth because of complicated, complex, and subtle ecological and environmental effects."

As can be readily seen, it is the "uncertain issues which are quite certain to arise as long as we and

7 *Government and the Nation's Resources* (Washington: U.S. Government Printing Office, December, 1976).

Table I

EIGHT BASICALLY SOLVABLE ISSUES*

These issues are at the center of current controversies and are thus very troublesome for the present and the immediate future. However, a surprisingly broad consensus concerning their nature and possible solution is probably attainable. Thus, the current debate is very misleading and drains off energies which could better be devoted to the real issues listed above. At the same time much current discussion discourages practical steps by assuming that they will be ineffective. If this potential consensus could be articulated and demonstrated, then the issues below could be addressed with greater effectiveness and, at the same time, more attention could be directed to the real issues.

1. Likelihood of population and GWP transition being caused more by "natural" limitation of demand than forced limitation of supply.
2. Overall demographic, land-use and income issues.
3. Agricultural and related food issues.
4. Energy issues.
5. Other resource issues.
6. Issues associated with clean air, clean water and aesthetic landscapes.
7. Partial images of the future, including images of the likely emergence of both the super- and the postindustrial economies.
8. An important and exciting role for space.

*Kahn, page 228.

Table II

EIGHT BASICALLY UNCERTAIN ISSUES*

These are the real issues of the future. Their general nature is sometimes clear; the exact shape they will take, the degree of danger and problems involved and their likely resolution are unclear.

1. Effects of U.S. superindustrial economy on environment, society and culture of the U.S. and the world.
2. Effects of U.S. postindustrial economy on environment, society and culture of the U.S and the world.
3. Parallel developments in other countries.
4. Political, institutional, international-security and arms-control issues.
5. Possible damage to earth because of complicated, complex and subtle ecological and environmental effects.
6. Issues relating to quality of life, attitudes, values, morals and morale for different nations and groups.
7. Images of the future and the likely problems and opportunities created by these images.
8. Degree and effects of bad luck and bad management.

*Kahn, page 227

the rest of the biological world remain more complex than even the most sophisticated computers. The world of universal affluence, based on "business as usual," might be achievable if mankind and the species on which he depends were programmable—which (for good or ill) they are not.

The section ends with two pieces. The first is a thoughtful and frustrated essay by Samuel Florman which moves forward the story of the Club of Rome. Covering the Club's Bicentennial meeting in Philadelphia, Florman finds its members attractive, idealistic, committed . . . and wistful. There is no arguing with the logic of his conclusion that we dare not wait for a fundamental change in human nature before we take action—that just because there *is* a crisis we must plan to meet it now with all the resources and intelligence that we presently possess.

Yet I read Florman's article not too long after I had read an article in *Science* about progress toward the development of what we have been promised will be the clean unlimited power of nuclear fusion.[8] The story pointed out that in the present (admittedly crude) reactor models, the "first wall" or inside layer of the shielding "blanket" of a tokamak reactor would be made out of stainless steel, and that it would have a useful life estimated at from 2 to 5 years, after which humankind would be faced with the problem of disposing of 500,000 kilograms (551 tons) of highly radio-active stainless steel! So much for clean energy.

And then I realized that the choice we were being offered was not really a choice between changing human nature or just going on as we are. The cornucopians all appear to assume an unlimited supply of energy, with nuclear energy, breeder reactors and fusion—figuring largely in their plans. What kinds of freedoms would such a nuclear world allow? Questions have already been raised in a number of European countries as to whether a plutonium state where "everything must be protected and everyone watched"[9] is compatible with the freedoms we have come to associate with Western democracy. Richard Falk, Professor of International Law at Princeton has pointed out the extreme difficulty—unlikelihood—of achieving complete technological reliability in nuclear construction, operation, fuel reprocessing, and waste storage. In the end, he concludes, even if "the reassurances could be taken at face value . . . even if we can imagine flawless technical 'fixes' . . . we can't envision social 'fixes' that would guard against the range of human failures over a period of many centuries. . . . What may turn out to be even worse, because of the pressure to take precautions commensurate with the risk, governments would have an ample rationale for citizen surveillance and generalized repression. . . . In this regard, nothing less than an 'anthropological fix' is required if we are to proceed with nuclear power in a prudent way."

Thus, although the cornucopians do not appear to be arguing for a change in human nature— merely for a continued pursuit of our own ends, there is implicit in their technological optimism a notion of a perfectable and regimentable humanity. It is reported that we now have in our underground defense installations men who sit and watch our missiles. They watch in pairs—each keeping one eye on the equipment and one eye on each other. Each has a gun to use if some aberrant enzyme in his companion's brain defects from duty and sends its owner amok. What kind of programmed, error-free human will the automated nuclear world of Kahn and Esfandiary require? Are we not in Falk's memorable phrase "the Wrong Species for Nuclear Power"?[10] Is it not true, as he argues, that "even if the equipment can work, the inherent character of nuclear technology is too difficult for the human species to handle given its present stage of development"?

"We dare not trust the future of our children to any scheme that insists upon a change in human

[8] "Fusion Research (II): Detailed Reactor Studies Identify More Problems," *Science* 193:38-40 (2 July 1976).
[9] Robert Jungk, quoted in "West Germany, The Case of the Bugged Physicist," *Time*, p. 28 (14 March 1977); Also see Nigel Hawkes, "Science in Europe/Benn and British Rethink Energy Policy," *Science* 196: 146-147 (8 April 1977).
[10] Richard Falk, "The Wrong Species for Nuclear Power," *Business and Society Review*, pp. 40-42 (Fall 1976).

nature," Florman writes about the humanistic optimism of the Club of Rome. But is it really less likely that men and women might evolve into more reliable machines? We cannot know the answer yet. The final selection in this chapter, published in the *New Yorker* around Christmas of 1975, argues for our redeemability.

CHAPTER 2

Food and People – Giving and Taking

The Golden Age

GEORG BORGSTROM

The food and people dilemma is the subject of this chapter and the title of the book from which this first selection is taken. The book is by Georg Borgstrom whose unique perspective as a geographer has long illumined discussions of the world food crisis. To those well-versed in world history, this account of the *European* population explosion will come as no surprise. More surprising to most "Westerners" will be Borgstrom's revelations about the sources of the food supply on which that early population explosion flourished.

Although man appeared on earth more than one million years ago, only in the post-glacial period did he emerge as a dominant species with world-wide distribution. At first his numbers increased at exceedingly slow rates. Human population amounted to only a quarter-billion (by recent estimates) at the beginning of the Christian era. It took sixteen centuries to double this number, the first billion being reached as late as 1820. The second billion was reached only 110 years later (1930). Then came the awesome acceleration; in 1960, only 30 years later, the third billion had been added. Unbelievably, mankind is now in the unprecedented situation of adding almost another billion during the single decade of the seventies.

The present global population upsurge had its counterpart in the European population explosion, which peaked about the opening of the 20th century but had its major spectacular growth in the 100-year period, 1850 to 1950. Experts frequently cite medical advances as the major stimulus for this upsurge in population, and most textbooks emphasize the following sanitary improvements: (1) the creation of waterworks coupled with sewage disposal facilities, (2) the introduction of mass vaccination, and (3) the compulsory measures taken for the pasteurization of milk. Unquestionably each of these innovations drastically reduced mortality, particularly among infants, and as the number of individuals surviving to adulthood increased, the potential number of humans likewise increased. Basically, however, medical advances and improved sanitation do not adequately explain this tremendous population growth, nor its explosive nature. Other forces, set in motion when Europeans swarmed over all corners of the globe and tapped into a world-wide support system, are far more significant. . . .

Europeans multiplied sixfold in three centuries, while the total of all other peoples was augmented only threefold. After representing only about 20 per cent of the world's population in 1650, Europeans had increased to almost 40 per cent by the year 1950, including descendants in other lands. The big splash occurred between 1850 and 1950, adding around 580 million more. . . .

The Great Migration (The Big Grab)

During the Golden Age (1850-1950), Europeans swarmed all over the globe. In the North American prairie they created a colony in tilled acreage, forest lands, and in mineral wealth far richer than the combined resources of all the

European countries from which they came. In addition, the South American pampas were earmarked for their use. White man, in the guise of these European emigrants, also grabbed major choice pieces of the highland soils of Africa and took power positions of trade along the African coast. During this process India became British; the East-Indies became Dutch. Furthermore, the entire continent of Australia and its invaluable satellite New Zealand had become part of the white man's booty. This world-wide grab induced the greatest migration in history. Nearly 100 million left the European continent, although about one-fourth eventually returned, for a net exodus of 75 million. These millions became the progenitors of hundreds of millions more of European descent around the globe, primarily in North America, Latin America, Oceania, and Siberia.

The European swarming was the greatest migration in human history. . . .

In 1907 the European migration peaked in the United States at a level of 1.2 million and remained close to that annual figure until 1913. This enormous influx of people created some of the most populous German, Polish, and Italian cities in the world. Interestingly enough, more people of Scandinavian ancestry now live in North America than in the Nordic countries.

The European imprint and impact affected the entire Western hemisphere. The Spanish and Portuguese broke into the Aztec and Inca empires in the 16th century and became the spearhead of the European push into the "new lands," bridging north and south. . . .

The Slave Trade

During his odyssey into the Western hemisphere, such enormous potentialities fell into the lap of the white man that at the time he could not take care of them, far less exploit them. So in the initial phases, prior to the great exploitation and fill-up after 1850, manpower was acquired from Africa through the infamous slave trade. Western man wrote some of the most disgraceful chapters of his entire social history by joining and expanding the hunting raids around Africa that had been initiated by the Arabs more than a millennium before. It has been estimated that some 40 to 50 million Africans were involved in this operation, with 15 million Africans being brought to the Americas. The wastage in human lives in the dispatching ports, on board the slave ships, in the receiving harbors and prior to the final settling was formidable.

Three points related to the food-and-people issue should be emphasized here. First, the influx of African labor dwindled in relative significance after the mid-19th century when the great European tidal wave started rising. Second, of the 15 million slaves brought to the Western hemisphere, only about one-half million reached the United States. Thus, in historical and biological perspective, one-half million Africans was minor in comparison to the 35 million European immigrants to the United States. This discrepancy is reflected even today in the lesser proportion of blacks (now increased to 12 per cent of the total population), many of whom carry European "blood." The third aspect of importance to the food-and-people issue is that African slave labor not only became instrumental but also indispensable to the development of the Western sugar empire in the Caribbean, led by Great Britain and France. This creation became a benefactor of Western man, but unquestionably a malefactor to the victimized slaves. The entire West Indies was organized to provide cheap and ample calories to the industrializing millions of Europe. The effect undoubtedly had an influence in pushing the European population figures upward and also in disassociating thinking, politics, and economy from awareness of the prime role of land and agriculture in the feeding of man and livestock. This sugar festival was the first "trip" in the European swindle of inebriation. The second, almost simultaneous, intoxicating drink was the great expansion of ocean fishing, in particular the long-distance hauling of codfish from the Grand Banks to provide inestimable high-rate protein. . . .

The Last Trail

There has been constant debate in sociological and economic studies of the relative significance of the forces exercising the greatest influence on the great European trek, whether it was the "pull"—the prospects for a better life—or the "push," as manifested in the growing land shortage of Europe and in imbalances there between industrialization and the degree and rate of employment. The push and the pull coincided, however, in the food and resource issue. Never in history did a group of men procure a greater bounty than those who came to the northern flank of the western hemisphere with its great resources in land, soils, forests, and minerals. The North American prairie has no counterpart in any other continent. The real exploitation of these riches was telescoped in time to not much more than one hundred years.

Americans tend to picture their accomplishments as a big sweep, spanning a whole continent, when the Anglo-French thrust from the North and Northwest finally joined hands with the Spanish from the South and Southeast and the Russian from the Northwest. Spain and Russia had both overexpanded, and California, Alaska, and later Hawaii, became swept up into the great Western thrust. The lesson to be drawn from this historical maneuver is that Western man opened up his last frontier, and in so doing, blazed his last trail.

The billions of people in the non-Western world cannot match this drive—there are no new continents to exploit. The populations of India, China, and the Middle East have no new America to turn to for food. Where would China or India find new lands, as Europe did in the prairie, from which to feed their forthwelling millions to the combined tune of almost 30 million people per year? The world could not possibly meet an overseas demand corresponding to that of present-day Europe. There is even less likelihood of these hungry nations following the Japanese model, still more excessively fed from extraterritorial sources.

China and India—Net Import of Cereals

1967-69	Net Import	Kilograms per capita
Europe	25.5	56.3
Japan	12.5	124.0
China & India	10.6	7.9

The conclusion, however, is the same for both sides of the Gap. The Western world has to apply the brakes on human growth in order to reduce its grand scale exploitation of the globe. It is also going to be forced to gain control of its growing numbers in order to avert further nutritional impairment or, even worse, to avoid mounting mortalities. Any gains that are made need to accrue to those now living and to the betterment of their lot.

The Golden Age of Western Man

The European branch of the human family not only staged the greatest migration in history but further improved its situation by (1) developing transoceanic and transcontinental transportation, (2) applying canning and refrigeration to food preservation, and finally (3) procuring higher yields through a massive input of science and technology.

Equally significant was the fact that these advances almost exclusively were mobilized, not to feed all of the world's people, but to provide for a select group of Europeans who felt the pressure of people and the need for expanded resources. Only vaguely was the dualism of this pressure recognized, namely the intertwining or even reversal of cause and effect. This whole upheaval may be described in technical terms as an explosion, but equally well and perhaps more adequately as biological gross dynamics, as a growth in numbers resulting from satisfactory feeding.

The Transportation Upheaval

The European reshaping of global transportation had a particularly dramatic effect upon the food scene. The emergence of the combustion engine and the discovery of easily handled liquid fuel (petroleum) introduced an entirely new concept—for the first time cities of a million people could be fed. Studies about early Asian cities, allegedly of that size, and previous statements to that effect about the city of Rome have not stood the test of renewed historical scrutiny. Their inhabitants numbered about 350,000 and never exceeded a half-million. The haulage of grains, rice from the Indonesian archipelago to the Asian mainland, and wheat and barley across the Mediterranean from the Nile Valley, Carthage, and later from Scythia (Ukraine), was limited in volume because of the small size of the vessels and the slow movement by oars and sails. Through clipper ships Europe and North America created a grand finale to this stage, and at the same time introduced the initial phase of what later became a large-scale global transfer of grain from Australia and the South American pampas to rapidly overfilling Europe.

The transportation revolution also contributed indirectly to the global creation of Western feeding bastions. Key features of this mercantilistic drive were the build-up of the Caribbean sugar empire, of the meat industry of Argentina and Uruguay, the butter and mutton potency of New Zealand, and not least, the plantation enterprises for cotton, oilseeds, bananas, cacao, and coffee.

The Golden Age saw the capacity of the vessels swell and the velocity rise. For the first time in history hunger vanished from the North American prairies and from the farmlands of Europe. As late as 1850 to 1870, years of hunger and starvation are documented in Scandinavia, Germany and France. The minor

classic, *Giants in the Earth* by O. E. Rolvaag (1927), about Norwegian pioneers in North Dakota in the latter part of the 19th century, vividly describes the equally harsh limitations of the prairies whenever drought, locusts, or frost hit. This is a salutary reminder of the shortages even the affluent West someday may face. It also illustrates the degree to which Western man commissioned the entire globe for his well-being with little concern until the 1950's for the legitimate needs of the other three-fourths of the world's people.

As in Europe, North American cities of a million or more exist only on the basis of long-distance hauling. Transcontinental railways and a vast network of highways spanning the North American and Eurasian continent constitute indispensable prerequisites for the feeding of these huge conglomerates, not to mention the enormous inputs of energy required for the haulage of at least one million pounds of food each day for every million inhabitants. Education has failed to convey to most Westerners, and in particular to each American, an awareness of this dependence on distant prairie soils, dairy farms, feed lots, and rangelands. This large-scale feeding from many thousands of miles away contributed drastically to the Western world's losing touch with ecological realities. In fact, it is a key factor of the present crisis. Technology has not changed in one iota man's basic dependence on soil, water, and food. . . .

Dispelling the Myths

History textbooks often blatantly reveal how poorly understand the European outflow is in biological and even historical terms. How Western man, almost for his exclusive survival, created huge beachheads around the world with little consideration for the world at large is disregarded. These vast supporting colonies were taken for granted as parts of the white man's domain, and the ensuing influx of food and feed is often considered evidence of the efficiency of the homeland agriculture rather than recognition of the enormous expansion in overseas real estate.

"The rationalization of husbandry resulted in an increase in output which ended once and for all the threat of famine. The last hunger in Europe came in the 1840's"—Yet millions of emigrants crossed the ocean to the Western hemisphere.

"The Agricultural Revolution insured an adequate food supply. Only when war or revolution disrupted the international market was there a serious danger of food shortage. This change in attitude was a measure of how swiftly the food supply of Europe had grown during the previous one hundred and fifty years. The production of food ceased to be the occupation of the great majority of Europeans. Basic changes in the forms of human employment were made possible by expanding surpluses in agriculture. Without these surpluses there could have been no shift of population from country to city, from husbandry to manufacturing."—Yet in several key countries the influx of food from transoceanic sources was an indispensable prerequisite for European urbanization in the wake of industrialization.

The monopolistic nature of these ventures is little heeded in historians' analyses: "The material welfare of mankind was increasingly based on a vast world market in which the interests of all nations converged and interacted." This statement mirrors in almost uncanny terms a gruesome and myopic ethnocentricity, or does it reflect callousness—that only Western man counts in history?

Some writers proudly point to the great improvements in ocean transportation, introduced during the 19th century, that made it possible for farmers overseas to feed and clothe the European consumer. "Wheat grown in the United States and Canada began to cross the Atlantic. Argentinian beef and Australian wool invaded the Continent. Subsistence farming everywhere retreated before commercial farming. Self-sufficiency became a mirage." Nowhere in this fairy tale is there a recognition of the colossal broadening of the European feeding base that took place to parallel the great migration. The whole emphasis is on technique, almost completely overlooking the Big Grab. . . .

Abridged from *The Food and People Dilemma* by Georg Borgstrom, pp. 1-12. Copyright 1973 by Wadsworth Publishing Company, Inc., Belmont CA 94002. Reprinted by permission of the publisher, Duxbury Press.

Triage. Who Shall Be Fed? Who Shall Starve?

WADE GREENE

Having secured our own "feeding base," as Borgstrom might put it, we are now troubled by dramatic upsurges in population in those very lands which—contrary to our myths—have helped to provision us. Wade Greene's article, published in the *New York Times Magazine* shortly after the 1974 World Food Conference, lays out clearly the dilemma which then apparently faced us: could we feed continually burgeoning numbers of people from our food surplusses, or should we "humanely" let them starve for the long-range good of the human race?

During the trench-warfare slaughters of World War I, a system for separating the wounded into three groups was practiced in Allied medical tents. The groups consisted of those likely to die no matter what was done for them, those who would probably recover even if untreated, and those who could survive only if cared for immediately. With supplies and manpower limited, the third group alone received attention. Such a practice was called triage—from the French verb *trier*, to sort. While it is still little discussed, triage has become a standard wartime procedure for making the most efficient use of scarce medical resources.

With severe food shortages in many parts of the world today, some people are advocating the unsentimental, morally uncomfortable practice of the medical tent for dealing with nations that are victims of the battle against starvation. The triage analogy is the basis of a scenario as bleak, as unthinkable, as any of those thoughts about life-after-holocaust that issued from the Hudson Institute in the nineteen-fifties:

Instead of floundering in nuclear ruin, the world is swept by famine as the populations of many regions outstrip their agricultural capacities. Only one nation, the United States, has a sizable surplus of food. And, with godlike finality, we dispense it, after systematically deciding which people are salvageable and should be fed, which will survive without help, and which are hopeless and should be left to the ravages of famine.

Unthinkable, perhaps, but no longer unthought. The idea has haunted recent discussions of mounting global food shortages. Some observers detected it in the halls of the recent World Food Conference in Rome. It has cropped up in graduate seminars and Congressional committees. ("Will you and I as American citizens some day have to participate in the choice of 'Food Triage'?" wondered a House agriculture subcommittee in a recent report.) And triage-type thinking was recently expressed by no less respectable a figure than the president of the American Academy of Sciences.

The current attention to the idea represents, in effect, a delayed reaction. Food triage was first proposed in 1967 in a book entitled "Famine—1975!" The authors, William and Paul Paddock, one an agronomist and the other a retired career officer of the Foreign Service, prescribed triage as a mode of U.S. food allocation in a coming time of widespread famine. With experts now estimating that as many as 10 million people may starve to death this year and that as many as half a billion are hovering on the brink of starvation, "Famine—1975!" may prove to have been precisely prescient. Whether its prescription for dealing with famine was equally inspired is another matter.

"Triage is not a system to cut off aid. It is not a system to reduce help," William Paddock said emphatically the other day when I talked by phone to him at his home on the Bahamian island of Eleuthera. "It's a system to make it more effective."

That may be, but the focus of attention has fallen on the morally disturbing notion that some countries should be cut off from food aid for the benefit of the rest. Which countries? The book describes them: "Nations in which the population growth trend has already passed the agricultural potential. This, combined with inadequate leadership and other divisive factors, makes catastrophic disasters inevitable. . . . To send food to them is to throw sand in the ocean." The book looks at a number of examples, invites the reader to do some triage reckoning himself, aided by three check boxes following each example, and gives the authors' own judgments at the end of the grim game. The biggest loser is India. " . . . Today's trends show it will be beyond the resources of the United States to keep famine out of India during the nineteen-seventies. Indian agriculture is too antiquated. Its present government is too inefficient to inaugurate long-range agricultural development programs. Its population tidal wave is too overwhelming, more than 11,800,000 are added each year to the current half-billion population."

If triage struck a responsive chord in some circles, it was not, predictably enough, well received in others. As the authors note in the book itself, some who read the manuscript before publication reacted with "complete horror." As for critical reaction after publication, "we were thoroughly clobbered," recalled William Paddock.

But for the most part, the book and the triage idea went relatively unnoticed outside of special-interest circles. The book had been written during a severe drought in India where famine was staved off only by the shipment of millions of tons of American grain. But the weather improved as the book appeared, and soon after the Green Revolution was proclaimed. Miracle rice and wonder wheats seemed to promise nearly limitless expansion of the world's food production. The Paddocks' dire projection and even direr prescription tended to be dismissed as crop yields did in fact increase and the threat of famine faded for a while.

At about the same time, however, anxiety over the unprecedented expansion of world populations began to inspire other proposals challenging traditional humanitarian values including Western respect for individual freedom, even the sanctity of life itself. Paul Ehrlich's *The Population Bomb* appeared (in 1968) a year after the Paddocks' book and approvingly referred to "triage" while also declaring that "many apparently brutal and heartless decisions" will have to be made in order to bring birth rates down. That same year, the hardest and most relentlessly reasoned thoughts about population appeared in the respected professional publication *Science*. The article was entitled "The Tragedy of the Commons," and its author—whose name among populationists has since become almost synonymous with thinking the unthinkable—was a University of California ecologist-biologist, Garrett Hardin.

I had lunch with Dr. Hardin the other day after watching him testify before a House subcommittee. He had calmly advised the lawmakers that we would be doing a favor to starving countries as well as ourselves if we refused to send them any more food. He seemed good-natured and was surprisingly humorous, however. "I'm supposed to be gloomy," he said at one point when we were talking about another member of what some in the New York- and Princeton-based population establishment call the "California camp." "But he's much gloomier than I am." Dr. Hardin wore a vasectomy pin in his lapel, a golden replica of the male symbol in biology with a chunk out of the circle. When I asked him about it, he said he had had himself vasectomized 20 years ago, after having had four children. "Just like in India," he said, an ironic allusion to the contention that many Indian men who have vasectomies in exchange for incentive payments or food bonuses already have as many children as they want.

Dr. Harding's writing is deadly earnest by comparison to the person at lunch, both in its style and in its message. "The Tragedy of the Commons" proposed compulsory birth control on the grounds that those who do not practice birth control will otherwise outbreed those who do to the detriment of an overpopulated society as a whole—just as a commons, a pasturing area open to all, will tend to be overgrazed because it is in each user's interest to put as many cattle on it as he can. "The only way we can preserve and nurture other and more precious freedoms is by relinquishing the freedom to breed, and that very soon," Dr. Hardin concluded. He drew broader social and moral implications, too, borrowing some thoughts from a recent book on "situation ethics." "The morality of an act," he wrote, "is a function of the state of the system at the time it is performed." In other words, freedom to have as many children as one wanted was properly valued in a sparsely populated planet but should be limited in an increasingly crowded one. Other values are changing as well in our heavily peopled world, he suggested.

The relativity of right and wrong was at the same time beginning to be argued by Jay Forrester, the management professor at the Massachusetts Institute of Technology, who invented the memory device central to the operation of digital computers and whose

disciples subsequently put together computerized projections of doom under the auspices of the Club of Rome. In turning his attention from corporations to social systems (which he has described as "multiple-loop, nonlinear feedback mechanisms"), Dr. Forrester looked first at the city of Boston, later at the world. And he came to the conclusion that we no longer intuitively understand the outcome of some societal actions, not because of population growth per se, but because of the increasing complexity of social systems. So what in the short run may seem to be an unqualified good may lead in the long run to undesirable—bad—results. Is the good then good?

Dr. Forrester espoused his gospel of moral complexity in 1971 in a speech before an unlikely audience, the Division of Overseas Ministries of the National Council of Churches. He advised the church group to reconsider traditional international humanitarianism in the light of what he regarded as the long-range inhumanities of some supposedly humane acts. "Consider a country that is overpopulated," he said. "Its standard of living is low, food is insufficient, health is poor, and misery abounds. . . . The country is operating in the overextended mode where all adversities are resolved by a rise in the death rate. The process is part of a natural mechanism for limiting further growth in population. But suppose that humanitarian impulses lead to massive relief efforts from the outside for each natural disaster. What is the long-term result? The people who are saved raise the population still higher. . . . Relief leads to more people in crisis, to still-greater need for relief, and, eventually, to a situation that even relief cannot handle." . . . "The church should begin to examine the limits and consequences of humanitarianism," the technologist advised the theists.

A doctoral student of Dr. Forrester, Dale Runge, later expanded this theme in an unpublished but widely-read paper, "The Ethics of Humanitarian Food Relief," in which, with the aid of computerized projections, he came to the conclusion that such relief is "not ethical" because by itself it creates more misery over the long run than it alleviates.

As this course of thinking developed in recent years, so did its relevancy. The climate, generally favorable for decades in the world's main agricultural areas, reverted to its haphazard ravages, drastically reducing crop yields in several parts of the world. Energy costs soared, and because of the Green Revolution's heavy dependence on energy (for pumping water and for petroleum-based fertilizer), the cost of food also soared—out of reach for millions in impoverished areas. Increasing cries for food relief have added an immediacy to proposals that we should not answer all, or perhaps any, such appeals. Other economic factors added an extra dimension to these proposals. Until recently, the U.S. found it quite painless to give or sell food cheaply to countries that needed it. We produced far more than we could use and were paying $1-million a day just to store excess grain. But U.S. grain reserves are gone now, mostly to Russia. Meantime, quadrupled oil prices have made us increasingly dependent on international food sales to maintain our balance of payments; these sales have grown from $8-billion to $21-billion annually in the last three years and now head the U.S. export list.

Doubts about our humanitarian impulses have been generally phrased in terms of whether these impulses were good for the "beneficiaries" or for the world as a whole; some doubters now feel it is appropriate also to ask whether they are good for us. Garrett Hardin, for one. His "Tragedy of the Commons" has been anthologized in no less than 48 different collections, and he revived and extended the commons theme last fall, reasoning that our generosity not only does no long-range good for others but imperils us in the process.

In articles in *Psychology Today* and *BioScience* magazines, he argues for an adjusted ethics of survival dominated by unsqueamish self-interest; lifeboat ethics, he calls it, in an analogy that has already begun to rival triage. The rich nations of the world, he writes, are adrift in lifeboats. "In the ocean outside each lifeboat swim the poor of the world, who would like to get in, or at least to share some of the wealth. What should the lifeboat passengers do?" We could try to take everyone aboard, but we would sink the lifeboat if we did, he says. "The boat swamps, everyone drowns. Complete justice, complete catastrophe." Because he thinks we have already exceeded the carrying capacity of our land in some ways, Dr. Hardin suggests that it would be prudent not to take anyone aboard. "For the foreseeable future," he concludes, "our survival demands that we govern our actions by the ethics of a lifeboat, harsh though they may be."

Harsh indeed in light of Americans' ingrained image of themselves as international benefactors and rescuers. The lifeboat ethic was denounced as an "obscene doctrine" in a guest editorial in November's *Science* by Roger Revelle, head of Harvard's Center of Population Studies. Dr. Hardin says that mail from his *Psychology Today* article has been running about 95 per cent against his doctrine, accusing him of "being a scoundrel."

Cutting off aid to starving nations was proposed recently from another more surprising source—Philip Handler, president of the National Academy of Sciences. But he adds a significant proviso that offers little moral comfort. We should not give food aid, he said, if we aren't *willing* to do enough to effect long-range solutions. Dr. Handler contended, in a speech in late September, that if we are going truly to help hungry countries, food aid has to be accompanied by further assistance aimed at setting those we help on the road to both agricultural self-sufficiency and lower population growth rates, which tend to fall as standards of living rise. Anything short of that, says Dr. Handler, with a clear echo of Forrester and Runge, is "probably intrinsically counterproductive," and only leads to later misery "on a larger scale."

"Cruel as it may sound," Dr. Handler said, "if the developed and affluent nations do not intend the colossal, all-out effort commensurate with this task"—and he indicated his doubts that they do—"then it may be wiser to 'let nature take its course.'" Asked later whether he was saying that a policy of triage should be considered, Dr. Handler replied: "That's what I was saying, gently."

Such are the major contours of the recent challenges to America's humanitarian instincts —or at least what we like to think are our instincts—toward the starving, suffering millions in the rest of the world. How persuasive are the analogies and the arguments?

In recent weeks I talked to most of the principle advocates involved, some of their supporters and some of their dissenters. These are gloomy times, of course, and the burden of proof in many situations rests almost wholly on those prophets who claim things are not bad and are not getting worse. Still, I found experts who have considered—and dismissed—the triage and lifeboat reasonings because they feel the world can and will surmount disparities between food supplies and population. People like the Paddocks, however, seem more convinced of their pessimistic premises than ever. "Everything is so much worse than when we wrote that book," said William Paddock. "You have a couple of hundred million more people to worry about, you've got the energy crisis, you've got inflation.... Another thing is that we have less land under production today than we did in 1967 due to losing land from salting and advancing deserts."

The facts are not all on one side or the other. To some extent, one's opinion about them and about the harsh measures being proposed depends on an *a priori* sense either that material progress and a little bit of luck are part of man's boundless destiny or, as many ecologists and philosophers and Forrester's computers contend, that nature sets firm limits, which we are approaching, on how much an ever-larger population can extract from a finite planet.

The major, recurrent argument I encountered against the triage concept was that, even if there are such limits, we are not close enough to them to justify triage—not while much of the world enjoys an overabundance of its fruits. This viewpoint was not limited to the U.S. It extended to other countries that produce or consume disproportionate amounts of food and energy—wealthy, food-surplus countries like Canada and Australia, the newly-rich oil-producing countries and Western Europe and Japan. Nonetheless, it was the U.S., according to this argument, with its unmatched capacity for food production and widely disproportionate consumption of global resources, which figuratively has the most fat to trim before it can justify dictating the starvation of others. It has been noted, for example, that if Americans cut their meat-consumption by only one-tenth, the saving in grain used for cattle feed would totally eliminate the estimated grain shortage of countries now verging on starvation.

"As long as the wealthy societies are consuming at the rate we are, I think there's an awful lot that can be done short of triage," says Roger Shimm, president of Union Theological Seminary and one of many religious leaders who are considering anew the dimensions of the age-old scriptural injunction to feed the hungry. And as long as cutting back on consumption is a possibility, he added, "I would find it extremely hard to say that I would deliberately consign people to starvation by any act, positive or negative."

But how much of a possibility is this, in terms of the will if not the way? The question arose at a recent three-day meeting near Baltimore, sponsored by the Aspen Institute, at which experts from government, private groups and the academy who have been concerned with food, population and ethics gathered to consider the world food situation. In one vigorous exchange, the protagonists were Jay Forrester, to whom many of the questions were directed, and Peter Henriot, a Jesuit, who works with the Center for Concern in Washington. Their disagreement grew out of a discussion of Dr. Hardin's lifeboat analogy. Dr. Forrester asked whether it would be moral to rescue the drowning poor if it meant swamping the boat. To which Peter Henriot replied that the moral thing to do would be first to make the boat more efficient—get rid of the excess baggage. That's just so much preaching, Dr. Forrester answered.

In any case, could the United States adopt a deliberate, explicit policy by which it determined which countries were to be helped and which left to the inexorable course of nature — a governmental version of the Paddocks' triage check list? I asked Representative John Dingell, before whose House subcommittee Garrett Hardin testified. "In terms of U.S. politics," Representative Dingell said, "we can't do it either morally or politically." But many policies aren't arrived at "clearly and explicitly . . . they sort of grow and evolve. And whether we make a conscious decision of the kind that Hardin has discussed in his papers, the hard fact of the matter is that nature is probably going to make those judgements for us. . . . Triage is going to come upon us whether we like it or not."

Some others say it already has, that we have begun practicing triage without declaring it. "There has always been a degree of triage in the world," said Dr. Forrester in the course of a recent scientific conference at the Franklin Institute in Philadelphia.

John Steinhart, professor of geology and geophysics at the University of Wisconsin, was more specific and less philosophic as he discussed the subject at Representative Dingell's hearings. "I guess I would argue," he said, "that we are already practicing triage, whether we call it by that name or not. The decision, for instance, that the President not respond to Secretary Butz's or Senator Humphrey's request for additional food for India, but, instead, supply some additional food to Syria means a triage decision. That decides that some Indians will die and some Syrians will live. It is as simple as that."

Both Dr. Forrester and Dr. Steinhart were using the term loosely, however. In the battlefield analogy, the triage decision is made on the basis of which sufferer will gain some decisive benefit. Our food allocation these days seems to be based almost entirely on how it benefits us—the donors rather than the recipients—either by helping our balance of payments through export sales or our balance of power, by keeping strategically important countries friendly. In fact, in recent years, most of our food aid, in the form of low-interest, long-term loans for food purchases, has gone to countries like South Vietnam, South Korea, Pakistan, Indonesia, Egypt, Syria and Israel. While this has had the effect of reducing "humanitarian" shipments to much needier countries, the effect seems to have been incidental rather than a result of the harsh logic of triage. That Washington policymakers may be moving toward a harder look at humanitarian food relief in its own right, however, was evidenced by a National Security Council representative's recent remark that "to give food aid to countries just because people are starving is a pretty weak reason."

Perhaps the ultimate obstacle to triage, or the lifeboat ethic, is a moral self-image with which Americans cannot tamper without severe, perhaps devastating, consequences. "I have certain moral feelings about letting some poor bastard starve," concedes Representative Dingell. Somewhat more elegantly, Ronald Jager, a professor of philosophy at Yale University, who took part in the Aspen Institute meeting, asks: "What happens to us, to our whole conception of what a moral life is, if we force ourselves to turn callously away? What happens when a nation does that, when a nation has to tell itself, when its leaders have to tell its people: this is what we must do, the moral thing to do is let Bangladesh disappear in anguish? . . . What you create is an internal situation which I think is just disintegrative."

I asked Garrett Hardin about this. "I'm not sure I can exactly answer you," he said, "but I've got a sort of reply. We have gotten ourselves into a difficult position in the last 25 years. . . . . The success of the Marshall Plan in Europe was one of the great motivations for embarking on

AID [Agency for International Development]. Now this was the first time that the nation ever embarked on such a project as trying to save the whole world. People have been starving to death for centuries—and even in large numbers. There's nothing new about that. But now, because of the feeling that has been built up over the last 25 years—that we somehow can, we have an obligation to, save the world— we're in a difficult position. That, coupled with television so that the person who is dying 8,000 miles away can be brought into our living room. . . . But quite apart from whether it's desirable or not, I think the realities are that we simply don't have the ability to take care of the rest of the world and we better adjust to that. I think we have a very hard psychological adjustment to make. My only point is that we don't have to go up against the sentiment of the ages, it's only the sentiment of the last 25 years."

Several people I talked to, however, said that they were not prepared to adjust to some realities. Richard Neuhaus, author of the book, "In Defense of People," and a Lutheran minister, said, "A world that would choose Garrett Hardin's options is a world in which I for one would not care to survive."

When I pressed Dr. Hardin on this point, he admitted that the question of whether we could live with ourselves by the values he is espousing was probably the strongest challenge to his case. "But I firmly believe that we can," he said. "I'm doing it. I don't think it's easy. But—it's like gravity. We may not like the law of gravity either. But once you know it's true, you don't sit down and cry about it. That's the way the world is."

Philosophers have been arguing the fundamental ethical question posed by triage at least since Plato: the weighing of "good" ends against "bad" means. This problem has cropped up in very concrete form throughout history, also. It has been solved notoriously in some cases—in Nazi atrocities, for example. Other solutions have been less easy to condemn, however, including a legally famous application of Dr. Hardin's lifeboat ethics, the case of United States

v. Holmes. Holmes was a sailor on a passenger ship that was wrecked on an iceberg in 1841. He and a number of passengers found themselves in a dangerously overloaded lifeboat, so Holmes directed that several passengers be thrown overboard. He and the rest were eventually rescued. Holmes was tried for manslaughter, convicted and then pardoned by President Tyler.

The ultimate course of the law in not punishing Holmes seems just in this case, and it may appear to offer some support to the ethics of food triage and of Dr. Hardin's lifeboat analogy. But, in the view of several people I talked to, the difference between a literal situation involving individuals and the analogous one involving nations may make precisely the difference between right and wrong.

In the Holmes case, the likelihood of everyone's dying unless a few were sacrificed was presumably immediate and total. But even with computer projections, the future is far from being absolutely predictable in the complex realm of food and population. Who can be sure that tens or hundreds of millions of people will eventually starve to death if we are not willing to write off a lesser number now—sure enough, that is, to make the decision to do so?

Another distinction generally acknowledged at the Aspen Institute meeting is that life and death terms don't apply to nations as they do to individuals. Gerald Barney of the Rockefeller Brothers Fund raised the point that nations don't die, they don't disappear. And not helping them does not eliminate them as a problem; it may even create a larger problem of prolonged social upheaval and violence.

Dr. Forrester, who had shown considerable interest in the triage concept when he came to the Baltimore meeting, seemed to have become disillusioned with it during the discussions, for when I talked with him afterwards, he was saying some of the same things Mr. Barney had said. He was far from abandoning his underlying moral arguments over whether help is really helpful, however. "There's an implication going along with the word [triage]," he said, "that there are those who, if you help them, will survive and some who, if you don't help them, won't. And neither of these is true. It seems to me that those we help are not going to be better off than those we don't help. In many ways the problems we see around us today are related to past attempts to help that haven't succeeded."

Part of the gloom of the times is the pervasiveness of at least one aspect of Dr. Forrester's viewpoint—the feeling that many social programs aren't working, at least not the way we want them to. But even he is said to have left the Aspen Institute meeting expressing the hope that his computers might still come up with ways of helping that really do help.

Meantime, there appears to be a great deal of soul-searching in and out of Government to try to determine just what we can and should do to stem the tide of hunger and famine, something more than muddling from crisis to crisis. Some people are quite happy to use the specter of triage as a moral prod.

Some, too, while deploring such a viewpoint, feel that the population explosion in some parts of the world may have pushed the search for answers beyond the framework of traditional liberal values. Several people I talked to mentioned China. Though I am sure these people view China's repressive society as intolerable, they still look at China's improving living standards and rapidly declining birth rate and find repression an acceptable alternative to the degradation and death of millions.

Many of the same people felt, however, that a great deal more to alleviate hunger could be done by the world's wealthy nations within their traditional humanitarian standards. Whether Americans, among others, have the will to do so is another matter. I encountered considerable doubt about that. Yet the feeling, frequently expressed, was that if we turn our backs on the world's starving because we have not summoned the will to provide effective help regardless of its cost, it will be at a bitter loss in self-esteem, no matter how sophisticated our ethical justifications. In such an event, as sociologist Daniel Patrick Moynihan has put it, "We are going to have to face up to the fact that we're a different people than we thought we were."

Reprinted with permission from *The New York Times Magazine*, pp. 9-11+ (5 January 1975). Copyright 1975 by The New York Times Company.

Lifeboat Ethics: The Case Against Helping the Poor

GARRETT HARDIN

The third paper in this section, "Lifeboat Ethics: The Case Against Helping the Poor," was first published in *Psychology Today* in September, 1974. Its author, Garrett Hardin, is a biologist on the faculty of the University of California at Santa Barbara. A villain to some, a hero to others, he is a man whom no one accuses of lacking the courage of his unpalatable conviction: that we must let the poor starve, since aiding them will only ensure the non-survival of the species. It is this argument that Hardin convincingly advances in this article.

Environmentalists use the metaphor of the earth as a "spaceship" in trying to persuade countries, industries and people to stop wasting and polluting our natural resources. Since we all share life on this planet, they argue, no single person or institution has the right to destroy, waste, or use more than a fair share of its resources.

But does everyone on earth have an equal right to an equal share of its resources? The spaceship metaphor can be dangerous when used by misguided idealists to justify suicidal policies for sharing our resources through uncontrolled immigration and foreign aid. In their enthusiastic but unrealistic generosity, they confuse the ethics of a spaceship with those of a lifeboat.

A true spaceship would have to be under the control of a captain, since no ship could possibly survive if its course were determined by committee. Spaceship Earth certainly has no captain; the United Nations is merely a toothless tiger, with little power to enforce any policy upon its bickering members.

If we divide the world crudely into rich nations and poor nations, two thirds of them are desperately poor, and only one third comparatively rich, with the United States the wealthiest of all. Metaphorically each rich nation can be seen as a lifeboat full of comparatively rich people. In the ocean outside each lifeboat swim the poor of the world, who would like to get in, or at least to share some of the wealth. What should the lifeboat passengers do?

First, we must recognize the limited capacity of any lifeboat. For example, a nation's land has a limited capacity to support a population and as the current energy crisis has shown us, in some ways we have already exceeded the carrying capacity of our land.

Adrift in a Moral Sea. So here we sit, say 50 people in our lifeboat. To be generous, let us assume it has room for 10 more, making a total capacity of 60. Suppose the 50 of us in the lifeboat see 100 others swimming in the water outside, begging for admission to our boat or for handouts. We have several options: we may be tempted to try to live by the Christian ideal of being "our brother's keeper," or by the Marxist ideal of "to each according to his needs." Since the needs of all in the water are the same, and since they can all be seen as "our brothers," we could take them all into our boat, making a total of 150 in a boat designed for 60. The boat swamps, everyone drowns. Complete justice, complete catastrophe.

Since the boat has an unused excess capacity of 10 more passengers, we could admit just 10 more to it. But which 10 do we let it? How do we choose? Do we pick the best 10, the neediest 10, "first come, first served"? And what do we say to the 90 we exclude? If we do let an extra 10 into our lifeboat, we will have lost our "safety factor," an engineering principle of critical importance. For example, if we don't leave room for excess capacity as a safety factor in our country's agriculture, a new plant disease or a bad change in the weather could have disastrous consequences.

Suppose we decide to preserve our small safety factor and admit no more to the lifeboat. Our survival is then possible, although we shall have to be constantly on guard against boarding parties.

While this last solution clearly offers the only means of our survival, it is morally abhorrent to many people. Some say they feel guilty about their good luck. My reply is simple: "Get out and yield your place to others." This may solve the problem of the guilt-ridden person's conscience, but it does not change the ethics of the lifeboat. The needy person to whom the guilt-ridden person yields his place will not himself feel guilty about his good luck. If he did, he would not climb aboard. The net result of conscience-stricken people giving up their unjustly held seats is the elimination of that sort of conscience from the lifeboat.

This is the basic metaphor within which we must work out our solutions. Let us now enrich the image, step by step, with substantive additions from the real world, a world that must solve real and pressing problems of overpopulation and hunger.

The harsh ethics of the lifeboat become even harsher when we consider the reproductive differences between the rich nations and the poor nations. The people inside the lifeboats are doubling in numbers every 87 years; those swimming around outside are doubling, on the average, every 35 years, more than twice as fast as the rich. And since the world's resources are dwindling, the difference in prosperity between the rich and the poor can only increase.

As of 1973, the U.S. had a population of 210 million people, who were increasing by 0.8 percent per year. Outside our lifeboat, let us imagine another 210 million people, (say the combined populations of Colombia, Ecuador, Venezuela, Morocco, Pakistan, Thailand and the Philippines) who are increasing at a rate of 3.3 percent per year. Put differently, the doubling time for this aggregate population is 21 years, compared to 87 years for the U.S.

Multiplying the Rich and the Poor. Now suppose the U.S. agreed to pool its resources with those seven countries, with everyone receiving an equal share. Initially the ratio of Americans to non-Americans in this model would be one-to-one. But consider what the ratio would be after 87 years, by which time the Americans would have doubled to a population of 420 million. By then, doubling every 21 years, the other group would have swollen to 354 billion. Each American would have to share the available resources with more than eight people.

But, one could argue, this discussion assumes that current population trends will continue, and they may not. Quite so. Most likely the rate of population increase will decline much faster in the U.S. than it will in the other countries, and there does not seem to be much we can do about it. In sharing with "each according to his needs," we must recognize that needs are determined by population size, which is determined by the rate of reproduction, which at present is regarded as a sovereign right of every nation, poor or not. This being so, the philanthropic load created by the sharing ethic of the spaceship can only increase.

The Tragedy of the Commons. The fundamental error of spaceship ethics, and the sharing it requires, is that it leads to what I call "the tragedy of the commons." Under a system of private property, the men who own property recognize their responsibility to care for it, for if they don't they will eventually suffer. A farmer, for instance, will allow no more cattle in a pasture than its carrying capacity justifies. If he overloads it, erosion sets in, weeds take over, and he loses the use of the pasture.

If a pasture becomes a commons open to all, the right of each to use it may not be matched by a corresponding responsibility to protect it. Asking everyone to use it with discretion will hardly do, for the considerate herdsman who refrains from overloading the commons suffers more than a selfish one who says his needs are greater. If everyone would restrain himself, all would be well; but it takes only one less than everyone to ruin a system of voluntary restraint. In a crowded world of less than perfect human beings, mutual ruin is inevitable if there are no controls. This is the tragedy of the the commons....

One of the major tasks of education today should be the creation of such an acute awareness of the dangers of the commons that people will recognize its many varieties. For example, the air and water have become polluted because they are treated as commons. Further growth in the population or per-capita conversion of natural resources into pollutants will only make the problem worse. The same holds true for the fish of the oceans. Fishing fleets have nearly disappeared in many parts of the world, technological improvements in the art of fishing are hastening the day of complete ruin. Only the replacement of the system of the commons with a responsible system of control will save the land, air, water and oceanic fisheries.

The World Food Bank. In recent years there has been a push to create a new commons called a World Food Bank, an international depository of food reserves to which nations would contribute according to their abilities and from which they would draw according to their needs. This humanitarian proposal has received support from many liberal international groups, and from such prominent citizens as Margaret Mead, U.N. Secretary General Kurt Waldheim, and Senators Edward Kennedy and George McGovern.

A world food bank appeals powerfully to our humanitarian impulses. But before we rush ahead with such a plan, let us recognize where the greatest political push comes from, lest we be disillusioned later. Our experience with the "Food for Peace program," or Public Law 480, gives us the answer. The program moved billions of dollars worth of U.S. surplus grain to food-short, population-long countries during the past two decades. But when P.L. 480 first became law, a headline in the business magazine *Forbes* revealed the real power behind it: "Feeding the World's Hungry Millions: How It Will Mean Billions for U.S. Business."

And indeed it did. In the years 1960 to 1970, U.S. taxpayers spent a total of $7.9 billion on the Food for Peace program. Between 1948 and 1970, they also paid an additional $50 billion for other economic-aid programs, some of which went for food and food-producing machinery and technology. Though all U.S. taxpayers were forced to contribute to the cost of P.L. 480, certain special interest groups gained handsomely under the program. Farmers did not have to contribute the grain; the Government, or rather the taxpayers, bought it from them at full market prices. The increased demand raised prices of farm products generally. The manufacturers of farm machinery, fertilizers and pesticides benefited by the farmers' extra efforts to grow more food. Grain elevators profited from storing the surplus until it could be shipped. Railroads made money hauling it to ports, and shipping lines profited from carrying it overseas. The implementation of P.L. 480 required the creation of a vast Government bureaucracy, which then acquired its own vested interest in continuing the program regardless of its merits.

Extracting Dollars. Those who proposed and defended the Food for Peace program in public rarely mentioned its importance to any of these special interests. The public emphasis was always on its humanitarian effects. The combination of silent selfish interests and highly vocal humanitarian apologists made a powerful and successful lobby for extracting money from taxpayers. We can expect the same lobby to push now for the creation of a World Food Bank.

However great the potential benefit to selfish interests, it should not be a decisive argument against a truly humanitarian program. We must ask if such a program would actually do more good than harm, not only momentarily but also in the long run. Those who propose the food bank usually refer to a current "emergency" or "crisis" in terms of world food supply. But what is an emergency? Although they may be infrequent and sudden, everyone knows that emergencies will occur from time to time. A well-run family, company, organization or country prepares for the likelihood of accidents and emergencies. It expects them, it budgets for them, it saves for them.

Learning the Hard Way. What happens if some organizations or countries budget for accidents and others do not? If each country is solely responsible for its own well-being, poorly managed ones will suffer. But they can learn from experience. They may mend their ways, and learn to budget for infrequent but certain emergencies. For example, the weather varies from year to year, and periodic crop failures are certain. A wise and competent government saves out of the production of the good years in anticipation of bad years to come. Joseph taught this policy to Pharaoh in Egypt more than 2,000 years ago. Yet the great majority of the governments in the world today do not follow such a policy. They lack either the wisdom or the competence, or both. Should those nations that do manage to put something aside be forced to come to the rescue each time an emergency occurs among the poor nations?

"But it isn't their fault!" Some kind-hearted liberals argue. "How can we blame the poor people who are caught in an emergency? Why must they suffer for the sins of their governments?" The concept of blame is simply not relevant here. The real question is, what are the operational consequences of establishing a world food bank? If it is open to every country every time a need develops, slovenly rulers will not be motivated to take Joseph's advice. Someone will always come to their aid. Some countries will deposit food in the world food bank, and others will withdraw it. There will be almost no overlap. As a result of such solutions to food shortage emergencies, the poor countries will not learn to mend their ways, and will suffer progressively greater emergencies as their populations grow.

Population Control the Crude Way. On the average, poor countries undergo a 2.5 percent increase in population each year; rich countries, about 0.8 percent. Only rich countries have anything in the way of food reserves set aside, and even they do not have as much as they should. Poor countries have none. If poor countries received no food from the outside, the rate of their population growth would be periodically checked by crop failures and famines. But if they can always draw on a world food bank in time of need, their population can continue to grow unchecked, and so will their "need" for aid. In the short run, a world food bank may diminish that need, but in the long run it actually increases the need without limit.

Without some system of worldwide food sharing, the proportion of people in the rich and poor nations might eventually stabilize. The overpopulated poor countries would decrease in numbers, while the rich countries that had room for more people would increase. But with a well-meaning system of sharing, such as a world food bank, the growth differential between the rich and the poor countries will not only persist, it will increase. Because of the higher rate of population growth in the poor countries of the world, 88 percent of today's children are born poor, and only 12 percent rich. Year by year the ratio becomes worse, as the fast-reproducing poor outnumber the slow-reproducing rich.

A world food bank is thus a commons in disguise. People will have more motivation to draw from it than to add to any common store. The less provident and less able will multiply at the expense of the abler and more provident, bringing eventual ruin upon all who share in the commons....

Chinese Fish and Miracle Rice. The modern approach to foreign aid stresses the export of technology and advice, rather than money and food. As an ancient Chinese proverb goes:"Give a man a fish and he will eat for a day; teach him how to fish and he will eat for the rest of his days." Acting on this advice, the Rockefeller and Ford Foundations have financed a number of programs for improving agriculture in the hungry nations. Known as the "Green Revolution," these programs have led to the development of "miracle rice" and "miracle wheat," new strains that offer bigger harvests and greater resistance to crop damage. Norman Borlaug, the Nobel Prize winning agronomist who, supported by the Rockefeller Foundation, developed "miracle wheat," is one of the most prominent advocates of a world food bank.

Whether or not the Green Revolution can increase food production as much as its champions claim is a debatable but possibly irrelevant point. Those who support this well-intended humanitarian effort should first consider some of the fundamentals of human ecology. Ironically, one man who did was the late Alan Gregg, a vice president of the Rockefeller Foundation. Two decades ago he expressed strong doubts about the wisdom of such attempts to increase food production. He likened the growth and spread of humanity over the surface of the earth to the spread of cancer in the human body, remarking that "cancerous growths demand food; but, as far as I know, they have never been cured by getting it."

Overloading the Environment. Every human born constitutes a draft on all aspects of the environment: food, air, water, forests, beaches, wildlife, scenery and solitude. Food can, perhaps, be significantly increased to meet a growing demand. But what about clean beaches, unspoiled forests, and solitude? If we satisfy a growing population's need for food, we necessarily decrease its per capita supply of the other resources needed by men.

India, for example, now has a population of 600 million, which increases by 15 million each year. This population already puts a huge load on a relatively impoverished environment. The country's forests are now only a small fraction of what they were three centuries ago, and floods and erosion continually destroy the insufficient farmland that remains. Every one of the 15 million new lives added to India's population puts an additional burden on the environment, and increases the economic and social costs of crowding. However humanitarian our intent, every Indian life saved through medical or nutritional assistance from abroad diminishes the quality of life for those who remain, and for subsequent generations. If rich countries make it possible, through foreign aid, for 600 million Indians to swell to 1.2 billion in a mere 28 years, as their current growth rate threatens, will future generations of Indians thank us for hastening the destruction of their environment? Will our good intentions be sufficient excuse for the consequences of our actions?

My final example of a commons in action is one for which the public has the least desire for rational discussion—immigration. Anyone who publicly questions the wisdom of current U.S. immigration policy is promptly charged with bigotry, prejudice, ethnocentrism, chauvinism, isolationism or selfishness. Rather than encounter such accusations, one would rather talk about other matters, leaving immigration policy to wallow in the crosscurrents of special interests that take no account of the good of the whole, or the interests of posterity.

Perhaps we still feel guilty about things we said in the past. Two generations ago the popular press frequently referred to Dagos, Wops, Polacks, Chinks and Krauts, in articles about how America was being "overrun" by foreigners of supposedly inferior genetic stock. But because the implied inferiority of foreigners was used then as justification for keeping them out, people now assume that restrictive policies

proportion of parents in those countries, large families are still economic assets.

Yes, it works. Parents in the low-income world will want smaller families only when they have very good reasons. The precondition is profound improvements in living conditions. In order for the desire for smaller families to be widespread, the benefits of development must also be widespread. This must come first.

Reprinted with permission from *The New Internationalist*, (32) p. 6 (October 1975).

The Poor Are Not Stupid....

TARZIE VITTACHI

Nothing short of a holocaust can stop the population of the planet doubling inside 30 years. The people who will go forth and multiply are already born.

How can the world sustain twice as many people when half its present population lacks the basic necessities of life? On present trends, it can't. There is a population crisis.

The World Population Conference in Bucharest last year was convened to examine this crisis. It was an honest conference: it admitted that many of the attempts made so far to deal with the population crisis had been mistaken. It was a useful conference: it publicly learnt and taught the lessons of those mistakes. It was also a turning point: for it shifted the focus of attention from the problems of population to the problems of people.

It is perhaps a measure of the condescension inherent in the approach to the population problem so far, that the biggest lesson that has had to be learnt is that poor people are not stupid; that they make rational decisions over their own lives; and that large families are very often an intelligent response to economic circumstances.

When poor people no longer need large families for security and help and opportunity and satisfaction in the struggle to live, then the family planning advice may be welcomed and the population 'explosion' may be defused.

It is a sign of hope and progress that this new analysis, with its new avenues for action, has now gained such widespread acceptance. As the recent appointed Minister of Health and Family Planning in the Indian government, Dr. Karan Singh, has said "Development is the best con-traceptive. Unless you can have a marked improvement in the living standards of the people ... family planning is simply not going to work."

It is at this point that the roots of the population problem reach down into the subsoil of the present economic order, and that genuine solutions must follow them and join in the search for a New Economic Order.

For in as much as the population problem is a function of poverty and under development, the failure to solve it reflects the failure of development.

The inadequacy of our past notions and strategies of development is clear, and continued population growth is only one proof of this. Another is the fact that there are now more malnourished, sick and illiterate people in the world than there were when the first Development Decade began 15 years ago.

No, the old solutions are visibly threadbare. The call for a New Economic Order is a call for new solutions, new concepts, and new strategies of world development. A response to this call is not only essential in itself to end the poverty which afflicts half the world today; it is also the only way of significantly slowing the world's population growth and preventing even more poverty in the future.

It is my belief that recent study of the population issue has much to offer in this search for a new development. For we have learnt that to a large extent the rate of population growth is an indicator of a people's sense of security and well being—of development in their own terms.

And the factors which now appear to be the main determinants of population growth—adequate nutrition, basic health care, employment, education, and more equal opportunities for women—could constitute the basis of a new definition and direction of development.

The meeting of these basic needs should be the goals of the 'new development,' to be aimed at directly as ends in themselves and not as side effects of modernization and economic growth.

To achieve this, I believe that redistribution of wealth and income, and especially of future opportunities for economic growth, will be essential. It is unlikely that the earth's resources could sustain, or that the earth's environment could tolerate, the achievement of these ends by pursuing present patterns of economic growth.

And in any case, the pattern of growth has already proved itself inadequate to the task of meeting the basic needs of the majority of the world's citizens. The institutions which generated it are not neutral with regard to its distribution and the process of 'trickle-down' has clearly become constipated.

The Old Economic Order, based on a market system which makes resources available to those who can afford them rather than those who need them, has been seen to be working against the aim of meeting the basic needs of all in favour of over consumption by the already rich.

It is in this way that our knowledge of population issues converges with our knowledge of other world problems to reinforce the present call for a New Economic Order.

Reprinted with permission from *The New Internationalist*, (32): p. 7 (October 1975).

Population and Food: Metaphors and the Reality

WILLIAM W. MURDOCH and ALLAN OATEN

Hardin's article "Living on a Lifeboat," a slightly longer version of "Lifeboat Ethics," was published in the journal *BioScience* in October of 1974. A year later, in the same journal, two of Hardin's fellow professors at Santa Barbara published this detailed criticism of their colleague's "Commons" and "Lifeboat" metaphors. Letting people starve, they point out, is somewhat less tidy—and a good deal less necessary—than it has been made to seem.

Should rich countries provide food, fertilizers, technical assistance, and other aid to poor countries? The obvious answer is "yes." It is natural to want to fight poverty, starvation, and disease, to help raise living standards and eliminate suffering.

Yet, after 25 years of aid, diets and living standards in many poor countries have improved little, owing partly to the population explosion that occurred during these same years. Death rates in poor countries dropped sharply in the 1940's and 1950's, to around 14/1,000 at present, while their birth rates declined very little, remaining near 40/1,000. Some populations are now growing faster than their food supply.

As a result an apparently powerful argument against aid is increasingly heard. Its premise is simply stated. "More food means more babies" (Hardin 1969). Our benevolence leads to a spiral that can result only in disaster: aid leads to increased populations, which requre more aid, which leads. . . . This premise mandates a radically new policy: rich countries can perhaps provide contraceptives to poor countries, but

they should not provide food, help increase food production, or help combat poverty or disease.

This policy would result in the agonizing deaths, by starvation and disease, of millions of people. Consequently, one expects its advocates to have arrived at it reluctantly, forced to suppress their humanitarian feelings by inexorable logic and the sheer weight of evidence. Its apparent brutality seems a sure guarantee of its realism and rationality.

We believe that this allegedly realistic "non-help" policy is in fact mistaken as well as callous; that the premise on which it is based is at best a half-truth; and that the arguments adduced in its support are not only erroneous, but often exhibit indifference to both the complexities of the problem and much of the available data. We also believe that the evidence shows better living standards and lower population growth rates to be complementary, not contradictory; that aid programs carefully designed to benefit the poorest people can help to achieve both of these ends; and that such programs, though difficult to devise and carry out, are not beyond either the resources or the ingenuity of the rich countries. . . .

Misleading Metaphors

The "lifeboat" article actually has two messages. The first is that our immigration policy is too generous. This will not concern us here. The second, and more important, is that by helping poor nations we will bring disaster to rich and poor alike:

Metaphorically, each rich nation amounts to a lifeboat full of comparatively rich people. The poor of the world are in other, much more crowded lifeboats. Continuously, so to speak, the poor fall out of their lifeboats and swim for a while in the water outside, hoping to be admitted to a rich lifeboat, or in some other way to benefit from the "goodies" on board. What should the passengers on a rich lifeboat do? This is the central problem of "the ethics of a lifeboat." (Hardin, 1974, p. 561)

Among these so-called "goodies" are food supplies and technical aid such as that which led to the Green Revolution. Hardin argues that we should withhold such resources from poor nations on the grounds that they help to maintain high rates of population increase, thereby making the problem worse. He foresees the continued supplying and increasing production of food as a process that will be "brought to an end only by the total collapse of the whole system, producing a catastrophe of scarcely imaginable proportions" (p. 564).

Turning to one particular mechanism for distributing these resources, Hardin claims that a world food bank is a commons—people have more motivation to draw from it than to add to it; it will have a ratchet or escalator effect on population because inputs from it will prevent population declines in over-populated countries. Thus "wealth can be steadily moved in one direction only, from the slowly-breeding rich to the rapidly-breeding poor, the process finally coming to a halt only when all countries are equally and miserably poor" (p. 565). Thus our

help will not only bring ultimate disaster to poor countries, but it will also be suicidal for us.

As for the "benign demographic transition" to low birth rates, which some aid supporters have predicted, Hardin states flatly that the weight of evidence is against this possibility.

Finally, Hardin claims that the plight of poor nations is partly their own fault: "wise sovereigns seem not to exist in the poor world today. The most anguishing problems are created by poor countries that are governed by rulers insufficiently wise and powerful." Establishing a world food bank will exacerbate this problem: "slovenly rulers" will escape the consequences of their incompetence—"Others will bail them out whenever they are in trouble"; "Far more difficult than the transfer of wealth from one country to another is the transfer of wisdom between sovereign powers or between generations" (p. 563).

What arguments does Hardin present in support of these opinions? Many involve metaphors: lifeboat, commons, and ratchet or escalator. These metaphors are crucial to his thesis, and it is, therefore, important for us to examine them critically.

The lifeboat is the major metaphor. It seems attractively simple, but it is in fact simplistic and obscures important issues. As soon as we try to use it to compare various policies, we find that most relevant details of the actual situation are either missing or distorted in the lifeboat metaphor. Let us list some of these details.

Most important, perhaps, Hardin's lifeboats barely interact. The rich lifeboats may drop some handouts over the side and perhaps repel a boarding party now and then, but generally they live their own lives. In the real world, nations interact a great deal, in ways that affect food supply and population size and growth, and the effect of rich nations on poor nations has been strong and not always benevolent.

First, by colonization and actual wars of commerce, and through the international marketplace, rich nations have arranged an exchange of goods that has maintained and even increased the economic imbalance between rich and poor nations. Until recently we have taken or otherwise obtained cheap raw material from poor nations and sold them expensive manufactured goods that they cannot make themselves. In the United States, the structure of tariffs and internal subsidies discriminates selectively against poor nations. In poor countries, the concentration on cash crops rather than on food crops, a legacy of colonial times, is now actively encouraged by western multinational corporations (Barraclough 1975). Indeed, it is claimed that in famine-stricken Sahelian Africa, multinational agribusiness has recently taken land out of food production for cash crops (Transnational Institute 1974). Although we often self-righteously take the "blame" for lowering the death rates of poor nations during the 1940's and 1950's, we are less inclined to accept responsibility for the effects of actions that help maintain poverty and hunger. Yet poverty directly contributes to the high birth rates that Hardin views with such alarm.

Second, U.S. foreign policy, including foreign aid programs, has favored "pro-Western" regimes, many of which govern in the interests of a wealthy elite and some of which are savagely repressive. Thus, it has often subsidized a gross maldistribution of income and has supported political leaders who have opposed most of the social changes that can lead to reduced birth rates. In this light, Hardin's pronouncements on the alleged wisdom gap between poor leaders and our own, and the difficulty of filling it, appear as a grim joke: our response to leaders with the power and wisdom Hardin yearns for has often been to try to replace them or their policies as soon as possible. Selective giving and withholding of both military and nonmilitary aid has been an important ingredient of our efforts to maintain political leaders we like and to remove those we do not. Brown (1974b), after noting that the withholding of U.S. food aid in 1973 contributed to the downfall of the Allende government in Chile, comments that "although Americans decry the use of petro-

leum as a political weapon, calling it 'political blackmail,' the United States has been using food aid for political purposes for twenty years—and describing this as 'enlightened diplomacy.'"

Both the quantity and the nature of the supplies on a lifeboat are fixed. In the real world, the quantity has strict limits, but these are far from having been reached (University of California Food Task Force 1974). Nor are we forced to devote fixed proportions of our efforts and energy to automobile travel, pet food, packaging, advertising, corn-fed beef, "defense" and other diversions, many of which cost far more than foreign aid does. The fact is that enough food is now produced to feed the world's population adequately. That people are malnourished is due to distribution and to economics, not to agricultural limits (United Nations Economic and Social Council 1974).

Hardin's lifeboats are divided merely into rich and poor, and it is difficult to talk about birth rates on either. In the real world, however, there are striking differences among the birth rates of the poor countries and even among the birth rates of different parts of single countries. These differences appear to be related to social conditions (also absent from lifeboats) and may guide us to effective aid policies.

Hardin's lifeboat metaphor not only conceals facts, but misleads about the effects of his proposals. The rich lifeboat can raise the ladder and sail away. But in real life, the problem will not necessarily go away just because it is ignored. In the real world, there are armies, raw materials in poor nations, and even outraged domestic dissidents prepared to sacrifice their own and others' lives to oppose policies they regard as immoral.

No doubt there are other objections. But even this list shows the lifeboat metaphor to be dangerously inappropriate for serious policy making because it obscures far more than it reveals. Lifeboats and "lifeboat ethics" may be useful topics for those who are shipwrecked; we believe they are worthless—indeed detrimental—in discussions of food-population questions.

The ratchet metaphor is equally flawed. It, too, ignores complex interactions between birth rates and social conditions (including diets), implying as it does that more food will simply mean more babies. Also, it obscures the fact that the decrease in death rates has been caused at least as much by developments such as DDT, improved sanitation, and medical advances, as by increased food supplies, so that cutting out food aid will not necessarily lead to population declines. . . .

The lifeboat article is strangely inadequate in other ways. For example, it shows an astonishing disregard for recent literature. The claim that we can expect no "benign demographic transition" is based on a review written more than a decade ago (Davis 1963). Yet, events and attitudes are changing rapidly in poor countries: for the first time in history, most poor people live in countries with birth control programs; with few exceptions, poor nations are somewhere on the demographic transition to lower birth rates (Demeny 1974); the population-food squeeze is now widely recognized, and governments of poor nations are aware of the relationship. Again, there is a considerable amount of evidence that birth rates can fall rapidly in poor countries given the proper social conditions (as we will discuss later); consequently, crude projections of current population growth rates are quite inadequate for policy making.

The Tragedy of the Commons

Throughout the lifeboat article, Hardin bolsters his assertions by reference to the "commons" (Hardin 1968). The thesis of the commons, therefore, needs critical evaluation.

Suppose several privately owned flocks, comprising 100 sheep altogether, are grazing on a public commons. They bring in an annual income of $1.00 per sheep. Fred, a herdsman, owns only one sheep. He decides to add another. But 101 is too many: the commons is overgrazed and produces less food. The sheep lose quality and income drops to 90¢ per sheep. Total income is now $90.90 instead of $100.00.

Adding the sheep has brought an overall loss. But Fred has gained: *his* income is $1.80 instead of $1.00. The gain from the additional sheep, which is his alone, outweighs the loss from overgrazing, which he shares. Thus he promotes his interest at the expense of the community.

This is the problem of the commons, which seems on the way to becoming an archetype. Hardin, in particular, is not inclined to underrate its importance: "One of the major tasks of education today is to create such an awareness of the dangers of the commons that people will be able to recognize its many varieties, however disguised" (Hardin 1974, p. 562) and "All this is terribly obvious once we are acutely aware of the pervasiveness and danger of the commons. But many people still lack this awareness. . ." (p.565).

The "commons" affords a handy way of classifying problems: the lifeboat article reveals that sharing, a generous immigration policy, world food banks, air, water, the fish populations of the ocean, and the western range lands are, or produce, a commons. It is also handy to be able to dispose of policies one does not like and "only a particular instance of a class of policies that are in error because they lead to the tragedy of the commons" (p. 561).

But no metaphor, even one as useful as this, should be treated with such awe. Such shorthand can be useful, but it can also mislead by discouraging thought and obscuring important detail. To dismiss a proposal by suggesting that "all you need to know about this proposal is that it institutes a commons and is, therefore, bad" is to assert that the proposed commons is worse than the original problem. This might be so if the problem of the commons were, indeed, a tragedy—that is, if it were insoluble. But it is not.

Hardin favors private ownership as the solution (either through private property or the selling of pollution rights). But, of course, there are solutions other than private ownership; and private ownership itself is no guarantee of carefully husbanded resources.

One alternative to private ownership of the commons is communal ownership of the sheep—or, in general, of the mechanisms and industries that exploit the resource—combined with communal planning for management. (Note, again, how the metaphor favors one solution: perhaps the "tragedy" lay not in the commons but in the sheep. "The Tragedy of the Privately Owned Sheep" lacks zing, unfortunately.) Public ownership of a commons has been tried in Peru to the benefit of the previously privately owned anchoveta fishery (Gulland 1975). The communally owned agriculture of China does not seem to have suffered any greater over-exploitation than that of other Asian nations.

Another alternative is cooperation combined with regulation. For example, Gulland (1975) has shown that Antarctic whale stocks (perhaps the epitome of a commons since they are internationally exploited and no one owns them) are now being properly managed, and stocks are increasing. This has been achieved through cooperation in the International Whaling Commission, which has by agreement set limits to the catch of each nation.

In passing, Hardin's private ownership argument is not generally applicable to nonrenewable resources. Given discount rates, technology substitutes, and no more than an average regard for posterity, privately owned nonrenewable resources, like oil, coal and minerals, are mined at rates that produce maximum profits, rather than at those rates that preserve them for future generations. . . .

On Malign Neglect

Hardin implies that nonhelp policies offer a solution to the world population-food problem. But what sort of solution would in fact occur?

Nonhelp policies would have several effects not clearly described in "Lifeboat" (Hardin 1974). First, it is not true that people in poor countries "convert extra food into extra babies" (p. 564). They convert it into longer lives.

Denying them food will not lower birth rates; it will increase death rates.

These increases might not take effect immediately after the withdrawal of aid. Increases in local food production and improvements in sanitation and medicine would probably allow populations to continue growing for some time. (Death rates would need to increase almost three-fold to stabilize them.) Thus, in the future we could expect much larger populations in poor countries, living in greater misery than today. The negative relation between well-being and family size could easily lead to even higher birth rates. A "solution" that puts us back to prewar birth and death rates, at even higher population levels, is certainly not a satisfactory permanent solution.

Second, the rich countries cannot remain indifferent to events in poor countries. A poor country or a group of poor countries that controls supplies of a vital raw material, for example, may well want to use this leverage to its advantage; it may be very uncompromising about it, especially if its need is desperate and its attitude resentful, as would be likely. Just how intolerable this situation would be to the rich countries can be guessed at by recent hints of war being an acceptable means for the United States to ensure itself adequate supplies of oil at a "reasonable" price.

War is an option open to poor countries, too. China and India have nuclear weapons; others can be expected to follow. With Hardin's policies, they may feel they have little to lose, and the rich countries have a great deal to lose.

Thus we could look forward to continuing, and probably increasing, interference in and manipulation of the increasingly miserable poor countries by the rich countries. We do not believe this is a stable situation. One or more poor countries will surely want to disrupt it; recent events show that our ability to prevent this is limited. Alternatively, in the future, one or more of the rich countries may decide to help poor countries reduce their birth rates, but will then be faced with an even greater problem than we face today. In sum, malign neglect of poor nations is not likely to cause the problem to go away.

If Hardin's proposals are so defective, why are they attractive to so many people? We have already discussed Hardin's use of oversimplified metaphors, but there are other temptations.

An obvious one is the presentation of false choices: either we continue what we are doing, or we do nothing. Aid is either effective or ineffective; much of our aid has been ineffective, so all aid is, and it always will be. Such absolute positions are tempting because they save thought, justify inaction, never need reconsideration, and convey an impression of sophisticated cynicism. But they do not conform to the facts. Intelligent and effective aid, though difficult, is possible.

The apparent callousness of Hardin's proposals is itself a temptation. There is an implication that these policies are so brutal that they would not be proposed without good reasons. Conversely, those who argue for increased aid can be dismissed as "highly vocal humanitarian apologists" or "guilt addicts" (Hardin 1974, pp. 563 and 562). The implication is that these views *could* arise from unreasoning emotion, so therefore they *must* arise this way. Proposals for increased aid are then "plaintive cries" produced by guilt, bad conscience, anxiety, and misplaced Christian or Marxist idealism. But such argument by association is plainly misleading. Benign policies can also be the most rational; callous policies can be foolish.

Birth Rates: An Alternative View

Is the food-population spiral inevitable? A more optimistic, if less comfortable, hypothesis, presented by Rich (1973) and Brown (1974a), is increasingly tenable: contrary to the "ratchet" projection, population growth rates are affected by many complex conditions beside food supply. In particular, a set of socioeconomic conditions can be identified that motivate parents to have fewer children; under these conditions, birth rates can fall quite rapidly, sometimes even before birth control technology is available. Thus, population growth can be controlled more effectively by intelligent human intervention that sets up the appropriate conditions than by doing nothing and trusting to "natural population cycles."

These conditions are: parental confidence about the future, an improved status of women, and literacy. They require low infant mortality rates, widely available rudimentary health care, increased income and employment, and an adequate diet above subsistence levels. Expenditure on schools (especially elementary schools), appropriate health services (especially rural paramedical services), and agricultural reform (especially aid to small farmers) will be needed, and foreign aid can help here. It is essential that these improvements be spread across the population; aid can help here, too, by concentrating on the poor nations' poorest people, encouraging necessary institutional and social reforms, and making it easier for poor nations to use their own resources and initiative to help themselves. It is *not* necessary that per capita GNP be very high, certainly not as high as that of the rich countries during their gradual demographic transition. In other words, low birth rates in poor countries are achievable long before the conditions exist that were present in the rich countries in the late 19th and early 20th centuries.

Twenty or thirty years is not long to discover and assess the factors affecting birth rates, but a body of evidence is now accumulating in favor of this hypothesis. Rich (1973) and Brown (1974a) show that at least 10 developing countries have managed to reduce their birth rates by an average of more than one birth per 1,000 population per year for periods of 5 to 16 years. A reduction of one birth per 1,000 per year would bring birth rates in poor countries to a rough replacement level of about 16/1,000 by the turn of the century, though age distribution effects would prevent a smooth population decline. We have listed these countries in Table 1,

TABLE 1. Declining birth rates and per capita income in selected developing countries. (These are crude birth rates, uncorrected for age distribution.)

| Country | Time span | Births/1,000/year | | |
		Ave. annual decline in crude birth rate	Crude birth rate 1972	$ per capita per year 1973
Barbados	1960-69	1.5	22	570
Taiwan	1955-71	1.2	24	390
Tunisia	1966-71	1.8	35	250
Mauritius	1961-71	1.5	25	240
Hong Kong	1960-72	1.4	19	970
Singapore	1955-72	1.2	23	920
Costa Rica	1963-72	1.5	32	560
South Korea	1960-70	1.2	29	250
Egypt	1966-70	1.7	37	210
Chile	1963-70	1.2	25	720
China			30	160
Cuba			27	530
Sri Lanka			30	110

together with three other nations, including China, that are poor and yet have brought their birth rates down to 30 or less, presumably from rates of over 40 a decade or so ago.

These data show that rapid reduction in birth rates is possible in the developing world. No doubt it can be argued that each of these cases is in some way special. Hong Kong and Singapore are relatively rich; they, Barbados, and Mauritius are also tiny. China is able to exert great social pressure on its citizens; but China is particularly significant. It is enormous; its per capita GNP is almost as low as India's; and it started out in 1949 with a terrible health system. Also, Egypt, Chile, Taiwan, Cuba, South Korea, and Sri Lanka are quite large, and they are poor or very poor (Table 1). In fact, these examples represent an enormous range of religion, political systems, and geography and suggest that such rates of decline in the birth rate can be achieved whenever the appropriate conditions are met. "The common factor in these countries is that the *majority* of the population has shared in the economic and social benefits of significant national progress. . . .[M]aking health, education and jobs more broadly available to lower income groups in poor countries contribute[s] significantly toward the motiva-

tion for smaller families that is the prerequisite of a major reduction in birth rates" (Rich 1973).

The converse is also true. In Latin America, Cuba (annual per capita income $530), Chile ($720), Uruguay ($820), and Argentina ($1,160) have moderate to truly equitable distribution of goods and services and relatively low birth rates (27, 26, 23, and 22, respectively). In contrast, Brazil ($420), Mexico ($670), and Venezuela ($980) have very unequal distribution of goods and services and high birth rates (38, 42, and 41, respectively). Fertility rates in poor and relatively poor nations seem unlikely to fall as long as the bulk of the population does not share in increased benefits. . . .

Costs, Gains, and Difficulties

We have neither the space nor the expertise to propose detailed food-population policies. Our main concern has been to help set the stage for serious discussion by disposing of simplistic proposals and irrelevant arguments, outlining some of the complexities of the problem, and indicating the existence of a large quantity of available data.

However, some kind of positive statement

seems called for, if only to provide a target for others. . . .

Brown (1974a) estimates that $5 billion per year could provide:

- family planning services to the poor nations (excluding China, which already provides them); the cost includes training personnel and providing transportation facilities and contraceptives;
- literacy for all adults and children (a five-year program); and
- a health care program for mothers and infants (again excluding China).

To this we could add the following:

- 10 million metric tons of grain at an annual cost of $2 billion;
- 1.5 million metric tons of fertilizer, which is the estimated amount of the "shortfall" last year in the poor countries (U.N. 1974); the cost, including transportation, is roughly $1 billion; and
- half of the estimated annual cost of providing "adequate" increases in the area of irrigated and cultivated land in the poor countries (U.N. 1974), about $2 billion.

. . . The total cost is $10 billion. Still, these estimates are very crude. Let us suppose the real cost is $20 billion. Other wealthy countries could (and should) provide at least half of this. This leaves about $10 billion to be provided by the United States. Can the United States afford it?

In the past, U.S. aid has not normally been free. Indeed, India is now a net exporter of capital to the United States because it pays back more interest and principal on previous aid loans than it receives in aid. However, even giving away $10 billion is likely to have only minor effects on the U.S. economy and standard of living. It is about 1% of the GNP, about 10% of current military expenditure. It would decrease present and future consumption of goods and services in the United States by slightly more than 1% (because the cost of government accounts for about 25% of the GNP). . . .

In short, although we must take care that the burden is equitably borne, the additional aid could be provided with only minor effects on the well-being of the U.S. population. Such a reduction in living standard is hardly "suicidal" or a matter of "human survival" in the United States, to use Hardin's terms. It is not a question of "them or us," as the lifeboat metaphor implies. This simple-minded dichotomy may account for the appeal of Hardin's views, but it bears no relation to reality.

The six measures suggested above should encourage economic growth as well as lower birth rates in poor countries. . . .

Will the aid in fact be used in ways that help reduce birth rates? As a disillusioning quarter-century of aid giving has shown, the obstacles to getting aid to those segments of the population most in need of it are enormous. Aid has typically benefitted a small rich segment of society, partly because of the way aid programs have been designed but also because of human and institutional factors in the poor nations themselves (Owens and Shaw 1972). With some notable exceptions, the distribution of income and services in poor nations is extremely skewed—much more uneven than in rich countries. Indeed, much of the population is essentially outside the economic system. Breaking this pattern will be extremely difficult. It will require not only aid that is designed specifically to benefit the rural poor, but also important institutional changes such as decentralization of decision making and the development of greater autonomy and stronger links to regional and national markets for local groups and industries such as cooperative farms.

Thus, two things are being asked of rich nations and of the United States in particular: to increase nonmilitary foreign aid, including food aid, and to give it in ways, and to governments, that will deliver it to the poorest people and will improve their access to national economic institutions. These are not easy tasks, particularly the second, and there is no guarantee that birth rates will come down quickly in all countries. Still, many poor countries have, in varying degrees, begun the process of reform, and recent evidence suggests that aid and reform together can do much to solve the twin problems of high birth rates and economic underdevelopment. The tasks are far from impossible. Based on the evidence, the policies dictated by a sense of decency are also the most realistic and rational.

Excerpted with permission from *BioScience,* 25 (9): 561-567 (September 1975) published by the American Institute of Biological Science.

Is It Time to End Food for Peace?

EMMA ROTHSCHILD

The dilemma re-emerges. Aid could be given, should be given perhaps. More food does reduce death rates; and reduced death rates ultimately do reduce population growth. We *should* send food, Murdoch and Oaten argue; and we should *also* send money. But if help is possible, why has our past help—our "astonishing" generosity of the post World War II era—not "paid off?" Emma Rothschild, a young British economist, here suggests some of the reasons why our past quarter century of "generosity" has failed to produce the results we had been led to expect.

Twenty-three years ago, the United States Congress wrote a law which has changed the diet and the political life of half the world. The law, known as Public Law 480 of the 83d Congress, or the Food for Peace act, provides for the United States to send food as aid to foreign countries. Its scope is vast. The United States Government has spent more than $30 billion on the program, sending food to 130 countries. In wheat alone, the United States has distributed enough grain to bake a hundred loaves of bread for every person alive today.

Yet P.L. 480 has been since its birth the subject of bitter political conflict. In the late 1970's, its shortcomings are ever more evident. The program has failed, first of all, in its humanitarian purpose of helping hungry people. During the world food crisis of 1973-74, the United States actually reduced its aid to many poor countries—above all, to Bangladesh at the time of the 1974 famine. In the second place, the program now seems obsolete, suited to an era which is gone forever. P.L. 480 was passed in 1954 as a way to get rid of surplus food and

fiber. Now, the United States Government no longer owns mountains of surplus wheat, and foreign aid is no longer an exciting adventure. . . .

There are at least four purposes to P.L. 480, as there have been since 1954. It is a way to get rid of surplus food, and a way to help hungry people, an instrument of political and military policy, and a way to create markets for American food. Each of these purposes corresponds to a phase in the history of the program, and in the postwar history of America. Yet each is preserved, the embodiment of earlier hopes. In the immediate drama of food aid, all are present, jostling to the fore.

The United States now spends a little over a billion dollars a year on food aid. More than three-quarters of the aid—mostly wheat and rice—is sent under the P.L. 480 program. Eighty countries receive some food aid from the United States, although most of the aid each year goes to four or so countries. Quite prosperous countries are eligible for aid. Israel was the leading recipient of United States food aid in the 1976 fiscal year. In 1975, the largest recipient was

India. South Vietnam was first in 1974 and 1973, and South Korea in 1972.

P.L. 480 has two main parts. Under Title I, the larger part of the law, the United States Government lends countries money to buy American farm products—mainly wheat, rice, cotton, tobacco and soybean oil. The countries then usually have 20 to 40 years in which to repay the loans, in most cases at three percent interest. Under Title II, the United States donates food either to foreign governments or to international relief organizations like CARE. The United States Government also sends some food aid outside P.L. 480, under the Agency for International Development's development assistance program. The A.I.D. shipments provide a Garden of Eden of exports: baby chicks and almonds, sugar and dried soup mixes. . . .

Surplus Disposal

P.L. 480 was devised in 1954 as a measure for the "disposition of agricultural surpluses." In the early years of the program, rich countries such as Britain and Poland received large amounts of aid, including, for example, products like tobacco, tallow and canned fruit juices. But the main surplus commodities were wheat and cotton. Since the New Deal, the United States Government had bought farm products to support agricultural prices. When prices fell after World War II, and again after the Korean War, farmers sold their products to the Government for want of a better buyer. It was these publicly-owned stocks of food and fiber that the United States planned in 1954 to export under the new aid program. The measure was meant to be temporary. In three years, the law's sponsors hoped, the United States could rid itself, once and for all, of its burdensome abundance.

As the program was extended time after time, it had less to do with surpluses. In the 1960's, P.L. 480 money was used to buy farm products that were neither "surplus" nor owned by the Government; the Government bought commodities for food aid on the open market.

(Three-quarters of all United States wheat exports and a third of the entire national wheat harvest was destined for P.L. 480 in the mid-1960's.) Yet the idea of surplus remains even now. All farm products used for P.L. 480 must be certified by the Secretary of Agriculture as being available beyond what is needed for domestic requirements, stocks and likely commercial exports.

In the mid-1950's, the P.L. 480 program captured the imaginations of several Democrats in Congress, above all of Senator Hubert Humphrey. In 1957, Senator Humphrey conducted a series of hearings on the program, eventually publishing a report with the inspiring title of "Food and Fiber as a Force for Freedom." . . . He suggested that the program should be seen as a persisting instrument of United States policy, both for political purposes and to develop new foreign markets for American food. . . .

Political and Military Aid

"I have heard here this morning that people may become dependent upon us for food," Humphrey said during the 1957 hearings. "I know that was not supposed to be good news," he went on. "To me that is good news, because before people will do anything, they have got to eat. And if you are really looking for a way to get people to lean on you and to be dependent upon you, in terms of their cooperation with you, it seems to me that food dependence would be terrific."

Senator Humphrey saw a close association between food and the political concerns of the time. He suggested that if America's allies could rely on food from Kansas or Oregon, they could take people out of agriculture to build an army. . . .

Most food aid in the 23 years of the program has gone to countries that were also military friends, such as Israel and Turkey in the 1950's, South Korea and Pakistan throughout, South Vietnam in the 1960's and 1970's. (Ten countries, including these, account for more than half of all P.L. 480 shipments. The others are

India, Egypt, Yugoslavia, Indonesia and Brazil.) Some countries were allowed to use the proceeds from selling P.L. 480 food for military purposes. Many aid agreements called for the countries to repay the United States in their local currencies. But the United States would often give the money back, to be used for "common defense." About 80 percent of all the money collected in South Korea was used in this way, and a similar proportion in Vietnam. . . .

Market Development

The other great advantage of P.L. 480 to Senator Humphrey and his colleagues, was that it helped to create new markets for American food. At the 1957 hearings, Minnesota's Senator Edward Thye explained: "If they ever develop the taste for powdered milk or for butter. . . or if they develop a strong habit for wheat, where they are rice consuming, then we will always have a market there. . . . We put these foods at their disposal for a period of six months or a year, after which they are always going to be looking for that type of a product." Humphrey noted that "Chedder cheese, for instance, was not the most desirable product in some parts of the world, but now they are beginning to like it."

The original P.L. 480 legislation provided that part of the money countries paid back to the United States, after they borrowed money to buy food, was to be used in "market development." But the activist Democrats in Congress believed that Eisenhower's Administration had been as timid here as in its political efforts. Witness after witness described prodigies of promotion, and was urged to ever greater exertions.

One executive testified that P.L. 480 money had been spent in Rome on an "American Way supermarket project," "sending a supermarket overseas as a working example of people's capitalism." (The "exact replica of its moderate size American counterpart," it featured frozen TV dinners, was praised by Pope Pius XII and attracted half a million Italian visitors.) Another

described the American Wheat Cup presented at the annual golf tournament of the Japanese Grain Importers Association. Perhaps the most constant theme concerned the education of bakers, from South Korea to Colombia. In Japan, the Oregon Wheat Growers League used P.L. 480 money to set up a "bakers' training school." Once adept, the baker cadres "return to their home prefectures [where] they in turn conduct classes" in the mysteries of wheat. . . .

And the enterprise continues. . . with baking classes and seminars around the world. "An evaluation of one such project in [South] Korea showed that housewives exposed to cooking demonstrations used an average of 16 percent more wheat in family meals. . . ." Throughout Asia and Latin America people were introduced to wheat, to the American way of eating, by the P.L. 480 program. Now American agricultural exports, all food aid aside, are worth more than $20 billion a year. Such countries as India and Brazil, South Korea and Japan are leading commercial customers, paying dollars for American food.

Food for Peace

. . .P.L. 480 was an important part of Kennedy's foreign policy in Asia and Latin America. It seemed to epitomize the sense that Americans had in the early 1960's that all things were possible, in a world growing daily richer and braver. . . .

Food for Peace had the merit, too, of pleasing the most diverse people. . . . Some congressmen saw it as aid to Kansas, and others as aid to Asia. Administration officials often seemed deliberately vague, seeking, perhaps, to preserve the program's multiple appeal.

Food for Development

The Kennedy and Johnson Administrations set out boldly to promote economic development around the world. P.L. 480 after 1966 was tied closely to development projects, and in particular to agricultural programs. Countries receiving Title I aid were required to practice "self-help" in agriculture. Yet these efforts were fraught with contradictions.

Food aid itself was a disincentive to agricultural production abroad. Since the early 1960's, almost a third of all United States official development assistance has been in the form of food aid. In such countries as South Korea, Brazil, even India, P.L. 480 helped to make it possible for governments to neglect their own farmers. The program served to reinforce the bias of development policies in favor of urban and industrial growth. In South Korea, for example, the Government received American food and kept local rice prices low. Industry flourished, while in the countryside, poor rice farmers found they could not make a living. They were forced into Seoul and other cities. Farmers who remained found that more and more people had acquired the taste for wheat from the cadres of bakers who surged across the country.

Successive U.S. Governments have tried to help the poorest people with food aid. But here again P.L. 480 proved a mixed blessing. Wheat is the leading food-aid commodity, and in many poor countries, particularly in rice- and corn-growing regions, wheat is sold largely to relatively prosperous consumers. . . .

The history of the United States Government's pork projects in Asia illustrates the conflicts of P.L. 480. . . . In South Vietnam, pig cooperatives were set up with "surplus American corn, eight sacks of cement for a pigsty, and three pigs for each participating family."

By 1968, senators reviewing P.L. 480 learned that South Vietnam had agreed to "pursue aggressively a policy of increasing pork production," and to "establish a selling price for imported corn which will encourage its expanded use as feed grain for pork production." That same year, U.S. aid experts undertook the most grandiose project of all, directed at the entire pig population of South Vietnam. As explained five years later in the P.L. 480 annual report, "1973 is regarded as the 'wrap-up' year of a long

range effort . . . to establish a viable commercial swine industry in South Vietnam. Through the introduction of U.S. technology and Vietnamese acceptance of the principle of self-help, the swine population has been changed from that of the rural-reared scavenger sway-back pig—an inefficient converter of feed to pork—to a meat-type pig."

Here, as elsewhere, efforts to use food aid to help foreign livestock producers left the farmers dependent upon American food and technology. In the case of the pork programs, the United States left in Vietnam a "population" of American-style pigs that was largely dependent on corn feed, long after American technologists had departed.

The Nixon Years

Under President Nixon, the United States turned away from foreign aid in general and from P.L. 480 in particular. Food aid had come to be associated with unrewarding projects (pig banks) and ungrateful recipients (India). The amounts of food shipped under P.L. 480 fell fairly steadily, from a high level of 18 million tons in 1966 to 11 million tons in 1970 and 3.3 million tons in 1974.

Describing the "Nixon Doctrine" in foreign policy, President Nixon wrote that "we need to replace the impulses of the previous era: both our instinct that we knew what was best for others and their temptation to lean on our prescriptions." Nixon's food-aid policy reflected to some extent this objective: It recognized that P.L. 480 required real money, and that the United States itself had real problems with inflation and with its balance of payments.

But there were other, less inspiring, themes in the Nixon food policy. The military element in P.L. 480 became stronger, in accordance with the Nixonian principle that foreign aid should be tied directly to national self-interest. . . .

The Nixon Administration, finally, did not begin to answer the new question of how the United States should act as the era of aid was succeeded by an era of commercial trade. By the 1970's, the long years of market development had been vindicated. Rich and poor developing countries had acquired the taste for imported food. But they found P.L. 480 limited. As Senator Thye had foreseen 15 years earlier, they went into commercial markets to buy American wheat for dollars. The change was sudden. In the 1972 fiscal year, United States aid-financed farm exports to developing countries were worth $1.1 billion, while commercial exports were worth $1.7 billion. By 1975, the aid exports were again worth $1.1 billion. But the value of commercial exports had quadrupled, to a value of $6.8 billion.

The Crisis

The world food crisis of 1973-74 came about, then, at a time when the United States food-aid program was in disarray. By the end of 1973, U.S. wheat exports cost three times as much per ton as they had little more than a year before. There were many reasons for the inflation: the worldwide economic boom, bad weather in several countries, the Russian purchase of American food, the efforts of the United States and other food-exporting countries to restrict farm production, the success, too, of United States market-development schemes. But the consequences were most serious in developing countries.

"An anomalous situation has developed over the past two years," a senior United States official, Thomas Enders, testified early in 1975: "At the very time that food aid was most needed, it turned out to be the hardest to get." Most countries found their P.L. 480 food shipments cut in 1974, the worst year of the world food crisis. When prices were high, the money spent on aid bought less food. The Title II donations program, to illustrate, was cut dramatically. Thirty-one million fewer people received Title II food in 1974 than in 1973. In Bangladesh alone, 13 million people were struck from the rolls.

P.L. 480, after 20 years, was tested in a worldwide crisis and found wanting. . . .

The Aftermath

In the period since the 1974 famines, the United States food-aid program has gone from scarcity to abundance and obesity. People in Asia were dying of starvation in 1974. A year later, in the same countries, rats choked on surplus American rice.

Many Americans became outraged, in the course of 1974, about the fiasco of food aid. Congress in December 1974, reacting to this concern, passed legislation requiring that most food-aid sales be reserved for very poor countries. (The requirement, which is still in force, now provides that 75 percent of all Title I P.L. 480 shipments go to countries with an average income per person of less than $300 a year.) Senator Hubert Humphrey, who has been consistent since 1954 in sustaining the humanitarian parts of the aid program, was a major force for the change.

In 1975, the United States more than doubled its food aid to the poorest countries. In part because of American aid, the food situation improved greatly. Yet the contradictions of the P.L. 480 program were not to be avoided. Many food shipments arrived too late, when the worst of the crisis was over. India received more food than it could store. Bangladesh was sent six times as much Title I grain in 1975 as had been dispatched in the famine year of 1974.

Meanwhile, the old agricultural interest in surplus disposal and market development returned. Agricultural prices have fallen, particularly prices of wheat and rice. Farmers in several states lobby to have their products bought for P.L. 480. The U.S. Government buys stocks of rice, peanuts and milk. Food aid, once more, seems commercially enticing. . . .

Ending Food for Peace

What is to be done with the food-aid program? My own view is that the time has come for the slow end of P.L. 480. The denouement will last for 10 to 20 years. But it should begin at once. . . .

In the period between now and, say, 1990, several very poor countries will continue to need food aid, particularly in their intermittent food crises. P.L. 480 procedures should be reformed so as to work better in such emergencies. Yet U.S. policy should try, eventually, to end the program. For P.L. 480 will continue to present serious problems "both to those who give and those who receive."

Congress itself should undertake an examination of P.L. 480. . . . One of the reasons for the food-aid fiasco of 1973-74 was that people concerned about humanitarian questions—church groups and others—did not find out what was happening until the worst was almost over. The Public Law 480 annual report, for example, is nearly inaccessible to most people and is published as much as two years after the events it describes. This document should be on sale in every United States Government bookstore. Short quarterly reports should also be widely distributed.

The procedure for deciding who gets food aid should be changed. The P.L. 480 apparatus, with its interagency committee, should eventually be moved from the Department of Agriculture to the State Department. This is not because one set of officials is likely to be more kindly or expeditious than the other. But the most important remaining functions of P.L. 480 will be humanitarian and political. The program should properly, therefore, belong to the foreign policy bureaucracies. . . .

The denouement of P.L. 480 will be without question enormously difficult. The different forces in P.L. 480 lie deep in United States political life and in the country's perception of itself. The P.L. 480 dilemma is part of a larger choice, of how the United States will act toward other countries while the economic order for which it was responsible comes to an end. The opportunity is to act justly and openly and with self-knowledge, as a new epoch begins.

Excerpted with permission from *The New York Times Magazine,* pp. 15+ (13 March 1977). Copyright 1977 by The New York Times Company.

Food First

FRANCES MOORE LAPPÉ and JOE COLLINS

If we change our behavior toward other countries in the coming decades as Rothschild and others in this chapter have suggested we should, we must then decide how we ought to behave. One of the influential thinkers on the subject has been Francis Moore Lappé, whose best-selling *Diet for a Small Planet* argued that we should stop feeding so much of our grain to animals and use it instead to feed the poor overseas. Now, like the other authors in this section, she has developed doubts about the beneficence of what we have done in the name of aid-giving. The article "Food First" here reproduced from *The New Internationalist*, is a brief summary of the book which she has recently written with Joe Collins, co-founder with Lappé of the Institute for Food and Development.

For the last several years we have struggled to answer the question "why hunger?" Analyses that call for more aid or for reducing our consumption so that the hungry might eat left us with gnawing doubts.

Here we want to share the six myths that kept us locked into a misunderstanding of the problem as well as the alternative view that emerged once we began to grasp the issues. Our hope is to help anchor the hunger movement with an unequivocal and cogent analysis. Only then will our collective potential no longer be dissipated.

Myth One: People are hungry because of scarcity—both of food and agricultural land.

Can scarcity seriously be considered the cause of hunger when even in the worst years of famine in the early 70's there was plenty to go around—enough in grain alone to provide everyone in the world with 3000 to 4000 calories a day, not counting all the beans, root crops, fruits, nuts, vegetables and non-grain-fed meat?

And what of land scarcity?

We looked at the most crowded countries in the world to see if we could find a correlation between land density and hunger. We could not. Bangladesh, for example, has just half the people per cultivated acre that Taiwan has. Yet Taiwan has no starvation while Bangladesh is thought of as the world's worst basketcase. China has twice as many people for each cultivated acre as India. Yet in China people are not hungry.

Finally, when the pattern of *what* is grown sank in, we simply could no longer subscribe to a "scarcity" diagnosis of hunger. In Central America and in the Caribbean, where as much as 70 percent of the children are undernourished, at least half of the agricultural land, and the best land at that, grows crops for export, not food for the local people. In the Sahelian countries for Sub-Saharan Africa, exports of cotton and peanuts in the early 1970's actually *increased* as drought and hunger loomed.

Next we asked: What solution emerges when the problem of hunger is defined as scarcity?

Most commonly, people see greater production as the answer. So techniques to increase production become the central focus: supplying the "modern" inputs—large scale irrigation, chemical fertilization, pesticides, machinery and the seeds dependent on these other inputs. All of this is designed to make the land produce more. But when a new agricultural technology enters a system shot through with power inequalities, it brings greater profit only to those who already have some combination of land, money, credit "worthiness" and political influence. This alone has barred most of the world's rural population and all the world's hungry from the benefits of 'producing more.'

More Production, More Hunger

Once agriculture is viewed as a growth industry in which the control of the basic inputs guarantees big money, a catastrophic chain of events is set into motion. Competition for land sends land values soaring (land values have jumped three to five times in the "Green Revolution" areas of India). Higher rents force tenants and sharecroppers into the ranks of the landless. With the new profits the powerful buy out small farmers who have gone bankrupt (in part through having been forced to double or triple their indebtedness trying to partake of the new technology). Moreover, faced with a short planting and harvest time for vast acreages planted uniformly with the most profitable crop, large commercial growers mechanize to avoid the troublesome mobilization of human labor. Those made landless by the production focus, finding ever fewer agricultural jobs, join an equally hopeless search for work in urban slums.

Fewer and fewer people gain control over more and more land. In Sonora, Mexico, the average farm before the Green Revolution was 400 acres. After 20 years of publicly funded modernization, the average has climbed to 2000 acres with some holdings running as large as 25,000 acres.

The poor pay the price. Total production per capita may be up yet so are the numbers who face hunger. A strategy to solve hunger by increasing production has led directly to increased inequality, in fact to the absolute decline in the welfare of the majority. A study

now being completed by the ILO shows that in the very South Asian countries—Pakistan, India, Thailand, Malaysia, Philippines and Indonesia—where the focus has been on production and where the GNP has risen, the majority of the rural population are worse off than before.

But if the scarcity diagnosis, with the implied solution of increasing production, by technical inputs, has taken us not forward but backward, what is the right diagnosis?

We could answer that question only after our research at IFDP led us to conclude that there is *no* country without sufficient agricultural resources for the people to feed themselves and then some. And if they are not doing so, you can be sure there are powerful obstacles in the way. The prime obstacle is not, however, inadequate production to be overcome by technical inputs. The obstacle is that the people do not control the productive resources. When control is in the hands of the producers, people will no longer appear as liabilities—as a drain on resources. People are potentially a country's most under-utilized resource and most valuable capital. People who know they are working for themselves will not only make the land produce but through their labour make it ever more productive.

Myth Two: A hungry world simply cannot afford the luxury of justice for the small farmer.

We are made to believe that, if we want to eat, we had better rely on the large landowners. Thus governments, international lending agencies and foreign assistance programs have passed over the small producers, believing that concentrating on the large holders was the quickest road to production gains. A study of 83 countries, revealing that just over 3 percent of the land holders control about 80 percent of the farmland, gave us some idea of how many of the world's farmers would be excluded by such a concentration.

Yet a study of Argentina, Brazil, Chile, Colombia, Ecuador and Guatemala found the small farmer to be three to fourteen times more productive per acre than the larger farmer. In Thailand plots of two to four acres yield almost 60 percent more rice per acre than farms of 140 acres or more. Other proof that justice for the small farmer increases production comes from the experience of countries in which the re-distribution of land and other basic agricultural resources like water has resulted in rapid growth in agricultural production: Japan, Taiwan, and China stand out.

But where has the grip of this myth led? As the large holders are reinforced, often with public subsidies, the small holders and laborers have been cut out of production through the twin process of increasing land concentration and mechanization. *To be cut out of production is to be cut out of consumption.*

Flowers not Food

As fewer and fewer have the wherewithal either to grow food or to buy food, the internal market for food stagnates or even shrinks. But large commercial farmers have not worried. They orient their production to high-paying markets—a few strata of urban dwellers and foreign consumers. Farmers in Sinaloa, Mexico, find they can make 20 times more growing tomatoes for Americans than corn for Mexicans. Development funds have irrigated the desert in Senegal so that multinational firms can grow eggplant and mangoes for air freighting to Europe's best tables. Colombian land-holders shift from wheat to carnations that bring 80 times greater return per acre. In Costa Rica the lucrative export beef business expands as the local consumption of meat and dairy products declines. Throughout the non-socialist countries we find a consistent pattern. Agriculture, once the livelihood for millions of self-provisioning farmers, is being turned into the production site of high-value non-essentials for the minority who can pay.

Moreover, entrusting agricultural production to the large farmers means invariably the loss of productive reinvestment in agriculture. Com-

monly profits of the large holders that might have gone to improve the land are spent instead on conspicuous consumption, investment in urban consumer industries or job-destroying mechanization. The control of the land by large holders for whom the land is not the basis of daily sustenance often means its underutilization. In Colombia, for example, the largest land owners control 70 percent of all agricultural land but actually cultivate only 6 percent.

It is not enough simply to deflate the myth that justice and production are incompatible. We must come to see clearly that the only solution to hunger is a conscious plan to reduce inequality at every level. The reality is that not only will the re-distribution of control of agricultural resources boost production but it is the only guarantee that today's hungry—the rural poor and the urban refugees—will eat.

Myth Three: We are now faced with a sad trade-off. A needed increase in food production can come only at the expense of the ecological integrity of our food base. Farming must be pushed onto marginal lands at the risk of irreparable erosion. And the use of pesticides will have to be increased even if the risk is great.

Is the need for food for a growing population the real pressure forcing people to farm lands that are easily destroyed?

Haiti offers a shocking picture of environmental destruction. The majority of the utterly impoverished peasants ravage the once-green mountain slopes in near-futile efforts to grow food to survive. Has food production for Haitians used up every easily cultivated acre so that only the mountain slopes are left? No. These mountain peasants must be seen as exiles from their birthright—some of the world's richest agricultural land. The rich valley lands belong to a handful of elites, who seek dollars in order to live an imported lifestyle, and to their American partners. These lands are thus made to produce largely low-nutrition and feed crops (sugar, coffee, cocoa, alfalfa for cattle) and exclusively for export. Grazing land is export-oriented too. Recently U.S. firms began to fly Texas cattle into Haiti for grazing and re-export to American franchised hamburger restaurants.

A World Bank study of Colombia states that "large numbers of farm families. . . . try to eke out an existence on too little land, often on slopes of 45 degrees or more. As a result, they exploit the land very severely, adding to erosion and other problems, and even so are not able to make a decent living." Overpopulation? No. Colombia's good level land is in the hands of absentee landlords who use it to graze cattle, raise animal feed and even flowers for export to the United States ($18 million worth in 1975).

During the Sahelian drought media coverage highlighted over-grazing as a cause of the encroachment of the desert. Too much demand for meat? No. Supressed FAO reports show that, while more than enough grain for everyone in the Sahel was produced during the drought, much of it was hoarded for speculation. Nomads found that one month they could exchange one head of cattle for four bags of millet while the next month one head was "worth" only a single bag of millet. One reason, therefore, the pastoralists tried to increase their herds was to survive in a food speculation economy. The tragedy was that everyone trying to have a herd large enough to survive resulted in the destruction of the means by which anyone could have any herd at all.

The Amazon is being rapidly de-forested. Is it the pressure of Brazil's exploding population? Brazil's ratio of cultivatable land to people (and that excludes the Amazon Forest) is slightly better than that of the United States. The Amazon forest is being destroyed not because of a shortage of farm land but because the military government refuses to break up the large estates that take up over 43 percent of the country's farmland. Instead the landless are offered the promise of future new frontiers in the Amazon basin even though most experts feel the tropical forest is not suited to permanent cropping. In addition, multinational corporations like Anderson Clayton, Goodyear, Volkswagen, Nestle, Liquigas, Borden, Mitsubishi and multibillionaire Daniel Ludwig's Uni-

verse Tank Ship Co. can get massive government subsidies to turn the Amazon into a major supplier of beef to Europe, the U.S. and Japan.

It is not, then, people's food needs that threaten to destroy the environment by other forces: land monopolizers that export non-food and luxury crops forcing the rural majority to abuse marginal lands; colonial patterns of cash cropping that continue today; hoarding and speculation on food; and irresponsible profit-seeking by both local and foreign elites. Cutting the number of the hungry in half tomorrow would not stop any of these forces.

The Real Pests

Still we found ourselves wondering whether people's legitimate need to grow food might not require injecting even more pesticides into our environment. In the emergency push to grow more food, won't we have to accept some level of damage from deadly chemicals?

First, just how pesticide-dependent is the world's current food production? In the U.S. about 1.2 billion pounds, a whopping six pounds for every American and 30 percent of the world's total, are dumped into the environment every year. Surely, we thought, such a staggering figure means that practically every acre of the nation's farmland is dosed with deadly poisons. U.S. food abundance therefore, appeared to us as the plus that comes from such a big minus. The facts, however, proved us wrong.

Fact one: Nearly half the pesticides are used not by farmland but by golf courses, parks and lawns.

Fact two: Only about 10 percent of the nations cropland is treated with insecticides, 30 percent with weedkillers and less than 1 percent with fungicides (the figures are halved if pastureland is included).

Fact three: Non-food crops account for over half of all insecticides used in U.S. agriculture. (Cotton alone received almost half of all insecticides used. Yet half of the total cotton acreage receives no insecticides at all.)

Fact four: The U.S. Department of Agriculture estimates that, even if all pesticides were eliminated, crop loss due to pests (insects, pathogens, weeds, mammals and birds) would rise only about seven percentage points, from 33.6 percent to 40.7 percent.

Fact five: Numerous studies show that where pesticides are used with ever greater intensity crop losses due to pests are frequently *increasing*.

What about the underdeveloped countries? Do pesticides there help produce food for hungry people?

In underdeveloped countries most pesticides are used for export crops, principally cotton, and to a lesser extent fruits and vegetables grown under plantation conditions for export. In effect, then, these enclaves of pesticide use in the underdeveloped world function as mere extensions of the agricultural systems of the industrialized countries. The quantities of pesticides injected into the world's environment have very little to do with the hungry's food needs.

The alternatives to chemical pesticides—crop rotation, mixed cropping, mulching, hand weeding, hoeing, collection of pest eggs, manipulation of natural predators, and so on are numerous and proven effective. In China, for example, pesticide use can be minimized because of a nationwide early warning system. In Shao-tung county in Honan Province, 10,000 youths make up watch teams that patrol the fields and report any sign of pathogenic change. Appropriately called the "barefoot doctors of agriculture," they have succeeded in reducing the damage of wheat rust and rice borer to less than 1 percent and have the locust invasions under control. But none of these safe techniques for pest control will be explored as long as the problem is in the hands of profit-oriented corporations. The alternatives require human involvement and the motivation of farmers who have the security of individual or collective tenure over the land they work.

Myth Four: Hunger is a contest between the Rich World and the Poor World.

Rather than seeing vertical stratified societies with hunger at the lower rungs in both so-called developed and underdeveloped countries, terms like "hungry world" and "poor world" make us think of uniformly hungry masses. Hunger becomes a place—and usually a place over there. Rather than being the result of a social process, hunger becomes a static fact, a geographic given.

Worse still, the all-inclusiveness of these labels leads us to assume that everyone living in a "hungry country" has a common interest in eliminating hunger. Thus we look at an underdeveloped country and assume its government officials represent the hungry majority. Well-meaning sympathizers in the industrialized countries then believe that concessions, to these governments, e.g. preference schemes or increased foreign investment, represent progress for the hungry when in fact the "progress" may be only for the elites and their partners—the multinational corporations.

Moreover, the "rich world" versus "poor world" scenario makes the hungry appear as a threat to the material well-being of the majority in the metropolitan countries. To average Americans or Europeans the hungry become the enemy who, in the words of Lyndon Johnson, "want what we got." In truth, however, hunger will never be addressed until the average citizen in the metropolitan countries can see that the hungry abroad are their allies, not their enemies.

The Grip of Agribusiness

What are the links between the plight of the average citizen in the metropolitan countries and the poor majority in the underdeveloped countries? There are many. One example is multinational agribusiness shifting production of luxury items—fresh vegetables, fruits, flowers and meat—out of the industrial countries in search of cheap land and labor in the underdeveloped countries. The result? Farmers and workers in the metropolitan countries lose their jobs while agricultural resources in the underdeveloped countries are increasingly diverted away from food for local people. The food supply of those in the metropolitan countries is being made dependent on the active maintenance of political and economic structures that block hungry people from growing food for themselves.

Nor should we conclude that consumers in the metropolitan countries at least get cheaper food. Are Ralston Purina's and Green Giant's mushrooms grown in Korea and Taiwan cheaper than those produced stateside? Not one cent, according to a U.S. government study. Del Monte and Dole Philippine pineapples actually cost the U.S. consumers more than those produced by a small company in Hawaii.

The common threat is the worldwide tightening control of wealth and power over the most basic human need, food. Multinational agribusiness firms right now are creating a single world agricultural system in which they exercise integrated control over all stages of production from farm to consumer. Once achieved, they will be able to effectively manipulate supply and prices for the first time on a world wide basis through well-established monopoly practices. As farmers, workers and consumers, people everywhere already are beginning to experience the cost in terms of food availability, prices and quality.

Myth Five: An underdeveloped country's best hope for development is to export those crops in which it has a natural advantage and use the earnings to import food and industrial goods.

There is nothing "natural" about the underdeveloped countries concentration on a few, largely low-nutrition crops. The same land that grows cocoa, coffee, rubber, tea and sugar could grow an incredible diversity of nutritious crops—grains, high-protein legumes, vegetables and fruits.

Nor is there any advantage. Reliance on a limited number of crops generates economic as well as political vulnerability. Extreme price fluctuations associated with tropical crops combine with the slow-maturing nature of plants themselves (many, for example, take two to ten years before the first harvest) to make development planning impossible.

Often-quoted illustrations showing how

much more coffee or bananas it takes to buy one tractor today than 20 years ago have indeed helped us appreciate that the value of agricultural exports have simply not kept pace with the inflating price of imported manufactured goods. But even if one considers only agricultural trade, the underdeveloped countries still come out the clear losers. Between 1961 and 1972 half of the industrialized countries increased their earnings from agricultural exports by 10 percent each year. By contrast, at least 18 underdeveloped countries are earning *less* from their agricultural exports than they did in 1961.

Another catch in the natural advantage theory is that the people who need food are not the same people who benefit from foreign exchange earned by agricultural exports. Even when part of the foreign earnings is used to import food, the food is not basic staples but items geared toward the eating habits of the better-off urban classes. In Senegal the choice land is used to grow peanuts and vegetables for export to Europe. Much of the foreign exchange earned is spent to import wheat for foreign-owned bakeries that turn out European-style bread for the urban dwellers. The country's rural majority goes hungry, deprived of land they need to grow millet and other traditional grains for themselves and local markets.

The very success of export agriculture can further undermine the position of the poor. When commodity prices go up, small self-provisioning farmers may be pushed off the land by cash crop producers seeking to profit on the higher commodity prices. Moreover, governments in underdeveloped countries, opting for a development track dependent on promoting agricultural exports, may actively suppress social reform. Minimum wage laws for agricultural laborers are not enacted, for example, because they might make the country's exports uncompetitive." Governments have been only too willing to exempt plantations from land reform in order to encourage their export production.

Finally, export-oriented agricultural operations invariably import capital-intensive technologies to maximize yields as well as to meet product and processing specifications. Relying on imported technologies then makes it likely that the production will be used to pay the bill— a vicious circle of dependency.

Land for Food

Just as export-oriented agriculture spells the divorce of agriculture and nutrition, food first policies would make the central question: How can this land best feed people? As obvious as it may seem, this policy of basing land use on nutritional output is practiced in only a few countries today; more commonly, commercial farmer and national planners make hit-and-miss calculations of which crop might have a few cents edge on the world market months or even years hence. With food first policies industrial crops (like cotton and rubber) and feed crops would be planted only after the people meet their basic needs. Livestock would not compete with people but graze on marginal lands or, like China's 240 million pigs, recycle farm and household wastes while producing fertilizer at the same time.

In most underdeveloped countries the rural population contributes much more to the national income than it receives. With food first policies agricultural development would be measured in the welfare of the people, not in export income. Priority would go to de-centralized industry at the service of labor-intensive agriculture. A commitment to food self-reliance would close the gap between rural and urban well-being, making the countryside a good place to live. Urban dwellers, too, like those volunteering to grow vegetables in Cuba's urban "green belts," would move toward self-reliance.

Food self-reliance is not isolationist. But trade would be seen, not as the one desperate hinge on which survival hangs, but as a way to widen choices once the basic needs have been met.

Myth Six: Hunger should be overcome by redistributing food.

Over and over again we hear that North America is the world's last remaining breadbasket. Food security is invariably measured in terms of reserves held by the metropolitan countries. We are made to feel the burden of feeding the world is squarely on us. Our overconsumption is tirelessly contrasted with the deprivation elsewhere with the implicit message being that we cause their hunger. No wonder that North Americans and Europeans feel burdened and thus resentful. "What did we do to cause their hunger?" they rightfully ask.

The problem lies in seeing redistribution as the solution to hunger. We have come to a different understanding. Distribution of food is but a reflection of the control of the resources that produce food. Who controls the land determines who can grow food, what is grown and where it goes. Who can grow: a few or all who need to? What is grown: luxury non-food or basic staples? Where does it go: to the hungry or the world's well-fed?

Thus redistribution programs like food aid or food stamps will never solve the problem of hunger. Instead we must face up to the real question: How can people everywhere begin to democratize the control of food resources?

Six Food First Principles

We can now counter these six myths with six positive principles that could ground a coherent and vital movement:

1. There is no country in the world in which the people could not feed themselves from their own resources. But hunger can only be overcome by the transformation of social relationships and is only made worse by the narrow focus on technical inputs to increase production.

2. Inequality is the greatest stumbling block to development.

3. Safeguarding the world's agricultural environment and people feeding themselves are complementary goals.

4. Our food security is not threatened by the hungry masses but by elites that span all capitalist economies profiting by the concentration and internationalization of control of food resources.

5. Agriculture must not be used as the means

to export income but as the way for people to produce food first for themselves.

6. Escape from hunger comes not through the redistribution of food but through the redistribution of control over food-producing resources.

What would an international campaign look like that took these truths to be self-evident?

If we begin with the knowledge that people can and will feed themselves if allowed to do so, the question for all of us living in the metropolitan countries is not "What can we do for them?" but "How can we remove the obstacles in the way of people taking control of the production process and feeding themselves?"

Since some of the key obstacles are being built with our taxes, in our name, and by corporations based in our economies, our task is very clear:

Stop any economic aid—government, multilateral or voluntary—that reinforces the use of land for export crops. Stop support for agribusiness penetration into food economies abroad through tax incentives and from governments and multilateral lending agencies. Stop military and counter-insurgency assistance to any underdeveloped country; more often than not it goes to oppose the changes

necessary for food self-reliance.

Work to build a more self-reliant food economy at home so that we become even less dependent on importing food from hungry people. Work for land reform at home. Support worker-managed producers, and distributors to counter the increasing concentration of control over our food resources.

Educate, showing the connections between the way government and corporate power works against the hungry abroad and the way it works against the food interests of the vast majority of people in the industrial countries.

Counter despair. Publicize the fact that 40 percent of all people living in underdeveloped countries live where hunger has been eliminated through common struggle. Learn and communicate the efforts of newly liberated countries in Africa and Asia to reconstruct their agriculture along the principles of food first self-reliance.

Most fundamentally, we all must recognize that we are not a "hunger" movement. Rather we all can become moulders of the future who have chosen to seize this historical moment. We have chosen to use the visible tragedy of hunger to reveal the utter failure of our current economic system to meet human needs.

Reprinted with permission from *The New Internationalist*, (42): 5-9 (August 1976).

There Is "A Morning's War"

BARBARA WARD (LADY JACKSON)

This section ends with a speech—given several years ago to the National Audubon Society—by economist Barbara Ward (Lady Jackson). Despite the rapidity with which the immediate issues in the world food/population crisis appear to change—as fluctuating weather patterns move us from short-term shortage to short-term glut—the continuing timeliness of Lady Jackson's paper makes clear both her prescience and the chronic nature of the hard continuing truths.

SCRIPT OF SPEECH TO THE NATIONAL AUDUBON SOCIETY

There is "a morning's war" in our minds these days between fear and hope. We are conscious of vast new risks that were almost unimaginable only a dozen years ago—population doubling to 7 billion in less than three decades, increases in food supplies lagging behind the explosion of people, energy falling short of basic needs as oil and gas reserves run out, the very integrity of the planet's airs and waters endangered by ever rising numbers making ever rising material claims.

But even as the prospects darken, we hear the counter voices of confident optimism. They tell us not to underestimate man's scientific and technological capacities. Miracle drugs will deal with fertility. Newer and greener revolutions will keep food ahead of population. Nuclear power will provide 15 billion people with the *per capita* energy consumption of modern America. And with this amount of energy, benefication of low grade ores, recycling techniques, and counter-pollutional technologies can be relied on to keep the planet well supplied and clean.

We feel the shadows recede. Then the warnings begin again. Given the youth of most of the world's peoples, populations will go on growing for at least four or five decades even after they achieve stability. And with an annual growth rate of 2.5 percent now, it would be bold indeed to predict no more than a replacement rate by the end of this century. Crash programs in agriculture tend to increase the risks of environmental disruption since a vast increase in fertilizers and pesticides is part of the package. Moreover, the demands on energy of sufficient nitrogen and effective mechanization are simply not compatible with the world's diminishing oil budget. True, there are nuclear alternatives for the industrial part of the program. But some of them—above all, the fast breeder reactor—pose all but inconceivable risks. The by-product of breeder reactors, plutonium 239, has a half life of nearly 25,000 years and experts suggest that a lethal dose for the whole human race need not be larger than an apple. Yet the program already mentioned—designed to satisfy the needs of 15 billion people—would produce 15,000 tons of plutonium a year. Where would we put all those stainless steel containers labeled: "do not open for 25,000 years"? Or, more immediately, how would we set up the safeguards needed to defeat the terrorist intentions of desperate men?

Such are the shafts of dark and light that fall

across our troubled minds. How are we to make sense of the contradictory arguments? How are we to find a path of reason between the doom-sayers and the techno-fixers? It is hard enough under any circumstances to assess dangers and consider alternatives in our violently changing world. It is all but impossible when one is being deafened by the rival cries of Cassandra and Pollyanna.

Perhaps a possible thread through the maze might be to follow one issue steadily through all the arguments and confrontations. It could be energy. It could be raw material supplies. It could be man's impact on climate. And, indeed, all these issues tend to be involved in each other, which is another reason for our confusion of thought. But let us try to see how optimists and pessimists shape their arguments when they discuss the central issue of food. We may not live by bread alone. But it is where we start and given any failure, where we finish. It is, arguably, the most serious issue of all. Where do we stand?

We have, of course, just come through a very alarming year. For the first time in twenty years, food supplies, which had been growing about one percent or so ahead of population, failed to keep pace and world stocks were pretty well cleaned out. Nor does this general picture give the full scale of the crisis. The distribution of food in the planet at large is in any case tragically skewed. Nearly a third of the world's peoples do not live much above the level of bare subsistence. Their children's diet lacks the indispensable ingredient of sufficient protein—indispensable, that is, to the full growth of the brain. Shorter supplies in the world at large raise prices which poor countries cannot afford and drastically reduce concessionary food exports, such as Food for Peace. The cushion vanished. As a result there were—and are—actual famines in Africa and severe shortages in parts of Asia. It is surely not entirely fanciful to see here the first sharp warning of a not so distant Malthusian future in which population will decisively outstrip the world's supply of food.

But the optimists will not accept any such gloomy conclusion. They believe that this year's excellent Atlantic harvests coupled with the increase in acreage planned for next year's planting in the Northern hemisphere will produce a surplus both of grain and soya bean—a critical source of protein. World stocks can be built up again and exports made available to deficient areas. Meanwhile, the news from Asia has improved, showing that the gains of the Green Revolution are not illusory. Indeed, current research may well produce breakthroughs as vital as the so-called miracle seeds. To hybrid grains which are short and sturdy enough not to fall over, scientists may be able to add the capacity to fix nitrogen; they may find ways of crossing barley and wheat to produce a new drought-resistant super-grain; they are increasing the protein content of grass juice and experimenting with recycling some forms of manure back into feedstuffs. These are just a few of the ongoing experiments. Ten years ago, who could have foreseen a doubling of wheat and rice yields from one harvest to the next? Why should there be skepticism now about the possibility of comparable scientific achievements?

And if these possibilities are admitted, another could follow. Successful farming and rising food supplies encourage modernization in the economy and with it more rapid stabilization of population. Of 47 developing countries providing complete registrations of births, 42 already showed falling birth rates in the Sixties. Once the trend sets in, it tends to accelerate. Confidence in the family's future seems to be a vital ingredient in the change.

But at this point we have to go back to the less hopeful voices—and the case is strong. There is, they claim, an immediate and possibly fatal flaw in the chain of progress. Stock-rebuilding and new surpluses now depend overwhelmingly on one geographical area—the Great Plains of North America. It produces two-thirds of the world's exportable surpluses of grain and 90 percent of exportable soya beans. Yet, as Dr. Walter Orr Roberts reminds us, this area is vulnerable to droughts which seem to occur on about a 25-year cycle. The last created the Dust Bowl of the 1930's. Another may be overdue. Should it coincide with bad harvests elsewhere, particularly in the Soviet Union or China, there would be no surplus of any kind. Starvation would set in in all the poorer deficit areas.

Behind the chance of immediate catastrophe, a slower crisis may be in the making. As affluence increases, the citizen wants to take his food in more appetizing forms by putting his cereals through those highly inefficient processors, beef cattle. In the developing world, people eat, *per capita,* about 350 to 400 pounds of grain a year directly. But in North America the equivalent of 1300 pounds of grain is eaten in high protein meats. Western Europe is not far behind with 800 to 900 pounds. Eastern Europe and Russia are in the 700-800 pound bracket. Indeed, one reason why in 1972 the Soviet Union purchased the totally unprecedented amount of 30 million tons of cereals from America and precipitated last year's food crisis was the Soviet leaders' determination that their people should go on getting meat and not revert to the direct eating of bread and potatoes.

But if this *is* the trend, the old buffer stocks of cereals look as if they will be absorbed by the wealthy countries' growing demand for more protein. Add the severe reduction of marine protein supplies and the question of how much more land can be planted to soya bean as an alternative and we can easily foresee a time when, as Dr. David Hopper has suggested, the superior purchasing power of rich countries may divert more and more of the world's food production away from basic biological needs— above all, the most basic need, protein in infancy—over to the luxury tastes of high consumption.

The trend would certainly seem to presage for developing peoples a much greater dependence on their own farming sectors. And there are problems here, too. Many of the present technologies associated with rapidly rising agricultural productivity demand heavy investment and eat up energy—in some areas, more energy is absorbed in fertilizer and mechanization than is released in food supplies. Some techniques are environmentally disruptive, involving the rise of excessive run-off of nutrients into watercourses and the use of biologically dangerous pesticides. Above all, the substitution of scarce capital for abundant labour favors the rich, accelerates the exodus from the land and bloats the swollen cities with rural migrants lacking skills and work. Overpopulation on the land is endemic anyway in many parts of the globe. The sudden introduction of high technology into farming aggravates all the factors of imbalance and contributes to the increasingly recognized phenomenon—a modernizing economy growing by ten percent a year and the entire gain reverting to the wealthiest ten to fifteen percent of the people. And it is in these economies that the highest rates of population growth—three percent a year and more—are to be found.

So in our seesaw swings of hope and discouragement must we once again veer to pessimism and accept the bleak fact that over the next three decades the prospect of balancing food and peoples will fade in many parts of the planet? Are the "Hungry Eighties," more devastating and global than last century's "Hungry Forties," irrevocably on the way?

The answer surely is that they *could* be on the way but there is nothing irresistible and irreversible about a trend. Strategies are available for an alternative future and are beginning to be seriously considered. Dr. Henry Kissinger has made the proposal that the United Nations should formally take up the issue of food supplies and devote a special conference to possible solutions. Mr. Maurice Strong, Executive Director of UNEP, has pointed out that, given the present level of reserves and the vulnerability of future supplies, the building up of buffer stocks, strategically placed, should be the world's first order of business. To this could be added a more organized disaster relief service for instant mobilization when the pressures begin to mount. And to counter the long slow disaster of children without protein, a world protein service, possibly guided by UNICEF and bringing in all the voluntary agencies, is almost as urgent as famine relief.

Also in the longer terms, the building up of agricultural capacity on a sound and sustainable basis in developing lands deserves the highest priority. Mr. Robert McNamara in his Presidential address this year at the World Bank meeting in Nairobi, challenged the governments to dedicate their funds, expertise and research to the small farm sector from which nearly a billion people draw their livelihood and millions more must be able to derive their food. Labour-intensive technology, credit for the cooperatives of small farmers, farming practices which use decentralized forms of energy—above all, solar power, fertilizer practices which carefully use all organic wastes, weeding and insect control which accept the availability of labour—these are the sorts of inputs of a new kind of Green Revolution and there is evidence now that economies with this type of emphasis—Mieji Japan at the turn of the century, mainland China, Taiwan, South Korea, parts of Mexico and Yugoslavia today—are in fact producing just as high an output as the more official "Green Revolutions" but within an infinitely sounder social and ecological environment.

Underpinned by vigorous popular participation, supported by appropriate labour intensive industries and handicrafts, linked to intermediate market centers and small towns where health, education and cultural opportunities are available, these societies are not only becoming more skilled and productive. Their social organization avoids the unsettling extremes of wealth and destitution and their population growth is slowing down. Even more important, they may be models of the only kind of effective modernization possible in an age of much more scarce and expensive energy and a smaller scale of mineral reserves. The megalopolis of the developed world is possible only at the expense of vast wastes of energy in running high rise center cities and commuting to lowspread suburbs. A quite different pattern of urbanism will almost certainly be dictated by material

restraints in the future—an issue which will be thoroughly explored at the U. N. Conference/Exposition on Human Settlements in Vancouver in 1976. It is perhaps the good fortune of the still developing lands that the urban patterns they cannot follow are increasingly seen as the heaviest, most costly and most anti-social burden the "over-developed" countries have to bear.

But there is, of course, a price attached to such a global strategy. The Food and Agricultural Organization some years ago made an estimate of some $8 billions as the extra annual capital sum needed to modernize world agriculture. If we add the cost of research, of new energy systems, more viable towns and transport networks, we could easily double the figure. Compared with the world's sacrilegious annual spending on arms—some $250-billions—the sum is nothing. But it is a third higher than all present transfers of wealth—public and private—from rich to poor countries. It is not clear that anything like such an infusion of vital funds can be mounted after the disillusions of the last decade.

It is perhaps at this point that we begin to realize that underlying the swings of the argument between the inevitability of world famine and the technical possibility of world abundance, we confront something rather different—not the question of "can" but the question of "ought." On balance it seems that the technical optimists and those who believe in possible solutions have a strong case. Capital and research can revolutionize agriculture. Modernized agriculture is the basis of general modernization—in industry, in health, education, in expectations—and hence, of slowing population growth. Experiments in decentralized productive balanced systems are beginning to appear. We have means. We have models. But what is much less certain is whether the moral and political will is available to turn "can" into "must."

Pessimism begins when we ask whether in fact the wealthy nations and the wealthy minorities in developing lands will mount an effective world strategy for food and proteins, whether buffer stocks will be built, the needed $16 to $20 billions invested, the research into low-impact, labour-intensive technologies, the the new urban and transport conferences and commitments. The citizens' response, on present showing, will be languid indeed.

And here, I believe, we have the clue to the larger debate between hope and despair. There *are* solutions. There *are* constructive ways forward. But they depend upon a radical change in the way in which we look at the world. We have been living for nearly four hundred years on vivid, intoxicating and potentially destructive energies. Big science getting control of nature by measurement and the application of power, economic growth thrust forward by human skill and greed, national drives claiming total sovereignty may have spun our planet forward on the most incredible journey of adventure and change ever undertaken by man. But today, the pessimists are right to remind us, ever more technology powered by ever more energy and applied with ever more singleminded drive to the ambitions of economic growth and political sovereignty can literally judder our small planet to disintegration. These are our *habits*. This is what we are used to. Can we stop and begin to change in time?

The profound moral issue is that all the solutions that do exist demand from us an end to many of our favourite bad habits. Take again the question of food supplies. The kind of research and technology needed for ecologically sane, labour-intensive farms and for decentral-ized towns and markets is small, patient, interconnected, respectful of fragilities, temperate in energy use. It is not the big bang-bang stuff. It does not "break through": it connects. The economics of small scale farming is not a drive for economic growth at all costs, concentrating wealth and high investment, increasing the gap between rich and poor. It is, on the contrary, the economics of cooperation, of participation, of greater equality and the building up of a million small achievements. And the political decisions needed for a world food policy are based on cooperation and sharing on a planetary community that is aware of limits, conscious of justice, alive to responsibility, fit, in a word, to survive.

So I think we must say in the end that the "morning's war" between hope and fear is not really a scientific, an economic or even a political debate. It transcends them all. It concerns our judgment of modern man's ethical response and his ability to turn his breathtaking and appalling energies from self-assertion—personal and collective—to a patient, cooperative search for the common good.

On his present course, he is in sober truth an "endangered species." No planet can carry indefinitely the fright of population, aspiration, consumption, destruction and exhaustion with which we threaten it. In fact, it is the planet itself that is desperately signaling to us the millenial lesson of all the world's prophets and poets—that "we must love each other or we must die." Survival is now simply the issue whether we can learn and change in time.

Reprinted with permission from Barbara Ward, Lady Jackson and the National Audubon Society. Acceptance speech as the 1973 Audubon Medalist, presented at the National Audubon Society's Annual Dinner, 8 November 1973.

Food and People— Giving and Taking

"Americans continually find themselves in the position of having killed someone to avoid sharing a meal which turns out to be too large to eat alone."[1]

Humankind's primary need is for enough simple food to live. How do *we* learn to understand that? As typical Americans (excluding, of course, the untypical American poor), we seldom experience even hunger—except when we are dieting—and know of starvation only by report. "I'm starving," we say, when what we mean is that we have forgotten to eat breakfast. Among far too many human beings, however, starvation is not a casual metaphor for a morning's hunger; in much of the world simply getting enough to eat is a lifetime's—albeit a sometimes sadly short lifetime's—occupation.

For Americans the food issue has been made relevant not in terms of hunger, but in terms of aid. Thus the articles in this section have largely explored the question of "aid"—its extent and its usefulness, its intentions and its effects.

We in America have been taught to perceive ourselves as generous, yet as Georg Borgstrom points out in the selection from *The Food and People Dilemma* reprinted here, we have remained persistently ignorant of our roles as consumers rather than providers of global food resources. Our self-centered educational system, he writes, has failed to make us all aware of the extent of our dependence upon vast reaches of Asian, African, and Latin American topsoil. When the European population explosion occurred in the middle of the last century, Europeans spread over the globe and began to send back to Europe the produce of other lands to support the growing population.

"Western man," Borgstrom writes, "commissioned the entire globe for his well-being with little concern until the 1950's for the legitimate needs of the other three-fourths of the world's people . . . It is not yet fully realized by the peoples of the industrialized nations of the West that their high standards of living have been—and in part are continuing to be—achieved by a massive exploitation of the world's total resources and a concomitant accumulation of capital." And now that those lands we have exploited are experiencing their own population explosion, we have left them no place to go; even their own croplands and coastal waters are often used to produce foods to meet not *their* legitimate *needs*, but *our wants*—tuna for cat food, carnations, coffee, cocoa, cotton.

And our vision of our own pecuniary generosity has been painfully altered by the revelation that we rank 14th out of the 17 "developed" nations in the percentage of our gross national product which we devote to aiding others less fortunate than ourselves. Yet there is no denying that our God-given productive potential and our agricultural prowess have made us over the last decades the source of much of the world's exportable food surplusses, surplusses which have helped stave off famine when crops have failed abroad.

Now we are apparently being asked to decide whether to continue our aid. Is it true, as some have

---

[1]   Philip Slater, *The Pursuit of Loneliness*, p. 103 (Boston: Beacon Press, 1976).

said, that our food aid only makes matters worse in the long run? If we continue to send "those people" grain will "they" just continue to convert it into children?

Wade Greene's article, "Triage," states the dilemma as it has come to be widely viewed (a view to which his article no doubt contributed). Can we continue to send food to countries which cannot—or will not—check their own population growth? And if we do not send food, can we live with ourselves? It was the Paddocks' book, *Famine, 1975!*, as Greene mentions, which first laid out in black and white the previously unmentionable possibility of abandoning certain countries as unsalvageable. *Famine, 1975!*, initially published in 1969, was recently reissued under the title *Time of Famine*, unchanged except for a new introduction and postscript. Ten years did not alter the Paddocks' view of the problem.

Greene himself concludes that one's approach to solving the food/population crisis depends largely on one's philosophical predisposition. "One's opinion about [the facts] and about the harsh measures being proposed depends on an *a priori* sense either that material progress and a little bit of luck are part of man's boundless destiny or, as many ecologists and philosophers and Forrester's computers contend, that nature sets firm limits, which we are approaching, on how much an ever-larger population can extract from a finite planet." We are, in other words, once again in a contest between the Cornucopians and the Malthusians—except that in this round, those who question the advisibility (or practicality) of unchecked material growth find themselves in the discomforting company of those who would withhold food from the starving.

Garrett Hardin is one of the latter. His eloquent arguments in favor of applying "Lifeboat Ethics" to the developing countries have been a source of outrage and anguish to many in the "hunger movement." We are all living in lifeboats, he says, while all about us in the water float increasing numbers of people who will shortly drown. If we take them all aboard the lifeboat, the craft will surely swamp and they—and we—will go down together. Essentially the article presents a detailed and disturbingly well-argued rationale for stopping food aid to overpopulated nations and for simultaneously stopping emigration from the poor to the rich countries.

Hardin's vision of a sort of fortress America, stuffed with her own food abundance, battling off the starving but insensately multiplying hordes, is offensive to many Americans—and to all developing countries. The question, however, is not whether it is offensive, but whether such an outcome is inevitable. In different ways, each of the articles which make up the rest of the chapter raises questions about the assumptions that underlie the Triage and Lifeboat positions. The two very short pieces which immediately follow Hardin's take sharp exception to his implied assumption that population expands simply because food is available. James Kocher points to evidence that population decline follows economic development—but only if the benefits of that development are widespread so that children become a liability rather than an asset. Vittachi, like Kocher, suggests that "The Poor Are Not Stupid" and argues that poor people in developing countries will continue to have babies despite the relative unavailability of food, as long as they perceive themselves to have good reasons for doing so. As Robert McNamara, President of the World Bank wrote recently: "It is a mistake to think that the poor have children mindlessly or without purpose or—in the light of their own personal value systems—irresponsibly. Quite the contrary. The poor, by the very fact of their poverty, have little margin for error. . . Poor people have large families for many reasons. But the point is, they do have reasons. . ."[2]

Murdoch and Oaten take issue with Hardin on a number of specific issues and on the over-riding fact that both the "lifeboats" and "commons" metaphors obscure reality and, by oversimplifying

---

[2] Robert S. McNamara, "Accelerating Population Stabilization Through Social and Economic Progress," p. 37 (Washington, D.C.: Overseas Development Council, Development Paper 24, August 1977).

what are complex problems, obviate the necessity for thought. Unlike Hardin's lifeboats, they point out, real countries interact. The frantically paddling poor are not likely to float quietly in the water while we sail away in our yachts without them. They have very little to lose, after all, if their boarding parties overturn our boats.

Moreover, it should be clear to any reader of this chapter that Hardin totally disregards the lesson Borgstrom teaches and Lappé and Collins document—namely the fact that the present hunger and poverty of many "underdeveloped" nations are the consequence not only of our *past* expropriation and exploitation, but of our present active involvement in maintaining the status quo. Those "slovenly rulers" Hardin castigates are all too often given our assistance to remain in office since they provide a secure "investment climate" for Western businesses. It is of some interest that Hardin fails to include among the slovenly, who do not put food away against a time of emergencies, the U.S., which sold off her own grain reserves (to maintain the Russian beef supply) just before a world-wide crop failure; or Russia herself; or the other Western nations which, despite the pleadings of World Food experts like Lord Boyd-Orr in 1945, have still not established a reliable grain reserve system—even for themselves.

Moreover, it is not true, as Hardin asserts, that poor people simply convert food into more babies. "They convert it into longer lives. Denying them food will not lower birth rates; it will increase death rates." It is the very cruelty of this solution, Murdoch and Oaten argue, which gains it adherents. "There is an implication that these policies are so brutal that they would not be proposed without good reasons."

As was pointed out in Chapter 1, the population "explosion" in developing countries did not result from people having *more* babies, but from people losing *fewer* babies. Less food will cause a rise in death rates among infants and children, the long-range result of which will be a desire on the part of those children's parents to have more children. McNamara[3] has pointed out that increasing numbers of developing countries have official family planning programs and growth rate reduction policies. When a country like Sri Lanka which has had marked success in reducing its rate of population growth loses out in food distribution programs motivated by military rather than humanitarian considerations, surely long-range goals are not well-served.

There are a number of other inconsistencies in the reasoning that leads to Hardin's final solution. Which countries can and ought to survive? There is an implication that it ought to be countries capable of taking care of themselves. In other words, as the Paddocks put it, those to be cut off are those in "which the population growth trend has already passed the agricultural potential." As Borgstrom has pointed out elsewhere, by these standards, the United Kingdom, Netherlands, Germany, Italy, Japan, among other countries are heavily overpopulated in that each "has too many people to be supplied by the inadequate basic resources of its territory." When three-fourths of the earth's crops are consumed by one-third of the earth's peoples, it is presumably the ability to *pay for food* and not mere self-sufficiency that would be Hardin's real criterion of salvageability.

Hardin's second suggestion, that we cut off immigration, may seem like an increasingly good idea in the face of rising U.S. unemployment, even if there were no food issue involved. However, given our inability to cut off the present flow of illegal immigrants across our extended borders and lengthy shorelines, it is a "solution" that, like atomic energy, suggests a level of police control which may be totally incompatible with what we are prepared to accept merely for the sake of continuing our present levels of overconsumption.

Yet if walling ourselves up with our food is not really feasible, what is the answer? Should Americans give food aid? Should Americans give economic aid? How can American abundance best

---

[3] McNamara, 1977.

be shared? Rothschild's "Is it Time to End Food for Peace?" argues that our largest and most "generous" aid program has been a failure, and suggests that the mixed motives behind our food programs are at least a part of the reason why. We have given, with highly mixed motives, seldom losing sight of the potential market advantages of creating world appetites for American grains and animal products. Thus, whether or not the American people have intended their food programs to be generous, Rothschild points out, they have often not worked to the advantage of the neediest countries.[4]

But given our own enormous comparative affluence, and given the impracticality (not to say inhumanity) of simply writing off poor countries, what can we do to help? It has been pointed out by a number of humanitarians through the centuries that there are at least two ways to help poor people: by giving them direct aid or by getting off their backs. The selection in this chapter from Lappé and Collins urges us individually and corporately to work toward the latter approach. As they analyze it, our tendency toward usurping the wealth of others—a tendency whose historical roots Borgstrom identified—continues to flourish unabated, despite our apparent intentions to do good. Lappé is best known to date for her best-selling *Diet for a Small Planet*, a book which argued for using American food producing potential to feed the hungry abroad rather than for fattening cattle in the U.S. Our meat-heavy diet, based as it was on cattle fattened on grain, was a kind of protein and energy sink into which were poured enormous quantities of food which might otherwise feed the poor. Collins was a contributor to *Global Reach*, the much quoted look at the power of multinational corporations around the world. "Food First," the paper reprinted here, is a summary of their new book by the same name, a book in which they have pulled together a vast body of data in order, as they say, to answer the question "Why hunger?"

Their analysis moves the understanding of the food/population problem well along from the simple notion that grew out of Lappé's first book: that we should eat one less hamburger and send the money saved to CARE. There is no reason *not* to take such actions, but as Lappé and Collins point out, the solution is a much broader one than that—it is to get the inputs necessary to grow their own food into the hands of those who need it most. One by one they deal with the "six myths that kept [them] locked into a misunderstanding of the problem." Their conclusion: that every country can, and should, feed itself; that food self-sufficiency is a real possibility for even the most "hopeless"; and that, at least for the time being, it is exploitation and not overpopulation that is the source of the present crisis.

In the last quarter of the 20th century, food has become not merely a source of sustenance, but a source of immense global power. That is, it is a source of power when it is scarce. When no major country suffers a crop failure, then the same farmers who were reaping bonus prices for their crops in 1974, are rolling their tractors up to the steps of the Capitol to protest low grain prices. The year 1977 saw a generous world cereal grain surplus (which did not mean that everyone had enough to eat, merely that there was enough grain to meet "effective demand"—*i.e.*, those who could pay could buy). The 1978 surplus may be even larger. And so the crisis leaves the front pages and fades from our minds—until some natural or man-made disaster, unfortunate weather or poor planning, calls attention once more to the underlying problem parson Malthus identified.

Thus, as Barbara Ward's brilliant concluding essay reminds us, we vacillate between fear and hope as to whether we can somehow bring the food and people equation into balance. Reviewing the arguments on both sides, she concludes that we do, in fact, have the means to solve the problem.

---

[4]   A very recent example reported in the press (Alan Riding, "U.S. Food Aid Seen Hurting Guatemala," *New York Times* 13 November 1977) involved our donation of 27,000 tons of grain to Guatemala—over the objections of the local government—after an earthquake had devastated a part of that country. Since local farmers had just harvested a bumper grain crop, undamaged by the quake, the sudden influx of surplus American grain destroyed the grain market, wreaking havoc on the local farm economy.

"But what is much less certain is whether the moral and political will is available to turn 'can' into 'must.'" The ultimate problem, once more, is not technical, but human. "In the end. . . the 'morning's war' between hope and fear is not really a scientific, and economic, or even a political debate. . . it concerns our judgement of modern man's ethical response and his ability to turn his breathtaking and appalling energies from self-assertion—personal and collective—to a patient, cooperative search for the common good." For one more of our dilemmas it seems, there is no technological fix.

Whatever Happened to Food
or
It Does Pay to Fool With Mother Nature

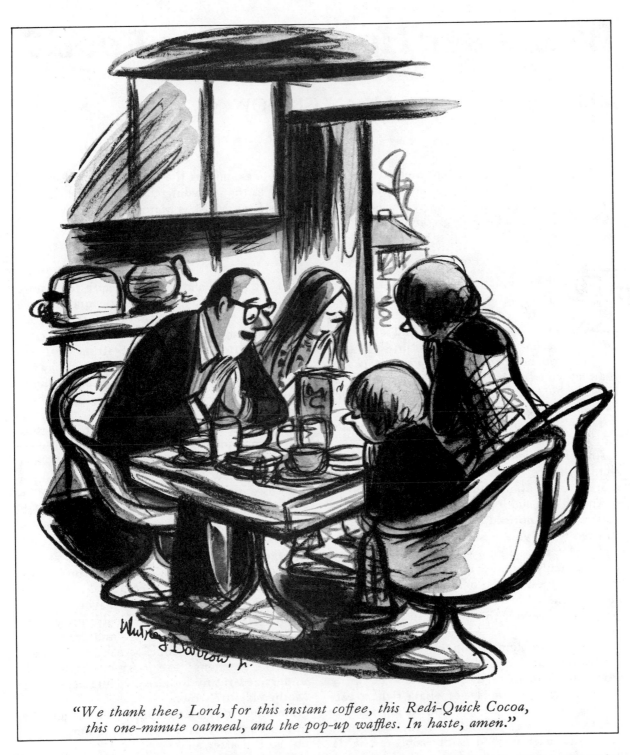

"We thank thee, Lord, for this instant coffee, this Redi-Quick Cocoa, this one-minute oatmeal, and the pop-up waffles. In haste, amen."

Reprinted with permission from *The New Yorker*, 49(17): 41 (16 June 1973). Drawing by Whitney Darrow, Jr.; copyright 1973 by **The New Yorker Magazine, Inc.**

Whatever Happened to Food?

MAUREEN MEYERS and JOAN GUSSOW

Chapter 3, "Whatever Happened to Food?" is devoted to examining the changing American food supply and its relationship to some of the issues raised in the preceding chapters. The title piece first appeared in 1971 in an early issue of the CAN newsletter. M. M. is Maureen Meyers who was at that time an advertising copywriter; J. G. is the present author.

Robert Finch says no. So even though cyclamates sounds more like a computer dating service than anything that could possibly be bad for you, all your diet sodas go down the drain.

Then you hear those nifty plastic packages that let you see both sides of the meat may be actually bad for your chuck steak (which isn't any too great to begin with).

There's mercury in fish. Dye in egg yolks. Not much to lean on in the staff of life.

And regardless of what Esther Williams thinks, that cereal she's eating isn't doing much more for her than her movies did for you.

And all of a sudden you begin to notice things you've never noticed before: strawberries that run red when you wash them; a cucumber that feels a lot more like a candle than something you'd actually pop in your mouth; a lot of crazy words on food labels; or worse still, no labels at all (which lets your imagination run wild). And the more you think about it, the worse it gets.

Now the problem is a double one. To graduate from synthetic food to *real* food. And to get from real food to really *good* food.

You've got a vague idea of what's right to eat. (Two green vegetables and one meat a day. Or is it the other way around?) But the food itself. . . . Is that beef as good as it possibly can be? Is that waxy squash really Mother Nature's own?

And are you willing to pay health food store prices for beef that isn't fed on questionable feed, and vegetables free of sprays and shellac?

It's not only expensive, it's difficult. You can't really be sure of what you're getting. You may have to travel miles to get it. And you may not get it when you get there. Supply being one of those things. And demand being something else.

So all you can do is do your best. And cook for your family as well as you can with what the not-so-supermarket has to offer. And when you're specially bugged you might whisper in the store manager's ear that it really would be nice if he'd take all the bottles back. And stock phosphate-free detergent. And more all-white paper products. And some uncarrageenaned cottage cheese, please? And he smiles at you benevolently some days. And treats you like the neighborhood pest on others. So you write to the store president. Well . . . maybe.

And when you get really frustrated, you go back to the health food store and splurge. (Is that frozen slab of chuck steak really better than the butcher's? Are those brown-spotted-undersized-funny-looking vegetables really Mother Nature's own?)

And then it's back to reality. The budget. The not-so-supermarket. Which is beginning to look not so bad after all.

If you read the labels.

If you know what you're looking for.

If you start matching price to nutritional value, and the absence of additives, and the number of ounces.

And you start eating better and you start feeling better and you know it's going to be all right.

If only you could stop smoking.

—M. M.

Who put the hydrolized plant protein in Mrs. Murphy's tomato soup? And what's it doing there, anyway? The explanation has more to do with economics and consumer psychology than with anything like nutrition or taste.

Whatever Happened to Food?

Many old-fashioned people are put off these days by the disappearance of food, despite the effort that food manufacturers have gone to to provide in its place an endless variety of quite authentic-appearing substitutes. Numbers of these attractive new items are available, often devised out of some basically nutritious substance such as wheat which has been pummeled, crushed, inflated, refined, "enriched," stabilized, emulsified, conditioned, homogenized, lyophilized, and otherwise transformed from a food into a "food product." Others are invented foods, synthesized *de novo* from simple laboratory chemicals.

Despite the widespread availability of these exciting and novel food products, there are some people who persist in worrying. Isn't it possible, they ask, that all this fooling around may take some things out of food that we need, or introduce some other things into food that we could better do without? For all these nervous people there is a straightforward answer. It comes from the government, the scientists, the food manufacturers, and others concerned about how Americans eat. The answer is: "We don't really know, but don't worry."

They don't *know?*

It's true, they *don't* know and they sincerely hope that what they don't know won't hurt you. This statement may come as a surprise to those who feel, quite justifiably, that someone ought to be in charge. Many other people won't even believe that knowledge does not exist. They believe that scientists and food manufacturers are in possession of proof, which they sinisterly refuse to divulge, that we are being poisoned by our food. There is no such proof. Moreover, despite all that isn't known, it's still safe to say that we're not in imminent danger of poisoning even if we can't afford to do our shopping in health food stores. But what this massive official ignorance *does* mean is that we can't blithely gobble up any old thing (or any new thing!) off the grocery shelf. We're simply not as protected as decades of optimistic bulletins from the FDA and the Department of Agriculture would have us believe.

Meanwhile, before our very eyes food is disappearing. Butter is replaced by margarine which is then supplanted by imitation margarine (!). Fruit juices are replaced by juice drinks which are replaced by Tang. Puddings made at home by mother from milk and eggs are replaced by puddings made from a box by adding milk and these are replaced by pudding-like plastics which come in slightly harder plastic containers in "your dairy case." With each step along the way the list of added chemicals—and hence of unanswered questions about safety—gets longer. Why is this happening to food? Are the food companies simply wicked to have so sorely corrupted the innocence of our food?

They are not wicked; they are merely businesses, dealing in a commodity which, as English researcher John Yudkin has pointed out, is unique in being consumable only within narrow limits: ". . . limits below which life cannot exist and above which even the most gluttonous cannot reach."

Food can be dressed up or down, made complex or simple, but there are rather strict limits beyond which it cannot be eaten.

What happens to a commodity for which there is a fixed rational market in an economic system which requires continual and accelerating growth?

The answer can be read in any supermarket. Such a commodity becomes irrational.

First, over-consumption must be encouraged. And second, non-caloric foods must be invented. These permit a sort of Dorian Gray approach to gluttony; aided by indigestible "bulking agents" like methyl cellulose, and non-caloric sweeteners like the cyclamates of fond memory, we can be tempted to consume far beyond need and yet avoid being *as fat* as our overindulgence would normally imply. (This delicate balancing process is insufficiently finely tuned at the moment. The best estimates are that by age 50, one-third of the men and one-half of the women in the United States are 20% or more over their best weight, i.e., fat.)

And finally, as a third measure to keep the market expanding even faster than the population, novelty and overprocessing must be used to coax people to buy less food value for more money.

Such an approach produces products like Jello 1-2-3 in which for about twice the price of regular Jello—no nutritional bargain to begin with—the customer is permitted to participate in a fascinating chemical experiment resulting in three layers of empty calories rather than one.

Along this line, perhaps the ultimate American cultural artifact is the frozen instant omelette.

At 79¢ for six eggs, three small plastic coated cartons, one larger carton to hold the three smaller ones, plus such assorted ingredients as milk, salt and "flavorings," instant omelettes would seem to represent no conceivable advance in either time-saving or convenience. And the ultimate in packaging pollution and profit.

Eggs are cheaper (you can get a dozen for well under the price of 3 plain instant omelettes). Whole eggs require no thawing, come in smaller biodegradable containers, and are, at an outside maximum, about 30 seconds less instant.

It is probably wishful thinking, but it would seem that with the instant omelette, the food manufacturers have gone about as far as they can go. As food becomes more inventive, more "processing" is required, more additives must be used, and the mixtures which must be kept intact through months of storage become more complex.

If what is being sold is irresistibility and ostensibly "convenience," the color, texture and flavor of a product become not merely *as* important, but more important than its contribution to health—especially since the customer is more likely to become aware of these things than she is to become aware of a product's nutritional virtues.

Food is becoming more artificial simply because, in order to stay in business, manufacturers feel they must sell more and more complex, more and more inventive, more and more novel food items with a longer and longer shelf life, at greater and greater profits. It's the American way.

It would be a vast mis-statement to imply, as many people now seem to be doing, that everything that's put into food hurts it. From a health standpoint it's probably better to have anti-oxidants in oil and oxygen interceptors in sausage, for example, than to have rancid oil and stale sausage. And when it comes to something like thiamine hydrocholoride, a vitamin, if they're going to take it out of grains in processing, they probably ought to put it back in.

But lots of things get put into food simply because they enhance certain mechanical characteristics important in the manufacturing (like how the food behaves while being handled by man or machine) and lots more get put in because the manufacturer decides they are important for sales appeal. *Food Technology,* the journal of the Institute of Food Technologists, is full of advertisements for synthetic flavors, synthetic colors, starches, gels, and wonderful things like "powdered cloud" to give your juice drinks "eye-appealing opacity."

As was suggested earlier, nobody at the moment is sure how much of this stuff really ought to be in our food supply. In fact, no one is even sure how much of it *is* in our food supply.

As the Panel on Food Safety of the White House Conference on Food, Nutrition and Health reported, we have no assessment of the "existing chemical burden" which we carry, nor would we know for sure what it meant if we did.

To decide whether something is safe to eat requires that you answer, among other questions, safe for whom? in what quantity? by what tests? over what period of time? combined with what other chemicals? We don't know very many of those answers about the foods themselves, to say nothing of what the manufacturers add to them.

Is there any relationship, for example, between our current epidemic of heart disease and the fact that over the last 50 years Americans have reduced by 25% their overall consumption of carbohydrates—largely cereals and potatoes—while simultaneously increasing by 25% their consumption of refined sugar products? We do not know. If we do not know the effect of such a massive dietary change—how much more difficult it is to assess the effect of the hundreds of smaller changes that take place constantly in our food supply.

In the face of our existing lack of knowledge, what can the consumer do?

The first thing the consumer can do is insist, by whatever means are available, that the recommendations of the Panel on Food Safety of the White House Conference on Food, Nutrition and Health be adopted immediately. Among other recommendations, the panel urged that there be continuous monitoring of the food supply; that there be regular surveys of the population to assess the effect of our increasing chemical burden from all sources; and that there be stringent testing of all additives, old as well as new, to make sure that they are not merely safe but necessary. Despite the difficulties involved, tests for safety of individual chemicals and of the food supply as a whole, can be conducted.

These recommendations, if put into effect, would go far toward guaranteeing us that our food supply was as safe as current scientific methodology could make it.

Second, the consumer can insist on accurate and complete food labeling.

We need really informative food labels which list not only all the food ingredients, but all the additives *and the purposes for which they are added.*

And we need to have them written in English plain enough for the shopper without a chemistry degree to understand.

Right at the moment the FDA is considering revised labeling regulations. But some time ago when they were considering proposals for the clearer labeling on fats and oils, they received 31 arguments *against* clear labeling (from representatives of the dairy industry) and a *single letter* (from a consumer) in support of it.

Industry won.

If you want more informative labeling, better let them hear about it.

In the meantime—and in the real world there is always a meantime—we can vote with our money to bring back food in the marketplace. Sometime in the balmy era before science promised to free us from all drudgery (it has—we have replaced drudgery with unmanageable anxiety which permits us to utilize another scientific triumph—the tranquilizer), we had something called skepticism. We've got to get back to asking that old question, "what's in it for me?" about the food on the grocer's shelf.

No one but the consumer can really convince the government and food manufacturers that people are concerned with nutrition and not with innovation—that we'd rather take our chances on mealtime boredom than see our food treated as if it were one more plastic novelty toy which becomes more and more "realistic" even as it becomes less and less real.

So long as the public remains enamoured of the technologically "new" in food, the food companies will compete to meet that demand—which they themselves have created.

—J. G.

Reprinted with permission from *Consumer Action Now*, pp. 1-2 (1971).

Dr. Dena Cederquist...
Questions and Answers

A contrasting view of the U. S. Food System is offered here by Michigan State nutritionist, Dr. Dena Cederquist. This positive look at consumer choice in America was published by the Kraft Food Company in a 1976 consumer newsletter.

Blessed with wry, good humor and honest religious conviction . . . it's easy to understand why nearly 700 Michigan State students attend her course in basic nutrition each year. Like any really good teacher, she has the ability to communicate deep, complex issues in clear, simple language.

"I talk straight with them," explains Dr. Dena Caroline Cederquist, Professor of Nutrition, Michigan State University.

"I'm really impressed with the large number of students—from all over the campus—that want to know the facts about food, facts that relate to their diets and their nutritional needs."

A student and teacher in nutrition and food education for the past 49 years, Dr. Cederquist is recognized as one of the nation's leading authorities on food.

On a recent Sunday afternoon on the MSU campus, she spoke to the "Consumer's Right to Know" about the serious food issues this country faces.

Q: Dr. Cederquist, our subject for this "Consumer's Right to Know" newsletter is Quality, specifically as the word relates to food and the food industry.

What is your opinion of the quality of the American food supply?

A: "There's such a variety of foods of very high quality. I was at the store yesterday, and there were cucumbers and tomatoes and cabbage . . . and a wide variety of citrus fruits. All of it looked appetizing and was clean and ready to eat. Now this is winter . . . in Michigan . . . could you imagine what would be available here naturally? Potatoes, carrots, turnips and rutabagas . . . and that would be pretty much it.

"I haven't been all around the world, but I remember going into a food store in Russia. It was in the summertime, and the only fresh things that were there were potatoes and apples. The potatoes weren't graded and the apples were spotted and had holes. Obviously they hadn't been sprayed. Most Americans wouldn't buy produce like that. But in Russia, that was all that was available.

"As you go from country-to-country, what's available to us in the U.S. is simply tremendous. I was in Guatemala last summer—my heart aches for them now—and they had these big food markets and absolutely no way to control quality.

"I can still see this big truck loaded with bananas, most of which were non-edible because of the way they were handled. There's such tremendous waste.

"The range of choices we have in this country is so remarkable. For example, let's say you're used to buying unsweetened pineapple chunks. You know without opening the can what you are going to get. The product you buy in New York or Chicago is just like the one you get in Des Moines or Denver. I think the general public doesn't know what goes on to insure that kind of quality. I think they take all of this for granted.

"What's especially important about quality and our food supply is that you can choose the particular quality you want and then consistently obtain it. I may think the only kind of cheese that should be consumed is good, old aged cheddar. Well then I don't have to buy Cheez Whiz. No one is forced to buy something they don't want. Cheez Whiz may be exactly what somebody else wants. That's what's great about our food supply. Quality isn't confined to expensive, elegant food. We expect and have high quality in less expensive food."

Q: Given all the positive aspects of the American food supply . . . then where does all the criticism of the food industry come from? And why?

A: "There is so much misinformation about food. I can't keep up with what people are going to say next about our food system. I can't say it's lack of intelligence, because some of the most intelligent people I know are often misled or mistaken about food and basic food facts. I think it's part of a larger pattern of distrust nowadays for government, industry, and each other. People just assume that if information comes from the food industry then it's not true. That the industry is trying to hide something, or put something over on the public.

"People just don't understand additives. All this hullabaloo about monosodium glutamate . . . a material that's been used by the Chinese as far back as we have any historical references. The Chinese have managed to survive.

"Anything used out of context can be harmful. Water can be harmful, if you drink it faster than the kidneys can excrete it. The mold that occurs in bread is the same compound deterrent that is found in certain cheeses. You eat it there, and nobody complains. But you take that same compound, put it in bread, and you're afraid of it.

"I was raised on an Iowa farm, and grew up on natural foods. Now I have prematurely gray hair, wear glasses, and have all my teeth filled. I had undulant fever as a child from drinking raw milk, and I've had major surgery for cancer. So, I'm delighted that milk is pasteurized, and that our food supply is of consistent, safe quality.

"We're surrounded by micro-organisms. I wish I could keep my own kitchen as clean as major food producers keep their plants. I wish we could get more people to understand what's involved. The food industry has done a tremendous job in safely preserving our food supply. We can depend on it.

"You can't have mass production without additives. We all like a roadside stand to pick up fresh fruits and vegetables, but there's no way that roadside stands are going to feed this nation. You must have additives. You must treat foods in certain ways. The idea that the food industry is trying to put something over on the consuming public by adulteration or contamination of the food supply to me is just unbelievable. Why would the food industry want to destroy its consuming public? I'm sure they'd like to keep us consuming for as long as possible."

Q: Hasn't the rise in food prices also contributed to the criticism?

A: "Yes, rising food prices are a big factor. The thing that people don't understand is that we spend the smallest amount of our total income for food than almost any other group of people in the world, as far as I know. If you read the history of agriculture in this country, you'll see historically that we've had inexpensive food at a terrific cost of human labor for which there was no reasonable rate of return. We expected a farmer to produce his crops for little or nothing. We've become accustomed to spending a small percentage on food so that we'd have money left over for two cars, two houses, and all the rest.

"Let's just talk about the rising cost of energy—fertilizer, transportation, equiment, labor . . . the price of energy in all forms has gone up. People know the gas they put in their tanks costs more, but they don't think of that in relation to the cost of food."

Q: How do you feel about the future, as it relates to nutrition?

A: "Really, the critics of our food system have done us a favor in that they've heightened consumer awareness in food and nutrition. My students now are really interested in the industry's efforts to improve food quality. People are into nutrition now . . . and we have a real responsibility to cash in on that now.

"We've done such a poor job in selling nutrition in this country. I ask my students: Could you guess what two of my favorite breakfast foods are? And they can't . . . because I love to eat strawberry shortcake and toasted cheese sandwiches. And why not? Many a morning in the summer I make a single biscuit and cover it with delicious fresh strawberries.

"And why can't I get my protein in the morning from the cheese in my sandwich? We've been so regimented in our thinking of what we eat and when we eat it."

Reprinted with permission from *The Consumer's Right to Know*, 1(IV): 1+. Copyright 1976 by Kraft, Inc.

In 1977 General Foods launched a major consumer information campaign. Like Mobil's energy campaign, the G. F. ads on additives, preservatives, processing and other areas of consumer concern, did not always serve to clear up confusion. In the ad reproduced here, the copywriter's dazzling sleight-of-hand almost succeeds in equating food processing with pea freezing.

"Dear General Foods, Nothing you do to a pea is going to make it a better pea. So why do anything?"

"Dear General Foods, Nothing you do to a pea is going to make it a better pea. So why do anything?"

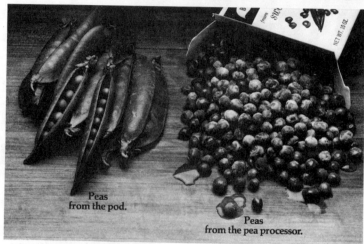

Peas
from the pod.

Peas
from the pea processor.

Nature makes sensational peas.

Unfortunately, Nature has a very limited pea distribution system. It's called a pod. Sure, the peas are right there in the pod for you to pick. But what if you don't live on a farm? Or what if it's February, and you live in North Dakota, and the only part of Nature still making peas is a thousand miles away?

What we do to foods to solve problems like this is called *food processing.* Freezing peas is one kind of processing. So is frying an egg or canning pears.

Of course, there are other kinds of food processing far more complicated than these. There are processed foods that weren't picked from any plant (imitation bacon, for example, or powdered orange drinks)—foods that weren't just *changed* by processing, but *created* by it. These are quite another story, too long to tell here. (We'll do it in a future ad.) The main point is that we're able to take for granted a ready supply of peas, orange drinks, and many other foods. But we wouldn't have anything like that ready supply if we didn't have food processing.

What's processed food?

Food processing is everything you do to food to make it easier to use, or better-tasting, or longer-lasting, or safer, or whatever.

Of course, it's impossible to process food without changing it in some way. The whole idea is to make sure that after the processing is over, more benefits than compromises have resulted from it.

Take breakfast cereals. Almost all major food companies, ourselves included, process their cereals—and as a result, you have flakes, puffed grains, and a variety of tastes and textures you might not have otherwise. But the same process that gives you this variety may also remove some of the vitamins from the grains. So as part of the processing of our Post® cereals, we restore the key vitamins that were taken out. (And then some: we add enough of several essential nutrients so that you get the amount breakfast should supply— 1/4 to 1/3 of your daily requirements of them.) The resulting cereal is good-tasting, available in many varieties, and nutritious—which is a greater array of benefits than might result from cereals made from the same unprocessed grain alone.

In short, processing can't work miracles. Once the grains have grown or the pears have ripened, all the miracles have already taken place. But processing *can* help deliver those miracles—and our Birds Eye® frozen peas are a good example.

What we do to the peas you eat.

From the day our peas are planted, careful records are kept of how much heat, sunlight, and rain they get. When the peas are almost mature, sampling teams check the fields constantly, to determine the precise time the peas will be ready. And at that time, they're picked.

Next the peas are shelled right in the field, and then rushed to the freezing station. Then they're tested for tenderness. Finally, they're washed, blanched, and frozen. The entire process is usually over within four hours. Unless you raise your own or live on a farm, it's almost impossible to get "fresh" peas that fresh.

This process results not only in fresh peas, but delicious ones. Peas contain a natural sugar that can begin to turn into starch shortly after they're picked. Since we freeze ours so quickly, they don't have much chance to lose flavor or get tough. And they don't suffer the nutrient loss that "fresh" peas can during distribution.

Whenever we process a food, we do it with the same concern for the food that we show towards our peas.

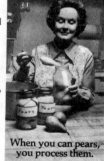

When you can pears, you process them.

Nobody makes food, peas included, the way Nature does. And getting you that food in its most delicious, nutritious and convenient form is what processing is all about.

For more information.

We hope this brief study of food processing gives you a better idea of how and why food gets processed.

If you have any questions about it, please ask us. Just write to Miss Peggy Kohl, V.P., Consumer Affairs, G.F. Consumer Center, White Plains, N.Y. 10625.

Our reasons for telling you all this are a mixture of helpfulness and pride in our products. The more you understand about food, the better off you'll be. And the more you understand about our food, the better off we'll be.

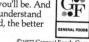

©1977 General Foods Corp.

Reprinted with permission from General Foods Corp. Copyright 1977 by General Foods Corp.

Food Processing: Search for Growth

ROBERT M. HADSELL

In 1971 Robert Hadsell, as assistant editor of *Chemical and Engineering News*, put together a special story on the food processing business. The article is excerpted here—still relevant because of the clarity with which it explains the economic thrust that underlies the ceaseless innovation of the U. S. food marketplace.

Concern for nutritive value, additives, convenience items, and new products, as well as diversification, mark this $90 billion industry.

The $90-billion food processing industry is noted for slow but steady sales growth and low profit margins. The amount of food consumed by each person in the U.S. has been increasing only slightly, if at all, and the U.S. population increases at a rate of only 1% a year. So executives of individual food companies face a continuing challenge to make their corporations grow faster and more profitably than the industry as a whole.

The introduction of new products is part of that challenge—foods that win consumer acceptance with more convenience, more nutrition, or more sensual appeal. Development of new products and shifting sales volumes of existing foods are of more than passing interest to many companies in the chemical industry which supply food additives and other food ingredients such as refined vegetable oils. In particular, the growing public and governmen-

tal interest in improving the nutritional value of foods presents the chemical industry with growing markets for vitamins, minerals, amino acids, and proteins.

Food companies are also growing by diversifying into new areas, both within and outside the food industry. One of the biggest areas for growth at present is the "food away from home," or institutional, market. Restaurants, drive-ins, snack bars, hospitals, and schools have always been an important part of the institutional food market, but food companies are becoming aware that institutional feeding presents opportunities for new products and food systems quite apart from the food-at-home grocery field.

The two trends toward nutritional improvement and institutional feeding have been brought together and given new impetus by the U.S. Department of Agriculture in the food programs it supports. USDA has recently set criteria for fortified and textured vegetable protein-supplemented food products in school feeding programs. This move is encouraging food companies to develop these foods by creating a market for them.

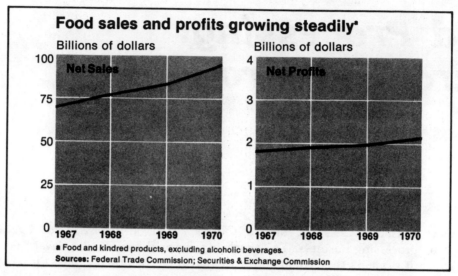

Food sales and profits growing steadily*

Billions of dollars

Net Sales

Billions of dollars

Net Profits

a Food and kindred products, excluding alcoholic beverages.
Sources: Federal Trade Commission; Securities & Exchange Commission

Sales. The food industry is one of the largest segments of the U.S. economy. Sales by manufacturers of food and kindred products, excluding alcoholic beverages, reached $91 billion in 1970, up 9% from $83.4 billion in 1969. (The gross national product in 1970 was $976 billion.) . . .

The Department of Commerce provides another handle on the food industry with values of shipments. Shipments of food products (excluding beverages) had a value of $87.6 billion in 1970, according to Commerce estimates. This figure is an increase of 6% from $82.8 billion in 1969. Commerce predicts average annual increases of 5% through 1980, giving shipments of $92 billion in 1971, $113 billion in 1975, and $147 billion by 1980. Bottled and canned soft drinks add $4.5 billion to the 1970 figure, up 14% from $3.9 billion in 1969. Shipments of soft drinks are predicted by Commerce to be $4.8 billion in 1971 (up 8%) and will increase at an average annual rate of 8.7% to reach $10.3 billion in 1980. In terms of value of shipments, the food industry is the largest single segment of manufacturers in the U.S.

The consumer encounters the food industry not at the factory but at the grocery store or restaurant. . . .

According to the Department of Commerce, total personal expenditures by U.S. consumers for food (excluding alcoholic beverages) were $114 billion in 1970. This amount is divided into $90.6 billion for food used at home and $23.4 billion for food consumed away from home. Thus about $1.00 out of every $5.00 for food was spent away from home in 1970. This has been the ratio since at least 1960. . . .

When viewed as a whole, the food industry lacks external forces for growth in the U.S. Slow annual growth in U.S. population is only a minor factor in growth of the food industry. Food consumption per person increased only about 5.5% between 1960 and 1969, according to USDA's food consumption index. By another USDA measure, the number of pounds of food consumed per capita underwent little change during the past decade; the amount was 1441 pounds in 1960, 1414 pounds in 1965, and about 1445 pounds in 1969.

Inflation not only accounts for much of the food industry's overall sales growth but also puts pressure on profit margins. Costs of labor, raw materials, and operations have all increased steeply during the past five or six years. Inflation comes on top of other long-standing pressures from intense competition and related costs for advertising and other forms of promotion. In addition, food processors stand in the middle of a distribution chain stretching from farmers through numerous brokers, wholesalers, and retailers, each pushing for a bigger share of the profits.

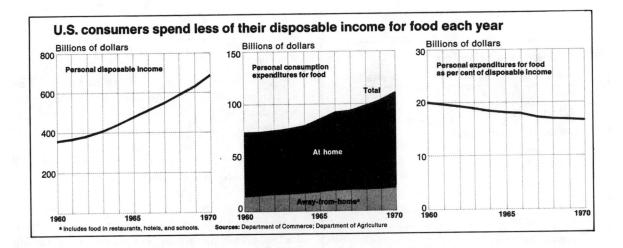

U.S. consumers spend less of their disposable income for food each year

Billions of dollars

Personal disposable income

Billions of dollars

Personal consumption expenditures for food

Total

At home

Away-from-home*

Billions of dollars

Personal expenditures for food as per cent of disposable income

* includes food in restaurants, hotels, and schools.   Sources: Department of Commerce; Department of Agriculture

In spite of these pressures, some food processors are presently enjoying growth in both sales and profits. This strength is particularly noticeable during the present period of economic doldrums, when companies in many other industries are struggling to even maintain sales and profits at current levels. . . .

At least some companies are finding ways to achieve rates of sales and profits growth beyond rates for the food industry as a whole. The introduction of new products is one critical factor in a company's growth, along with increasing public acceptance of existing products. Although per capita consumption of food may be increasing only slightly, there are continuing shifts in the composition of consumer's diets.

Some food commodities gradually have been declining in the average diet. In terms of USDA's figures for per capita consumption, food categories that have become a smaller portion of diets during the past decade include eggs, dairy products, fresh fruits and vegetables, wheat flour, and animal fat and oil.

Per capita consumption of cheese and vegetable fat and oil, on the other hand, each increased by nearly 40% during the past 10 years. Consumption of meat and poultry has also been climbing. The popularity of chicken has undoubtedly been helped by chicken prices, which have remained fairly constant during the past 10 years. In contrast, meat prices in 1970 were 35% higher than in 1960, with most of the

increase (25%) coming since 1965.

The trend toward convenience foods—foods that require less preparation before serving—has long been gospel in the food industry. The growing consumption of meat and poultry certainly runs counter to that trend, but other evidence supports it. Per capita consumption figures for canned and frozen vegetables and frozen fruits all increased during the past decade.

Other figures on convenience foods come from *Supermarketing* magazine, which says that frozen prepared foods, for instance, gained 10.6% from 1968 to 1969 in value of total domestic consumption ($1.28 billion in 1969). Frozen prepared foods include TV dinners, meat and chicken potpies, and frozen soups. The value of total domestic consumption of frozen foods in general was $5.60 billion in 1969, up 5.4% from 1968.

Snack foods, convenient, ready-to-eat foods, are probably best defined as between-meal foods, eaten for pleasure or to satisfy hunger pangs at odd hours. At the level of sales by manufacturers, *Snack Food* magazine estimates total snack food sales for 1969 to be $3.45 billion, up 5.2% from $3.28 billion in 1968. The average annual increase in manufacturers' sales since 1960 has been 5.9%.

At the retail level, the value of total domestic consumption of biscuits, cookies, potato chips, and crackers in 1969 was $2.44 billion, up only

Snack sales booming

Million of dollars	1969 SALES
Cookies, crackers	$1484
Potato chips	749
Snack nut meats	552
Frozen snacks, including pizza	145
Corn chips	130
Pretzels	130
Meat snacks	60
Toaster pastries	59
Prepackaged popcorn	9.2
Other snacks[a]	128
Total	**$3446**

a Includes extruded and expanded products, such as General Mills' Bugles and Whistles.

Source: Snack Food magazine

3.8% from 1969, according to *Supermarketing* magazine. Consumption of potato chips, however, jumped 8.4% to $997 million.

These trends by food category still don't tell the story of what is happening to sales and profits of individual products at the company level. As Nabisco, Inc., president Robert M. Schaeberle points out, snacks are volatile items; innovations and fads come and go, and products may be profitable only briefly—although Mr. Schaeberle points out that old standards such as Ritz crackers and Triscuit wafers just keep right on growing.

Chemicals. Trends in new products are important to the many chemical companies that supply food processors with food additives and other ingredients. Refiners of vegetable oils, for instance, are happy about the shift from animal to vegetable sources of oils and fats. In addition to vitamins, minerals, and proteins, chemical companies provide food additives used as flavors, colors, sweeteners, acidulants, preservatives, thickeners, emulsifiers, or sequestrants.

Nutritional improvement is only one of several trends that are opening up new markets

for food additives. In the field of convenience foods, additives make possible products that only require heating before serving. The additional step of defrosting is no longer necessary with some of these foods, which are stable on the shelves of supermarkets or institutional kitchens.

The increasing use of food additives will continue to meet with some measure of resistance, however. Consumers' uncertainty about the safety of some food additives is one factor. And food companies are not eager to increase the costs of their products by adding more ingredients.

Use of food additives in the U.S in 1970 was about $485 million, according to Richard L. Hughes of Arthur D. Little, Inc. This represents about 5 pounds per capita, he estimates. Use of food additives in 1980 will rise to about $756 million, when more than half of the foods sold will be prepared foods containing additives. By then, per capita consumption of food additives will have risen to about 6 pounds. . . .

For many companies in the food processing industry, growth involves more than just developing new food products. Especially during the past five or six years, food companies have been moving to broaden their bases of operations by diversification into new

Flavors lead additives

Millions of dollars	DEMAND FOR FOOD ADDITIVES	
	1970	1980
Flavorings	$150	$225
Stabilizers, thickeners	100	150
Surfactants	50	70
Antioxidants	22	45
Flavor enhancers	24	45
Acidulants	30	48
Nutrient supplements	10	15
Others	99	158
Total	**$485**	**$756**

Source: Arthur D. Little, Inc.

areas. Acquisitions have offered the fastest route to diversification. For some companies, the quest for greater sales and profits has taken food processors into such diverse areas as cosmetics, toys, travel trailers, or banking.

General Foods Corp., for example, entered the direct-sale cosmetics business in December 1969 with the acquisition of California-based Viviane Woodard Corp. In October 1970 it acquired Kohner Bros., Inc., a producer of toys for infants and pre-school children. The following month, General Foods added the W. Atlee Burpee seed company to its group of nonfood divisions.

"We are a company that deals primarily in convenience consumer products," says A. S. Clausi, General Foods vice president and director of corporate research. General Foods is supplying consumers with "products and services that are consistent with our life style," he adds. The company also notes in its 1971 annual report that the nonfood units open up new channels of distribution for General Foods products. . . .

Guidelines. The philosophical shift from food company to consumer products company is only one of various guidelines for diversification. . . .

Diversification of Nabisco, Inc., is being guided by the company's existing system of distribution through food outlets, according to president Robert M. Schaeberle. Supermarkets sell more than food, however, so this guideline covers not only Nabisco's acquisition of Freezer Queen Foods, Inc., in May 1970, but also the acquisition of Aurora Products Corp. (toys and hobbies) in May 1971 and the proposed acquisition of J. B. Williams Co., a manufacturer of men's toiletries and pharmaceuticals, including Geritol, Sominex, and Aqua Velva. . . .

Vertical integration is a variation on the diversification theme and can be an end in itself. Some food processors are integrating backward to control sources of ingredients and raw materials, or moving forward toward food outlets such as restaurants. Because profits are divided all along the lengthy chain of food distribution, vertical integration can give processors a bigger share of the profits on the products involved.

The Heinz U.S.A. division of H. J. Heinz Co. presents a typical example of vertical integration. Heinz does not own any farms, Heinz U.S.A. president J. Richard Grieb says, but does supply assistance to farmers, including equipment and new breeds of plants. Heinz manufactures a major portion of its cans but buys the tinplate. Heinz is the third largest user of glass in the U.S., Mr. Grieb says, but it owns no glass companies—although ownership may become tempting if glass prices keep increasing, he adds. Heinz is becoming self-sufficient in capmaking.

Heinz U.S.A. will not integrate forward into areas where Heinz U.S.A. has customers, such as supermarkets and institutional brokerage houses, Mr. Grieb says. Other divisions of Heinz, however, are already entering the fast-food field: Star-Kist Foods, Inc., operates Good-Time Charlie's Fish & Chips on the West Coast, and Heinz's Australian subsidiary is opening a chain of Clancy's restaurants.

Other food companies are wholeheartedly in the restaurant business, particularly the fast-food, limited menu variety. General Foods own the Burger Chef chain. Pillsbury owns Burger King. General Mills owns Red Lobster Inns of America, Inc., and is experimenting with two other chains—Betty Crocker Tree House Restaurant & Bake Shop and Betty Crocker's Pie Shop and Ice Cream Parlor. The General Mills restaurants are not of the conventional fast-food type, chairman McFarland says, but are in niches where there is room for expansion.

Restaurant owners also include CPC International, Inc. (Dutch Pantry, Kettle & Keg) and United Brands Co. (A&W International, Inc., Baskin-Robbins, Inc.). Four'n 20 Pies, a chain of pie and sandwich shops launched by Baskin-Robbins in 1969, has been well received, according to G. Burke Wright, United Brands vice president for planning. United Brands was formed in 1970 by a consolidation of the United Fruit Co. and AMK Corp., whose subsidiaries

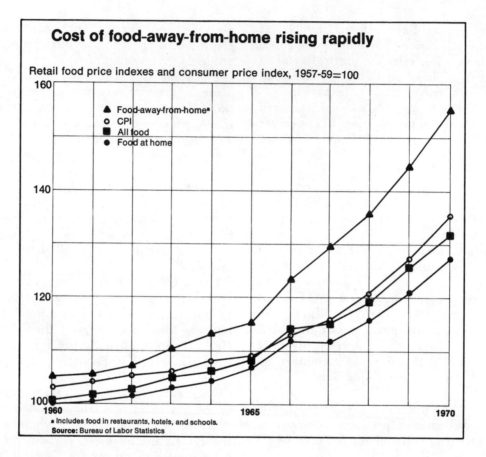

Cost of food-away-from-home rising rapidly

Retail food price indexes and consumer price index, 1957-59=100

▲ Food-away-from-home^a
○ CPI
■ All food
● Food at home

a Includes food in restaurants, hotels, and schools.
Source: Bureau of Labor Statistics

included both United Fruit and John Morrell & Co. meat packers.

Integration. Food processors can also be the target of vertical integration by suppliers of food ingredients. In 1970, Archer Daniels Midland Co. acquired Gooch Food Products Co., a regional producer of macaroni, spaghetti, and packaged dinners. Now called Gooch Foods, Inc., this division marks ADM's entry into the sale of consumer foods. ADM, which also acquired the National City Bank of Minneapolis in 1969, is chiefly involved in wheat milling, vegetable oil refining, and processing of soybeans, flax, and corn. ADM markets a line of soy protein ingredients, including textured soy protein made by extrusion in a 3000 ton-per-month plant at Decatur, Ill. . . .

Competition with customers can be a major limitation of forward integration, however. A food ingredient company that moves into food processing can find itself making foods in competition with other firms that buy the company's ingredients, notes Thomas W. Wilson, Jr., a consultant with McKinsey & Co., international management consultants.

This constraint may be a factor at ADM, which makes a textured soy protein product resembling bits of bacon but sells the product to other food companies to market. Central Soya's chemurgy division is developing new food products that include soy protein, says Dr. Joseph Rakosky, director of technical marketing service, but takes the prototypes to other food companies to develop into their own products.

Many of the soybean processors have a sizable portion of their sales in animal feeds. At least one such company has refrained from developing soy protein as meat extenders to avoid irritating its feed customers. However, two of the biggest meat companies, Swift and

Armour, are developing meat products that include soy protein. Swift is itself a producer of soy proteins, including textured proteins.

Institutional. Restaurants are more than just another type of acquisition for food processors. Restaurants are part of the food-away-from-home market, an area in which food companies see bright opportunities for expansion. The new emphasis on institutional markets and products may be due to the slowdown in growth rates in the traditional retail grocery channels, according to McKinsey's Mr. Wilson. Another factor may be the relative ease of introducing new products with fewer regulatory restrictions, as USDA's Gallimore points out.

In the view of Swift vice president Herbert Robinson, labor problems in the restaurant business are the key factor. The cost of labor is climbing, and good chefs are hard to find. The consequence is that owners of all but the top-level restaurants want pre-cooked meals that can be heated and served. In addition, less food is wasted when meals—including meats—are supplied to restaurants or other institutions in controlled portions.

Thus there exists a demand for convenience foods in institutional markets comparable to the demand in the grocery field. And lessons learned in the former market may be useful in the development of new products for the latter. William A. Schroeder, vice president of CPC International and president of its Best Foods subsidiary, speaks for other food executives as well when he says "Dutch Pantry is a tremendous research laboratory for what consumers like and don't like."

General Foods, which owns the Burger Chef restaurant chain, is actively trying to expand its institutional food service business, vice president Clausi says. He places an emphasis on tailormaking products specifically for institutional use. Restaurants need foods that are less perishable, for instance. Cool Whip, he notes, is superior to whipped cream in this respect. . . .

Nutrition. The institutional segment of the food market is becoming the arena for the development of nutritionally improved foods and foods that substitute one source of protein—soy, typically—for another, such as meat. Commercial success of such foods depends on consumer acceptance and governmental permission, in addition to costs of production. A number of forces are combining to make fortified and extended food products more acceptable. . . .

The popularity of organic or health foods may be an indication that consumers are becoming more concerned about the nutritional quality of food, although a desire to avoid food

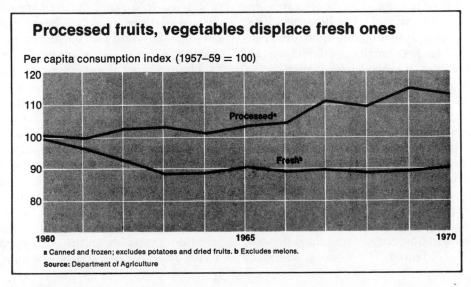

Processed fruits, vegetables displace fresh ones

Per capita consumption index (1957–59 = 100)

a Canned and frozen; excludes potatoes and dried fruits. b Excludes melons.
Source: Department of Agriculture

additives is also a factor. Food industry executives generally feel that consumers are becoming more aware of nutrition, but that taste and appearance are still more important in determining a product's success.

The nutritional value of food is already subject to manipulation. Vitamin D is added to milk, and iodine is added to salt. Enriched flour is used to make bread. Nabisco, Inc., for instance, uses enriched flour in all of its wheat-based cookie, cracker, and other snack products. ITT Continental Baking Co. adds thiamine, riboflavin, niacin, and iron to its major snack items to give levels comparable to enriched bread on a weight-for-weight basis. (Because the snacks contain only about one third as much flour as bread, these B vitamins and iron are at levels three times greater than if enriched flour were used.) Breakfast cereals that claim to provide 100% of the minimum daily requirements for vitamins and iron are common. . . .

Consumer acceptance is necessary for the success of fortified or vegetable protein-extended foods, but economic considerations are providing much of the real impetus. The costs of food and food preparation squeeze tightest in institutions, so it is in this segment of the food market that pressure is greatest for the introduction of new approaches. The greatest pressures exist in programs for feeding children in schools. Public demands for nutritionally adequate lunches and breakfasts have come up against small school budgets and a lack of facilities for food preparation.

As a result, USDA has set criteria for fortified and extended foods that can be used in its school feeding programs. These food products are intended to not only improve nutrition and lower costs, but also provide a market that the food industry has previously lacked. Foods developed for the government-subsidized school programs may then be able to succeed commercially. Thus one purpose of the new criteria is to encourage the food industry to improve nutrition for the public in general, according to Edward H. Koenig, assistant director of the nutrition and technical services staff of USDA's Food and Nutrition Service. In fact, products approved for use in the school feeding programs must be available commercially, or at least intended for the commercial market.

Criteria. Criteria have been established for three types of new products. A fortified baked product with creamed filling can be used in school breakfasts as a replacement for fruit or juice and bread or cereal. The product might be in the form of a cakelike sandwich. A breakfast of the product with one half pint of milk should supply one fourth to one third of the recommended daily dietary allowances for a 10- to 12-year-old boy or girl.

In school lunches, a protein-fortified, enriched macaroni-type product can be used to replace 1 ounce of the 2-ounce requirement for meat, poultry, cheese, or fish. Other meat alternates have previously been allowed in lunches, including 2 ounces of cheese, one egg, a half cup of cooked dry beans or peas, or 4 tablespoons of peanut butter. At least one food processor has developed a fortified peanut spread that may soon be permitted in the lunch program.

The third type of food product is meat extended with textured vegetable protein. The textured protein—generally soy protein—can be added to ground or diced meat, poultry, or fish in portions up to 30% by weight (hydrated). The combination can be served in the form of patties, sauces, stews, or meat loaves.

The textured vegetable protein products are intended to cut costs. Nutritional quality of the extended meats will not be decreased and may even be increased. A meat hamburger patty costs about 12 cents, Mr. Koenig says, but a patty with 30% soy protein will cost only 9 to 10 cents. At a saving of 25%, serving the textured soy protein product twice a week in 20 million lunches would give savings of as much as $36 million annually.

Many food processors are interested in providing products in the school programs' new categories. More than 50 companies are

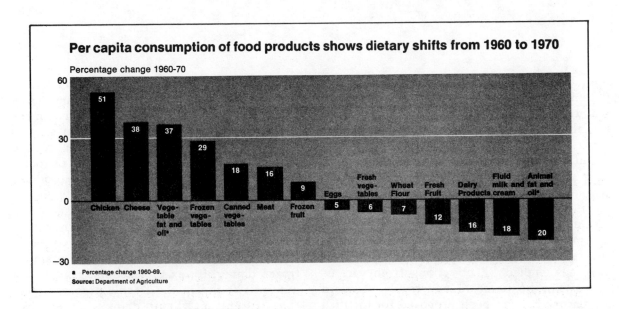

Per capita consumption of food products shows dietary shifts from 1960 to 1970

Percentage change 1960-70

Chicken 51, Cheese 38, Vegetable fat and oil* 37, Frozen vegetables 29, Canned vegetables 18, Meat 16, Frozen fruit 9, Eggs −5, Fresh vegetables −6, Wheat Flour −7, Fresh Fruit −12, Dairy Products −16, Fluid milk and cream −18, Animal fat and oil* −20

a Percentage change 1960-69.
Source: Department of Agriculture

working on products with a Rutgers University program headed by Dr. Paul A. LaChance, associate professor of nutritional physiology. The program, funded by USDA and the Office of Economic Opportunity, is conducting research to increase the effectiveness of school feeding in two major areas, Dr. LaChance says. Many schools have no feeding programs at all, for a variety of reasons. In schools that do have feeding programs, the number of students who participate needs to be increased. The appeal of food products is a major factor in this latter area.

Soy. Several food companies have already been supplying soy protein or soy-extended meat to individual schools, and it appears that this type of product will be used widely in schools sooner than the fortified macaroni and baked products. Although not necessarily related to the school programs, it is indicative of corporate interest that nearly 50 major food companies have been using pilot-plant quantities of Ralston Purina Co.'s soy isolate this past year, says Paul H. Hatfield, division vice president in Ralston Purina's protein division.

Development of and approval for fortified baked and macaroni products are moving more slowly. ITT Continental Bakeries has devel-oped several fortified versions of its Twinkies product, and a specification for the fortified baked product with creamed filling was developed with the fortified Twinkies in mind. ITT Continental's fortified product, called Astrofood, has been approved for school breakfasts and has been used in schools during the past year.

There are at least two fortified macaroni-type products: Golden Elbow macaroni (a blend of corn, soy, and wheat) from General Foods and a semolina-soy blended macaroni from ADM. Golden Elbow macaroni has been available under a temporary marketing permit since 1969; and ADM's macaroni will be offered to schools this fall.

Other fortified food products have failed so far to receive USDA's approval. Cost is one reason, or failure to meet specifications for nutrient content or weight.

Standards of identity are also slowing the introduction of the fortified macaroni-type products and will present a problem for the introduction of other fortified foods as well. CPC International, for instance, manufactures Skippy peanut butter through its Best Foods division and has developed a peanut butter product fortified with milk protein, vitamins, and minerals. CPC International has applied for a temporary permit to make the fortified peanut butter, in order to make the product available for the school lunch program. Standards of identity exist for both macaroni and peanut butter, and new or changed standards are necessary before permanent approval can be given for marketing of products with different ingredients but still identified as "macaroni" or "peanut butter." A new standard of identity was proposed for fortified macaroni by FDA in November 1970, but acceptance of the standard has been stalled by objections from various interests in the macaroni industry. No standard of identity has yet been proposed for fortified peanut butter.

Guidelines. The absence of nutritional guidelines is another factor that is making food processors cautious in upgrading the nutritional quality of their products. A wide variety of approaches have been proposed and debated. At one extreme are suggestions that certain foods—hamburgers, for instance, or snack items—should be fortified to provide 100% of a person's daily dietary requirements. At the other extreme would be a policy of no fortification, relying instead on nutritional labeling and education to guide consumers in selecting foods for a proper diet. Dr. LaChance at Rutgers favors an approach he terms "nutrification," adding nutrients to certain foods on the basis of calories from protein to make the foods provide the same percentage of all required nutrients.

The situation is due to be cleared up within the next year or so. FDA has requested the Food and Nutrition Board of the National Academy of Sciences/National Research Council to recommend guidelines for nutrient levels in many classes of foods. The first recommendation, on frozen dinners, have been sent to FDA. Dr. Ogden Johnson, director of the division of nutrition in FDA's bureau of foods, does not favor the creation of food products that claim to provide 100% of the daily dietary requirements, or even some percentage of all nutrients. Instead, he says, the nutrient content of a food product should be based on what the consumer expects it to contain. A frozen dinner, for example, should contain the nutrients found in the freshly prepared meat that it replaces. Fruit drinks, as another example, are used interchangeably with orange juice and thus should contain comparable levels of vitamin C. In the case of food products that have no clearly defined place in people's diets, more information is needed on dietary patterns before nutritional guidelines can be established.

In spite of present difficulties, food processors seem committed to improving the nutritional quality of their products wherever possible. And Paul LaChance, from his vantage point as head of the Rutgers program, is encouraged with the progress that food companies are making. One reason is that the fortified products are unexpectedly turning out to have improved technical properties and stabilities as bonuses to improved nutrition. "The food companies are doing things they didn't think they could do," Dr. LaChance says. Furthermore, he adds, "Schools have the tightest economics of any feeding system. If you can make a go there, you can make a go in any market."

Excerpted with permission from *Chemical & Engineering News,* 49:17-25 (23 August 1971).

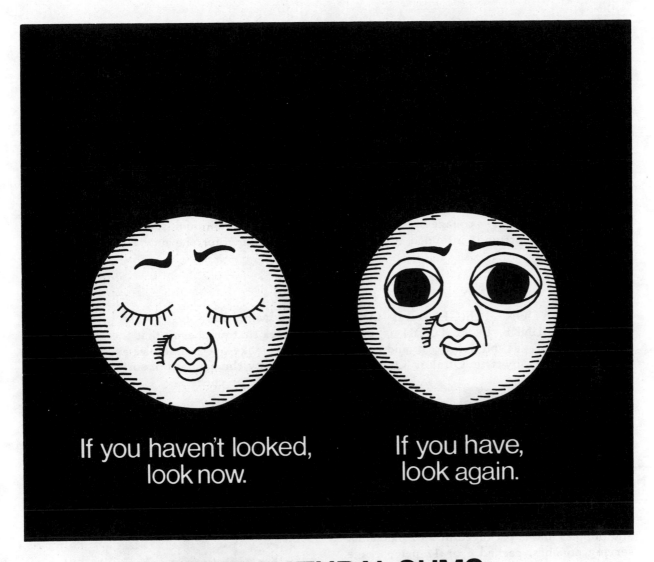

MEER NATURAL GUMS
AND OLEORESINS

If you need to find substitutes for your substitutes, look at Meer. What you will see may be an ideal solution to your problems: a reliable source of natural, dependable, quality materials to do all kinds of things. To stabilize. To emulsify. To flavor and to color. To disperse and to add gel strength and control viscosity.

And as the largest source of many of the 2,000 fine ingredients we offer, Meer is also uniquely equipped to help you with their application for your particular needs. Gums are available regular or spray dried; spices in regular or oleoresin form; flavor extracts in various concentrations; natural colors.

These products are all carefully processed with the most modern equipment, subjected to painstaking quality control by the most advanced techniques.

In these trying times, you could well find things looking up when you look into Meer natural gums, oleoresins and extracts.

Meer Corporation

9500 Railroad Avenue, North Bergen, N.J. 07047 / (201) 861-9500 / Chicago • Philadelphia • Los Angeles

Reprinted with permission from Meer Corporation, North Bergen NJ.

New Consumer Products

On the next few pages, a collage of items: advertisements, magazine columns, news-stories—a not-quite-random assortment intended to give the reader a feeling for the new rules of the food processing game.

KEN-L RATION BURGER and LIVER FLAVOR CHUNKS DOG FOOD is being introduced in Texas, New Mexico, and east of the Mississippi by the Quaker Oats Co.,

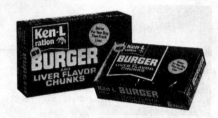

Chicago, Ill. The semi-moist dog food is said to be 100% nutritionally complete for adult dogs and puppies and is packaged in 6-oz individual-serving pouches, packed 6 or 12 per package.

HAMBURGER HELPER® main dish mixes marketed nationally by General Mills, Minne-

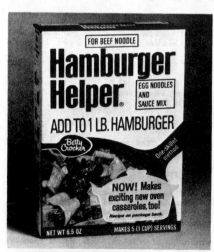

apolis, Minn., are being sold in redesigned packages that emphasize that the mixes can be used to make oven casseroles as well as skillet dinners, by the addition of such ingredients as eggs, milk, or cheese.

Italian-style salad cubes—croutons seasoned with a cheese and spice flavoring and packaged in easy-opening 3-oz metal cans—are being test-marketed in the midwest, east, and Florida by the Apollo Wheat Germ Co., Flint, Mich.

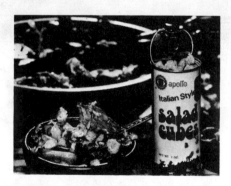

The metal cans—supplied by American Can Co., Greenwich, Conn.—feature a ring-pull, full-panel opening end and a plastic reclosure cap and are said to reduce rancidity and increase shelf life compared to croutons packaged in conventional paperboard containers.

Low-sodium products for salt-restricted diets being introduced nationally in single-serving cans by the Campbell Soup Co., Camden, N.J.,

include Chunky Beef Soup, Chunky Chicken
Soup, and Chili Con Carne with Beans.

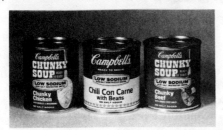

Reprinted with permission from *Food Technology*, 29(12): 68 (December 1975). Copyright 1975 by Institute of Food Technologists.

Breakfast Bestseller

Bacon and eggs, toast, waffles, pancakes have their devotees, but the most popular American breakfast is cold cereal with milk. So, at least, say cereal makers, and they have some figures to back up their claim. From 1967 through 1972, cereal sales hardly grew at all, but since then they have been rising rapidly—by 13% in 1973, 8% in 1974 and nearly 6% last year, to 1.8 billion lbs. In those three years, dollar sales have risen from $1.1 billion to $1.7 billion, and per capita consumption of cereal has expanded almost a third, from about 6 lbs. in 1972 to nearly 8 lbs. in 1975.

The years of the boom have been a period first of roaring inflation, then of deep recession, and those misfortunes seem to have increased the main appeal of breakfast cereals: economy. Says Kellogg's Corporate Publications Manager Rolfe Jenkins: "People on tight budgets have found cold cereal a good buy." With reason: the Cereal Institute, Inc., calculates the cost of an average 1-oz. serving of cereal and 4 oz. of milk at just under 11¢, even after the price rises of recent times. In addition, more and more married women are working outside the home; husbands and children who have to make their own breakfasts are increasingly inclined to reach for a box of cereal. Manufacturers also have make cereals more nutritious, partly in response to testimony by diet experts who in 1970 told a Senate subcommittee that many widely sold cereals had little or no nutritional value. The year before those hearings, only 16% of cold cereals were fortified with vitamins and iron; by 1973, 85% were.

Though prosperous, the cereal market remains a turbulent one in which no fewer than 156 brands, produced by about 55 manufacturers, fight for sales. The count changes

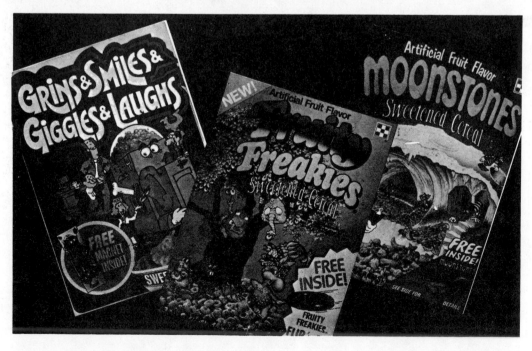

constantly, because cereal makers keep bringing out new brands—usually spending $3 to $5 million on advertising to introduce them—in order to catch the buyer's attention.

A Lot of Puff? The competition is hottest in presweetened cereals, which captured 31% of sales last year. Falling sugar prices are encouraging manufacturers to step up introductions of new brands: General Mills is bringing out Fruit Brutes, aiming to win kids away from Kellogg's Fruit Loops, and Ralston Purina is offering Fruity Freakies. Later this year Ralston will introduce Moonstones, a fruit-flavored cereal in crescent, star, and sphere shapes, and Grins & Smiles & Giggles & Laughs, which (so kids will be told) stream from the mouth of a "computer-type monster" named Cecil when his "funny bone" is tickled. New brands of presweetened cereals frequent-

ly have a short life: Post's Pink Panther Flakes, Quaker Oats' Quake Quangaroos and General Mills' Baron von Redberry have all been introduced and then dropped in the past four years.

Curiously, cereal makers are rather reticent in talking about their recent sales successes. Reason: a Federal Trade Commission investigation that began in 1972 and is likely to wind up in a few months. The FTC is seeking to determine whether Kellogg's, General Mills, General Foods (which markets Post cereals) and Quaker Oats have monopolized the market by flooding it with similar brands and advertising them on a scale that smaller competitors cannot match. The FTC, in other words, suspects that the competition is all a lot of puff; to the cereal makers, it seems only too real.

Reprinted with permission from *Time,* The Weekly Newsmagazine, 107 (12):61 (22 March 1976). Copyright 1976 by Time Inc.

Pringle's Vs. the Real Thing

JOHN EGERTON

Is the Lowly Potato Chip A Match for P.&G.?

NASHVILLE—The chips are down. In one corner is a corporate Goliath, the nation's largest advertiser with the distributive know-how and power to shove its products onto merchant's shelves—and juggle prices until it can build a market.

In the other corner is a scattered group of companies, 100 or so and including some giants, but mostly small, local manufacturers.

The struggle, of course, is between Procter & Gamble Company and its Pringle's "new fangled potato chips" (which aren't exactly potato chips) and the old line makers of honest-to-goodness chips.

P. & G. hasn't actually made a better tasting chip, but it's made a great leap forward in synthesizing, manufacturing and packaging—areas where cost-cutting turns into profit. The competition can just say they're making the same old good-tasting product that's pleased Americans for a century and even won the enthusiasm and praise of the late Nikita Khrushchev (who ordered chip production in the Soviet Union).

Don't bet against Goliath.

Just last week P. & G. won a major victory when the Food and Drug Administration said that after December, 1977—two years from now—Pringle's-like chips made from dehydrated potatoes must be identified as "potato chips made from dried potatoes" in lettering on the label "not less than one-half the size of the largest type in which the words 'potato chips' appear." The lettering now is smaller than this.

The key to the Government decision is that it allows Procter & Gamble to call its Pringle's "potato chips," which by dictionary definition they aren't (Webster's defines the potato chip as "thin slices of raw potato fried in deep fat").

The stakes in that decision are big: Just how big the potato chip market is and what share Procter & Gamble has won is guesswork. P. & G. as usual isn't saying. But it's estimated that chip sales volume will be about $1.5 billion this year and Pringle's has grabbed 10 percent of it. The F.D.A. says these "new fangled" chips, largely Pringle's, already have captured as much as 25 percent of the market in some areas.

At the Potato Chip Institute International in Euclid, Ohio, Lawrence Burch, executive vice president, admits the F.D.A. ruling is a setback for makers of real potato chips.

"For 65 years Webster's dictionary has defined a potato chip as a thin slice of raw potato, fried crisp and then salted. The F.D.A. held to that definition until 1969, when Procter & Gamble began to test-market Pringle's. Then, without notice to anyone, the F.D.A. gave Procter & Gamble permission to go ahead with the use of the words 'potato chips' on its product," Mr. Burch said.

P. & G. won't discuss its manufacturing process, but basically its potatoes are dehydrated, then turned into a mush and pressed and fried. It's believed Procter & Gamble, the nation's leading manufacturer of laundry detergents, shampoos, toothpaste, shortening, disposable diapers and toilet paper (sales were $4.9 billion and profits were $317 million in 1974) spent 10 years and $70 million to research, develop, manufacture and market its first Pringle's.

But their development went a long way toward solving a basic potato-chip problem, one that had kept any one manufacturer from dominating the market.

The natural chips are easily broken, which means they don't get shipped very far—and shipping natural potato chips means paying for shipping a lot of air because of their haphazard shape. What's more, they spoil and can't be kept on a grocery shelf more than a few months. But the uniform shape of Pringle's means easy packing and shipping in sealed, tennis ball-like containers which, combined with the use of preservatives, extended shelf life to a year.

There are essentially two views of Pringle's.

One is that they are an ever-crisp, tasty product that will dominate the market. The other is that they are another ersatz product shot through with chemical preservatives, symbolic of industry's debasement of American food.

"What P. & G. engineers have done with Pringle's," wrote food industry critic John Hightower in his recent book "Eat Your Heart Out," is to "devise an acceptable chip-like structure that makes potato chip oligopoly possible for the first time." He also charges the new product with trying to capture a consumer market with an inferior product, an adulterated one made from cheaper grades of potatoes but costing more than regular chips.

The F.D.A. in its announcement acknowledged the "intra-industry competitive struggle" and said "making potato chips from dried potato granules instead of from raw potato slices effects a change in the basic integrity of the product." But the agency also said that adding the phrase "made from dried potatoes" accurately describes the restructured product.

Pringle's already has passed many smaller manufacturers in sales even though it's been marketed nationally only since May. Wise Potato Chips, a unit of Borden, Inc., and Frito-Lay, made by Pepsico Inc., still are ahead of Pringle's.

At the first Pringle's plant, in Jackson, Tenn., visitors are definitely unwelcome. The production of 800 employees is kept secret, although it is put at 300 million canisters a year by some observers.

"They are very security minded," said Larry D. Welch, executive director of the Jackson Chamber of Commerce, who didn't want to say anything about the operation. This year P. & G. opened a second plant in Greenville, N.C.

"We've long believed," chairman Edward G. Harness has told an interviewer, "that there's nothing to be gained by telling our competitors how we do things. We'd rather have them spend the time trying to find out."

Why do shoppers buy Pringle's?

A spot check at supermarkets in Jackson, and in nearby Tennessee cities show the price to be the same as for regular potato chips in some stores and as much as 13 cents higher in others. That's true elsewhere, too. In Upper Montclair, N.J., for example, a 9-ounce package of Pringle's sells for 99 cents, or 11 cents an ounce, while A. & P.'s 10-ounce box of Jane Parker chips sells for 85 cents, or 8.5 cents an ounce. Two other brands—Wise and Valley Maid—are priced at 79 cents for 8-ounce bags, or 9.9 cents an ounce.

One Jackson market manager noted that price markdowns, special displays and advertising campaigns for Pringle's are the rule rather than the exception.

"They put on a lot of special promotions for Pringle's and during those weeks they sell as well as all other chips combined. But when there's no special on, the regular chips outsell Pringle's four or five to one," he said.

P. & G.'s competitors have decided to join them: At least three—Frito-Lay, Laura Scudder (made by Pet Inc.) and Planters (Standard Brands Inc.) have come up with similar products in look-alike cans.

The remainder of the industry, seeing the cost of potatoes and cooking oil soaring and the consumption of chips leveling off, can only hope customers will choose the traditional taste over the taste of Pringle's and its imitators.

"In terms of flavor and texture," says Mr. Burch of the Potato Chip Institute, "there is no question that Pringle's are an inferior product."

But shoppers may be saying something else and in the words of Mr. Harness of Procter & Gamble, "The essence of consumerism is giving them what they want."

Reprinted with permission from *The New York Times*, Sect. 3:1+ (30 November 1975). Copyright 1975 by the New York Times Company.

Potato Chip Makers Anticipate a "New" Pringle's; Better Flavor?

LARRY EDWARDS

CHICAGO — Pringle's vs. the real thing—the potato chip war—is far from over.

Makers of "real" chips, especially the strong regional brands, await Procter & Gamble's next moves with its dehydrated chip entry, meanwhile refining the comparison advertising approaches with which they have successfully fought off the heavy P&G ad attack.

Standard Brands has cut into Pringle's sales in the Southeast with its Planters potato chips, similarly formulated, stacked and packaged. In the same region, a canister-packed "real" french fried potato called Daddy Crisp has done even better than Planters, reports say, and is gearing up for national expansion. And Frito-Lay, the leading corn chipper, has taken a new tack which may broaden the battle—introduction of a stacked corn chip into test.

It has been seven years since Procter & Gamble upset the potato chip industry by moving into test with "newfangled" Pringle's potato chips—fabricated, the "real" chippers say; loaded with additives. But Pringle's offered several advantages: Long shelf life, warehouse distribution, uniform shape, unbroken chips, packaged in unique, convenient canisters (tennis ball cans, say the "real" chippers).

Concluding its slow national rollout last spring with an expensive push into the New York and Southern California areas, P&G's Pringle's has earned an estimated annual sales of $150,000,000. But in an expanded $1.5 billion business, that falls short of the 25% market share the product attained in early markets, and probably somewhat short of what P&G had hoped to maintain.

P&G also won its equally long legal hassle over whether it could, in fact, call Pringle's a potato chip, when the Food & Drug Administration concluded recently that it could—with the stipulation that by 1977 labeling play up more prominently the term "made from dried potatoes" (AA, Dec. 1).

(At the time of that ruling, not only the trade and business press, but newsweeklies, daily newspapers, even public tv—which gave it a half-hour on WNET, New York—have summed up the effects of P&G's revolutionary development.)

Today the food industry is busy anticipating the battle lines to be drawn. Some industry sources expect P&G to launch a ridged chip, like the Planters entry and Frito-Lay's well established Ruffles brand.

Yet the strongest speculation, which takes into account a classic P&G approach, plus what has been cited as Pringle's major weakness, is that P&G will be launching a "new, improved" version of its chip. According to reliable reports, the company has patented a "potato flavor enhancer," which sources say will be the essence of an improved Pringle's. P&G's main problem with its brand is repeat, not trial, purchases. And that comes down to taste, if not price.

At the Advertising Research Foundation's annual conference in New York Nov. 10, John Adler of AdTel gave a presentation on tv advertising frequency and purchasing behavior, comparing three potato chip brands—Pringle's, Ruffles and Lay's. The study involved a 56-week period using AdTel's regular weekly purchase diary (a 28-week pre-test period and 28-week test period).

Standing out in the results: Pringle's gained 4.1% total market share points among pre-test non-users, but lost 7.9% total market share points among families who were pre-test users of Pringle's. "Clearly," Mr. Adler's report stated, "Pringle's had a problem in maintaining share among its users." During the last 28-week period, the study noted, Pringle's ran twice as many commercials as the other two brands combined.

In a summary conclusion on advertising, the report said: "Pringle's advertising was either at saturation levels or relatively ineffective in retaining share among established buyers."

Nationally, sources put Pringle's share of the potato chip market at from 10% to 15%, below the 20% to 25% share widely reported previous to its concluding expansion moves. Broadcast ad expenditures, in the first nine months of '75, hit just over $6,500,000, mostly in spot tv.

Competitors, meanwhile, have been hammering away at the taste angle, through an over-all, major theme of natural ingredients as opposed to Pringle's additives.

Largely credited as the first regional chipper to launch that attack is Jay Foods, Chicago. With well over 50% of the potato chip market here, Jay's responded aggressively with its "We're for real" ad campaign (via Marsteller Inc.) when Pringle's entered this market in 1973.

The head-on comparison of real chips vs. dehydrated chips was picked up by other regionals as Pringle's rolled eastward, and undoubtedly helped the local No.1's retain their positions. In fact, preparatory to Pringle's New York invasion, the No.1 chip there—Wise—requested Jay's materials as a guide for its own campaign, handled by Needham, Harper & Steers.

Smaller brands, of course, have been hurt by Pringle's. Lay's potato chips apparently is one of them. Although it is a national entry, in many markets the Frito-Lay chip is No. 2 or lower.

Frito-Lay earlier responded to the P&G entry with a test of its own Crunch Barrel, a dehydrated potato-based, stackable, canister-packaged chip (AA, Aug. 12, '74). The Dallas marketer even tried warehouse distribution for the entry, a system many retailers prefer. Crunch Barrel has since been withdrawn.

Now F-L is making a new bid. Within the last few weeks, it moved into Columbia, S.C., and one other market with Sun Chips, a flat, round, uniformly shaped corn chip. Packaging is pure Pringle's: Twin canisters of 4½ oz. each, with resealable plastic lids. The company is, however, using its store-door distribution system for the corn chip.

A series of tv commercials out of Foote, Cone & Belding, New York, will support Sun Chips. The name was earlier used for a regular potato chip tested by the company in Memphis (AA, Feb. 18, '74), handled by Young & Rubicam.

If Pringle's is struggling with taste, its packaging and distribution innovations are accorded due credit throughout the industry. One chipper conducted research which revealed that many households buy both Pringle's and "the real thing"—the latter for immediate use and a can of Pringle's which is kept in reserve for unexpected guests.

The strongest direct challenger to Pringle's thus far appears to be Planters potato chips, from Standard Brands (AA, Nov. 11, '74). Planters has rolled out in the Southeast, and according to reports has made some inroads into the Pringle's business in that area. Also "made from dried potatoes," also in 4½-oz. canisters, the entry has been getting heavy tv, newspaper and couponing support. (The account recently shifted from J. Walter Thompson Co. to Benton & Bowles, along with other Standard Brands business.) Ads play up taste: "The new stackable chip with the perfect taste. A taste you've never experienced in any other stackable chip."

Other marketers who have adopted the dehydrated, stacked approach include Laura Scudder's Dittos on the West Coast and Mrs. Bumby's from General Mills, recently expanded into

Houston from a Lima, O., test.

Ad copy for Mrs. Bumby's notes, "It's the new potato chip sensation with the sensational potato chip taste. People tell us they taste better than chips in a can." Dancer-Fitzgerald-Sample, New York, is now handling the entry, which had been at Wells, Rich, Greene.

Using the Pringle's packaging idea but opting for the "real thing" has been the Daddy Crisp french fries entry, marketed by Daddy Crisp Co., Atlanta, in a joint venture with Intex Products. The product has achieved a 10% or better market share in its southeastern markets since introduction last summer, and the company has gone on stream with a second plant.

Daddy Crisp, recently moved into Cleveland as a test, is expected to begin rolling national by spring. Weltin Advertising is handling the product, getting tv, print and couponing support.

Reprinted with permission from *Advertising Age.* 47(3):3 (19 January 1976). Copyright 1976 by Crain Communications, Inc.

Pringle's Status Secure; Chippers Opt for Protest

ATLANTA — After two stormy sessions at an annual conference here last week, the Potato Chip Institute International decided to send a "protest letter" to the Food & Drug Administration, calling on FDA chief Alexander Schmidt to rescind the decision of seven years ago allowing Procter & Gamble Co.'s Pringle's to be called a potato chip.

The action is considered by many sources as indication that the group finally has given up its long fight against Pringle's. The closed-door meetings were described as "heated," with many members wanting to go to court in an effort to overturn FDA, and in the end losing out to a more moderate faction.

PCII's letter also attacks the FDA ruling of November, 1975, which requires labeling changes for the fabricated chips (AA, Dec.1) with the term "made from dried potatoes" to be printed in type half the size of the words "potato chips." The group is asking that this ruling become effective in 90 days, rather than the end of 1977.

According to PCII, "the regulation permits mislabeling to continue for another two years, all without a semblance of justification." It asked FDA "to fulfill its statutory duty by taking action to prohibit continued marketing of these misbranded products."

The group said the use of "dual-size type permitted by regulation is unprecedented, unlawful and unwarranted under the circumstances."

Meanwhile, stackable, fabricated chips continue to make news. General Mills, Minneapolis, is planning continued expansion of its Mrs. Bumby's potato chips, soon moving into the Denver market. The product, first introduced into test in Lima, O., in mid-74, was expanded into Houston last fall. Dancer-Fitzgerald-Sample, New York, handles.

Pet Inc.'s Laura Scudder division, a West Coast region chipper, has revamped its Dittos brand stack chips. Laura Scudder was the first marketer to copy the Pringle's canister packaging, but now it has gone back to foil-wrapped packages while continuing to stack the uniformly shaped chips. Agency for Dittos is Siteman/Brodhead, Beverly Hills, Cal.

Reprinted with permission from *Advertising Age*. 47(6):2 (9 February 1976). Copyright 1976 by Crain Communications, Inc.

Pringle's Loses Some Skirmishes

ANNE COLAMOSCA

The Great Potato Chip War that broke out last year when Procter & Gamble opened its national marketing campaign for Pringle's in their tube-shaped red packages is still going strong—and the big and highly regarded company has been taking some lumps.

Pringle's, nationally advertised as the "new-fangled" potato chips, battled it out gallantly with the small but hearty Clover Club in Utah markets and lost miserably. Large batteries of advertising cannons were brought out in Philadelphia against Wise, but again Pringle's took a severe beating. In Chicago Pringle's was firmly trounced by local potato chip czar Leonard Japp and his Jay Foods.

When Procter & Gamble, the nation's largest advertiser and marketer of packaged products, decided to move into the potato chip market 11 years ago no one at P. & G. thought they'd take over the market immediately. Procter & Gamble doesn't work that way.

The company, with scores of marketing successes in the past, is methodical, cautious and deliberate. For 10 years it struggled to produce a potato chip that could be shipped anywhere in the country—unlike any other potato chip on the market—and not crumble to bits or turn rancid in the process.

Researchers worked to develop a product that would not be mistaken for something else—like, for example, a snack food that would account for no more than a small percentage of the extremely profitable, $1.5 billion potato chip business. "They slaved and slaved over this concept," says one former P. & G. man. "Not too thin, not too thick. That's why it took an entire decade."

Now, the year after Pringle's glittering $15 million advertising debut, many food industry experts are calling the effort a "washout" and a "bomb." From a respectable 18 percent of the market, Pringle's has slipped to 10 percent over the last several months—a modest share of the market considering P. & G.'s mighty marketing clout and elaborate distribution system.

"It's doing lousy. We just can't sell the stuff," says John Catsimitdis of New York City's Red Apple supermarket chain. "Our store managers don't want it cluttering up their shelves. It costs them too much money."

Until Pringle's came into the picture, the potato chip industry was dominated by a handful of strong regional chains, most of which have been bought up by larger corporations over the years but which still operate with considerable autonomy and are regarded as local industry. Among the largest of the 100 or so companies in the chip business are Borden's Wise Potato Chips, headquartered in Berwick, Pa.; Pet's Laura Scudder division in southern California, Pepsico's Frito-Lay division in Texas and the independent Jay Foods in Chicago.

Leonard Japp, president of Jay Foods in Chicago, claims his share of the local market has jumped a couple of points, to 82%. Pringle's hit the Chicago market in 1973 before going national, when Jay, like the rest of the industry, was already in a tough position because of record potato shortages and soaring costs. Nevertheless Jay dove into an expensive direct advertising blitz that promptly shattered Pringle's.

Although there's been steady growth in the larger companies like Jay Foods, the business remained basically regional because potato chips have short, six-week shelf lives and must be shipped by local distributors to each supermarket. Pringle's, on the other hand, was created to overcome this problem. Made from dehydrated potato mash mixed with mono- and di-glycerides and butylated hydroxyanisole—as competitors are quick to point out—Pringle's has a two-year shelf life.

Curious customers across the country swarmed to stores to buy the novel potato chips, but evidently many stopped coming after they got through the first couple of cans. The most commonly repeated slur against Pringle's is that they "taste like cardboard."

"Pringle's is a major brand and we estimate that it is about tied for the lead in the U.S. potato chip market," said a Procter & Gamble spokesman. "Our volume has shown recent growth." Industry experts estimate that, at best, Pringle's will sell $150 million—a very substantial volume—in 1976, not far behind the $225 million of the top-selling brand, Frito's.

Meanwhile, at the same time that traditional potato chip manufacturers have been berating P. & G. over the airwaves for churning out a fabricated product, they have been test marketing and researching their own brands of fabricated chips, just in case the market swings that way.

The whole potato chip project has been costly for P. & G. Its highly automated Tennessee plant is estimated to have cost about $70 million, and there is a second, smaller plant in North Carolina. But despite the fact that it seems to be losing right now, P. & G. has time and money on its side. For, most important of all, the artificial chip is cheaper to produce and distribute over the long run. "The cost factor will be extremely important over the next couple of years," says Ed Jones, vice president of Mitchell, Hutchins Inc., the Wall Street firm. "P. & G. can keep bringing in new versions of Pringle's with different tastes and keep cutting prices."

Moreover, P. & G. has obviously convinced a consortium of European food firms that prefabricated potato chips are the way to go for Common Market countries too. The first of the now familiar canister-packed chips called "Chipsletten" went on the market in German grocery stores last May.

"Those people who think Pringle's is washed up don't know P. & G. very well," says Hercules Segalas, analyst and senior vice president of Drexel Burnham Lambert, another big investment house. "It will take a lot more to get them to throw in the towel."

Reprinted with permission from *The New York Times*, Sect. F: 13 (14 November 1976). Copyright 1976 by The New York Times Company.

Food Brokers Hear of 'Convenience' Challenge

SAN FRANCISCO—Grant C. Gentry, president of the Great Atlantic & Pacific Tea Co., told the National Food Brokers Assn. convention here that he believes consumers will be looking for more small convenience stores in the future.

These stores will offer a limited number of products—perhaps as few as 500 or less, rather than the thousands currently found in a suburban supermarket, Mr. Gentry said, as he examined areas of mutual retailer and broker interest.

"Ironically, such smaller stores have begun to flourish as a kind of pilot fish to the supermarket whale. The consumer seems to be telling us that this is the size store she wants when she's *not* having a 'one-stop shopping' experience."

Consumers will want these smaller stores while at the same time also wanting more of the large, "one-stop" stores offering general merchandise, pharmaceuticals and other products in addition to groceries. Consumers will be looking for the stocking of an "ever broader variety of products, both national and company brands, but perhaps in sizes more suitable to individual needs," he added.

One of the greatest challenges the industry faces in the next decade is to give the consumer palatable packaged and frozen food at competitive prices that can be easily reconstituted in conventional and microwave ovens so that people will continue to eat at home instead of the nearest fast-food operation, he said.

"If there is any one single opportunity that faces us today, it is the disposition of people to eat away from home. We can and must, if we are to survive, meet this challenge *now*," Mr. Gentry said.

Inflation has undoubtedly increased the incidence of failure in retailing, Mr. Gentry said. It has led consumers to alter shopping patterns and it also has made A&P "very conscious of protecting margins, a fact of marketing life that has a direct bearing on our mutual operations. We're put in the position of having to move merchandise through our system with greater velocity and are less likely to dilly-dally over new products, insisting instead that they prove their salability with all speed."

Noting that A&P has undertaken what will be a five-year, $500,000,000 revamping program, Mr. Gentry said the program has included an altering of the merchandising mix, "with greater shelf space allotted to national brands and nonfood merchandise. Our many new, larger supermarkets will have more than 25% of shelf space given over to general merchandise," he said. A&P's ad and promotion programs have been "dramatically increased," he noted, with greater emphasis on local tie-ins.

Donald R. McCurry, executive vp. A. C. Nielson Co., suggested to the NFBA convention that "within our much publicized 'flat' population trend, there are many subcurrents that represent sales and marketing opportunities—growth in young marrieds, infants and senior citizens; renewed vigor in rural areas, and steady movement from one place to another.

The "working wife ratio" in 1975 was 44%, up from the 1950 level of 24%, he pointed out. This statistic should "make us seriously question whether the swing away from convenience foods that occurred during the last recession—

in 1974 and 1975—is permanent. With this kind of a working wife ratio, I maintain that the need for high-quality convenience food will continue to grow long term," he said.

Private label or controlled brands should maintain their present market share of 28% to 29% of some 35 packaged grocery product categories, a share that has held steady over the past five years, he said.

Reprinted with permission from *Advertising Age.* 47 (50): 3 (13 December 1976). Copyright 1976 by Crain Communications, Inc.

USDA Proposes Snack Of Fortified Milkshake

USDA's Food and Nutrition Service (FNS) has proposed regulations allowing use of a "formulated, fortified milk-based product" as an alternative to the two-component snack now served in some summer feeding projects.

Summer feeding projects may serve up to three full meals daily plus mid-morning and mid-afternoon snacks. The proposed beverage would replace snacks consisting of a serving of milk, juice, fruit or vegetable, and a serving of bread or equivalent.

The FNS proposal...represents an attempt to give full legitimacy to products that the Department has allowed into summer feeding projects on a pilot basis since 1972. The proposed beverage is patterned after the Mead-Johnson product "Sustical," which is currently used in about 200 projects nation-wide, mostly in the South. The largest summer project using Sustical is in Savannah, Georgia, and feeds about 6,000 children, according to Mead-Johnson officials.

Kermit Bird, an FNS nutrition and technical services official, told CNI Weekly Report that the fortified milkshakes, which are stored in cans, offer convenience and good nutrition at a slightly higher cost than conventional foods to projects that wish to save on labor or handling costs.

Robert Fay, government affairs director for Mead-Johnson, told CNI Weekly Report that Sustical costs 19 cents for a six-ounce serving as against 17 cents for a minimal bread-and-milk snack. Summer feeding programs are now allowed 21.25 cents in federal reimbursement for snacks and between-meal supplements.

Fay said Mead-Johnson had originally promoted Sustical to physicians for use in hospitals, but the product found its way into day care and summer feeding projects. "We seem to do better in the South, where the summer programs are smaller in size," he said. "The larger programs don't usually serve a snack; food vendors usually don't want to be bothered. Savannah wanted a snack but it was afraid of wastage and spoilage. With Sustical, there are no litter problems, no waste and no spoilage And the kids like it."

Fay noted that Sustical is low in fat and in lactose, the milk sugar that often causes indigestion in black children and adults.

Fay said Mead-Johnson does not recommend Sustical for daily use, only one or two days per week to add flexibility to the snack pattern. "Perhaps on Mondays when the staff is pressed or on Friday with the weekend coming up," Fay said. "Or, if a project has it on hand, they can just open up a few cans if extra kids show up that day."

Not everyone is sold on Sustical or its proposed counterpart. Such products are generally high in sugar and fat so as to provide a high level of calories and palatability. The USDA proposal also raises the issue of whether a fortified milkshake in a can represents appropriate nutrition education for children.

Reprinted with permission from CNI Weekly Report, VI (31):4-5 (29 July 1976).

Restaurant Food: Frozen, Cooked, Then Refrozen and Recooked

JOHN L. HESS

"They ate frozen meat, frozen fried potatoes and frozen peas. Blindfolded one could not have identified the peas, and the only flavor the potatoes had was the flavor of soap. It was the monotonous fare of the beseiged . . . but . . . where was the enemy?

—*John Cheever in*
"The Wapshot Scandal" (1963)

When Mr. and Mrs. America step out to dine by candlelight, the chances are growing that they will eat the same sort of thing they left at home: TV dinners. The quality will be the same, but the price will be considerably higher.

Frozen foods have already taken over the quick-service industry. Now they are making inroads into the luxury trade. An executive selling equipment to the industry said the other day, "I think 1973 is the year of the breakthrough."

The extent of the breakthrough is difficult to measure. As a food supplier to luxury restaurants explained, "You won't get them to admit it, for obvious reasons."

Obviously, the clientele will not want to pay luxury prices for vending-machine food. But that is precisely what is happening.

Precooked frozen foods are not as good as well-prepared dishes made to order from well-chosen raw materials nor, in the long run, are they as cheap.

Under the best prevailing industrial techniques, such as flash freezing and drying at minus 52 degrees, cell walls are destroyed and texture and flavor damaged. Cryogenic freezing, at more than 300 degrees below zero, is better but requires large and costly equipment, and its advocates can only claim that it is "almost as good" as fresh.

Many foods, notably fish, are now frozen in bulk, then thawed and precooked, then frozen again, suffering further damage. In shipment and storage before consumption, they frequently are permitted to rise to temperatures where deterioration is speeded, despite the "Mark of Zero" campaign by the industry to encourage handlers to keep foods at zero.

In store and home refrigerators, these vulnerable foods often reach dangerously high temperatures. Finally, the product is usually thawed—in restaurants this is sometimes called "slushing down"—to 38 or 40 degrees before the final recooking. This again poses problems.

A majority of restaurants now own microwave or convection pressure ovens or other equipment especially designed for frozen foods. A handicap of precooked dishes is that each component has its own specific reaction to such heating, so that part cooks too fast, part too slow—and all in an unnatural manner.

This explains a recent experience in an expensive and famous Connecticut inn, where a rack of lamb ordered rare arrived at table cold.

To bring the precooked lamb up to proper temperature would have required serving it well-done. The only solution was to tell the client that rare lamb had to be cold, a patent absurdity.

A recent survey by Quick Frozen Foods, a trade publication, found that a majority of restaurants use some prepared frozen foods and plan to use more. The survey also showed that up to 80 per cent and even more of the fare sold by many chains and industrial feeders has been at least partly precooked.

$9 for 'Frozen' Filet Mignon

Tom Finnegan, a senior editor, commented: "It is not unusual to dine in a first-class 'steak house' in New York's theater district and pay $9 for a filet mignon that was delivered in a frozen state.

"Some processors have developed excellent precooked beef roasts that can be finished to the rareness requested by patrons," he went on. "Frozen turkey breasts, with the natural skin attached, can be finished to look like turkeys made from scratch. . . . The popularity of Surf 'n' Turf, combining lobster tails and filet mignon, has done much to hike the use of frozen seafood and meat.

"Breaded shrimp, oysters, crab meat, specialties, lobster Newburg and pompano are packed in attractive packages with four-color illustrations and tend to make a chef proud of preparing a gourmet entreé," Mr. Finnegan reported.

Many restaurant owners say the shortage and high price of skilled help are major reasons they turn to frozen foods. But kitchen wages are among the lowest in all industries, and the shortage of help may be a result, rather than a cause, of conditions in the trade.

A reader says his wife applied for a job with the Stouffer's chain and was told that they didn't need any cooks, only "thawer-outers." An executive acknowledged that the chain was "not a chef system but a food management system."

Mr. Finnegan wrote that the independents, who have yielded only belatedly to the $8-billion-a-year frozen-food movement, were being forced out of business by, among other things, high rentals on express highways and in new skyscrapers, where the chains install "in" dining spots at several levels, all served by a central thawing point.

He said that there had been some friction between the food packers, who prefer large "economy" packages, and the small restaurant operators, who want individual portions to reduce spoilage. He explained:

"Their reasoning is that if an item that costs them $1 is increased by a few cents for packaging, it's better to lose the extra cost in the kitchen rather than lose the $5 the item can bring at the table, if it fails to satisfy the customer."

The figures are revealing. Normally, the industry figures that the cost of food represents 30 to 40 per cent of the bill to the customer. The markup on prepared foods is much larger, the work and care minimal.

Food Processing, another trade journal, remarks that for quick-food chains, a sack of frozen French fries costs 5 cents and is sold for 20 cents. "Only soft drinks yield a greater percentage of profit," it says.

Mushiness in French Fries

Even the best cryogenically frozen precooked French fries, crisped in hot fat before serving, have a telltale mushiness inside. Several managers of moderately expensive restaurants were asked why it made more sense to maintain a complex industry with freezing plants, packaging, refrigerated trucks and special restaurant equipment, than to peel and fry spuds the proper, old-fashioned way.

"I swear you can't tell the difference," one of them said. "The frozen costs more, but what you don't use keeps, and you don't have to peel the potatoes, and keep them dry, and so on."

Amateurism in restaurant management was given as another reason: the inability to organize kitchen work and keep a staff busy.

The ignorance of the public was also cited.

The sudden appearance everywhere of "homemade" loaves of sweet bread is an example. Actually, they are made from frozen dough, and are fairly sad nourishment.

"Reconstituted, these have the appearance of homemade bread," Mr. Finnegan writes. "When brought to table on a cutting board, along with a sharp knife and generous amounts of butter or margarine, the loaves serve as an 'icebreaker' in gaining the patron's confidence in the restaurant's food and service."

Restaurant owners boast that many clients take leftover bread home, and buy more at the counter as they leave. Frozen baked goods are driving many bakers out of the trade.

Precooked Vegetables Due

Also nearly universal in restaurants now are frozen or synthetic juices, frozen fish sticks and nondairy or sterilized "cream." Coming up fast are precooked vegetables, seafood and frozen "gourmet" dishes and grilled meats in Pliofilm bags.

Now being test-marketed are frozen breakfasts on a tray, with fruit slices, French toast and roll. Omelets and scrambled eggs will be added later—the technicians have not yet solved the mystery of eggs sunny side up.

Frank M. Barrett, a group vice president of Howard Johnson's, recently summarized the philosophy of the movement in an interview on productivity, in *Fast Foods* magazine:

"I think anybody who's not using convenience foods is out of it. And some of the prepared food around today is top quality. You'd never know the difference. We're going to open a restaurant a week this year, and where could we get cooks and chefs for this kind of expansion? Even if we could get them we couldn't train them fast enough."

Reprinted with permission from *The New York Times*, Sect.1:30 (16 August 1973). Copyright 1973 by The New York Times Company.

A World of 'Idiot Proof' Crepes and Pseudo-Delicatessen Meat

MIMI SHERATON

CHICAGO—Food well seasoned with mendacity seems to be the specialty of an ever-increasing number of restaurants around the country. For while most of the public still naively assumes the food served in a restaurant was actually prepared on the premises by a resident chef or cook, more and more restaurateurs, eager to cut labor costs and to simplify their lives in general, are buying prepared convenience foods and palming them off as their own creations.

That, at least, is the conclusion one has to draw after seeing food exhibited last week at the National Restaurant Association's annual trade show here.

Grist for the Mill

The record crowd of 100,000 visitors (restaurant owners, hotel and institutional food service managers, dealers and franchise chain operators) who viewed the 907 exhibits saw, in addition to a phantasmagorical array of kitchen equipment and dining-room appointments, a dreary larder of convenience foods in varying stages of preparation, from meats that were merely pre-cut and frozen though raw, to fully cooked entrées that need only be reheated.

Exponents of so-called truth-in-dining legislation, aimed at forcing restaurant owners to tell on their menus which dishes were not made in their kitchen, would have found plenty of grist for their mills at this show.

The big news was crepes, with easy-to-use mixes substituting for fresh eggs and milk, and crepemaking machinery of varying types, all designed to be what is known in the trade as "idiot-proof." Not one of the half-dozen crepes tested was anything but pasty, tasteless and sticky.

Now that turkey no longer tastes like turkey, there's a big push on to make it taste like something else. The result is a group of pseudo-delicatessen meats called turkey-salami, turkey pastrami, turkey-ham and turkey bologna, made entirely of turkey, colored, spiced, smoked and textured to simulate the costlier, fattier originals. Although made by three or four different processors, all of the versions tasted were identically damp, limp, salty and more or less peppery.

A number of meats looked less than promising, including pre-sliced, sandwich portions of delicatessen meats sealed in boiling bags and accounting for much of the steamy, gray pastrami and corned beef sandwiches one is served these days in coffee shops and roadside chain eateries. Frozen-precooked steaks and hamburgers with grid marks that were seared or painted on and rubbery, frozen, cooked sausage patties seemed bad enough to make one give up eating altogether.

Oscar Mayer introduced "special tenderloin steaks," formed of two tenderloins dusted with tripolyphosphate so they stay together after being sealed in casings and frozen.

A company salesman showed them off, saying proudly, "Don't they look like hockey pucks?" I had to admit they did.

Swift's canned cooked bacon had a handy

feature, pointed out by a representative: "The bacon has to be heated if you want it crisp. But lots of schools use it cold, right from the can, when making bacon, tomato and lettuce sandwiches."

Dried Lettuce

There was nothing surprising or remarkable about the vinyl gardens full of frozen or canned vegetables, but I was not quite prepared for dried lettuce and salad greens, processed by Fresh Foods Inc. and Orval Kent, "The Salad People."

Shredded lettuce is spun-dried in a centrifuge, then packed in plastic bags and cartons and sent out to fast food chains for burgers, as well as to countless restaurants for their salad bars. Both slaw and lettuce, treated this way, looked like slightly moistened, pale-green excelsior.

Frying was by far the most popular method of cooking and by noon each day the air was cloudy with rising grease and steam. Almost everything that was fried was breaded, good news to the people at Golden Dipt, the company that makes most of the batters and breadings used by restaurants and institutions.

"If it's edible, it's breadable," was their motto, and looking around the hall it was hard to doubt the claim.

It is hard to recall just how many crisp, golden tubes of deep-fried air I sampled, but there were at least three dozen, in the guises of onion rings, shrimp or potatoes, all made from pastes, powders or dicings that cooked hollow and were virtually indiscernible from each other.

Potatoes took, perhaps, the worst beating of all, in metallic tasting potato pancake mixes (Tato-mix), or, grimmer yet, in French's Automash, a dispenser that spews forth "hot-buttery-flavored mashed potatoes." Press the button and what comes out is a milky-gray stream of mush which thickens as it stands. "In just seven seconds it's all set," said the demonstrator and she was right.

Any chef working with instant mashed potatoes is, of course, stuck when he wants to make stuffed baked potatoes because he has no shells. To come to his rescue Keebler has devised Tater Shells, small brown oval boats that look as though they were formed of stiffened brown wrapping paper but made, wildly enough, from Idaho potatoes. "An edible potato shell!" the brochure for these exclaims as though that were such a brand new idea.

The Bridgford Food Corporation of Anaheim, Calif., had tables stacked with at least 50 kinds of breads, coffee cakes and rolls, all made of the exact same sweet white bread dough. And it's their "ready-dough" that takes all the "scratch work" out of breadbaking and enables restaurants to serve those cute little hot loaves of bread on cutting boards. The one basic dough is reshaped and topped in the restaurant kitchen, homeshaped if not homemade.

Clams of a Sort

For all-around general miserableness, few new foods could compete with the canned clam cocktail put up by American Original Foods. Described as "tasty, succulent deep-sea clams," they are, in fact, chunks of the tough, fibrous abductor muscle of large sea clams, looking like stale rubbery scallops and leaving a thready residue on the tongue when chewed. The sauce, if it matters, is a sweet-acidy tomato-spice combination that does help the "clams" slide down, if nothing else.

"Spud 'n Salad Saver" is a powdered concoction designed to keep peeled raw potatoes and salad greens from changing color and texture, only one of many such products developed by the Pittsburgh Chemical Laboratory, which advises potential customers to "Chemicalize and up-up & up profits."

Sara Lee's minimally acceptable institutional cakes and pies were by comparison the Cadillacs of the show, and fortunately they did not repeat the advice given to restaurant owners a few months ago in an advertisement for their French cream cheese cake that appeared in *Institutions* magazine: "Tell them your French chef makes it," it suggested.

And if truth-in-dining advocates insist on

having menus list all of the ingredients used in various dishes, users of Sexton's Old Country Style Chicken Fricassee gravy better be ready for large menus.

The old country ingredients in this canned treat consist of chicken broth, chicken fat, wheat flour, partly hydrogenated vegetable oil base, corn syrup solids, soy protein isolate, dipotassium phosphate, sodium silico aluminate, tricalcium phosphate, .0076% BHA antioxidant, modified food starch, salt, lipolyzed butter fat, monosodium glutamate, hydrolized plant protein, vegetable oil, polysorbate 80, turmeric extractive, disodium inosinate and turmeric.

Suggested uses in addition to the obvious turkey and chicken gravies included orange or Montmorency sauce for duck, sweet and sour sauce for anything, red burgundy or curry sauce, and chop suey.

Reprinted with permission from *The New York Times*, Sect. 1:43 (1 June 1976). Copyright 1976 by The New York Times Company.

Science Has Spoiled My Supper

PHILIP WYLIE

Here, out of the food jungle stumbles Philip Wylie. And who, many of you may ask, is Philip Wylie? Everyone of my generation knew. He was the abrasive free-lance author of *Generation of Vipers*, and the inventor of momism, who told us that that dear little old lady wasn't always a friend. Nevertheless, he tells us here, her cooking could beat out Science's cooking even a quarter of a century ago. Things in the marketplace weren't so hot even before Freakies, Twinkies and Pringles.

I am a fan for Science. My education is scientific and I have, in one field, contributed a monograph to a scientific journal. Science, to my mind, is applied honesty, the one reliable means we have to find out truth. That is why, when error is committed in the name of Science, I feel the way a man would if his favorite uncle had taken to drink.

Over the years, I have come to feel that way about what science has done to food. I agree that America can set as good a table as any nation in the world. I agree that our food is nutritious and that the diet of most of us is well-balanced. What America eats is handsomely packaged; it is usually clean and pure; it is excellently preserved. The only trouble with it is this: year by year it grows less good to eat. It appeals increasingly to the eye. But who eats with his eyes? Almost everything used to taste better when I was a kid. For quite a long time I thought that observation was merely another index of advancing age. But some years ago I married a girl whose mother is an expert cook of the kind called "old-fashioned." This gifted woman's daughter (my wife) was taught by her mother's venerable skills. The mother lives in the country and still plants an old-fashioned garden. She still buys dairy products from the neighbors and, in so far as possible, she uses the same materials her mother and grandmother did—to prepare meals that are superior. They are just as good, in this Year of Grace, as I recall them from my courtship. After eating for a while at the table of my mother-in-law, it is sad to go back to eating with my friends—even the alleged "good cooks" among them. And it is a gruesome experience to have meals at the best big-city restaurants.

Take cheese, for instance. Here and there, in big cities, small stores and delicatessens specialize in cheese. At such places, one can buy at least some of the first-rate cheeses that we used to eat—such as those we had with pie and in macaroni. The latter were sharp but not too sharp. They were a little crumbly. We called them American cheeses, or even rat cheese; actually, they were Cheddars. Long ago, this cheese began to be supplanted by a material called "cheese foods." Some cheese foods and "processed" cheese are fairly edible; but not one comes within miles of the old kinds—for flavor.

A grocer used to be very fussy about his cheese. Cheddar was made and sold by hundreds of little factories. Representatives of the factories had particular customers, and cheese was prepared by hand to suit the grocers, who knew precisely what their patrons wanted in rat cheese, pie cheese, American and other cheeses. Some liked them sharper; some liked them yellower; some liked anise seeds in cheese, or caraway.

What happened? Science—or what is called science—stepped in. The old-fashioned cheeses didn't ship well enough. They crumbled, became moldy, dried out. "Scientific" tests disclosed that a great majority of the people will buy a less-good-tasting cheese if that's all they can get. "Scientific marketing" then took effect. Its motto is "Give the people the least quality they'll stand for." In food, as in many other things, the "scientific marketers" regard quality as secondary so long as they can sell most persons anyhow; what they are after is "durability" or "shippability."

It is not possible to make the very best cheese in vast quantities at a low average cost. "Scientific sampling" got in its statistically nasty work. It was found that the largest number of people will buy something that is bland and rather tasteless. Those who prefer a product of a pronounced and individualistic flavor have a variety of preferences. Nobody is altogether pleased by bland foodstuff, in other words; but nobody is very violently put off. The result is that a "reason" has been found for turning out zillions of packages of something that will "do" for nearly all and isn't even imagined to be superlatively good by a single soul!

Economics entered. It is possible to turn out in quantity a bland, impersonal, practically imperishable substance more or less resembling, say, cheese—at lower cost than cheese. Chain groceries shut out the independent stores and "standardization" became a principal means of cutting costs.

Imitations also came into the cheese business. There are American duplications of most of the celebrated European cheeses, mass-produced and cheaper by far than the imports. They would cause European food-lovers to gag or guffaw—but generally the imitations are all that's available in the supermarkets. People buy them and eat them.

Perhaps you don't like cheese—so the fact that decent cheese is hardly ever served in America any more, or used in cooking, doesn't matter to you. Well, take bread. There has been

(and still is) something of a hullabaloo about bread. In fact, in the last few years, a few big bakeries have taken to making a fairly good imitation of real bread. It costs much more than what is nowadays called bread, but it is edible. Most persons, however, now eat as "bread" a substance so full of chemicals and so barren of cereals that it approaches a synthetic.

Most bakers are interested mainly in how a loaf of bread looks. They are concerned with how little stuff they can put in it—to get how much money. They are deeply interested in using chemicals that will keep bread from molding, make it seem "fresh" for the longest possible time, and so render it marketable and shippable. They have been at this monkeyshine for a generation. Today a loaf of "bread" looks deceptively real; but it is made from heaven knows what and it resembles, as food, a solidified bubble bath. Some months ago I bought a loaf of the stuff and, experimentally, began pressing it together, like an accordian. With a little effort, I squeezed the whole loaf to a length of about one inch!

Yesterday, at the home of my mother-in-law, I ate with country-churned butter and home-canned wild strawberry jam several slices of actual bread, the same thing we used to have every day at home. People who have eaten actual bread will know what I mean. They will know that the material commonly called bread is not even related to real bread, except in name.

2

For years, I couldn't figure out what had happened to vegetables. I knew, of course, that most vegetables, to be enjoyed in their full deliciousness, must be picked fresh and cooked at once. I knew that vegetables cannot be overcooked and remain even edible, in the best sense. They cannot stand on the stove. That set of facts makes it impossible, of course, for any American restaurant—or, indeed, any city-dweller separated from supply by more than a few hours—to have decent fresh vegetables. The Parisians manage by getting their vegetables picked at dawn and rushed in farmers' carts to market, where no middleman or marketman delays produce on its way to the pot.

Our vegetables, however, come to us through a long chain of command. There are merchants of several sorts—wholesalers before the retailers, commission men, and so on—with the result that what were once edible products become, in transit, mere wilted leaves and withered tubers.

Homes and restaurants do what they can with this stuff—which my mother-in-law would discard on the spot. I have long thought that the famed blindfold test for cigarettes should be applied to city vegetables. For I am sure that if you pureed them and ate them blindfolded, you couldn't tell the beans from the peas, the turnips from the squash, the Brussels sprouts from the broccoli.

It is only lately that I have found how much science has had to do with this reduction of noble victuals to pottage. Here the science of genetics is involved. Agronomists and the like have taken to breeding all sorts of vegetables and fruits—changing their original nature. This sounds wonderful and often is insane. For the scientists have not as a rule taken any interest whatsoever in the taste of the things they've tampered with!

What they've done is to develop "improved" strains of things for every purpose but eating. They work out, say, peas that will ripen all at once. The farmer can then harvest his peas and thresh them and be done with them. It is extremely profitable because it is efficient. What matter if such peas taste like boiled paper wads?

Geneticists have gone crazy over such "opportunities." They've developed string beans that are straight instead of curved, and all one length. This makes them easier to pack in cans, even if, when eating them, you can't tell them from tender string. Ripening time and identity of size and shape are, nowadays, more important in carrots than the fact that they taste like carrots. Personally, I don't care if they hybridize onions till they are as big as your head and come up through the snow; but, in doing so, they are producing onions that only vaguely and feebly remind you of onions. We are getting some

varieties, in fact, that have less flavor than the water off last week's leeks. Yet, if people don't eat onions because they taste like onions, what in the name of Luther Burbank do they eat them for?

The women's magazines are about one third dedicated to clothes, one third to mild comment on sex, and the other third to recipes and pictures of handsome salads, desserts, and main courses. "Institutes" exist to experiment and tell housewives how to cook attractive meals and how to turn leftovers into works of art. The food thus pictured looks like famous paintings of still life. The only trouble is it's tasteless. It leaves appetite unquenched and merely serves to stave off famine.

I wonder if this blandness of our diet doesn't explain why so many of us are overweight and even dangerously so. When things had flavor, we knew what we were eating all the while—and it satisfied us. A teaspoonful of my mother-in-law's wild strawberry jam will not just provide a gastronome's ecstasy: it will entirely satisfy your jam desire. But, of the average tinned or glass-packed strawberry jam, you need half a cupful to get the idea of what you're eating. A slice of my mother-in-law's apple pie will satiate you far better than a whole bakery pie.

That thought is worthy of investigation—of genuine scientific investigation. It is merely a hypothesis, so far, and my own. But people—and their ancestors—have been eating according to flavor for upwards of a billion years. The need to satisfy the sense of taste may be innate and important. When food is merely a pretty cascade of viands, with the texture of boiled cardboard and the flavor of library paste, it may be the instinct of *genus homo* to go on eating in the unconscious hope of finally satisfying the ageless craving of the frustrated taste buds. In the days when good-tasting food was the rule in the American home, obesity wasn't such a national curse.

How can you feel you've eaten if you haven't tasted, and fully enjoyed tasting? Why (since science is ever so ready to answer the beck and call of mankind) don't people who want to reduce merely give up eating and get the nourishment they must have in measured doses shot into their arms at hospitals? One ready answer to that question suggests that my theory of overeating is sound: people like to taste! In eating, they try to satisfy that like.

The scientific war against deliciousness has been stepped up enormously in the last decade. Some infernal genius found a way to make a biscuit batter keep. Housewives began to buy this premixed stuff. It saved work, of course. But any normally intelligent person can learn, in a short period, how to prepare superb baking powder biscuits. I can make better biscuits, myself, than can be made from patent batters. Yet soon after this fiasco became an American staple, it was discovered that a half-baked substitute for all sorts of breads, pastries, rolls, and the like could be mass-manufactured, frozen—and sold for polishing off in the home oven. None of these two-stage creations is as good as even a fair sample of the thing it imitates. A man of taste, who had eaten one of my wife's cinnamon buns, might use the premixed sort to throw at starlings—but not to eat! Cake mixes, too, come ready-prepared—like cement and not much better-tasting compared with true cake.

It is, however, "deep-freezing" that has really rung down the curtain on American cookery. Nothing is improved by the process. I have yet to taste a deep-frozen victual that measures up, in flavor, to the fresh, unfrosted original. And most foods, cooked or uncooked, are destroyed in the deep freeze for all people of sense and sensibility. Vegetables with crisp and crackling texture emerge as mush, slippery and stringy as hair nets simmered in Vaseline. The essential oils that make peas peas—and cabbage cabbage—must undergo fission and fusion in freezers. Anyhow, they vanish. Some meats turn to leather. Others to wood pulp. Everything, pretty much, tastes like the mosses of tundra, dug up in midwinter. Even the appearance changes, oftentimes. Handsome comestibles you put down in the summer come out looking very much like the corpses of woolly mammoths recovered from the last Ice Age.

Of course, all this scientific "food handling" tends to save money. It certainly preserves food longer. It reduces work at home. But these facts, and especially the last, imply that the first purpose of living is to avoid work—at home, anyhow.

Without thinking, we are making an important confession about ourselves as a nation. We are abandoning quality—even, to some extent, the quality of people. The "best" is becoming too good for us. We are suckling ourselves on machine-made mediocrity. It is bad for our souls, our minds, and our digestion. It is the way our wiser and calmer forebears fed, not people, but hogs: as much as possible and as fast as possible, with no standard of quality.

The Germans say, "*Mann ist was er isst*—Man is what he eats." If this be true, the people of the U.S.A. are well on their way to becoming a faceless mob of mediocrities, of robots. And if we apply to other attributes the criteria we apply these days to the appetite, that is what would happen! We would not want bright children anymore; we'd merely want them to look bright—and get through school fast. We wouldn't be interested in beautiful women—just a good paint job. And we'd be opposed to the most precious quality of man: his individuality, his differentness from the mob.

There are some people—sociologists and psychologists among them—who say that is exactly what we Americans are doing, are becoming. Mass man, they say, is on the increase. Conformity, standardization, similarity—all on a cheap and vulgar level—are replacing the great American ideas of colorful liberty and dignified individualism. If this is so, the process may well begin, like most human behavior, in the home—in those homes where a good meal has been replaced by something-to-eat-in-a-hurry. By something not very good to eat, prepared by a mother without very much to do, for a family that doesn't feel it amounts to much anyhow.

I call, here, for rebellion.

Reprinted with permission from *The Atlantic Monthly*, 193: 45-47 (April 1954) and Harold Ober Associates Incorporated. Copyright 1954 by The Atlantic Monthly Company, Boston MA.

Apples that Eve never even thought of.

Pillsbury Cobblers made with apple pieces shaped, colored and flavored to please the most discriminating taste. Three tempting flavors: apple, peach and raspberry.

Easier than the proverbial pie. Just pour a little water, stir with a spoon, and bake. No peeling, no paring, the fruit's in the mix. Short on clean-up time because no mixer is needed.

People love 'em, plain or topped with whipped cream. And you can alter the basic mixes for greater variety. Order today from your Pillsbury distributor.

Serves you right!

Reprinted with permission from the Pillsbury Company.

Stalking Nature's Secrets

Researcher sees rapid growth for fabricated foods

NEW YORK—The development of fabricated foods is one of the paths chosen by food companies in a search for greater profitability, according to a study by researcher Frost & Sullivan.

The 190-page study on the fabricated food market predicts that such foods will account for 60% of the nation's annual food bill before 1983, or $27 billion of the food budget. Such foods now account for about 13% of the total.

By fabricated foods, the industry means items made from cotton seed, alfalfa protein, peanut flour, triticale and algae; dairy substitutes instead of dairy products; dehydrated potatoes instead of raw potatoes and vegetable protein meat analogs instead of meat cuts.

To the consumer, these foods offer convenience, speed in preparation and probably lower costs. Also finding their way into restaurants, fabricated foods offer accurate portion control, no-waste, time-saving efficiency, convenience and a reduction in otherwise necessary manpower, Frost said.

Since the food-away-from-home market is expected to account for 50% of the over-all consumer food budget by 1985 (up from 30% today), restaurants are moving rapidly to use fabricated foods, the study said. Another advantage of such items is that once the customers accept them in restaurants, they purchase them for home use.

The only hurdle foreseen for fabricated foods is government regulation. Because companies fall under the jurisdiction of several different governmental agencies, they find total compliance difficult, due to contradictory rules.

Tomato Taste Study Begun

DAVIS, Calif., July 31 (UPI)—California growers are spending $60,000 to find out why store-bought tomatoes do not seem to taste as good as those grown in backyard gardens.

Today the Strawberry, Tomorrow...

RUTH ROSENBAUM

If food doesn't taste like it used to, surely it cannot be the fault of the flavorists whose astonishing range of accomplishments Ruth Rosenbaum chronicles in this article first published in the *New Times* in June of 1976.

Nature, roll over—with an artful mix of chemicals, master flavorists are now reproducing the taste of just about every food. For most Americans, a favorite meat or vegetable may soon exist only as an essence.

They call them creative flavorists. In the entire world there are only 13 great creative flavorists and no more than 150 others who have what it takes to be considered part of their select society. Shielded from the public eye, these high priests of the multimillion-dollar flavor industry invoke the chemical elements and create from them the counterfeit flavors that are in three-quarters of the products on our supermarket shelves.

Advertisements in food industry journals boast of their masterpieces: take chocolate flavor that tastes and smells just like "the dark expensive stuff made from imported South American cocoa beans"; synthetic chicken flavor that *"feels* more like chicken than any other chicken flavor you have ever tasted"; "right off the bush" imitation strawberry flavor; imitation coconut flavor that "tastes more like coconuts than coconuts"; three species of artificial potato flavor—"European Bintje, green earthy Idaho and popular King Edward".... Though nature still clutches a few last secrets (the flavor and odor of fresh-baked bread and fresh-ground coffee are the most elusive), it cannot be long before the remaining untouched edibles are transformed by the alchemical powers that be.

Flavorists have even managed to go beyond nature with their artificial *canned* tomato and *canned* tomato paste flavors that give people the tinny taste they have become accustomed to. And then artificial fruit flavors infused with "burnt or scorched nuances" match the effect that processing has on the real thing.

But more than simply replicating all natural and industrial tastes within our experience, flavorists will soon be able to create primal taste-experiences and provide an individual with flavor landmarks from cradle, or even pre-cradle, to grave.

Researchers are investigating the possibility

of actually flavoring the amniotic fluid; they have found that if a pregnant woman is fed especially well-flavored food, the fetus knows and will consume more of the fluid.

At International Flavors and Fragrances, Inc. (IFF—the largest international flavor seller, based in New York), flavorists had perfected an artificial human breast-milk flavor as early as 1968. How did they do it? "We brought some mothers into the lab, squeezed the milk from them and then managed to simulate it," a flavorist fondly recalls. IFF also invests in Masters and Johnson's Reproductive Biology Research Center. "It can't hurt to know what we can do to improve man's sexual urge," said one IFF researcher.

Even death has been conquered. A flavorist at Norda, Inc., another large New York-based flavor house, successfully reproduced the odor of a cadaver, although flies put to the test seemed to prefer an artificial strawberry aroma.

Heavy steel doors guard the entrance to the flavorists' laboratories. Inside, the old guard of herbal extracts, essential oils and flower absolutes from all over the world are being pushed aside on vast shelves by hundreds of bottles of wood- and petroleum-derived chemicals. Powerful odors pervade the long corridors, changing outside each laboratory: air pockets of cheddar cheese, maple, onion and garlic, fried hamburger, brown gravy. . . . Magical changes, as there is not a telltale sign of the sites of creation, no steaming vials, no bubbling test tubes, just rows of unanimated bottles of multicolored powders and liquids.

The formulas conceived in these labs are locked away and guarded with greatest care and expense. Even flavorists within the same company may be denied access to one another's formulas. There is talk of secret labs in remote mountainous regions. According to one flavorist I spoke to, kidnapping has become a real menace in the industry. He dares not tell his wife and children even the names of the food manufacturers his company sells its flavors to, so they will have nothing to say to potential extortionists.

The center of artificial flavor intrigue and creation is the New York-New Jersey area, where most of the handful of companies that account for nearly all U.S. flavor sales are based. These include Fritzsche-Dodge & Olcott Inc., IFF, Givaudan Corp., Firmenich, Inc., Norda, Inc., Monsanto Flavor/Essence Inc., H. Kohnstamm & Co., Felton International, Inc., and Ungerer & Co. Major exceptions are McCormick Industrial Flavor Division in Maryland, and Warner-Jenkinson in St. Louis, Mo.

Each day these companies send out drums containing up to 50 gallons of precious formula (hand-mixed by employees who often know only code names for the chemicals they combine) not only to U.S. food manufacturers but to companies in almost every country of the world.

Cutthroat competition among flavor houses has forced executives to seek out, bid for and woo top creative flavorists who can conjure unique tastes for their customers' products. One New Jersey company with a newly formed flavor division managed to attract a master flavorist who had previously worked at IFF. "It was like the culmination of a two-year romance," the president told me proudly.

Romanticism is the core of the flavorist's profession. To "capture in a formula the essence of what I perceive with my own nose and tongue," is how one flavorist describes his ambition. Another calls God his "toughest competitor."

As I went from flavor lab to flavor lab, I found that they practice a distinctive art form with its own romantic aesthetic, and that they are themselves the gourmet chefs of the world of convenience foods.

People in the industry compare flavorists equally to sculptors, composers, painters and writers ("Shakespeare created great literature, we create great flavors," runs one ad), but the spirit of flavor creation seems closest to that of music composition. Even the vocabularies of the two arts converge at several points. The "note" is the basic unit of flavor vocabulary, and the desk at which the flavorist creates his chemical harmonies is called a "console."

No bigger than an average office desk, the

console has several tiers of shelves above it, placing at the flavorist's fingertips the chemicals he considers most essential. (Chemicals used in flavors are called "flavomatics.")

Let's say a flavorist wants to create an artificial strawberry flavor. First he has to have the "notes" of a real strawberry clear in his mind. Every flavorist will perceive them differently, but the "dominant notes" in strawberry that almost everyone agrees on are the "straw or hay notes," "sour notes," a "sweet note" often appearing as a "sweet green note," "ester notes" and "green butter notes," as well as "rose effects" and a "decidedly balsamic character." These vary according to the kind of product the flavor is destined for. With strawberry preserves, for example, the flavorist will play up the "rose and honey notes" and cool it on the "butter-balsam." For taffy candy, he'd tone down the "green notes." Once at his console, the flavorist's fingers fly to the flavomatics he knows, through years of experience, to yield basic strawberry notes.

Then one by one he chooses others, blending, smelling, tasting, adding a bit more of one, smelling and tasting again, trying another, refining the flavor each time until it is complete—with "supporting notes," "background notes" and "interest notes" as well as the basics.

In all, there are about 2,000 raw materials for the flavorist to choose from, each one with several characteristic notes. As the flavorist composes at his console, he must be able to envision how the notes of each material he adds will "sound" with every other note in the final flavor composition. (All materials have to be chemically attuned as well.) Flavor creation requires a great deal of delicacy. A change in a single ingredient at the ratio of a few parts per million in the final product could result in "off-flavors," or could even make the difference between the product's tasting like sweat or like coconut.

The number of ingredients in an artificial flavor varies from 25 to 100 or more, depending on the flavorist's style.

"With some of these newfangled mixed fruit and punch flavors, my colleagues'll use 200,

even 300 ingredients. I personally prefer to keep things simpler," said one flavorist.

As with strawberry, each particular flavor has a few indispensable notes. Normal milk, for example, has a "minute note of the body odor of the cow" and a slight "feedy note." You won't find beer or honey without their "horsey notes," nor apple without its "pip note." "Tingle notes," as in mint and anise, go into mouthwash and toothpaste flavors.

In my efforts to find out about the chemical concertos many of us consume at every meal, I came across a sinister unruly underworld of flavor notes, the minor key of the flavomatic scale.

"Oily Tonka-bean undertones" find their way into nut, cheese, vanilla and caramel flavors, and "sweat-like notes" into imitation rum, chocolate, pecan and butterscotch flavors. A flavomatic with "tarry-repulsive" and "choking" notes is used in making artificial cheese, coffee, chocolate, grapefruit and nut flavors. "Gassy notes" crop up in fruit, wine, brandy and nut flavors.

And there it was—the "fecal note." The chemical that brings us this note is commonly called Skatole—appropriately like scatology and skata ("shit" in Greek)—and is used in cheese, fruit and nut flavors. One author writes, "The use of Skatole in flavors may come as a surprise to some perfumers who find it hard to believe that we can 'eat' this odor."

"Overripe bass notes," "fresh metallic top-notes," "piercing apricot-like notes," "ethereal winey overtones"—the beat goes on as the flavorist, alone at his console, orchestrates everything into final flavor harmony.

"I am known in the industry as the creator of strawberry," says C. Strawberry, a senior flavorist at an important New Jersey flavor house who prefers that his real name remain confidential. His strawberry is called a "classic"; it is in every kind of pink-flavored food or drink you can imagine, and it has made millions for his company.

But ask C. Strawberry how *he* feels about it. "I'm not satisfied. It's still not what I have in mind. Strawberry has been my pet flavor since I was a child, and I want to examine it more, delve into it, see what makes it flash."

The technique of examining a flavor when he first began, over 30 years ago, and of examining one today are as different as "making fire with flint or making it with a match," says Mr. Strawberry. In the flint era, it first took a ton of strawberry, say, to get a half-pound of extractive of strawberry. The flavorist then had to separate out as many of the chemical constituents as possible through traditional chemical analysis (he might have obtained 10 or 12 for all his trouble) and then sniff for clues to the chemicals that yielded flavor notes.

Now, with the gas liquid chromatographer (GLC) that was used in most U.S. flavor companies by the early sixties, he can inject 5 millionths of a liter of strawberry oil into the GLC and, within minutes, obtain a long chart with a series of peaks that can be used to identify about 200 of the chemical constituents of the oil. Of these, the flavorist may be able to find 50 or 60 that contribute to natural strawberry flavor and that give him a broader range of definite "notes" from which to compose his flavors.

Flavorists don't hesitate to tell you what a tremendous aid the GLC has been to them, as long as you know who's still boss. And they make sure you know.

"I don't know how many times I've had to correct that thing," one said in mock exasperation. "You see, it confuses structurally similar chemicals, but if *I* go over and put my nose to the exhaust board, I can distinguish them as they separate out." No, flavorists do not feel technology is anywhere ready to replace them. What does worry them is that a new breed of flavorist, with undue respect for machinery and not much romantic motivation, may eventually degrade the profession.

J. J. Broderick, manager of H. Kohnstamm & Co.'s flavor division in New York City and author of *The Apricot—A Disappearing Art?* seemed sincerely concerned as he spoke about the problem: "What will happen to the industry if there are no more flavorists who know how to rely on

their own creativity and sense of perception? No flavor has ever been created from 100 percent technical know-how."

"You have these young men coming from all these universities and centers of education and so forth; well, they have a lot of knowledge of instruments, but so many of them have no imagination." C. Strawberry's tone was sad and a little scornful. "What they have yet to realize is that this is a very slow-going profession. Even now with the instruments, it takes a lifetime to really get to know all the raw materials and to get close enough to nature to be able to emulate her creations. You see, no instrument can ever achieve what the human nose and tongue can achieve."

The Monsanto Flavor Library in Montvale, New Jersey. A large room filled with tall cases, several shelves high, with rows four and five deep of brown-tinted bottles, each containing an achievement of the human nose and tongue.

"You just have to smell our watermelon. That's my favorite. Let's see, I think it's in the 8000's."

I follow my guide, Joe Jacobs, head of Monsanto's Flavor Application Laboratories, to the sixth aisle, where he begins looking among the early 8000's, reading off the selections.

"Lemon special, Formosan mushroom, celery, guava, bacon. . . ." It's like being in an uncatalogued bookstore where you can find *Twelfth Night* next to *Helter Skelter* and you never know what to expect next. ". . . Deer tongue, blackberry, cherry tobacco, black pepper. . . ." Still no watermelon.

Mr. Jacobs calls an invisible librarian and asks for help. A few seconds later we hear, from beyond the last set of shelves, perhaps from an adjacent room: "Try #8794 and #8999." First 8999, Imitation Watermelon. Joe unscrews the bottle and waves it in front of my nose. Perfect—watermelon at the reddest part, far from the rind. Next to this, Imitation Watermelon #8794 is very disappointing—a vague fruity sweet-sour odor, probably used in hard candies.

We move through the stacks, stopping in almost every aisle, spending the lunch hour sniffing whatever looks good—imitation ham and beef flavors, barbecue sauce flavors, three kinds of artificial mushroom flavor, imitation Yago Sant'gria, butter, sour cream, green pepper, boiled milk, Parmesan cheese, white wine and mango flavors. All these were satisfying, but what I really recommend is their Cucumber #7035—the artificial odor itself carries the impression of crunchiness, moisture and seeds, as well as real cucumber flavor.

For dessert I order artificial cheesecake flavor. A quick call to the librarian, who calls back "6002," and in seconds I have it before my nose.

One-quarter of the 11,000 flavors in Monsanto's library were created in the past eight years; so were approximately one-quarter of the 103,000 flavor formulas (dating from 1920) in the library of Fritzsche-Dodge & Olcott, one of the leading U.S. flavor companies. Most of the new stock is synthetic in these and other companies equally prolific.

Synthetic flavors were first widely used in the U.S. about 1880. They were mostly imported from Germany—imitation pear, cherry, melon, mulberry, quince, apricot, rum, and cognac flavors used to replace part of the natural flavor in food, wines and brandies. When World War I brought a stop to the importation of these delights, the U.S. began to cultivate its own garden, then mostly overrun with natural flavors.

From this time until almost 1960, fruit flavors, vanilla, maple and imitation spices (mostly developed during World War II) were the only synthetic produce. Not only that, the flavors were used either to add a dimension to a food with an unrelated flavor (artificial vanilla flavor used in making chocolate), or they were used to give a cheap boost to the natural flavor, as in ice cream or beverages. But except for certain classes of foods, like gelatin desserts and hard candy, artificial flavors were not used to replace totally the natural, nor to give a food its fundamental taste.

In the early sixties, however, flavorists armed with new flavor chemicals and with a mandate from the food manufacturers stormed the barnyard, the sea, the orchards, supplanting the first set of creations with their own. One company now offers 41 varieties of imitation meat and meat gravy flavors. There is an artificial "gulf-fresh shrimp" flavor, imitation tuna fish, scallop and crab flavors, and an all-round "crustacean flavor." What is significant is that more and more of the flavors are being used to replace entirely the real things. Soon the hamburger will not simply be helped, it will be relieved of all duties, dismissed completely. There already are meat-like products made from vegetable protein and artificial flavoring, and there are many more flavors waiting in the aisles of flavor company libraries for the proper product to come along. If manufacturers manage to mold a chicken shape from vegetable protein, they can dress it immediately with imitation chicken breast flavor, chicken fat flavor, chicken skin flavor and basic chicken flavor.

Fruit flavors have reached such a state of perfection that food manufacturers have been inspired to come up with totally artificial dried apricots and artificial "chopped strawberries" used in muffin mixes, both complete with flavor, aroma and texture of the real thing.

I was impressed to learn that it is often the flavorist himself who instills his flavor with texture, or as they call it, "mouthfeel" (or "how it chews"). They can bring to life whole families of flavors, each member having a different "bite". A chocolate flavor, say, could come in five different mouthfeels, ranging from a pulpy sauce to "a crispy bit typified by a crouton."

The vegetable patch was nature's last stronghold against the flavorists' advances. Not until the late sixties did the imitations begin to sprout. Tomato was first, followed by potato (baked and French fried), green bean, celery, parsley, pea, cucumber, carrot and mushroom. Most of these, with tomato the main exception, are not yet good enough to replace a natural flavor completely and may simply add "vegetable interest" to dressings, dips and sauces. (Even the Monsanto cucumber flavor that smelled so perfect is probably only capable of "enhancing cucumber character.")

But serious forages into vegetable territory began only within the last decade; there is not much doubt about what will happen in the next.

Having watched its army of artists triumph over almost every individual edible creation, the flavor industry was ripe for an assault on nature itself.

Earlier, in the fifties, companies would talk of their flavor conquests somewhat apologetically, embarrassed. "We are proud to announce our new improved cherry flavor; of course it is still no match for Mother Nature's," a company bulletin read.

In the early sixties, there was open boast of the flavorist's knowledge of nature and his ability to duplicate her. Everybody was doing it; there was no point in maintaining Victorian modesty. Still, Mother Nature was respected as *the* standard of excellence. Just a few years later, however, the campaign began subtly, and the quality of her flavors was to be cast in doubt maybe forever.

I first suspected foul play when, in the journals of the same companies that only ten years earlier were eating humble pie, I found whole articles devoted to character assassination. A pear, for example, is described as "temperamental, demanding to be picked while it hangs still imperfectly colored upon the tree"; otherwise it is "tasteless and gritty." No such problems with *synthetic* pear flavor.

Then the digs began to appear in ads. "Mother Nature is fickle," one says. "Profuse with her blessings one day, then turns on a flood, drought or blight the next." Why put up with these humiliations when a constant synthetic can give you "flavor that nature envies"? Another company points out that its artificial tomato flavors don't "leak, bruise or take up space." Above the comment is a picture of some fat, dented, overripe tomatoes made by you-know-who.

You see, nature only reminds of Eden, synthetic flavors actually bring it to you. No death, no change, no fickleness. So if you want "foreign particles, shell fragments, molds, off-flavors and shriveled pieces"—go ahead, eat real

nuts instead of new nutmeat substitutes that come in four flavors: pecan, black walnut, English walnut and almond.

In fact, the very idea of eating certain of nature's creations is enough to make you shudder. A recent IFF annual report warns its shareholders that "natural foods" are "a wild mixture of substances created by plants and organisms for completely different nonfood purposes—their survival and reproduction,"and that they "came to be consumed by humans at their own risk." W. C. Fields was more succinct—"Don't drink the water, fish fuck in it."

Although flavorists have become instruments of the industry's Faustian ambitions, they are themselves very likable characters, still in love with their work and driven by their own gentler ambitions.

"My cherry flavor is better than the natural, and without a single cocoa bean I make a chocolate flavor, so exquisite, so beautiful..." As Shlomo Reiss speaks, his wife, sitting next to him, watches him admiringly, nodding occasionally at me as if to reassure me that, as incredible as it seems, what he says is true.

Chief and only senior flavorist at Ungerer & Co.'s labs in New Jersey, Mr. Reiss began his career 40 years ago at the age of 15. His appealing accent derives from German, Polish, and Ukranian, the languages of his childhood.

"When I can go back to the bottle that has, say, my raspberry flavor in it—my raspberry is perfect—when I can go back to the bottle, sniff the flavor, taste it and honestly say, 'Ah, *this* is beautiful,' the pleasure at that moment is... Mr. Reiss pauses, looking out ahead of him, imagining, then continues, "...It is indescribable." Mrs. Reiss nods....

"It's time to come back to natural flavor. Remember the real taste of luscious golden apricots or ripe juicy pineapples? Your customers do—And they are asking for real flavor. They want ingredients that are natural."

Ralph Nader breaking into the flavor biz?

The *National Enquirer* of the food industry?

It's actually from an ad by H. Kohnstamm & Co. in a 1972 issue of *Food Technology* amidst rave reviews of artificial breakthroughs and articles warning against natural foods.

Flavor people are furious at the big food manufacturers for trying to capitalize on consumer and health food movements. "Instead of using their advertising power to assure people that there is nothing unsafe about artificial food additives, they come out with their own line of natural cereals and what-have-you. It's bound to make people wonder what's wrong with the other 80 percent of their food," one flavor researcher complained.

They are furious, but since they are not at the top of the food chain, survival means catering to the food manufacturing monopolies. So flavor companies now are pushing their natural flavors, as well as synthetic, hoping the ill wind will soon blow over.

If it doesn't, it could be the flavorist who suffers most, since his work is most dependent on the use of synthetic materials. Asking a great flavorist to create natural flavors is like asking a great painter to paint by number.

"They're no fun, no challenge. Making a natural flavor is basically an engineering job," one creative flavorist said.

Most flavor people try to downplay the force of the natural counterrevolution and to appear confident and unthreatened.

"Lower- and middle-class Americans—they're the main market for artificially flavored products, and they couldn't give a damn if a package says 'artificial' or 'natural.'" But apparently, the dam has already given. The industry's paranoia and fear of unfavorable public judgment are phenomenal.

To gain entry to some companies I had to go through a long clearance process, which involved speaking and writing to several people assuring them that my objective was not to stir the fires of the artificial-natural debate (which, in fact, it wasn't). At a few industrial fortresses, when I finally arrived, I was asked outright if I was a vegetarian, if I bought health foods, if I was a friend of Ralph Nader's. It got to the point where, if someone walked toward me, I expected to be frisked for sunflower seeds.

There seemed to be no way *not* to stir fires.

I called an executive at IFF to ask about "mouthfeel," and the first thing he said was, "I hope you're going to make it clear to everyone that this desire for 'natural' foods (pronounce 'natural' with a sneer on the first syllable) is down right stupid."

I innocently asked a flavorist what percent of raw materials used today is synthetic and what percent is natural. Immediately he started in: "First, let's get one thing straight—there is nothing bad about synthetic food additives. We are all made of chemicals, and all our food is made of chemicals. This 'no artificial anything,' 'no chemicals used' business is absolutely ridiculous. Let's face it—a chemical is a chemical is a chemical."

During lunch with three flavorists, one of them mentioned something about a flavorist getting ulcers. Quickly a second followed with, "If some of us do get ulcers, I can assure you it's only because of the tension involved every day in our work. The chemicals we work with are ABSOLUTELY safe. Every single one of them is on the government's GRAS list. G-R-A-S. Generally Recognized As Safe."

So what's everyone getting so upset about?

To its critics, the Generally Recognized as Safe (GRAS) list is generally recognized as suspect. Created in 1958 as part of the Food Additives Amendment, all substances listed on it have the privilege of unrestricted use in foods.

James Turner, author of *The Chemical Feast* (Ralph Nader's Study Group Report on the FDA), offers evidence that many of the substances have yet to be proved safe, that the FDA composed the list haphazardly, nelecting the stipulations it had itself set up. From what many critics say, it seems that some GRAS-listed chemicals should already have been sent to Flavomatic Heaven, by way of the Delaney Clause. (This clause, also part of the 1958 Food Additives Amendment, requires the banning of any additive that causes cancer when ingested by animal or man.) Other GRAS or regulated additives (the latter allowed in food only in certain specified amounts) may, critics fear, be teratogenic (causing birth defects) or mutagenic (causing gene damage). Even though these additives are used at very low levels in food, the argument is that cancer and mutagenesis are more likely to be caused by longrange daily exposure to tiny amounts of hazardous substances than by single or occasional large doses.

Dangerous chemicals remain in our food, critics say, because the various food industries supervise the FDA rather than vice-versa, as it should be. In the case of the flavor industry, its powerful lobbying force in Washington, the Flavor and Extract Manufacturing Association (FEMA), has had its own GRAS list since 1961. It now lists 1,476 substances, over 300 of which are not on the FDA list. The FEMA list is subject to FDA scrutiny but apparently is not often subjected to this scrutiny. According to one FDA official, decisions about flavoring additives are left pretty much up to the FEMA'S handpicked, high-paid panel of experts. "There are only one or two people on our [FDA] staff who are involved with the flavor industry," he said.

One of industry's main defenses against its critics is the benefit-risk concept. One flavorist asked indignantly. "How can people expect us to ward off starvation in this world [by trying to flavor algae, bacteria, manure and other cheap but unpalatable sources of protein] and yet expect that everything we use will be 100 percent safe 100 percent of the time?"

Flavorists present themselves as live evidence of the safety of the chemicals they use. "Look at me," one said. "Before all the regulations came about, I used to taste every single compound that came into the fragrance or the flavor division to see if it could be used in a flavor, and I'm fine."

The various pacts and sects, the ins and outs of chemicals on the GRAS list—these are, in the long run, of little consequence to the flavorist sitting at his console, taking upon himself the mysteries of flavor. It is just the Third Day of artificial flavor creation—a long time before the creators rest, or are laid to rest by their critics.

And tremendous forces, favorable to continuing creation, have aligned.

Food manufacturers now spend more for artificial flavoring than for any other group of synthetic food additives (including preservatives, stabilizers, colors, thickeners, anti-oxidants, etc.). The sales value of food, beverages and tobacco containing synthetic flavors, in the U.S. alone, is close to $80 billion per year. (This is a conservative estimate based on figures obtained from IFF.) Unless you religiously buy all your food from health food stores or raise it yourself, and unless you refrain from smoking and from drinking most liqueurs, fruit brandies and even some wines, you have assimilated the gospel of the new artificial order.

Synthetic flavors have created desires that they alone can fulfill. Take vanilla: if high cost were not a problem and we could have all the vanilla grown in the world, it would not be enough to satisfy the vanilla-cravings of Americans.

As an increasing number of Mother Nature's flavors fade from the marketplace because of high cost or scarcity, flavor companies are not waiting to see if we can wean ourselves and do without, or with less of them. They have already come up with addictive new flavor archetypes that will reign even if nature's become more accessible again. One company touts a cherry flavor that is typical of "neither the raw nor the processed cherry, nor of any special variety of cherries." This kind of flavor may be the key to addiction—"If you can't pin it down, you won't put it down," I was told.

Some flavorists look forward gleefully to the gradual elimination of their major competition. "In 20 years," one said, "I'll bet you that only 5 percent of the people will have tasted fresh strawberry, so whether we like it or not , we people in the flavor industry will really be defining what the next generation thinks is strawberry. And the same goes for a lot of other foods that will soon be out of the average consumer's reach. "Under the guise of democratizing taste experiences—making everything available to everyone—the flavor industry will dictate more and more eating habits that can only be supported by its artificial flavors.

Americans have the most "educated" tastes so far, but people in nearly every country of the world are being gradually mouthwashed. Firmenich, Inc. in Princeton, N.J. (known in the industry for its fruit and peanut butter flavors), has over 90 companies and agencies worldwide. In 1972, 60 percent of IFF's sales were outside the U.S., 75 percent is projected for 1982. They have discovered a great market in countries where the economic outlook is bleakest. An IFF executive cheerfully reports that "the poorer the malnutritioned are, the more likely they are to spend a disproportionate amount of whatever they have . . . on some simple luxury," like a flavored drink or smoke.

They call it the "Titanic Syndrome." If the boat is going down, you blow all your money on what seems most attractive at the moment. Also, lax or nonexistent food additive and labeling laws in many of these countries make it very easy on the flavor company.

While flavorists study the food preferences of poorer cultures so they can create seductive flavors for their last "rites," they positively confront the problem of starvation by trying to flavor inexpensive protein sources with the tastes each population is used to.

"What we want to do is get the chicken feathers back to the chickens," an IFFer told me. It sounded like a quote from a sequel to *Animal Farm* until he explained. Flavorists are working on a flavor to be added to recycled chicken feathers (very high in protein) so that they can be used as animal feed, leaving the grain for people.

Firestone Tire and Rubber Co. discovered a few years ago that a very nutritious strain of yeast grows magically on discarded rubber tires. (Enter: deus ex flavor company to make the yeast taste good.)

The roles that the flavorist may be called on to play in the next several decades are limitless. Each idea being researched now holds in itself incredible possibilities. Like the idea that the fetus is sensitive to the flavor of the amniotic fluid. When your great-grandchild is born, the type of flavoring given to his mother may be marked on his birth certificate along with his sex and blood type: e.g., Boysenberry L-243, library of Monsanto No. 591. 2219. Later in life, if the child has problems that a large chocolate-flavored ice cream soda won't solve, rather than submit himself to the psychoanalytical cult leaders of his time, he will simply go to one of many buildings filled with warm padded rooms, pay a single fee and enter the room filled with Boysenberry L-243 aroma for instant return to the womb.

Excerpted with permission from *New Times*, 6 (12): 45-52 (11 June 1976).

The way to a woman's heart is through their stomachs.

Unfortunately foods that are "good for you" do not necessarily taste good. Mothers know this only too well, who have to press and cajole their children into finishing their spinach or drinking more milk.

To make proteins and vitamins appealing, you must give them an appealing flavor.

Firmenich knows all about flavors. And about vitamins. And children. Our research is intensive and worldwide. Our knowledge and experience are matched only by our creativity and technical skills.

We know that dealing with flavors means dealing with realities. Because fruit and vegetables and meats are realities. And so are consumer demands and preferences.

This is why Firmenich is so often ready ahead of time. Ready for new markets, new products, new tastes. And new needs.

So with all the care you put into your food products, think of putting in a little something for Mother. The delicious, pure flavors that will help her give her children the health and body-building foods they need.

Let's get together. And we will turn you into Mother's favorite any day.

Isn't that something to look forward to?

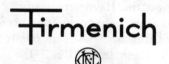

Forward planning in flavors.

CIRCLE 313

Firmenich Incorporated, 277, Park Avenue, New York, N.Y. 10017   Bogotá   Buenos Aires   Caracas   Chicago   Genève   Guayaquil   Köln   Limá
London   Los Angeles   Melbourne   Mexico   New York   Osaka   Paris   Quito   São Paulo   Sydney   Tokyo   Toronto

Reprinted with permission from Firmenich Incorporated.

On Parade: The Taste and Nonsmell of Un-Food

MIMI SHERATON

Mimi Sheraton, here reporting for *The New York Times* on the 1977 Institute of Food Technologists meeting, makes one wonder where all those flavors went. The man who patented *(really)* "fatty fried flavor" appears to have beaten out the lot of them.

PHILADELPHIA, June 6—The 37th annual meeting of the Institute of Food Technologists opened here last night with 240 exhibitors displaying their wares in an atmosphere that some visitors found disturbingly free of any food smells whatever.

In all, 7,000 to 8,000 people are expected to attend the convention, which ends Wednesday at the Civic Center. Most of them will be members of the food processing industry, and those attending last night's session were cheered by the words of the opening speaker, Senator Robert Dole.

The Republican Senator from Kansas said that he would vote against President Carter's proposed consumer protection agency because he believed that the interests of the American consumer were already being served.

"If the American people are given adequate information about the products they buy and the food they eat," he said, "they are intelligent enough to act sensibly without the intrusion of more bureaucrats operating as advocates."

Senator Dole told the group that Congress was now convinced that the rising cost of public health was due primarily to the unhealthy diet patterns and food habits of the people.

This country's food policies and programs, he added, will be determined "first and foremost by the degree to which they contribute to sound nutritional health."

Meanwhile, the convention's 450 display booths were dedicated to the latest developments in synthetic foods, chemical additives, artificial colorings and flavorings, extenders, emulsifiers, and products intended to increase the shelf-life of packaged foods.

Samples Offered

Many of the exhibitors offered samples to passers-by, and some of them led easily to the impression that the chemists' quest for artificial chocolate is equal only to the alchemists' quest for artificial gold.

Whether the product tasted was Cho-coa-lot extender made by the Food Materials Corporation, counterfeit chocolate by William M. Bell Company, or simple artificial chocolate from Fries and Fries (the flavor makers), Chocolm III by Ritter International, or Chocolate Nib by the National Food Ingredients Company ("We'll put a rainbow in your mouth"), all tasted identically medicinal and coagulated on the tongue.

Chocolate was one of the flavors Pillsbury

added to its Bitsyn (synthetic bits) line along with bacon, cheese, onion, garlic and already existing pecans and black walnuts. Formed of wheat germ, sodium cascanate and hydrogenated vegetable oils, sweet Bitsyn are used in such products as cakes, confections and ice cream, while bacon, onion, cheese flavors go into salad dressings, soups, crackers, and breads.

Archer Daniels Midland gave out samples of fabricated fish fillets blended with Haarman Reimer's fish flavor 94750, Ardex 700 F, textured vegetable protein and minced fish— each a spongy, soggy triangular fried fillet.

Frankfurter Pretzels

Fries and Fries handed out samples of frankfurter-flavored pretzels seasoned with liquid frankfurter flavoring, even as technologists from Washington State University were announcing the development of frankfurters in which the usual meat fillings were replaced in part by hake, an inexpensive fish under-utilized as food. The university report stated that if only 15 percent of the fish filling was used, the frankfurters could be kept four weeks before developing fish odor and flavor.

R.W. French ("We make your life delicious") had new powdered seasoning for flavoring potato chips. Sour cream and green garden barbecue were typical flavors, all of which were said to make dips unnecessary since the flavor was already in the chips.

Amoco Food Company, a division of the petroleum company, introduced a low-calorie creamy garlic dressing made with Torutein-50,

which it said "mimics fat mouth feel" -- which it certainly did. It was a cloying final result that stuck to the tongue and palate if not to the hips and waistline.

Fidco, a subsidiary of the Nestle Company, promoted Great Pretenders—artificial mushrooms, ham and bacon flavoring, to give meat and broth roast-meat flavor—and still other products to simulate flavors of seafood, charcoal-broiled meat, a pork-like taste and Type MB, a bittersweet blend designed for Bloody Mary mixes.

Riches Products Corporation introduced a tasteless tan powder, Bee Rich-Dry. A company spokesman said it contained a blend of molasses, corn syrup solids and just enough honey so that it could be declared honey in an ingredients list on a label.

Slogans around the room were as disturbing as the odorless, tasteless food. The I.C.I. Corporation, producers of artificial flavors and fragrance, asked "Hocus pocus a new food opus?" Durkee announced that it was into encapsulation—encapsulated cinnamon, citric acids, fumaric acid and vitamins for more efficient and economical use in manufacturing of food products.

Even pet food came in for a share of improving from Globe Extracts Incorporated, developers of artificial flavors such as bacon, beef, chicken, garlic, ham, hamburger, lamb chops and four cheese flavors, blue, cheddar, parmesan and romano. Asked why such flavors were necessary in food that appeals to pets, Leonard Weiner, a spokesman for the company, said "That's the only way to get pets to eat the garbage they put into that food."

Reprinted with permission from *The New York Times*, Sect L: 45 (7 June 1977). Copyright 1977 by The New York Times Company.

Our Diets Have Changed But Not for the Best

MICHAEL JACOBSON

In this article, originally written for the *Smithsonian* magazine, scientist and food critic Michael Jacobson raises questions about the U.S. diet which are somewhat more serious than whether it tastes bad or costs too much. It's unhealthy, he asserts, and explains why.

If the bromide, "You are what you eat," is true, we could all end up being very different people from our ancestors. Modern science and agriculture have freed the United States and many other nations from traditional diets based largely on natural farm products. New varieties of crops, transcontinental shipping, a wide spectrum of food additives, and new food-processing techniques have led, for better or worse, to diets different from any previously consumed by human populations. But these dietary changes reflect the decisions of business executives and investors, rather than nutritionists and public health officials.

The United States, not surprisingly, has been the leader in the genetic engineering of food crops and in the laboratory creation of new foods. Benjamin Franklin and Abraham Lincoln, if they could visit us, would probably have some difficulty distinguishing between a toy store and a supermarket. They would not even recognize as foods such products as artificial whipped cream in its pressurized can, or some of the breakfast "cereals" that are almost half sugar and bear little resemblance to cereal grains. Franklin and Lincoln world probably feel much more at home in the homey "natural foods" stores that are popping up everywhere than they would in the 10,000 item supermarkets. Many of the new foods do save us time and trouble, but they are often costly, in terms of both dollars and, ultimately, health.

"Modern" eating practices start young, often with the tiny infant. Most pediatricians agree that good old-fashioned breast-feeding is the best way to feed a baby, but all too often mothers are persuaded by cultural and commercial pressures—or because of their work schedule—to bottle-feed with canned baby formula. Only about one in four infants enjoys the nutritional (and psychological) benefits of breast-feeding.

Until the 1930's solid baby food was prepared at home by the mother. Now, however, commercially prepared strained baby foods are the rule and are being introduced into a baby's diet at an increasingly early age. Mothers often compete with one another on the basis of how early little Johnny or Susie starts to eat solid food. Many researchers believe that feeding a baby solid foods too early can lead to both overfeeding and allergic reactions.

Some pediatricians and researchers worry about the health consequences of commercial baby foods. In the past 20 years canned formula has become the most popular food for infants. Although this is probably superior to the old-fashioned formulas based on evaporated milk and corn syrup, it is still a pale imitation of human breast milk. For instance, it lacks the antibodies and enzymes that help ward off disease and the "bifidus factor" that promotes the growth of favorable intestinal bacteria. Because it is based on cow's milk, infants may have allergic reactions. Differences include higher levels of sodium and unsaturated fats and lower levels of cholesterol as compared to breast milk.

A researcher at the University of Iowa, Dr. Samuel J. Fomon, suggests that formula feeding may be more likely than breast-feeding to lead to obesity in later life. He reasons that the formula-fed infant is expected to finish the last drop in the bottle, while the breastfed baby stops when he has had enough. Fomon and his colleague, Dr. Thomas A. Anderson (who once worked for Heinz, a major baby food manufacturer), have also suggested that early introduction of solid foods may lead to overfeeding—the infant often is expected to finish the last spoonful in the dish.

Pediatricians also wonder about strained baby foods. Although as yet they have little solid evidence, some fear that the salt and sugar used so freely as flavorings establish taste patterns that remain with a person throughout life.

In 1969 a Congressional committee held hearings that focused on the high salt content of baby food. This attention led the manufacturers to reduce voluntarily the salt levels in baby foods, but many products still contain up to ten times as much sodium (mainly from added salt) as does breast milk. Salt is of great concern to doctors and nutritionists because too much of it in the diet of adults contributes to high blood pressure (hypertension), which is the primary cause of about 20,000 deaths a year and is the major underlying factor in some 900,000 deaths a year from stroke and cardiovascular disease. Dr. Jean Mayer, Professor of Nutrition at Harvard University and probably the most influential nutritionist in the country, has said that "preventing hypertension would

be much better than finding it and treating it—and a critical step in prevention is so easy: Just eat less salt."

For a child whose taste buds were initiated on blueberry buckle, raspberry cobbler and other sweetened and salted baby foods, the step to artificially colored and flavored sugar-coated breakfast "cereals" is a small and natural one. Many of these products, which could be called candies, are 30 to 50 percent sugar. One widely known children's cereal, for instance, contains a higher percentage of sugar (approximately 50 percent) than a chocolate bar (40 percent).

Highly sweetened foods encourage young children to develop a taste for sugar, of which the average American consumes approximately 100 pounds per year. Dental researchers have proved that sugar is a major cause of tooth decay. In addition, sugar's "empty calories" displace nutritious foods and contribute to obesity, diabetes and heart disease.

While the Food and Drug Administration has not taken any action on the high sugar content of some cereals, Dr. Lloyd Tepper, Associate Commissioner for Science at FDA, said this at a 1973 Senate hearing on nutrition:

"I don't think you have to be a great scientist to appreciate the fact that a highly sweetened, sucrose-containing material, which is naturally tacky when it gets wet, is going to be a troublemaker. And I would not prescribe this particular food component for my own children, not on the basis of scientific studies, but because I do not believe that prolonged exposure of tooth surfaces to a sucrose-containing material is beneficial."

While tooth decay is certainly not a deadly disease, it can be both painful and costly. Army surveys indicate that, on the average, every 100 inductees require 600 fillings, 112 extractions, 40 bridges, 21 crowns, 18 partial dentures and one full denture. Although Americans currently pay dentists about $2 billion a year for treating decayed teeth, Dr. Abraham E. Nizel, of the Tufts University School of Dental Medicine, has estimated that we would be paying $8 billion a year if everyone went to the dentist and had all his dental needs taken care of. It is Dr. Nizel's impression that tooth decay is so rampant that even "if all the 100,000 dentists in the United States restored decayed teeth day and night, 365 days a year, as many new cavities would have formed at the end of the year as were just restored during the previous year."

As children grow older and more independent, most of the messages they get from the adult world encourage them to eat food that is not best for their health. School cafeterias frequently serve meals rich in fat and low in whole grains. Television commercials employ the latest ad agency techniques to promote sugar-coated cereals and snack foods. The U.S. Department of Agriculture—over the objection of many nutritionists—allows schools to serve children nutrient-fortified cupcakes for breakfast in place of cereal and orange juice. Vending machines invite children (and adults) to buy soda pop, candy and gum. Fast-food outlets specialize in meals that are almost devoid of vitamins A and C, two of the vitamins that many Americans consume too little of. Living in this kind of environment, children may be confused when their health teacher admonishes them to "eat good foods."

America's eating habits are epitomized by what is served at our standard celebrations: baseball games, carnivals and picnics. What child would be caught at one of those affairs without a hot dog and soda pop? The child does not realize (and is not told), of course, that a diet with too high a fat content (including, for example, too many hot dogs) can contribute to the epidemic of heart disease and obesity with which this country is saddled.

Obesity is a serious medical problem. Dr. Ogden Johnson, former Director of Nutrition at FDA, has estimated that 40 million Americans are overweight or obese. In addition to being a severe social and psychological handicap, obesity is a major factor in cardiovascular diseases, mentioned earlier.

The fluffy white bun in which the hot dog is served is made from white flour, which lacks some of the nutrients that are present in whole wheat flour. Fiber is one substance that is almost entirely eliminated when the flour is refined. For several decades most researchers ignored this indigestible carbohydrate, disdaining it as mere "roughage." But evidence is mounting rapidly that fiber plays a crucial role in maintaining the health of the gastrointestinal tract (particularly the large intestine), in controlling calorie intake and in excreting cholesterol.

British physicians, notably Drs. Denis Burkitt, Thomas Cleave, G. D. Campbell and Hubert Trowell, have led the campaign to awaken the medical world to the importance of fiber. On the basis of field experience and laboratory studies, they maintain that people who consume too little fiber—and too much sugar—stand a high risk of developing obesity, diverticulosis, appendicitis, hemorrhoids, constipation, peptic ulcer, diabetes, heart disease and cancer of the colon.

Although Americans do get a substantial amount of fiber from fruits and vegetables, Burkitt and Trowell believe that this fiber is not nearly as effective in maintaining health as that found in whole grains and legumes. Many physicians and nutritionists in the United States are now urging Americans to base a larger part of their diet on whole grains, nuts, bran and other fiber-rich foods.

In their middle years, most Americans consume a diet that is reasonably complete as far as vitamins, minerals and protein are concerned. The typical diet usually reflects eating habits formed in childhood, however, and is hazardously high in calories, sugar, fat, cholesterol and salt, and hazardously low in fiber. Still, aside from dental problems and obesity, this diet usually causes no overt problems during the middle 20 to 30 years of most people's lives. Scurvy, pellagra, beri-beri and other nutritional-deficiency diseases are almost unknown in the United States. After about age 40 or 50, however, the changes within the body that have been gradually and silently occurring over the decades begin to make themselves felt.

A heart attack or stroke is often the first sign

that something is wrong. After the fact, physicians often urge dietary (and other) changes to prevent recurrences. The patient is ordered to lose weight and eat less cholesterol and less fat—especially the saturated fat found in meat and dairy products. The person who is around to make these changes in eating habits should consider himself lucky. The American Heart Association recommends reducing fat consumption and body weight *before* a heart attack drives home the message.

As old age approaches, signs frequently show up first—and painfully—in the large intestine. Every television watcher who suffers through the incessant commercials for laxatives surely knows that constipation or, euphemistically, "irregularity" affects millions of people. The commercials push brand-name panaceas, but vegetables, whole grain breads and cereals, and fiber-rich bran (which you can get in bulk from health food stores or as one of the all-bran cereals) can do the trick equally well. Of course, eating an adequate amount of fiber-containing foods all along would have helped prevent constipation from developing.

Many elderly Americans suffer from diverticulosis of the colon, and every year approximately 170,000 people are hospitalized for treatment. This often painful illness develops when pressure builds up within the large intestine, causing outpouchings, which frequently become infected. The prescription for prevention or treatment is the same: a diet high in fiber-rich foods.

To complete our description of a lifetime of eating, we return to baby food. This time around, though, the consumers are not infants, but the elderly who have lost their teeth as a result of decay and gum disease and can eat only semi-solid strained foods. About 18 percent of all American adults have no teeth.

Ironically, some of the same companies that manufacture the foods that contribute to heart disease, constipation, and other illnesses of middle and old age have special lines catering to the sufferers of these illnesses. Individuals who have become constipated partly through eating

sugar-coated flakes can switch to all-bran. Did high blood pressure result partly from heavily salted soups? The hypertensive patient can turn to dietetic low-salt soups (and pay a little extra for *not* having salt). Diabetics who once loved fruit canned in heavy sugar syrup must pay a premium price for fruit packed in water.

Despite the close relationship between diet and disease, no person, governmental agency or private organization in the United States has had the mission or authority to develop a broad national food policy that would consider nutritional value as a top priority in the way our food is grown, processed and distributed. As it is, our agricultural practices and eating habits have developed with little guidance from health professionals.

The importance of developing a coherent national food policy has gained much high-level support in the past year, largely because of rising food prices and an increasing awareness of nutrition. Famine overseas has also awakened many people to the moral obligations of the wealthy nations. The development of a food policy was given a boost last June, when the Senate Select Committee on Nutrition and Human Needs held a hearing on a national nutrition policy.

Heard time and time again at the Senate hearing was the need for us to base a larger part of our diet on vegetables than we now do. As Frances Moore Lappé explained so eloquently in *Diet for a Small Planet*, growing soybeans and grain to feed livestock and then eating the livestock is a much less efficient way of producing food than eating the vegetable crops (see *Smithsonian*, January 1975). Huge amounts of fertilizer, energy and food would be saved if Americans ate less grain-fed meat. More food could go to nations in short supply.

Serving as one cornerstone of a food policy should be the vast amount of knowledge that the world's researchers have produced in recent decades. We need to *apply* the findings of this research. One way of facilitating this would be to establish a Federal Nutrition Advocacy Agency, which could disseminate information to the public and professionals, and prod other governmental agencies to employ their resources to encourage better nutrition.

While awaiting the creation of such an agency, we can easily improve our own diets. For most of us, that means eating less fat, sugar, refined flour and salt—and more fiber. In terms of foods, that translates into more whole grain foods, fruits, nuts, beans and vegetables, and less meat and snack foods. A change to this kind of diet would mean better health for Americans and more food for the rest of the world and would give us less cause to worry about becoming what we eat.

Reprinted with permission from *Smithsonian*, 6: 96-102 (April 1975). Copyright 1975 by Smithsonian Institute.

The Social Implications of Food Technology

MAGNUS PYKE, F.R.S.E.

If we do, as Jacobson reiterates, become what we eat, we may lose more than our health and our sense of taste if things go on as they are going. Magnus Pyke's always literate and sometimes mordantly witty analysis of the effect of food technology on world social patterns raises, in a new context, some fundamental questions about the relationships between food and society.

(Address given at the annual meeting of Phi Tau Sigma, San Francisco Civic Auditorium, May 27, 1970)

THE SOCIALLY DIVISIVE INFLUENCE OF FOOD TECHNOLOGY

...In no area of modern life does the rapid advance of science and technology impinge more directly on social behaviour than it does on our dietary habits. New articles appear on the supermarket shelves every day and although to the unreflecting observer of the passing scene the production of a new food commodity might seem to be a trivial matter unworthy of serious consideration, this is not necessarily so. The technological expertise upon which any one item depends may require the full depth of scientific understanding. To produce frozen chicken wrapped in plastic, genetical science must be brought to bear to develop a purebred strain of chicks to be hatched in their thousands on appropriate days to fit the logistics of the master plan by which they are to be grown on a diet of exact nutritional composition, delivered at the correct weight as a steady flow of raw material to the processing plant, killed, mechanically plucked, cooled, dressed, wrapped, frozen and distributed to a thousand addresses. To fill the cans of delicate tender carrots, at which the housewife barely gives a hurried glance, an agricultural botanist has caused a carrot to grow exactly the shape and size to fit the manufacturer's standard can.

All this is admirable. It demonstrates the command that the food technologist has acquired over Nature—that he can propagate oranges without pits and get dried peas undried again when someone wants to eat them—and the housewife and the caterer alike can enjoy the convenience of "convenience" foods. But there is more to it than the mere exercise of technological virtuosity. Food plays a central part in social life and the rapid progress of food technology exercises a more profound social function than its protagonists have so far foreseen.

Social Fragmentation

It is of the nature of scientific technology to fragment the communities who practice it and detribalise their society. The division of labour is the doctrine, possessing almost the force of an article of faith, upon which modern industrial activity is based. Inevitably, those taking part in it cease to be diverse men and women and become units of the labour force. The same principle is also applied to other types of activity besides manufacture. A general medical practitioner no longer essays to cure his patient. He sends him to a cardiologist for his heart, to a neurologist for his nerves, to a pediatrician if he is young and to a geriatrician if he is over sixty. Besides the professions, which like trade and industry have been divided into internationally uniform parts, so too is the community itself split up and packaged.

Babies are no longer born at home surrounded by their grandmothers, aunts and neighbors. They are born among professionally qualified strangers in institutions designed for the purpose, although it should be added that pains are still taken to insure that among so many superficially standard infants each individual mother is given on leaving the baby she came in with. At three or four years of age the infant has become a pre-school child under the scientific tutelage of a child-guidance expert. Next, a well run comprehensive school takes charge of the children during term times and they spend the break between terms in educational cruises or camps. Teenagers and students can clearly be seen to be a separate sub-section of the community from which other sub-groups—taxpayers, trades unionists, unmarried mothers and the like—branch off. Later on, come the penultimate category of old-age pensioners and finally, there is another purpose-built institution to house the problem group of the dying.

The Influence of Food Technology on Domestic Life

The matter to which we are now directing our attention is the particular significance which food and food technology exert in providing—or ceasing to provide—coherence within the fabric of society which our industrialized and inevitably materialist system is so obviously putting under strain. Every anthropologist is aware of the peculiar importance within a viable social group of shared meals. In the past, the preparation of a meal—Sunday dinner, for example—was an elaborate undertaking. A series of complex operations, some of which required prolonged preparation, all had to be organized so that they reached their culmination simultaneously. A chicken, let us say, had to be killed and plucked as long as a week beforehand. The stock pot for soup needed attention long in advance. Vegetables had to be brought in from the garden, washed, prepared and cooked. A whole diversity of activities were concerned involving a high degree of mutual co-operation and good planning. Finally, all was ready. The family and guests gathered together: it was meal time.

"Convenience" foods, the prime achievement of food technology, have up till the present retained, at least to some degree, a function as part of a meal. Frozen and dehydrated peas, mashed potato powder and "instant" porridge save the housewife from the trouble and waste of shelling fresh peas, peeling potatoes and waiting for them to boil, and from the laborious business of putting porridge to cook in a double saucepan overnight. Nevertheless, although their use reduces the degree of social co-operation required, they are still intended to be employed as components of meals to be consumed by family groups. As food technology advances, however, I see the comparatively moderate convenience of "convenience" foods—after all, while a wrapped, sliced loaf is a popular commodity, the labour of cutting bread one's self is not very exacting—becoming more extreme. And it would not be so very large a technological step forward for the bite-sized dehydrated portions of fricasseed chicken, cheese sandwiches, pumpkin pie and the like already formulated for the sustenance of astronauts becoming the prototypes of the "chocolate bars" of the immediate future. At present, the manufacturers of chocolate bars claim how nourishing they are—that they "fill the gap" or top up the energy of their consumers. But so far they are not in fact a substitute for a meal.

Tomorrow, wrapped bars that are in every sense the equivalent of a sitdown affair will be on the market and real meals will have become a dietetic irrelevance. . . .

The Influence of Technology on the Social Attributes of Food Distribution

The supermarket has been the essential handmaiden of modern food technology. In no other way could the diversity of packets and products be exhibited. Little wonder that the number of supermarkets multiplied in the technologically active years of the 1960's[1]. It is not always appreciated, however, that supermarkets exert a significant social impact on both the people using them and the people working in them. A man or woman working in a family grocers is engaged in a diversity of jobs and at the same time is in close human contact with the owner's family, of which he is often a member and with the idiosyncrasies of the people who come to buy, with most of whom he will also be pretty well acquainted. Most of the workers in a supermarket, on the other hand, labour out of sight for fixed hours on what amounts to factory work, wrapping, packaging, slicing or loading trolleys. Such an employee is a member of a large staff many of whom he may hardly know and has as little contact with the customers on the other side of the partition as has an operative in a crematorium with the mourners. An indication of the social breakdown brought about by the impersonality of self-service marketing, technologically efficient though it may be, is that it is recognized that as supermarkets become larger the rate of pilferage increases, and this in spite of a proliferation of technological devices, closed-circuit television and the like. The customer in a neighborhood grocers shop is a member of a structured social group in which his knowledge of his own function and its recognition by others restrains him from stealing. Whereas, in the fragmented anonymous atmosphere of a supermarket these restraints do not apply.

The Influence of Technological Processing on Food Producers

Margarine If the disruptive social influence of food technology can be seen to affect the domestic life of a community and the communal activities of buying and selling food, this same influence affects those who produce food. Margarine can be taken as one of the major successes of food technology. Within a hundred years of its conception in 1869, the technology of its manufacture had achieved a high degree of sophistication and the annual production of margarine had reached five million tons[2]. The social consequences of this technological achievement were considerable. Let me cite one. In the main areas of West Africa where palm oil was traditionally produced, the land was owned by the community as a whole. In some places it was recognized that a man who planted a tree was entitled to enjoy its produce as long as he lived. In other places the accepted custom was that the crops a man grew on land cleared around the tree belonged to him but the disposal of the palm kernels was a perquisite of his wife. The incursion of Western technologists intent on setting up plantations for the large-scale production of palm oil for the manufacture of margarine as a "convenience" food for the industrial citizens of Europe and America destroyed the fragile and complex social system of the non-industrial Africans who produced the oil from which the margarine was made.

Bananas It is curious to recall that in 1870 when Z.D. Baker brought the first bananas to the United States from Jamaica more than half the habitable surface of the earth had yet to be penetrated by Europeans. In the following thirty years, in parallel with the acceptance of modern technology as a philosophy of behaviour, the entire planet, with the exception of the extreme polar regions, had been traversed by white men, its economic resources and potentialities catalogued, Africa had been parcelled

[1] McClelland, W.G., "Studies in Retailing", (Blackwell), Oxford, 1963.
[2] van Stuyvenberg, J.H., ed., "Margarine: an economic, social and scientific history, 1869-1969", Liverpool U. Press, 1969.

out, Oceania and Australia appropriated and spheres of interest demarcated in Asia and Latin America. By 1900, the total export of bananas from the Latin American republics, the Caribbean and Mexico was already nearly 20 million bunches. The figure reached 50 million bunches in 1913 and nearly 88 million bunches by 1932. And of this amount 67 million bunches, or 76 per cent[3], were handled by two great companies whose operations were organized entirely outside the countries in which the bananas were grown and whose operators had no interest in the people who lived where the bananas grew. The principles upon which this very substantial exercise in food technology was based were two-fold. The first was a single scientific fact, namely, that bananas can only be successfully transported from the tropical areas in which they grow to the markets of the Temperate Zone if their temperature is not permitted to fall below 13°C. (i.e. 55°F.). The second was the command of ships, railroads and the heavy equipment to build them, telephone and telegraph systems, an up-to-date medical service and, in fact, all the complex technology needed to support a major industrial undertaking.

The price of the plentiful supply of bananas to the populations of the developed countries of the world was the almost complete subordination of the social organization of the indigenous peoples—Spanish Americans, American Indians together with the negros of African stock—by the dominant, single-minded ethos of the United Fruit Company. One does not compliment a community by describing it as a "banana republic"....

Western "Agribusiness"

The social changes brought about by the advances in food technology have affected the rural populations of advanced industrialized communities every bit as drastically as they have those of developing countries. Indeed, the agricultural revolution brought about by two lines of advance, that is, by the development of new technology on the one hand and by the intellectual conception of telescoping agriculture and food processing into the single operation of "agribusiness" on the other has been dramatically abrupt. In my own memory, tomatoes were once a seasonal luxury. Today, tomato soup and tomato ketchup are standard products, distributed almost all over the world. Scientific plant breeding can already supply a variety which will stand up to machine harvesting and on which the fruit is tough enough to come to no harm. The agricultural engineers[4] have already designed a machine capable of cutting off plants at ground level, shaking off the fruit, discharging the vines off the back and conveying the tomatoes along a series of belts into a bin to be taken direct to the factory to undergo the next stage of the manufacturing process. Within three years of their first introduction, these monster "combines" were harvesting 24 per cent of the California tomato crop. By 1968, 800 of them were in operation handling 80 per cent of the crop. By 1969, almost all the tomatoes in the United States were being picked mechanically. And what can be done for tomatoes can be done for almost anything else. For example, a lettuce-harvesting machine has been designed to pick four rows of lettuces at a time. According to C. F. Kelly[4], however, this machine has not yet been put on the market for the odd reason that it is too technologically efficient. This implies that only about 600 altogether would be needed to harvest all the lettuces in the world. The big engineering firms consequently feel that it is hardly worth their while bothering to go into business for so small a number.

Oranges, apples, cherries, peaches, apricots and raspberries—all can be harvested mechanically by the combined researches of the plant breeders who raise appropriate strains of trees and canes and the engineers who devise means of shaking the fruit off and catching it without

---

[3] Kepner, C.D. and Soothill, J.H., "The Banana Empire", (Russell), New York, 1935.
[4] Kelly, C.F., Sci American, 216, 50, Aug. 1967.

its coming to harm. And there is little need for me to describe in detail the intensive "factory" methods which have been perfected for raising livestock economically and efficiently to meet the needs of the food technologist who shares with the grower a hand in the single operation of agribusiness."

Who can doubt that food technology has changed social life down on the farm? Haymaking was once a social occasion. The farmer, his son, the hired man, often a neighbor as well were there and as the work went on in the hot sun, the women came out to the fields with jugs of cider. The fragrant delights of getting in the hay harvest were described with zest by Roman writers two thousand years ago. But already the automatic baler developed in 1940 is becoming obsolete. In its place, a huge machine has been developed with which one man, throbbing backwards and forwards across the field, can pick up the hay and compress it under high pressure, not into 150 lb. bales, but into little cubes, occupying far less space than baled hay and capable of running down a chute directly into the hopper feeding the cows.

THE LIMITS OF FOOD TECHNOLOGY

It seems to me to be rational to accept the principle enunciated by Buzzell and Nourse[5] that an innovation introduced by a food technologist is only successful if it fills a social need. This is why so many of the numerous product innovations introduced each year after a short fitful life fade away never to be heard of more. Ingenious and technically successful though its manufacture may be, if the product itself does not fit into the social behaviour of the community as this behaviour evolves, it will not succeed. In 1948, much study was given to the design of an automated "conveyor cafeterior," as it was called[6]. This was a device in which the customers sitting in a row were carried sideways on a slowly moving conveyor with their dinners in front of them moving at the same speed. This speed was calculated so that the average eater reached his first "station" exactly as he swallowed the last mouthful of his first course. At this station his dirty plate passed away in one direction, his predetermined second course emerged in front of him and they travelled on together. Finally, at the end of the programmed period of travel the horizontal conveyor came to an end gently depositing the satisfied customer on his feet: the meal was over. This system was not only ideally suited for the dispensing of appropriately processed foods, it was also designed to overcome such undesirable factors as "voluntary customer movement," that is, the tendency of people in cafeterias to get out of line. The apparatus also made provision for umbrellas and parcels to be carried along with the diners and for a "siding" for those customers whose rate of eating deviated markedly from the average.

My purpose in describing this apparatus is to point out that it proved in practice to be comparatively unsuccessful. Apparently it represented a degree of technology beyond the limit of what people were prepared to accept. . . .

It has been the custom in any general review of food technology to assert that its basic importance as a meaningful human activity is not merely to find an innocuous means of preventing orange squash from depositing an oily ring in the neck of the bottle or of developing a plastic yet chunky canned pet food but to make an essential contribution to the diet of the starving inhabitants of the developing nations. It is now becoming apparent, however, that... the impact of food science on society...is, in fact, limited. Food technologists are very good at making fish fingers and frozen dinners, they are not so good at making a leaf-protein concentrate that the citizens of a distant country, no matter how impoverished, will willingly eat. It will be observed that I have now reached a point in my argument when I have presented evidence to show that food technology has exerted a powerful effect on society, on the one hand

[5] Buzzell, R.D. and Nourse, R.E.R., "Product innovation in food processing 1954-64", (Harvard), Boston, 1967.
[6] Pyke, M., "Automation: its purpose and future", (Hutchinson), London, 1956.

tending to break down the domestic family structure of those who consume its products, to de-personalize the role of those who distribute them and to destroy the entire community structure of those rural societies who produce its raw materials. But in spite of the impact of advanced food processing on community behaviour, in spite of the attractiveness and convenience of breakfast cereals edible without cooking straight from the box, of dehydrated potato ready in a trice without scrubbing or peeling, of fish fingers free from bones, skin, head, tail and entrails—in spite of the enthusiasm with which such products are embraced, the social impact of food technology though strong is not limitless and, is indeed, less strong than the deep powerful forces by which human behaviour is essentially controlled....It is, therefore, not unreasonable to foresee that the interplay of social forces by which we are buffeted today on every hand may represent the the shock leading to the establishment of a different equilibrium and that, rather than technological progress going on and on without end, the tide may turn, the sea of fish fingers and dehydrated baby food recede and the contribution made by the social warmth of a meal take its place side by side with the technological factors, the calorific value, chemical composition, color, aroma and rheological characteristics of its ingredients with which we concern ourselves almost exclusively today.

TOWARDS A TWO-TIER TECHNOLOGY

I am not suggesting that the social trend which I foresee presages the end of food technology as it is now practiced. Because the citizens of a town object to sonic booms it does not follow that they decline to make use of the convenience of air travel. Neither does it follow that the existence of parents who feel that neither the table manners of their children nor their need for love and affection are likely to benefit from their being given their mid-day meal by a vending machine implies that they will refuse to eat canned salmon or use instant coffee....

The change in intellectual climate to which I am drawing attention comes when the benevolent food technologist urges that a million dollars-worth of produce be sent from the plenty of the technologically efficient producers of the developed countries to remedy the want among the poor developing countries of Asia, Africa, and Latin America. Then he stops to take thought, this benevolent food technologist, and finds himself compelled to admit that, in as much as his food technology is an extension of the expertise of the efficient and highly mechanized activities of the developed world's agriculturalists he is neither benevolent nor efficient. An examination of the facts demonstrates, firstly, that want in the developing world is far better served by improvements in economic status there and an increase in food supplies rather than by Multi Purpose Food, or fish protein concentrate, and, secondly—which is the hardest blow of all—that the productivity of agriculture in many developing areas is higher than that of the wealthy developed nations, otherwise why do the developed peoples, even with all their technology, protect themselves with tariffs, guaranteed prices, subsidies, support buying organizations and a big share of domestic quotas—and against whom? . . .

The Ebb and Flow of Technology

The technological revolution had its antecedents, it happened and is, indeed, still happening. In a little while as history unfolds it will dwindle into the perspective of the past. The people of the future having built their motorways will not give up their motor cars. They are, however, already building pedestrian precincts. Similarly, the food technologists will still find a demand for "convenience" foods of advanced technological food manufacture—excellet, nutritious, sanitary but inevitably uniform. The number of products will extend beyond the several thousand items already provided for the supermarket shelves and even beyond the local dishes of Italy, Greece, India and Latin America already being processed. How extensive this basic industrially manufactured infrastructure of future eating will be is perhaps indicated by the cannery set up at Whale Cove on Hudson Bay[7] producing canned whale heart in gravy, whale meat balls, seal flipper, seal liver in gravy, and a product rather like tripe made from white whale cut into strips and called "mukluk." It is even proposed to market canned Eskimo pet food based on walrus flesh which, it appears, is particularly esteemed by husky dogs.

But as well as all these one can forsee two developments about which the food technologist could well reflect. Already the sophisticated expertise and efficiency of the supermarket, in which foods are presented packaged to attract the eye as well as preserve the contents, is being overtaken by the discount store or "cash-and-carry" where little or no attention is given to presentation. Is this perhaps the birthplace of the new "inconvenience" foods? The wheel of social evolution having turned from the village store with its barrels and sacks, to the chain grocery with the first packaged and branded articles and thence to the supermarket is now going full circle to the trading post of the discount house from whence the housewife hauls away in her truck, not only a dozen packets of cornflakes but perhaps a sack of beans as well to tide her over the month's strike of electricity generator workers which she forsees looming up just as her grandmother foresaw a hard winter....

Perhaps the food technologist, while continuing to pursue technological progress leading to the ever-more sophisticated "convenience" product, flavoured, coloured, stabilized, rich in protein and vitamins or, on the contrary, the ultimate "non-food" about which I have written elsewhere[8], ideally suited for consumption by the non-hungry in the "bunny" places dedicated to non-sex, should also be prepared to supply a demand for food technology at a different level. This might be a return, as nearly as modern conditions allow, to unprocessed foods for people who enjoy the creative art of cooking and the social warmth to be enjoyed round a hospitable table.

Excerpted with permission from *The Food Scientist*, 9 (1) (Fall 1971).

---

[7] Anon., The Times, London, 31st Oct. 1968.
[8] Pyke, M., "Synthetic food", (Murray), London, 1970.

Who's Going to Eat the Breakfast of Champions?

JOAN GUSSOW

Breakfast of Champions is the title of a Kurt Vonnegut novel which helped inspire the speech from which the following essay has been excerpted. Vonnegut's "breakfast" was a martini; mine, in this essay, is Peruvian algae. The message is that food technology will not solve the world food crisis. Part of the speech was previously published under the same title in *CNI Weekly Report* in June of 1974.

In a book called *Breakfast of Champions*, one of Kurt Vonnegut's characters arrives on a planet where all animal and plant life except for the humanoids has been killed by pollution. The people on this planet now eat food made from petroleum and coal. They also spend a lot of time going to dirty movies, and they take the hero to one. Here is his description of it:

> The theater went dark and the curtains opened. At first there wasn't any picture. There were slurps and moans from loudspeakers. Then the picture itself appeared. It was a high quality film of a male humanoid eating what looked like a pear. The camera zoomed in on his lips and tongue and teeth which glistened with saliva. He took his time about eating the pear. When the last of it had disappeared into his slurpy mouth, the camera focussed on his Adam's apple. His Adam's apple bobbed obscenely. He belched contentedly, and then these words appeared on the screen, but in the language of the planet:

> THE END
> It was all faked, of course. There weren't any pears anymore.[1]

In one or the mythical planets Kurt Vonnegut invented in *Breakfast of Champions*, all of the food was made from petroleum and coal. (Obviously, he wrote before the fuel crisis.) On our very real planet—if the world portrayed for us by optimistic scientists comes into being—man's burgeoning population will ultimately be supported gastronomically by a tasty array of mock foods made from algae, from fish protein concentrate, from single-cell protein grown on petroleum byproducts, animal wastes or wood, or, ultimately, from simple chemicals made up into carbohydrates, fats and proteins through miracles of modern chemistry. These substances, designed to nourish the body of not the spirit, are—so we are told—the foods of the future.

Instant Salvation

Recently, a student gave me one of those

[1] Kurt Vonnegut, Jr., *Breakfast of Champions*, p. 60 (New York: Delacorte Press, 1973).

instantaneous salvation articles headlined, "New Plant Falls Between Milk and Eggs in Protein."

"On the sunny slopes of Lima, Peru," it began, "Peruvian and West German scientists are busy with a project that will help feed a hungry world when the day comes that conventional agriculture can no longer do the job, even for the affluent." The story goes on to comment that futurologists are predicting that within 70 years available agricultural land will not be sufficient to produce food for the hungry millions. Hence, projects such as this one involving the growing of algae in basins of water. The "crop" of algae is harvested by centrifuge and dried to produce a kind of leaf-colored flour. This novel substance is a protein of a quality somewhere between eggs and milk—in other words, very good. The article goes on to point out that one acre devoted to producing algal "flour" can produce almost 22 thousand percent more protein in a year than the same area assigned to milk production, almost 16,000 percent more protein than an acre planted with wheat, and 4,400 percent more protein than an acre of soybeans.

I'm somewhat skeptical of those figures. But the fact is that growing algal protein is clearly a much much more efficient use of land area than using the same area to graze cattle. In fact, since the pans full of water can presumably be set on stony ground or on solid rock, such processes ought to enable us to grow protein where no protein at all is presently produced. Now this particular product is green, so that its use presents certain aesthetic problems to those who wish to think of it as flour—and, as previous attempts to produce and market miracle protein foods have revealed, producing a product is one thing, getting people to use it—especially people in traditional societies—is another.

For the moment, however, let us assume that acceptability problems can be overcome—a large assumption. Are revolutionary sources of protein the "solution" to the world food prob-

lem? At least until recently, many proposed calculations—a serious mistake when energy is coming to be understood as the common coin of the environmental crisis.

Energy Costs

...In any world of the future, we cannot ignore the cost of energy, so all these amazing food-producing schemes need to be examined for their energy relationships. They may turn out to be highly impractical in an energy-conserving world. Not only are many of the processes proposed energy-intensive—synthesis of food materials in the laboratory, for example—but they require machinery complexes which are themselves energy demanding. And to bring them up to a scale which will make them truly economical they must often be very large, thus requiring large capital inputs which make them highly impractical for the poor countries which they are designed to help.

Growing algae may appear to make energy sense, since algae make use of the "free" energy of the sun. But even on a pilot scale, as they are being grown in Peru, they have to be centrifuged (an energy-costing process) and dried (another energy-demanding process). And those who have carefully studied the algal schemes from an energy point of view have concluded that when these projects are replicated on a true production scale, they may not turn out to provide the net gain of energy which they seem to promise.

Fertilizer Needed

Even more critically, perhaps, algae do not live on nothing. They must be fertilized or they die, which means that such projects would have to compete with conventional agriculture for the world's presently limited supply of fertilizers.

Just for the sake of argument, however, to satisfy those who say that science can always find a way, let's disregard these technical problems and ask whether such foods, in the real world, make human sense—if their energy and nutrient demands can be accommodated. Are special novel proteins really the solution to the hunger of those people now closest to starvation?

Let me very briefly suggest some of the other areas of difficulty. We have already spoken of acceptability problems. There are also some nutritional problems involved. We do not know enough to keep man alive, generation after generation, on a totally synthetic diet, nor are our research methods sophisticated enough to measure the long-range effects of subtle deleterious changes in food composition. The only diets with which we have long-range experience are those made up of various combinations of the world's animal, vegetable and mineral substances—as they have been selected out over the centuries by people in different parts of the world.

Moral Problems

While the acceptability factor *may* be overcome and the nutrition factor *may* be a risk worth taking if it is offered as an alternative to starvation, the more critical problem inherent in the new foods lies in what I would call the fairness factor. The appeal of magical solutions is that they do not require us to change *our* behavior—they only require other people to change theirs.

Bluntly, the world is not likely to permit us privileged few to go on eating steak while the great hungry majority of mankind is eating algal soup. The real problems are not scientific—they are moral.

If present trends continue unchanged, we can easily predict what will really happen to most of the new foods. Here is the last sentence of that article on the miraculous Peruvian algae. "The possibilities are almost unlimited," its West German developer commented. "They range from baby foods for infants, to cookies for preschool children, to green noodles for pasta

lovers, to protein drinks for weight watchers." It is the sad and ironic truth that in terms of marketing realities, these miraculous new foods are not likely to feed the starving millions who cannot provide a worthwhile "market" for them. If they sell at all, they are more likely to end up in American diet soft drinks, providing unneeded protein for some fat American who already has too much to eat.

If miracle foods cannot solve the problem of growing world hunger, what can be done? What can *we* do? We can urge our leadership—as soon as we have some again—to increase our contribution to carefully planned local development projects which will enable countries to help themselves both to feed their present populations and to cut down their projected future populations. For, in the long run, it is perfectly clear that we have to stop world population growth. If we do not, nature will do it for us. The carrying power of the earth is simply limited.

Short-run Solutions

But that is not a short-run solution. In the short run, no matter what we do, there will be twice as many people on earth by the time I am 71 as there are today—and all of them will wish to eat. There are several things Americans in particular can do immediately—and individually—to increase the world's supply of food.

We can eat less, we can waste less, and we can live lower down on the food chain. In the face of the world food crisis, we could eliminate obesity in this country, with a purpose. A purpose more worthy than personal vanity—or even personal health. Or we wouldn't have to go so far. There are 210 million Americans. If each of them ate 100 less calories per day, we would save 21 billion calories every day, enough to keep ten million people alive and well. Some of us could cut down our intake more than 100 calories a day to make up for those people who are not getting enough to eat in *this* country.

We could waste less. Our garbage pails would

certainly feed another 100 million people at a minimum. The waste built into our food system alone would, if eliminated, produce a tremendous multiplication of available food. For example, there is a simply staggering loss in the quality and quantity of food inherent in taking a nutritious cereal grain containing all the vitamins and minerals necessary for its own metabolism and turning it into a breakfast confection—to tempt the ruined palates of our overfed children.

And, finally, we can eat more vegetable and less animal protein. I am sure most of you are aware—perhaps some of you as belatedly as I—that meat is not necessary to life or health, that the majority of the world's people live largely on vegetable protein, and that the raising of animals as they are raised in this country— much of the time on grains and not on grass—is a terribly wasteful way of producing food.

If, however, we insist on continuing to eat as high on the cow as our budgets will allow, the rest of the world will go hungrier. If we do not voluntarily reduce our demand on world food supplies, we are going to be watching people die on television—in living color—while we sit and eat our TV dinners. What this will do to us morally, I care not to contemplate. But make no mistake, people making $200 a year cannot compete for food on the open market—as Agriculture Secretary Butz is urging them to do— with people making $200 a week.

Of course, we can go on as we are—on the odds that no one can make us change. The odds are fairly bad, however. Alternative scenarios are available to the one which has one-quarter of the world barricaded behind our indifference while three-quarters of the world goes hungry. A number of observers consider nuclear blackmail a highly likely prospect. And when the world equivalent of the Symbionese Liberation Army asks for ransom, they are not going to want our single-cell proteins or our algal soup. They will want food of the kind they are used to eating; or perhaps—moving up in the world— they will want food of the kind *we* are used to eating.

I think that before that time comes we would be well advised to take our heads out of the sands, to stop waiting for science to make it all better and to begin making use of what economist Herman Daly has called our "scarce moral resources." As persons knowledgeable about food and nutrition we are uniquely qualified to help people distinguish between wants and needs where food is concerned. Let us begin by teaching ourselves the painful relationship between American wants and the world's needs and see where it takes us. In the coming world struggle, the challenge for Americans is not survival—*we* have enough food to survive. It is survival with honor. None of the choices will be easy.

Red Meat Decadence

RUSSELL BAKER

In the eyes of many New Yorkers, persons without access to *The New York Times* are deprived. Not the least of their deprivations is regular *Times'* columnist Russell Baker, especially when he is serious. The column reproduced here was first published in April of 1973 when we were "boycotting" meat because the price had gone up. In it he is very serious indeed.

Nobody who remembers the Depression of the nineteen-thirties will be impressed by the heroism of boycotting meat for a single week. During all the years of that era, there must have been one or two pieces of beef, a pan-fried steak somewhere in 1934 or 1935 surely, but if so it left no imprint in memory.

Canned salmon, on the other hand, remains vivid in memory over almost forty years. It must have been ridiculously cheap then—ten or eleven cents for a big can. It now costs ten times as much, as does chipped beef, which was another staple of the Depression diet.

With chipped-beef gravy one night and fried salmon cakes another, we were eating fairly well, the meat boycotters might say. We certainly thought so. We did not even feel deprived on the third night when the main course was macaroni and cheese.

Chicken was the luxury meal at our house, as in a great many American households of the time, and this treat was invariably served on Sunday. Sunday was the day for noble dining in America and most of us who were children then probably grew up believing that when some fancy writer referred to "a Lucullan feast," he was talking about chicken, mashed potatoes, gravy and peas.

The chicken was always either fried or roasted. Fried was best. Roasted meant it was going to be leathery, and the elders at the table who remembered the glorious eating of the nineteen-twenties would make jokes about its being rooster.

Looking back, one realized that they may not have been joking, that the leathery fowls really may have been roosters, but there was so much joking at that table—joking with gaiety in it and not the embittered undercurrent that distinguishes the humor of our present age of decadence—that a child's memory of the period hears laughter everywhere.

That is a mystery still. It was such a bad time. What were they laughing about? Yet we heard it. They had one foot in the serene stability of the Edwardian age and the other in the mess of 1914-1929. They had been badly wrenched out of one time into another, but with nothing really damaged much. Perhaps their survival had left them permanently delighted.

Our children will probably not, at ages 40 and 50, hear us laughing in their memories. Oh, we are a glum bunch! Where did it come from, that glumness of ours that already echoes from our children's music and in the mission of moral uplift to which so many have dedicated themselves?

Those are deep questions, and on the theory that a deep question deserves a frivolous answer, I would suggest that the gloom we exude comes not from our Depression childhoods, but from our turning in early adulthood into a generation of beefeaters.

This beef madness began during World War II when richly fatted beef was force-fed into every putative warrior. Meat 21 meals a week was the formula for beating the Axis, although the men who really did the job, of course, were living on good old Depression foods, like Spam, while they were at work.

After the war there was no tapering off. We had become a nation of beef-a-holics. By the nineteen-fifties the smell of barbecued beef hung like smog over 100,000 American suburbs. A social crisis was no longer your relief check's failure to arrive before the rent was due, but the arrival of a steak cooked medium rare when you had ordered it rare.

This was not a crisis met with a gay smile on the lips, and a joke. Tension prevailed over that table. One was aware that his manhood had been challenged by the chef. Did one dare to threaten nuclear retaliation by demanding to see the manager? Would one lose face if....

One sweated.

One? We all sweated. It was the age of sweating. When people were relaxed, which was rare, they acknowledged it by saying, "no sweat." And beef and all those other meats every day of the year—they kept us sweating, and grim.

Nowadays if you want to hear laughter, you must think of macaroni and cheese and listen very carefully, and it may—just may, mind you—come dimly through the beef-clotted memory.

Reprinted with permission from *The New York Times*, Sect. L: 43 (3 April 1973). Copyright 1973 by The New York Times Company.

NAME OF ORGANIZATION: "ON SECOND THOUGHT"
PUBLIC SERVICE MESSAGES

SUBJECT: OVER-SNACKING

30 SECONDS

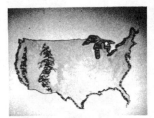

1. (MUSIC UNDER THROUGHOUT) (VO): America,

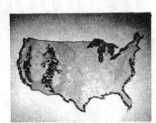

2. you have more good food to eat than any country in the world.

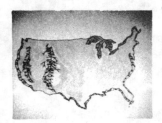

3. And what do you choose to eat?

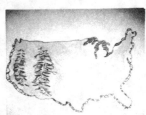

4. Potato chips,

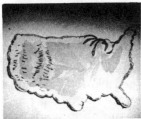

5. french fries, candy,

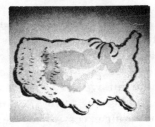

6. cookies, cake,

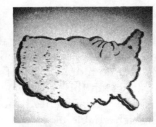

7. sodas, snacks.

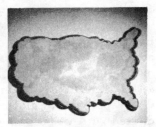

8. America, you're under-nourished and overweight.

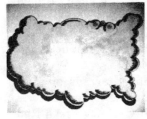

9. America,

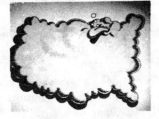

10. (SFX: LOUD BURP COMES FROM GREAT LAKES REGION ON MAP)

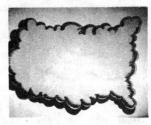

11. look what you're doing to yourself!

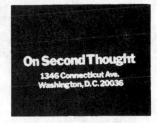

On Second Thought
1346 Connecticut Ave.
Washington, D.C. 20036

12. (SILENT)

Reprinted with permission from Council on Children, Media and Merchandising, Washington D.C.

Whatever Happened to Food? or It Does Pay to Fool with Mother Nature

In this "...land of the Cluett/Shirt Boston Garter and Spearmint/Girl With The Wrigley Eyes.../land above all of Just Add Hot Water and Serve..."[1] the problem is not scarcity but abundance. The American experience, as anthropologist Margaret Mead is fond of pointing out, is of having to *refuse* food. "Please, no more, I'm stuffed"; "Just a tiny piece. I'm on a diet!"; "Oh, what a *wicked* dessert." As the first article in this section points out, we have even designed a kind of Dorian Gray approach to gluttony; we have invented foods—diet soft drinks, calorie-free cookies, bread diluted with wood pulp—which enable us to continue our excessive calorie consumption without visibly exaggerating our tendency to overweight.

Perhaps the most obvious effect of this food excess is that it makes other people's hunger hard to believe. Faced with the temptations of those brightly-lit aisles, those floor-to-ceiling shelves filled with Pop-Tarts, Kool-Aid, Cap'n Crunch, and Screaming Yellow Zonkers, it is hard to remember that in much of the world millions are thankful for one real meal a day—each day's meal very like that of the day before; perhaps nothing more than a portion of grain or starchy tuber, seasoned with vegetables and, with luck, perhaps a scrap of chicken or fish.

No unsweetened pineapple chunks in rows of identical cans, no foil-wrapped arrays of margarines, distinguishable from one another only by their imaginative names and their precise levels of polyunsaturates; no Flintstones Yabba Dabba Dew Orange Drink, no Hi-C Dairy Fresh Red Punch (*red* punch? *dairy* fresh?); no arrays of breakfast cereals—"Norman," "Frute Brute," "Grins & Smiles & Giggles & Laughs"—dazzlingly flavored and colored to appeal to a newly emergent "child market"; no textured vegetable protein rendered into mock bacon and sausage products (what the British in their wisdom call "knitted meats") designed to assuage the anxieties of the fat-avoiders and cholesterol-phobes.

With increasing frequency, the American food supply of which these products are a part, has come under attack. There are those who say it is tasteless and absurd; that it is killingly unhealthy for *us* and immorally wasteful and exploitative in relation to the rest of the world. Its defenders call these charges alarmist, pointing to the fact that there is no place in the world where consumers have such choice and abundance, defending processing on the ground that it serves to preserve food that in less developed countries might be wasted.

Perhaps the critical question to be addressed in this volume is the following: If there *is* a world food and population and resource problem—and there is—is our food supply part of that problem or

---

[1]E.E.Cummings, "Poem or Beauty Hurts Mr. Vinal," *The Oxford Book of American Verse*, p. 926 (New York: Oxford University Press, 1950).

part of its solution, or neither? It seems appropriate to begin examining that topic by breaking it down into some simpler questions: where is our food supply now, where is it going, and why?

This section began by giving two contrasting answers. The first, called "Whatever Happened to Food?", is a brief and lightheartedly serious look at how the food product situation appeared in 1971 to two of its critics. What is remarkable about rereading "Whatever happened. . ." at several years remove is how little things seem to have changed. The head of HEW at the time was Robert Finch who had just seen one of his FDA Commissioners shot down over the too-slow banning of cyclamates as possible carcinogens. Only recently the FDA, under another new leader, created a congressional uproar by proposing a ban on the only remaining non-caloric sweetener, saccharin, as a possible carcinogen. There is still no continuous monitoring of the food supply or of the nutritional status of the population. There is still no requirement that additives be "necessary" for anything but the producer's convenience, though our per capita consumption of them has increased. We still don't know the total added "chemical burden" our food carries. We still don't have complete ingredient labeling, and consumers still appear confused—and mis-informed, in a 10,000-plus item food supply.

All of these criticisms seem silly at best, and at worst destructive, to Dr. Dena Cederquist as she talks with the Kraft Food Company. She praises the range of choices and the consistency of the food products available to Americans from one end of the country to the other. She admires the presence of fresh summer vegetables in mid-winter Michigan and argues that what we have gained from food industry efforts is cheaper, higher quality food and the opportunity to buy, for example, Cheez Whiz if we want it.

In the copy-filled ad that follows, General Foods agrees. Arguing that the principal purpose of "processing" is to make food "easier to use, or better-tasting, or longer-lasting, or safer, or whatever," GF goes on to launch a spirited defense of the frozen pea. There are few critics—even those most intemperate in their attacks on the American food supply—to whom the freezing of a green pea, picked at the peak of freshness, would seem an anti-social or anti-nutritional act. That is not the real problem. General Foods states the real problem perfectly in its own ad copy: "Nobody makes food, peas included, the way nature does." That is an undeniable truth. Nobody does, or can, make foods the way Nature does. But an increasing number of people appear to be trying.

Clearly, the argument between the defenders and the attackers of the food supply in the past decades has not been waged over the virtues of canned applesauce and frozen peas, but over the introduction into the marketplace of thousands of "food novelties," everything from fish-shaped crackers for people, to cracker-shaped fish for dogs. How and *why* all these curious food objects have come to be invented is the topic of Hadsell's by now almost historic article on the food industry's search for growth through processing and diversification. The article lays out with great clarity the importance of the new product and the new product line to the growth and profitability of the food business.

I used Hadsell's "old" article to make the point because my students—and I assume other people of their generation(s)—tend to think that nothing more than five years old can possibly be worth reading—or any longer true. A reading of Hadsell reinforces the important understanding that a correct identification of the forces underlying a particular change *remains* correct over time—and enables one to predict the manner in which alteration of those forces may (over time) alter the character or the direction of change.

By 1976, the economics of food were quite different than they had been in 1971. And in March of that year *Business Week* ran an article in its Marketing Section titled "The Hard Road of the Food Processors." In it, Stephen A. Greyser, Director of the Marketing Science Institute, is quoted as fearing the "staggering consequences" of higher food prices, including perhaps "less impulse buying, less eagerness to try new products, and less interest in expensive convenience and snack foods." Data in the article confirm the fact that new product introductions were indeed lower in 1973 than in 1972. But does this indicate a trend back to "basics"? Away from processing? Quite the contrary.

For the chronic problem is the inability of the consumer to consume much more than 1500 pounds of food a year. Therefore, if the goal is to keep the food industry growing, then the unchanged necessity is to induce the consumer to pay more and more for the same amount of food. And if commodity prices go up, as they have in the 70's, then one can predict that there will be an accelerating move to produce "food" products which do not rely heavily on "food" materials.

This is precisely what Arthur D. Little, Inc. was recommending to the Food and Agribusiness Industries in the wake of the energy crunch in May of 1974. One strategy, they wrote, "for weathering times of shortage and high prices, is development of products with relatively complex formulations and/or high value added, such as convenience foods. Standard low-value-added-food products—quasi-commodities—are not easily reformulated without loss of identity. Moreover, their profit margins are generally not large enough to cushion rises in raw material costs. Processors of more complex food products have much greater latitude in the raw material selection process... *The further a product's identity moves from a specific raw material—that is, the more processing steps involved—the less vulnerable is its processor.*" (Italics, J.G.) Or, as the Meer Corporation (whose ad is reproduced on page 141) might put it, "If you need to find substitutes for your substitutes..."

Thus it would not have been hard to predict that among the new products of the seventies would be Hamburger Helper—a relatively high priced box of pasta, seasonings and additives originally "positioned" (in marketers' lingo) as a "skillet dinner" (using *your* hamburger), and subsequently "repositioned" (still using *your* hamburger) as a source of casserole dinners as well; or Pringles, the virtually immortal potato snack, no longer dependent—for its existence or its price—on the fresh potato.

It would have been easy to predict that when sugar prices dropped, novelty cereals for children would be big again—since they contain less of the valuable grain raw material than "adult cereals," and command a premium price. (One might *not* have predicted—as too absurd to imagine—a product like French Toast Batter Mix in which the customer, using *her* bowl, *her* milk, *her* bread and *her* frying pan, replaces the "inconvenience" of beating a couple of eggs into the milk with the "convenience" of beating-in the contents of a 25¢ packet of "sugar, whey solids, wheat flour, whole egg solids, tapioca, starch, dextrose, hydrogenated vegetable oil, salt, baking powder, lactose and artificial color.")

Recognizing the economics of food processing, it would not have been difficult to anticipate an attempt (ultimately unsuccessful) to introduce into the government's feeding programs a formulated liquid originally designed for hospital diets. By this means children could be weaned early from those unreliable creations of mother nature: milk, juice, fruits and vegetables. And finally, as the brief news stories indicate, the "search for growth" was bound to lead processors to put even "faster" foods into the supermarkets in answer to the "eating out" trend, just as it was bound to have as its ultimate outcome the decline in the use of freshly prepared food, even in "high class" restaurants.

Thus it is clear that whether or not increasingly processed and formulated foods really meet consumer demand, they are (and will continue to be—in the absence of a food policy that alters the economics of the situation—or a consumer revolt) essential to food companies who wish to present an attractive profit picture to their stockholders. Does the American *consumer* profit from the variety which this adds to the marketplace? Dena Cederquist argues that s/he does. A number of the authors in this chapter have argued that s/he does not.

Philip Wylie, in "Science Has Spoiled My Supper," reminds those of us over forty that those somewhat younger have a less firm memory of the taste of ordinary "food," since science had by their infancies already begun converting food into "products." The American people, Wylie marvels, will stand for lots of things, will, finally, *settle* for something that will "do" if it is presented to them in the name of novelty and progress. One wonders what Wylie, profane denouncer of "momism," might have thought of Pringles, or of mock peach and raspberry cobblers made of apples, or of the "creative flavorists" whose activities Ruth Rosenbaum chronicles in her article, "Today the Strawberry, Tomorrow. . ." According to Rosenbaum, the flavorists' attitude toward Mother Nature has moved from modest imitation (flavors that were "no match for Mother Nature") to outright hostility: i.e. a recent IFF annual report which "warns its shareholders that 'natural foods' are 'a wild mixture of substances created by plants and organisms for completely different non-food purposes—their survival and reproduction,' and that they 'came to be consumed by humans at their own risk.'" In short, beware of the broccoli, for its function is to flower.

Near the end of her article Rosenbaum takes note of the argument most often used in defense of our move toward the synthetic—that it is necessary if we are to feed the world's hungry. There will never be enough "natural" flavors or enough "natural" food to meet our demand, the argument goes; thus we must begin using "novel" food sources and make them taste like the foods people are used to eating. Hadsell suggested as much in discussing soy protein analogues; the flavorists cite world hunger as one important justification for their activities.

While it would be difficult for anyone who has recently tasted a fresh raspberry (home grown, of course—progress has eliminated them from the normal channels of commerce) to swallow the idea that anybody's raspberry flavor is "perfect," it is troublesome to imagine that such nostalgia is holding back advances that may solve the world food problem. That issue is dealt with in "Who's Going to Eat the Breakfast of Champions?", an excerpt from a speech delivered at the 44th Annual Meeting of the New York Dietetic Association. The essay is an attempt to answer a number of arguments that have been advanced to support the usefulness of "novel" food sources in meeting the world food crisis. What is often not taken into account, I point out, is that given the necessary inputs of water, fertilizer and energy, most of these magic solutions turn out to be too expensive for the hungry poor of the world to buy—so that soy protein analogues are more likely to end up as Baco's than as survival rations.

The same is true in this country, of course. Highly processed foods are *not* really cheap—they cannot be, for someone has to pay for the processing. That French Toast Batter Mix, which contains more sugar, whey solids and wheat flour than egg solids, costs more—and provides less food value—than the eggs it presumes to replace.

The customer is the one who pays for processing, as the saga of Pringles—here documented in press clippings—so clearly demonstrates. It is a fascinating tale indeed, showing the determination that lies behind product introductions with the potential profit of these paraboloid potato corpses. Given the extent of consumer resistance to their disappointing flavor and high price, it is hard to argue that such a product was designed to meet consumer needs, wants—or even whims. Rather this is clearly a product designed to meet *company* needs, into which great energies (and vast amounts of capital) have been poured in an attempt to *create* a consumer demand. (Keep Pringles in mind when you read the next chapter, in which is examined that singularly American art form, advertising, the motive force behind the marketplace this chapter is exploring.)

Yet taken all in all, it could be argued that these Baroque outcroppings of the food supply are merely silly, merely the extravagant price we pay for our abundance. Perhaps a culture which prefers Cool Whip to whipped cream, because it is more durable, is merely pointless in its excesses—not harmful, but amusing. Three of the selections in this chapter have suggested that the changes in our food supply are more sinister than silly. Michael Jacobson, in "Our Diets Have Changed But Not for the Best," points out (in a somewhat tempered version of the no-holds-barred style for which he is noted) that in moving away from foods to food products, we have done much more than permit the continued growth of the food companies. And our high meat diets, our apparently insatiable appetite for beef, are not only increasing our demand on world food supplies but straining our health as well. We have, he shows, changed the nutrient composition of our diets in a way that appears to be related to our increasing vulnerability to degenerative disease. Our diet is unhealthy, and apparently getting more so, and we have as yet no federal, state or local policies to impede its decay.

Moreover, argues Magnus Pyke in a brilliantly inclusive essay, food technology has impacted more than just us and our diets. His article, first published (like Hadsell's) in 1971, is astonishingly up-to-date. Only his prediction that "tomorrow" we will have "wrapped bars that are in every nutritional sense the equivalent of a sitdown affair" has been overtaken by time. What was tomorrow in 1971 is today, today. Breakfast Bars, that "terrible tasting product," as one General Mills' executive characterized them[2], are obviously intended to be the nutritional equivalent of a meal.

Like their manufacturers, Pyke has somewhat more faith in technology's ability to achieve exact nutritional equivalence than some of the rest of us. Nevertheless, his article effectively and literately pulls together a number of other objections to technological foods that had already been raised: that such foods are not the answer to the hunger of the developing countries, that productivity in those countries is higher than in our own, and food prices therefore lower, and that many of our problems are not technological, to be solved by technological advances, but human. His unique perception is of the manner in which we are all being changed by the food environments which the contemporary American food supply has created. (Keep in mind Pyke's observations about the pilferage in large supermarkets when you reach the chapter where it is argued that the basic failure of large solutions is that they always require large police forces.)

The chapter ends with a selection from *New York Times'* columnist Russell Baker, supplying, as he says, "a frivolous answer" to a serious question. The answer is "meat"—the question to which it is the answer is, "What has made us stop laughing?" It is a more serious answer than it appears to be though not, clearly, than it intends to be.

---

[2] The Hard Road of the Food Processors," *Business Week* (March 1971).

CHAPTER 4

Selling It!

Advertising as a Philosophical System

JULES HENRY

Sociologist Jules Henry, whose angry yet elegant critique of advertising begins this chapter, included "Advertising as a Philosophical System" in his book titled *Culture Against Man*. As far as I am concerned, there is no single other piece in the book which so vividly defines *our* problem.

Advertising is an expression of an irrational economy that has depended for survival on a fantastically high standard of living incorporated into the American mind as a moral imperative. Yet a moral imperative cannot of itself give direction; there must be some institution or agency to constantly direct and redirect the mind and emotions to it. This function is served for the high-rising living standard by advertising which, day and night, with increasing pressure reminds us of what there is to buy; and if money accumulates for one instant in our bank accounts, advertising reminds us that it must be spent and tells us how to do it. As a quasi-moral institution advertising, like any other basic cultural institution anywhere, must have a philosophy and a method of thinking. the purpose of this chapter is to demonstrate the character of advertising thought, and to show how it relates to other aspects of our culture. In order to make this relationship manifest at the outset I have dubbed this method of thought *pecuniary philosophy*.

The Problem

Since the problem of truth is central to all

philosophy, the reader is asked to ask himself, while perusing the following advertising, "Is it literally true that..."

...everybody's talking about the new *Starfire* [automobile]?

...*Alpine* cigarettes "put the men in menthol smoking"?

...a woman in *Distinction* foundations is so beautiful that all other women want to kill her?...

...one will "get the smoothest, safest ride of your life on tires of *Butyl*"? ...

...*Pango Peach* color by Revlon comes "from east of the sun...west of the moon where each tomorrow dawns"...is "succulent on your lips" and "sizzling on your finger tips (And on your toes, goodness knows)" and so will be one's "adventure in paradise"?...

...when the Confederate General Basil Duke arrived in New York at the end of the Civil War "*Old Crow* [whiskey] quite naturally would be served"?

...*Bayer* aspirin provides "the fastest, most gentle to the stomach relief you can get from pain"?

Are these statements, bits of advertising copy, true or false? Are they merely "harmless exaggeration or puffing"[1] as the Federal Trade Commission calls it? Are they simply para-poetic hyperboles—exotic fruits of Madison Avenue creativity? Perhaps they are fragments of a new language, expressing a revolutionary pecuniary truth that derives authority from a phantasmic advertising universe. In the following pages I try to get some clarity on this difficult and murky matter by teasing out of the language of advertising some of the components of pecuniary philosophy I perceive there.

Pecuniary Pseudo-Truth. No sane American would think that literally everybody is "talking about the new *Starfire*," that Alpine cigarettes literally "put the men in menthol smoking" or that a woman wearing a *Distinction* foundation garment becomes so beautiful that her sisters literally want to kill her. Since he will not take these burblings literally, he will not call them lies, even though they are all manifestly untrue. Ergo, a new kind of truth has emerged—*pecuniary pseudo-truth*—which may be defined as a false statement made as if it were true, but not intended to be believed. No proof is offered for a pecuniary pseudo-truth, and no one looks for it. Its proof is that it sells merchandise; if it does not, it is false.

Para-Poetic Hyperbole. Revlon's rhapsodies on *Pango Peach* . . . and similar poesies are called para-poetic hyperbole because they are something like poetry, with high-flown figures of speech, though they are not poetry. Note, however, that they are also pecuniary pseudo-truths because nobody is expected to believe them.

Pecuniary Logic. When we read the advertisements for *Butyl* and *Old Crow* it begins to look as if *Butyl* and *Old Crow* really *want* us to believe, for they try to prove that what they say is true. *Butyl*, for example, asserts that "major tire marketers . . . are now bringing you tires made of this remarkable material"; and *Old Crow*

says that the reason it "would quite naturally be served" to General Duke in New York was because he "esteemed it 'the most famous [whiskey] ever made in Kentucky.'" When one is asked to accept the literal message of a product on the basis of shadowy evidence, I dub it *pecuniary logic.* In other words, pecuniary logic is a proof that is not a proof but is intended to be so for commercial purposes.

There is nothing basically novel in pecuniary logic, for most people use it at times in their everyday life. What business has done is adopt one of the commoner elements of folk thought and use it for selling products to people who think this way all the time. This kind of thinking—which accepts proof that is not proof—is an *essential* intellectual factor in our economy, for if people were careful thinkers it would be difficult to sell anything. From this it follows that in order for our economy to continue in its present form people must learn to be fuzzy-minded and impulsive, for if they were clear-headed and deliberate they would rarely put their hands in their pockets; or if they did, they would leave them there. If we were all logicians the economy could not survive, and herein lies a terrifying paradox, for *in order to exist economically as we are we must try by might and main to remain stupid.* . . .

Pecuniary Truth

Most people are not obsessive truth-seekers; they do not yearn to get to the bottom of things; they are willing to let absurd or merely ambiguous statements pass. And this unde-mandingness that does not insist that the world stand up and prove that it is real, this air of relaxed wooly-mindedness, is a necessary condition for the development of the revolutionary mode of thought herein called *pecuniary philosophy.* The relaxed attitude toward veracity (or mendacity, depending on the point of view) and its complement, pecuniary philosophy, are important to the American economy, for they

---

[1]An expression used by the Federal Trade Commission in dismissing a complaint against a company for using extreme methods in its advertising.

make possible an enormous amount of selling that could not otherwise take place. . . .

We turn now to a more central theme of the pecuniary system, *pecuniary psychology.*

Pecuniary Psychology

The fundamental concepts of pecuniary psychology are the "brain box" or, more simply, "the head," and "penetration." The head is a repository for advertising "claims" or "messages," and these enter the head by virtue of their penetrating power.... Thus pecuniary psychology pivots, like any system of thought, on a conception of the mind.

Other important concepts are: the advertiser's "claim," "finiteness" of head content, "measurability" of head content, transitoriness. Transitoriness is really an implicit underlying idea or parameter. . . . Fundamentally it implies impermanence, instability, evanescence—disloyalty, so to speak, of consumers, for consumers are viewed (rather ungratefully, I think) as being constantly on the verge of deserting one product for another.... Not "product loyalty" but product *dis*loyalty is the foundation of our economy. After all, if everyone stuck with a product once he had tried it, how would dozens of other manufacturers enter the field with identical ones? . . .

The conception of the head or "box" involves the hidden assumption of mental passivity, for the brain box is conceived of as an inert receptacle which the advertiser enters by penetration, i.e., his "campaign" gets a claim inside the box. . . .

Monetization

Since values like love, truth, the sacredness of high office, God, the Bible, motherhood, generosity, solicitude for others, and so on are the foundation of Western culture, anything that weakens or distorts them shakes traditional life. The traditional values are part of traditional philosophy, but pecuniary philosophy, far from being at odds with them appears to embrace

them with fervor. This is the embrace of a grizzly bear, for as it embraces the traditional values pecuniary philosophy chokes them to death. The specific choking mechanism is *monetization.*

Let us consider the following advertisement for a popular women's magazine: Against a black sky covering almost an entire page in the *New York Times* of June 2, 1960 is chalked the following from the New Testament: "Children, love ye one another." Below, the advertising copy tells us that *McCall's* magazine will carry in its next issue parables from five faiths, and that

> [s]uch spiritual splendor, such profound mystical insight, seem perfectly at home in the pages of *McCall's,* where the editorial approach is all-inclusive, universal, matching the infinite variety of today's existence.

Guilt by association is familiar enough to the American people through the work of various sedulous agencies of Government. *McCall's,* however, has discovered its opposite—*glory* by association, or, in the language of this work, pecuniary transfiguration. Since "spiritual splendor" and "mystical insight" are traits of holy books, and since examples of these are printed in *McCall's,* it is by that fact a kind of holy book. This is what I mean by the use of values for pecuniary purposes; this is value distortion through monetization.

Consider now the following report from the *New York Times,* July 27, 1961:

> It is understood that President Kennedy for the first time has authorized the use of his name and photograph in an advertisement.
>
> The ad will be one of a series of institutional advertisements run in behalf of the magazine industry. The President's picture will appear together with a statement discussing the role of magazines in American life.
>
> An element of controversy has surrounded the use of President Kennedy's name and photograph in advertising. Last week the National Better Business Bureau criticized the unauthorized use of the President's name and

likeness and warned that White House policy forbade such practices. The bureau noted such items as a "Kennedy Special" fish stew, J.F.K. rocking chairs and so forth.

The reason certain forms of logic are abandoned is not because they are wrong, but rather because they have proved inadequate to new problems and new knowledge. The old logics cannot make distinctions that must now be made, or they make distinctions that are no longer necessary. In the *Times* article we perceive such a situation, for obviously practitioners of pecuniary logic have somehow used the President's name inappropriately in naming a fish stew after him. Consider the following imaginary slogans:

John F. Kennedy, President of the United States, endorses the American way of life.

John F. Kennedy, President of the United States, endorses our fish stew.

John F. Kennedy, President of the United States, endorses American magazines.

One can see instantly that endorsement of the American way of life by the President would make one feel comfortable, whereas presidential endorsement of fish stew would cause one to feel vaguely unhappy and perhaps a little sick. The third statement might merely stimulate a little wonder that the President could do anything so brash. However, if magazines can be linked by pecuniary transfiguration to a basic value like "the American way of life," then it becomes reasonable to bring in the President. Herein lies the genius of the Madison Avenue logicians—the wave of the future—for though in the present case they have avoided the worst pitfalls of pecuniary logic, they have remained true to its spirit. The failure of pecuniary logic in the fish stew case lies in its inability to make a distinction between something of high cultural value ("the American way of life") and something of little or no cultural

value (fish stew). This failure can be referred to the inadequacy of the basic premise, "anything that sells a product is right." In the present instance the premise was not right because it brought pecuniary thinking into collision with tradition as embodied in the Better Business Bureau. The magazine men were smarter.

Consider now the following imaginary brands:

"George Washington" Corn Chowder.
"Abe Lincoln" Blackstrap Molasses.

The reader will not very likely take offense at either of these because (a) Washington and Lincoln are dead; (b) corn chowder and blackstrap molasses have a primordial, earthy, American atmosphere about them. The fish, however, is a deprecated, rather low-caste animal in American culture, in spite of the enamoured pursuit of it by millions of week-end fishermen. Furthermore, though *fried* fish has higher status, fish *stew* sounds plebian and even hateful to many people. One can now begin to understand the instinctive revulsion of the BBB to attachment of the President's name to fish stew. Fundamentally it has nothing to do with the monetization of a national symbol. Basically BBB recoiled at the degradation of the symbol through association with fish, and at the connection of a *living* president with a commercial product. (It would not be so bad if he were dead.)

Though Americans have traditionally shown little respect for public office, some men, like the Founding Fathers and Abraham Lincoln, have become almost sacred, and their memories are still rallying points for the forces of traditional ethics in American life. Hence their names and likenesses, *downgraded,* perhaps, are yet useful for advertising many things, from banks to whiskey. This being the case, we can surmise that the reason we do not protest the use, for pecuniary purposes, of passages from the New Testament, or the widespread monetization of values is because *traditional values are losing the respect and the allegiance of the people,* even though Madison Avenue can still transmute into cash what residues of veneration they yet evoke. An important social function of the Franklin, Lincoln, and Washington sagas is to make Americans ready to patronize any institution or buy any product bearing their names. One might say, "Sell a kid on the cherry tree and you can sell him cherries the rest of his life."

In their wars of survival pecuniary adversaries will use anything for ammunition—space, time, the President, the Holy Bible, and all the traditional values. Monetization waters down values, wears them out by slow attrition, makes them banal and, in the long run, helps Americans to become indifferent to them and even cynical. . . .

Pecuniary Philosophy as Cradle Snatcher

> The Flower-eyed Wonderment of Babes;
> The Phantasy of Their Play;
> The Joy of Christmas
>
> > The brand-image created on
> > television and embedded in
> > the minds of children assures
> > good volume for these items. . . .[1]

Homo sapiens trains his children for the roles they will fill as adults. This is as true of the Eskimo three-year-old who is encouraged to stick his little spear into a dead polar bear as it is of an American child of the same age who turns on TV to absorb commercials; the one will be a skilled hunter, the other a virtuoso consumer.

In contemporary America children must be trained to *insatiable* consumption of *impulsive* choice and *infinite variety*. These attributes, once instilled, are converted into cash by advertising directed at children. It works on the assumption that the claim that gets into the child's brain box first is most likely to stay there, and that since in contemporary America children manage parents, the former's brain box is the antechamber to the brain box of the latter.

In their relations with children manufacturers and advertising agencies are dedicated cultural surrogates, like any other teacher, for since the central aims of our culture are to sell goods and create consumers, they educate children to buy. What should businessmen do, sit in their offices and dream, while millions of product-ignorant children go uninstructed? This would be an abdication of responsibility. Besides, the businessmen might go bankrupt. The argument that advertising campaigns beamed at young children are somehow sickening because such campaigns take advantage of the impulsiveness and the unformed judgment of the child is old-fashioned squeamishness, somehow reminiscent of the fight against vivisection. Time and again we have had to fight off crackpots who do not understand that animals must be sacrificed to human welfare, and that because of anesthetics vivesection is now painless. So it is with the child versus the gross national product: what individual child is more important than the gross national product? And is it not true that TV is an anesthetic?

Let us now look at a few reports on advertising directed to children.

> In a span of time few things have greater memorability than a brand name learned in childhood.
>
> As a result, many large advertisers are using toys to get their products into the hands of children. Many of the companies are providing the merchandise free or below production cost to a Pennsylvania toy manufacturer, who then sells miniature sets of products for children. . . .
>
> John White, Jr., sales promotion manager of Chesebrough Ponds, Inc., explains:
>
> "This is just about the only medium that affords us direct contact with future users of our products. We're very much aware of the importance of preselling the youngsters. . . . I think there's no doubt that the company whose product has been used as a play item during the impressionable years of childhood, has just that much edge on a competitor who does not engage in this type of promotion. . . ."
>
> There was another favorable comment from

---

[1]*New York Times*, November 11, 1960.

Winton May, vice president of the Chicopee Manufacturing Company, whose Miracloth dishcloths are included in one of the toy sets. He said:

"This is an especially good medium for establishing brand images."[1]

[The H.J. Heinz Company has just floated a campaign aimed at the back to school trade], which they say will put "the whole world" in the hands of school children while putting Heinz tomato soup in their mouths.

The "whole world" turns out to be a plastic globe, 12-inches in diameter. The student may get the globe by sending $2 in cash to Heinz along with three Heinz tomato soup labels.[2]

A Share for Johnny

Like a stone cast in water that makes wider and wider concentric ripples, stock market enthusiasm is reaching a wider and wider public. But recently Cadre Industries Corporation of Endicott, N.Y., decided that children had not yet been reached effectively.

To mark its tenth anniversary, the company has published a booklet called A Share for Johnny.[3]

Educating a child to buy stocks is not, of course, the same as inspiring him to buy soup or pie, but the general principle is the same: training the young mind in spending money.

A Pie for Billy

Youngsters like pie. Pies usually are made in grown-up sizes. If they are made in children's sizes, more will be sold to children.

The Wagner Baking Corporation of Newark, N.J., has been following this reasoning and the result is the introduction of a snack-size Billy Wagner Pie, which will be promoted to children as a confection for meals, between meals and for school lunch boxes (to be eaten on the way to school).[4]

It would be narrow, fanatical, eggheaded legalism to urge that business is merely *legally* innocent of coercion in such advertising. After all, what is the tender-eyed innocence of children for? Is it not for gazing spellbound and uncritical on the doubtful wonders of the culture?

Is it not better that American children engage in productive play such as manipulating standard brands in miniature cans, than waste their time and energy in mindless games of jacks? The outstanding characteristic of children's play in all societies has been preparation for adult life. We were deviant in this respect until advertising put us back on the right path. The charge that pitching advertisements to youngsters, *conditioning* them before they have a chance to *think*, is an arrogant and brutal *invasion of the function of judgment*, is hysterical. It reminds one of 1984. The idea that Campbell's, Heinz, Chicopee, Texaco, et cetera, could become like "big brothers" to our children is laughable. Absurd to imagine that my grandchild, as he swings his jet-propelled road-skooter into the nearest Shell station should feel as if a speaker went off in his head saying gently, "Texaco! Remember?" And that he should then wheel away, heading guiltily for the next Texaco service station! Preposterous! . . .

Deprive business of its capacity to appeal to children *over the heads of their parents* and what would happen to most of the cereals, some of the drugs, and many toys? If advertising has invaded the judgment of children, it has also forced its way into the family, an insolent usurper of parental function, degrading parents to mere intermediaries between their children

---

[1]*New York Times*, August 3, 1960.
[2]*Ibid.*, July 18, 1960.
[3]*Ibid.*, October 6, 1961. I would not wish to give the impression that Americans are the only ones with progressive ideas. The *New York Times* of November 4, 1961 reports that Lord Ritchie of Dundee, chairman of the London Stock Exchange recommended that children be instructed in school on "how the stock market operates" so that "when they were older it would seem natural for them to invest in the future prosperity of their country...."
[4]*Ibid.*, August 17, 1960.

and the market. This indeed is a social revolution in our time!

Meanwhile this arrogance is terrifyingly reminiscent of another appeal to children over the heads of their parents: that of the Nazi Youth movement, for it too usurped parental function. The way the Nazis did it was by making society state-centered. What we have done is to combine product-centeredness with child-centeredness to produce a unique American amalgam, consumption-centeredness: a cemetery of brain boxes filled with the bones of pecuniary claims....

In analyzing monetization I said that "in their wars of survival pecuniary adversaries will use anything for ammunition—space, time, the President, the Holy Bible and all the traditional values"—a discovery that led to the conclusion that the erosion of traditional values was due in no small part to fear of competition.

The modes of thought and the view of man entertained by pecuniary philosophy have been shown to derive in great part from fear and contempt. Thus we have discovered that an industry now contributing nearly 12 billion dollars to the gross national product derives much of its dynamism from contempt and fear. It has also the most radical conception of *Homo sapiens* that has ever been proposed.

Shame and Degradation

> The pretty girl is probably the marketing man's best friend. At least he depends on her more than anything else to catch the eye of the public....
>
> The college co-ed is quite an effective marketing tool....
>
> The suburban socialite type of model...is a good saleswoman for products involving self-indulgence....[1]

There ought to be a section of this report dealing with *parts* of the female that are the best "marketing tools." For example, I have an advertisement for a popular automobile showing a blonde, bottom up, on the roof of it. The lower part of her is clad in scarlet tights and glows arrestingly against the warm browns and yellows of the autumn background.[2] Another ad is a closeup color photo of a lovely young woman on ice skates coming to a spectacular, braking, "swoosh" of a stop. Since the camera is shooting from below upward and the girl is wearing tautly stretched tights and a tiny skirt that conceals practically nothing, the view of the buttocks, flung sideways at the lens by the sizzling half-turn is unparalleled.[3] How many points the GNP has risen on the feminine buttock is an interesting question.

I once showed several advertisements to a class of advanced graduate students in business administration, in order to illustrate how women are used by advertising in our culture. When I came to a Japanese student he glanced at the red-tights ad but quickly averted his eyes. This is *shame.* Shame seems still to live in Japan, hence the averted eyes; for the Japanese could never confront his inner self if he permitted himself to look brazenly on the publicly flaunting buttocks of a woman, even in a photograph.

The female has lost her *shame functions* in our culture; impulse has broken through the wall of shame and advertising has been quick to see the pecuniary value. I am not saying that advertising has caused a breakdown in the shame functions of women. Rather I am urging that since women have already lost their shame functions, advertising merely exploits the consequences.

By *shame function,* I mean the following: In some cultures the culturally central emotions tend to be embodied in one sex or the other, and that sex becomes the symbol of the emotion. From Lorca and Pitt-Rivers[4] we know the importance of *sangre y verguenza* in Spain: man the embodiment of courage and violence (*sangre*),

---

[1] Report on a study done by Social Research, Inc., a commercial outfit of high-power University of Chicago social scientists. From the *New York Times,* April 11, 1961.
[2] *Esquire,* July 1960.
[3] *Life,* January 20, 1961.
[4] See Pitt-Rivers, *People of the Sierra.*

women the repository of shame (*verguenza*). Together they are the emotional underpinning of
Spanish peasant culture and social life. The
blood and brooding night of Lorca's plays flow
from the peril to these in the Spanish villages of
which he wrote. It was not so different in our
own culture not too long ago, except that the
ferocity of the defense and the darkly oppressive quality of these feelings found in Spain
were not present in America. With the transformation of American culture into a consuming one, all inhibitory emotions, all feelings that
contribute in any way to an austere view of life
and to the constriction of impulse, had to go.
Female shame, and masculine respect for female
shame, are casualties of the era of impulse
release and fun in the United States. As usual,
advertising merely converts the casualty into
cash. In doing so, however, it drives the message home: *shame has lost its force in American life,*
and women, having turned their backs, lead the
retreat....

Advertising's use of female ecstasy is, perhaps, the most imaginative monetization of
woman. Campaigns for undergarments, soaps,
sanitary tissues and napkins, perfumes, and
cigarettes have pictured women swooning or-
gastically under the spell cast by the product.
The prophetic, though unarticulated, message
in the advertisements is that men and women
have become so estranged from one another
and from themselves that for many the love-
climax has become *socially* meaningless. When
an orgasm is self-centered, a narcissistic experience only, and does not unite one overwhelmingly to another human being, there is no
particular reason why it should not be pinched
off, mimicked, monetized, and used to sell anything.

"Are we wasting women?" queries *Life* editorially.[1] The answer is, Of course not! No nation

on earth has ever used them to greater advantage! Without the pecuniary uses of women—
their hair, their faces, their legs and all the
wondrous variety of their personality and ana-
tomy—the economy would perish. Even the
armaments race would not save it, nor could we
eat enough nostrums to make up for the loss of
the monetized female! But along with monetization, along with this power to hurl the
economy to unimagined heights,[2] woman has
been degraded. How can she permit advertising
to portray her as it does? Why does she not rise
up in rage? Perhaps her idealization of herself
prevents the American woman from perceiving
what is actually happening to her. . . .

Advertising, Consumption Autarchy, and the Self

Consumption autarchy is the term I have coined
for the condition in which a country consumes
all it produces. In 1960 the United States exported 4 per cent of its gross national product.[3]
This closeness to consumption autarchy is made
necessary by the low purchasing power of much
of the rest of the world and by reduction to a
mere trickle of exports to the communist countries. Thus advertising's extreme behavior is
inseparably connected with the *world* consumption pattern and fear-ridden international relations.

Advertising methods are related also, however, to a first tenet of American business:
profits must increase without limit. Given consumption autarchy and the tenet of limitless
increase, only the wooly-minded consumer,
trained to insatiability, can put the tenet into
effect; and advertising alone can excite him to
the heroic deeds of consumption necessary to
make of the tenet a concrete reality.

In the background of all of this is the collective Self of the American people which has been

---

[1]July 28, 1961.

[2]In 1947 projected gross national product for 1960 was $202 billion at 1944 prices. See *America's Needs and Resources* by J. Frederic Dewhurst and Associates. New York:
The Twentieth Century Fund, 1947, p. 24. Correcting for about a 70 per cent price rise since 1947, this would give around $350 billion for 1960-61. Thus the
projection erred by almost 40 per cent!

[3]United States Department of Commerce, World Trade Information Service. *Statistical Reports.* Part 3. No. 60-30. September 1960. 4.1 per cent, the actual figure given
by the Department of Commerce, includes military supplies and equipment and other forms of foreign aid.

educated to put the high-rising living standard in the place of true Self-realization. Consumption autarchy, the drive toward higher profits, and alienation from Self are the factors that account for advertising. To ignore these while considering America's problems of production, consumption, and advertising is to ignore the ocean while studying the tides.

Excerpted with permission from *Culture Against Man*, pp. 45-99 (Random House, Inc., 1965).

Random Notes from Madison Avenue

Advertisers attending the 1977 annual meeting of the Association of National Advertisers heard one speaker suggest that consumer boycotts of the products of manufacturers who sponsored violent TV shows were equivalent to acts of kidnapping by terrorist groups.

A communications student has written to *Advertising Age* suggesting that among the outgrowths of the coming science of "advertology" already in existence was "event engineering...techniques for the creation and designing of artificial events that can maximize audience attention levels for TV commercials...."

As part of a special promotion *The Wall Street Journal* ran off an issue that included the headline, "World's end catches Americans by surprise, disrupts many plans." Its success exceeded expectations.

Granola Again 'Hot'—Now As Solid Snacks, Breakfast Bars

LARRY EDWARDS

What does the food industry do with a product that *doesn't* sell? It "repositions" it, sometimes "reformulates" it, probing for a different weakness in the consumer, investing in the neighborhood of two-million dollars in three months to seek a place in the "brain box." That's what Groucho Marx would have called a very classy neighborhood.

CHICAGO—Granola is back in the boom business. This time compacted into new form, it has helped turn a declining instant breakfast category into one of the hottest sections of the supermarket.

While the category may seem narrow, the competitive implications are actually broad because the two "hot" entries—General Mills' Nature Valley granola bars and Crunchola bars from Sunfield Foods—are being positioned and promoted as snacks. Regardless, it is clear that the quick-meal set finally is being given a solid food alternative and apparently liking it.

Food industry sources report that the category is up 50% over last year, with much of the growth coming during the first quarter of '76. "It is now a $100,000,000 business and that growth is directly tied to the bar activity," one exec said, adding that "powders were declining at a 15% rate before the bars came in."

Positioning has been key to success, apparently. "The smart ones are calling themselves a snack, and getting use as a snack, a quick lunch and a fast breakfast," one marketer said. To solidify that observation, reports are that the original solid instant breakfast—General Mills' Breakfast Squares—has fallen into a rapid sales decline as has (to a lesser degree) Carnation Breakfast Bar, which rolled out in January, 1975, with three granola varieties.

By the end of the year, sources say, Breakfast Squares and the Carnation entry each held a 40% share of the segment, but were trending down while Crunchola, at about 13%, was on its way up.

Crunchola, introduced in mid-'75, is a candy bar-like combination of peanut butter and granola. Sunfield Foods is a relatively new division of Sunmark Cos., St. Louis candy and confections marketer. The company put about $750,000 in media ad support behind it in late '75, via Vinyard & Lee & Partners in St. Louis, but, apparently realizing the potential it had tapped, moved its account to Doyle Dane Bernbach, New York, earlier this year. DDB's efforts for the brand—"the delicious, crunchy, wholesome snack"—began airing in April.

The biggest push has come from General Mills. Nature Valley granola bars were launched nationally in January, and according to most reports it has become the No. 1 product in the category—with the help of an estimated $2,000,000 media ad expenditure during February, March and April.

Sunfield's budget for Crunchola is not known, and industry execs do not expect General Mills to continue spending at that pace for Nature Valley. However, total ad spending in the category is sure to increase because other marketers are getting ready to jump in with new products.

Nabisco, having failed to get out of test market twice with an instant breakfast bar, is in test again with a unique bid for a piece of the business—Fast Break Breakfast Loaf. The new entry, in Seattle and other markets, is a banana nut loaf, apple raisin loaf or chocolate chip loaf, of which two half-inch slices and a glass of milk "gives you all the nutrition you need for breakfast."

Kellogg is in St. Louis test with its entry, "all natural" Oatnut Bars, being billed as a toaster snack but which do not need to be toasted. Like the Nature Valley bars, the product is an offshoot from a natural cereal, in this case Country Morning. It is made of rolled oats, honey and almonds, and packaged similarly to the company's Pop-Tarts. Indications are that Kellogg may be rolling out the product soon.

The influx of solid product into a liquid category has been well received in another area, too. Pillsbury Co., whose Figurines diet bars have captured a 50% share of the $70,000,000 meal replacement market at the expense of Carnation's Slender and Pet's Sego, will soon face new competition.

Next month, Pet reportedly will move its own Sego diet bars into about 35% of the country. The company's earlier bid for extending the Sego name to a more solid product—Spoon-Up pudding—failed to capture a position in the market.

Sources say Spoon-Up has about a 3% share, giving Pet an estimated 18% total share when combined with Sego liquid. Carnation is said to be down to about 35% now, behind Figurines. The company commanded a 45% share one year ago.

Reprinted with permission from *Advertising Age*, 47 (24): 1+ (14 June 1977). Copyright 1977 by Crain Communications, Inc.

Counternutritional Messages of TV Ads Aimed at Children

JOAN GUSSOW

"Counternutritional Messages of TV Ads Aimed at Children" is the published version of testimony given before a Senate Sub-committee concerned over the effects of advertising to children. It followed by a year and a half some much more highly publicized testimony given by a Washington activist, Robert Choate, on the poor nutritional quality of breakfast cereals advertised to children. The study here reprinted was an attempt to explore further what it was children might be learning about nutrition from Saturday and Sunday morning TV.

Over the years that I have gone to the supermarket, I have watched it turn from a food store into an amusement park. I watched juice drinks, juice cocktails, and dry powdered breakfast mixes crowd out fruit juices on the grocery shelf. I watched the frozen food cabinets expand to fill aisle after aisle, offering the casual shopper everything from a frozen instant omelette for breakfast to a frozen hero sandwich for lunch and frozen chow mein for dinner.

I saw the shelves fill up with an overwhelming array of cookies, crackers, breakfast cereals, soft drinks—and snacks and snacks and snacks. Everything from Bugles to Funions, from On-yums to Screaming Yellow Zonkers—and fake bacon made out of bargain basement soybeans to sell at Fifth Avenue prices. I have since learned that the number of items in the average supermarket went from around 900 in 1928—the year I was born—to over 7,500 in 1968. Large supermarkets now carry more than 10,000 items. . . .

I found I had to ask myself where people were actually learning what to eat. On what basis did the shoppers who walked down the aisles of supermarkets make their decisions on what to choose from among those 10,000 items? . . . That is what led me to advertising. For it is an article of faith among nutritionists that the reason we have so much trouble altering people's diets for the better is because eating habits, once established, are hard to change. Yet somehow, between 1928 and 1968, people had learned to eat thousands of new food items. Some change agent much more persuasive than we were must have been at work.

. . . We have *begun* by looking at the *television* advertising of foods in order to find out what foods are advertised to whom, how they are advertised, and whether the total advertising message is working for or against good nutrition.

Saturday Morning Ads

The project involved eight masters' degree students, myself, and Ruthe Eshleman, a dietitian and nutritionist with over 20 years of experience. For this portion of the study, we viewed Saturday morning children's TV...in the last week of January, 1972....

We already knew that food, drink, and vitamin products were much more heavily advertised to children than to adults. Robert Choate had previously reported[1] that during the week of April 11, 1971, food, drink, and vitamin ads—which accounted for 26% of all commercials on adult television—accounted for 64% of the commercials to children. Since then, however, things have gotten considerably worse. When we checked the total listings for the week we monitored, we found that out of 388 network commercials run during 29 hours of children's television, 82% were for ingestible items—food, drink, candy, gum, or vitamin pills.

These percentage figures are actually low because they omit local spot announcements which are heavily weighted toward food. NBC also lowers the average since it carries only about one-third as many commercials on its children's hours as do the other networks. On the Saturday morning we monitored, for example, NBC ran only 44 ads—33 of them for edible products—in five hours of children's programming. In the same time period, ABC ran 112 commercials, of which 87% were for food, drinks, or vitamins—that is, only 15 ads in five hours were for anything you couldn't eat. In six hours that same Saturday, CBS ran 126 commercials, of which 87% were once again for edible products.

If a child had gotten up at 8:00 that morning and turned on CBS, he would have seen no commercials for anything except food and vitamins until after 9:00. In other words, by the time his folks crawled out of bed to feed him breakfast, he would have already been subjected to 27 ardent salesmen trying to tempt him to eat their products.

Which Products?

We have now analyzed distribution of the 319 network food commercials which ran on the 29 hours of children's TV during the week we sampled. The chart I have here shows the distribution of ads into product categories.

Breakfast cereals	38½%
Cookies, candy, gum, popcorn, and other snacks	17%
Vitamins	15%
Beverages and beverage mixes	8%
Frozen waffles and pop-tarts	7½%
Canned pasta	5%
Canned desserts, frozen dinners, drive-ins, peanut butter, oranges	9%

This distribution is really no surprise. With minor variations, it is virtually indistinguishable from what one could have found by looking at children's television any time over the last year or so, as I have done. Since my long acquaintance had made me something of a biased witness, I wanted the nutrition students to tell me what the impact of this barrage of commercials would be on them....

On the Saturday morning we monitored, one of the students began her morning by logging 21 food commercials between 9:17 and 10:25, starting with Quake (a cereal) and ending with Pals, shaped and colored vitamins. When she reached ad number 22 for Kellogg's Rice Krispies, she wrote, under "general reaction," "I can't believe it. There are millions of Kellogg's commercials." On ad number 23, her comment was "sick and tired," and by number 25 she was up to "disbelief." By the 33rd food commercial, we felt obliged to relieve her. Watching children's television if one likes and respects food—and children—is sickening.

Food Habits: Learned, not Inborn

Nourishing ourselves is a learned skill. The ingestion of food and drink is a physiologic survival behavior which, unlike other physiologic behaviors such as breathing and sleeping, must be taught. (If you doubt that eating be-

[1]Choate, R. B., Testimony before the House Select Committee on Small Business, June 11, 1971.

havior has to be taught, remember that a one-year-old human will eagerly swallow a bottle of aspirin tablets or a cigarette butt.) Human beings have always had to discover how to select from all those things they could potentially swallow, those substances which would sustain life and health. And this nutritional wisdom, once discovered by trial and error, has traditionally been passed on from one generation to the next as rules about what is good to eat.

Children left to their own devices *cannot* choose a nutritious diet, though an early study by a researcher named Clara Davis[2] is widely misquoted to defend the notion that they can. Dr. Davis took a number of newly weaned children who had never eaten solid food and exposed them to a variety of foods, which were served unseasoned and unmixed. Even salt was not added to foods but was served separately in a dish. No sugar was available at all. The table below shows the list of foods offered.

1. *Meats* (muscle cuts)
   Beef
   Lamb
   Chicken

2. *Glandular Organs*
   Liver
   Kidney
   Brains
   Sweetbreads (thymus)

3. *Sea Food*
   Sea fish (haddock)

4. *Cereals*
   Whole wheat
   Oatmeal (Scotch)
   Barley (whole grains)
   Corn meal (yellow)
   Rye (Ry-Krisp)

5. *Bone Products*
   Bone marrow (beef and veal)
   Bone jelly (soluble bone subst.)

6. *Eggs*

7. *Milks*
   Grade A raw milk
   Grade A raw whole lactic milk

8. *Fruits*
   Apples
   Oranges
   Bananas
   Tomatoes
   Peaches or pineapples

9. *Vegetables*
   Lettuce
   Cabbage
   Spinach
   Cauliflower
   Peas
   Beets
   Carrots
   Turnips
   Potatoes

10. *Incidentals*
    Sea salt

As you can see from the table, the diet offered consisted basically of various meats and eggs, milks, fruit and vegetables, and grains. These, not by accident, are what nutritionists call the four food groups. They are the foods from which we say children ought to have some servings every day in order to get the nutrients which they need. Given a choice of *only* these foods, Dr. Davis found that children could select a well-balanced diet.

Note that among the foods offered, however, there was not one snack food, not a single rich dessert, not a single soda, candy bar, or colored sugared breakfast cereal. The diet *offered* by Dr. Davis was so nutritious that it would have been hard for a child to go very far wrong. The diet *sold* to children by television, on the other hand, is so impoverished that it makes it impossible for a child *not* to go wrong.

Thus, whatever one may think of individual

[2]Davis, C., Self-selection of diet by newly weaned infants, Amer. J. Diseases Child., 36:651, 1928.

products or of individual commercials, it is clear that the diet children's television commercials are promoting is an imbalanced one. Yet most advertisers deny that they are teaching nutrition—they point out, in fact, that nutritional messages do not move the product.

TV's Implicit Messages

Assessing television's impact as a teaching medium is a trap. Traditionally, when television is attacked for failing to live up to its potential, we are told that it is not a good medium for teaching—and we are given examples of its failure to teach. To suggest that television does not teach anything to small children who sit in front of it for up to six hours a day is, of course, arrant nonsense—a fact which the success of *Sesame Street* has tended to underscore. To say that we have not yet learned to measure all that it teaches appears to be true. What is misleading, I think, is that we often fail to look at the right messages. The most powerful messages television delivers are its implicit ones—the things it sells us when we don't even know we are being sold. The heavy advertising of beer and soft drinks, for example, delivers a message far more potent than the urging to buy any single product. In terms of this message it doesn't really matter whether someone going to the refrigerator gets out a Pepsi or a Coke, a 7-Up or a Budweiser. What matters is that a thirsty American in the 1970s goes to the refrigerator to open up a container rather than to the sink to open up the tap. That behavior has been sold to us.

What is a nutritional message? On public television's *Sesame Street*, one of the most popular characters is a Cookie Monster, which predictably and amusingly devours boxes of cookies. The Cookie Monster is a nutrition message—and one which puts *Sesame Street* in the same *nutritional* league with other children's programming.

On commercial TV it is a nutrition message—and a positive one—when the Campbell's Soup Company in advertising its products shows them as part of a complete meal whose nutritional value has been considered in planning the ad. It is a negative nutrition message when 15% of all the commercials aimed at children advertise vitamins—"to keep you growing right even if you don't eat right." It is nonsense to say that the companies who advertise ingestible products to children do not or cannot give nutrition messages; they are doing so all the time, and many of them are, at least by implication, lies.

One of the messages delivered by children's television commercials has to do with what is *not* advertised. As we have seen, the four food groups are very poorly represented at the table television sets for children. There is no milk (though there are things to make milk "palatable"), and except for hot cocoa mixes there are no milk products—not even ice cream. There are no eggs, no meat, no cheese, no vegetables, and—but only of late—just a single fruit. That is a nutrition message. That tells little children what kinds of foods we do not think it is important to excite them about.

To a nutrition educator, plain old food—not food products but food—is conspicuous by its absence from the children's hours. When I asked the students to sum up what they thought a child would learn about food from all this, one of them said "If a child had to depend on television to know what food was, he'd never know."

There are thousands of good and nutritious and valuable products on the grocery shelves. Unfortunately, these products are seldom promoted with any nutritional sophistication even to adults, and, so far as we have been able to determine, they are almost *never* promoted to children, informatively or otherwise.... For every advertiser, the decision on what and where to advertise is, of course, based on marketing wisdom, not nutritional wisdom. Unfortunately, the combined impact of all these *marketing* decisions delivers a rather stunningly counternutritional message to our children. We may notice what foods are absent. To a child what is present is insistent.

Findings and Comments

Our intention when we looked at commercials was to pick out the bad or misleading ones. What we found was that the whole was considerably worse and more misleading than the sum of the parts. But some of the parts are misleading too—and I will comment very briefly on a few of them.

Something aproaching 40% of children's food commercials are for cereals.... Cereals on children's television are oversweetened, overpriced, and overpromoted, and, I think, at times overenriched.

Nutritionists as a group have what I think is an unfair reputation as pleasure prohibitionists. ... I hope I can make it clear that no one opposes sweets as a nutritionally minor component in a diet otherwise composed of nourishing foods.

What we really object to is the strong implication that *only* sweet things taste good—and unfortunately within the present context of children's television the advertising of candy becomes part of the chorus of chocolatey sweetness. So do the ads for chocolate powders and syrups to mix with milk. That is an unnecessary corruption of a basically good food....

We were also offended by the notion that Hershey's chocolate syrup ought to be poured over and into everything. "It makes even milk a dessert" the copy says—as if milk needed to be a dessert. Another ad for Hershey's Instant shows a lot of cows against the background of what appears to be San Francisco. They are leaving the country, a voice says, because kids have stopped drinking their milk. Chocolate saves the day, of course. Now that we have Hershey's Instant which makes milk taste like a Hershey Bar, all the cows are going back to the farms. Kids shouldn't be sold on the idea that milk, as milk, is unacceptable. We don't think milk has to taste like a Hershey Bar in order to taste good—and, what is probably more important, children

don't think so either unless someone has taught them to.

There are some good commercials for orange juice on television now—unfortunately they do not run on children's television. On children's TV, the closest approach to "fruit juice" is a Hi-C, Hawaiian Punch, Tang, and Kool Aid. None of these is a fruit juice, though some of them contain fruit juice.

I had an experience recently which is relevant here. I had talked to a group of high school girls and, after the talk, a girl of about 17 came up to me and asked what she should drink since she didn't like bottled soda. She said she drank a lot of Tang, and asked if that was all right. I said "Well, you might just as well drink a glass of water and take a vitamin pill. It would have more nutrition, less additives, and less sugar." But, I said, she'd really be better off drinking fruit juice. It turned out that she wasn't really sure what fruit juice was—that is, she asked me if I meant "Orange Plus"—one of those half-synthetic, half-natural fruit juice products which are proliferating like rabbits in your grocer's freezer and on his shelves. It's probably not surprising—it's getting harder and harder to find fruit juice in the market even if you *know* what it is; but the incident is depressing. We in nutrition don't really know the nutritional implications of this increasing dependence on progressively more synthetic products. If we are going to raise a generation of children who do not know what fruit juice is, hadn't we better make that decision ourselves and not leave it up to the advertisers to make it for us?...

It was difficult choosing the most offensive vitamin ad—they're all nutritionally outrageous. Their overall message—that vitamin pills make up for poor eating habits—is a lie. If it weren't so misleading, such a message would be actually funny, coming as it does hard on the heels of all those commercials selling poor eating habits....

Ads: How Effective?

So much for the commercials. What our survey has told us is that nutrition messages are numerous on children's television, that few of them even hint at proper eating habits, and that altogether they encourage poor eating habits. A few of them, especially the vitamin ads, are directly misleading. In short, the messages are there but are they effective? What are children learning from them?...

How does a child decide what tastes good? Clara Davis' study—which I mentioned earlier —demonstrates that children find a surprisingly large number of tastes attractive, even some we would consider strong or unusual, if their appetites are uncorrupted....

However,... the foods advertised to children tout a curiously limited range of flavors—from a kind of fruity to a kind of chocolatey sweetness—what I would call a dessert taste. No food on children's television is crisply fresh like an apple or a salad. Nothing on children's television is tart, or spicy, or meaty. Everything is fun, sweet, sparkly, gay, colorful, thick and chocolatey, magicky, or crunchily delicious. The appeal is repeatedly a sweet one. It's either a chocolatey mouthful or, in the words of one particularly revolting commercial, a "frootful snootful."

It is possible to stand fast against this if one is nutritionally informed, stubborn as a mule, and as morally self-righteous as I am. But how does a mother stand against it who is unsure of herself nutritionally and trying hard to be a good—and popular—mother? How especially does she stand against it when products as outrageous as Count Chocula and Frankenberry carry proudly on their boxes the admonition to mothers: "This is a nutritious cereal...it provides eight of the essential vitamins and iron..." etc?

I would like to believe that children and their mothers are not being sold by these insistent messages. I would like to believe it, but the profit pictures of the heaviest advertisers and the evidence of my own eyes in the marketplace

convince me that it isn't true. I am also convinced by some rather astonishing recent statistics accumulated by Scott Ward and his associates at the Harvard Graduate School of Business Administration on the effects of television advertising on children.[3] Dr. Ward found, among other things, that attention to commercials was greatest among the youngest children and that they were most concerned with products which "relate to immediate impulsive needs." But few preschoolers do the shopping. How do they satisfy their "impulsive needs?" Dr. Ward has a table which he entitles "Percent of Mothers 'Usually' Yielding to Child's Purchase Influence Attempts." For five- to seven-year old children, the following were the percentages of mothers "usually" yielding.

Breakfast cereals	88%
Snack foods	52%
Candy	40%
Soft drinks	38%

By the time children were 8 to 10, 91% of the mothers were yielding to their children's influence on which cereal to purchase. Advertisers are not so dumb!

Who is Responsible?

We do not really know who is teaching adults whatever they know about choosing foods for themselves and their children. Television undoubtedly has a role. Advertising in other media may have a larger role. Certainly we have no evidence that nutrition educators are making much headway. What is, in any case, obvious is that children—when they are still young enough to be forming their notions of what is good to eat—are being urged on television to eat foods which produce neither present good health nor healthful lifetime food habits.

What is equally clear is that parents are failing to stem the tide of Devil Dogs, Kool Aid,

[3]Ward, S. and Wackman, D. B., Television Advertising and Intra-family Influence: Children's Purchase Influence Attempts and Parental Yielding, unpublished paper, June, 1971.

Hostess Twinkies, and Frankenberry which are rotting their children's teeth, setting them up for obesity, and building up in them a taste for sugar which will force these same children as overweight adults to indulge in whatever non-caloric sweetener is then in vogue to satisfy their insatiable craving for sweets.

There is one last thing I should like to say. Two years ago...I wrote something which I should like to close with now:

"The growingly poor diets of many affluent Americans are—in the context of a world much more poorly fed in spite of itself—irrelevant, immaterial, and not worth worrying about were it not for the example we set to the world of what is an advisible end point of technological and material progress. Moreover, in a world context the attitude of some American food manufacturers toward food—that it is just one more of the world's raw materials to be played with and manipulated for our amusement and for the greater delight of that 'consuming prince' the American—is immoral."

Excerpted with permission from *Journal of Nutrition Education*, 4(2): 48-52 (Spring 1972).

Cereal Fighting for Shelf Space

PHILIP H. DOUGHERTY

Nowhere are the battles for the brain box more fierce than in the breakfast cereal market. Some of the mind-boggling statistics are presented by *New York Times* advertising columnist Philip H. Dougherty in this article originally published in February of 1976.

Ralston-Purina, which has already delivered Freakies and Fruity Freakies to an eager young populace, has now developed Grins & Smiles & Giggles & Laughs. This, too, is a presweetened ready-to-eat cereal. Its special benefit is that on each crunchy, round, corn-based piece are two eyes and a smiling mouth.

The new cereal is being prepared for market now, and its advertising agency is Wells, Rich, Greene. Next comes the battle to get and keep the product's segment of shelf space in the supermarkets of America—space that depends strictly on survival of the fittest.

Other recent national cereal entries are Punch Crunch from Quaker Oats and Frosted Rice from Kellogg, which is also understood to have Corny Snaps in test market. General Foods is testing a C.W. Post brand.

The new entries have joined the more than 150 brands of ready-to-eat cereals that, according to Sales Area Marketing Inc., are available in two or more market areas.

(There are also 83 brands of hot cereals.)

The space devoted to them by the retailers has been steadily growing, according to the A.C. Nielsen Company. It calculates that the average supermarket devoted 91 linear feet of shelf space to them in 1972 and 107 feet last year. That compares with last year's 169 feet for soft drinks and 182 feet for dog food and cat food.

Nevertheless, according to a supermarket

source, the retail food chains like dry cereals because, although they are in the medium-price range, there is very fast movement, bringing in a lot of dollars. "Fast movement" is probably the key phrase; the chains certainly don't want to stock a brand that gathers dust.

Usually the chains make their judgments on the basis of data available from SAMI and Nielsen on best-selling brands, their own historical sales data and, in the case of new products, the national advertising and promotion plans.

The big companies with proven track records have an edge.

More than $118 million was spent on advertising in all measured media for cold and hot cereals in 1974, with $105 million of that figure in television.

Television advertising in the first nine months of last year was $76.2 million, down $2 million from the similar period of 1974.

That might reflect an earlier softness in part of the cereal market—specifically the presweetened segment—catching up with advertising budgets.

However, Wall Street and industry sources say the cereal market for the whole year was very good, with sales (on a weight basis) up 5 percent in 1975 to 1.82 billion pounds.

Earlier, rising sugar prices drove up the cost of the presweetened brands. But in 1975 for the most part, industry sources say, the consumer apparently considered most dry cereals a more economic alternative for breakfast than many other types of food.

Presweetened cereals accounted for 30.9 percent of the tonnage in 1975, about the same as in the previous year. The all-family brands, however, showed a 14 percent growth to a 63 percent share of the market. The natural cereals, which at their height had about a 10 percent share, were down to 6.1 percent last year.

(The negative comments of consumer advocates about presweetened cereals seemingly have not affected their sales. "Mothers buy what their kids will eat," an industry source said.) However, positive stories about the need for high-fiber diets apparently gave a lift to sales of bran-based cereals.

Retail sales of ready-to-eat cereals are put at $1.7 billion by Sales Area Marketing Inc., which estimates Kellogg's share at 41.6 percent, General Mills at 19 percent, General Foods at 17.8 percent, Quaker at 8.3 percent and Ralston-Purina at 3.4 percent.

There seems to have been no slackening in the use of premium promotions, despite the proposed banning of advertising of such promotions by the Federal Trade Commission a couple of years back. That proposal is still going through regular channels. It may even be in limbo.

Reprinted with permission from *The New York Times*, p. 45 (6 February 1976). Copyright 1976 by The New York Times Company.

Kids, It's Saturday TV Again!
Shut Up and Eat Your Chocolate-Chip Ravioli!

JOHN H. CORCORAN, Jr. with JOHN H. CORCORAN III

The National Observer first published this depressingly amusing account of one father's morning with his son in the kid-vid ghetto. The questions he raises (almost offhandedly) about the rationality of it all are the questions the regulatory agencies must wrestle with in the teeth of powerful industry pressures.

Let me take a moment to introduce my new assistant. John H. Corcoran III, or Supercritic, will occasionally be lending his expertise to this column. His first assignment was to help his old man watch the Saturday-morning kiddie shows. Supercritic was 6 days old at the time, and while he slept and burped his way through most of the morning, his first comment was a telling one: How better to sum up the state of Saturday-morning television than by forcing Daddy to learn the manly art of diaper changing?

I hadn't watched a TV cartoon show since *George of the Jungle* klutzed up the tube in the late '60s. George communicated at two levels: There was broad slapstick for the kids and some sophisticated adult satire for grown ups. George himself was a clumsy Tarzan who called his pet elephant "Nice Doggie," and he was helped out by a British-accented gorilla, a fat-headed race driver, and Superchicken, a heroic fowl. The program was brightly written and genuinely funny. I seldom missed an episode.

So last Saturday, with Supercritic on lap, I searched for a new *George of the Jungle* and ended up, instead, with a jungle of junk. Together we watched or slept through a dozen kiddie shows, five dozen commercials, and a sea of tripe. A report:

Pass the Pepto. If we do not become a nation of Shmoos, it will be through no fault of the Saturday-morning ghetto. By actual count, 32 of the 59 commercials I saw in a four-hour period were for junk food. There were ads for chocolate-chip cookies, canned ravioli, peanut-butter cups, candy bars, fast-food chains, and enough carbohydrates to supply the minimum daily requirements of a small nation. Any kiddie plotzed in front of the tube on Saturday morning risks audio-visual diabetes.

Take It All Off

One cereal, in a tease worthy of Blaze Starr, offered scratch and sniff cartoon riddles in every box. Two junior hucksters sniffed the riddle, smiled deliriously, and were about to spill the beans when a third warned, "Shhh! Don't tell them!" Nothing like peddling cereal by frustrating the young.

In the midst of all this, there was a single public-service spot by the Advertising Council. Eat *other* foods first, the Cookie Monster advised; then he was deluged by thousands of cookies. Final score: Junk Food 32. Cookie Monster 1.

Among the 18 ads for toys and dolls was one for "Nerf" footballs—those sponge-rubber superlight balls appropriate, one supposes, for kids too weakened from junk food to heft a real football. While I saw no ads for toy guns, there was a beaut for a commando team apparently spawned by the Marquis de Sade out of Sam Pekinpah. Four—count 'em, four—fighting dolls, including one who uses a whip, one who fires arows, one called "Mr. Steel," who presumably crushes the enemy to death, and their leader, Big Jim. Very Macho.

For the girls, there are dolls who eat, drink, speak, wet, sneeze, and do everything except earn a college scholarship. The crowning effort is a little girl doll called "Growing Up Skipper," who grows taller in front of your eyes. All you do is turn her arm and watch her grow. Something else grows, and while the ad didn't mention it, viewers could see her change from a flat-chested pre-pubescent into one of the Gabor sisters. Very feminine.

King Kong Karate

As for the programs themselves, the ones I could watch between diaper changes and lullabies were homogenized and mostly humorless. There has been a trend in recent years away from the cartoons to "live people" programming. Ruth Buzzi and Jim Nabors star, for instance, in a silly and relatively harmless effort called *The Lost Saucer.* The show has an occasional zinger thrown in for daddies: "Don't touch my buttons," Ms. Buzzi warns Nabors in a voice implying all *entendres* shall be double.

Strange and weird animals and beasts abound in both cartoon and live efforts. Sampling the shows on a single network (ABC), we encountered *Grape Ape,* a purple King Kong look-alike who appears to have fallen into a vat of vino, *Hong Kong Phooey,* an Amos 'n' Andy-voiced janitor-dog who turns into a karate-chopping

crime-fighter; the *Pink Panther;* and old standbys *Tom and Jerry,* now fighting off a horde of termites resembling a Nazi motorcycle club. Fun shows.

In the coincidence department, there is *Land of the Lost,* a Sid and Marty Kroft production that boasts the hokiest special effects this side of *Godzilla Meets the Tidy Bowl Man.* Two of the dinosaurs in the show, nicknamed "Grumpy" and "Dopey," appear just before a commercial for a re-release of—what else?—*Snow White and the Seven Dwarfs.*

Summing Up

All in all, Saturday-morning television offers lots of nonsense, a little violence, and a continuous message to eat, eat, eat. I can't draw final conclusions from one quick, baby-distracted viewing, but I do have definite impressions, and they aren't good. The Saturday-morning kiddie show is a dangerous baby sitter. That danger is not in any single advertisement, but in their cumulative effect: Consume, eat, pop glop into your mouth. It's fun, it's neat, it's popular. Your friends do it. Your heroes do it. You should do it.

Some adults have argued that Saturday-morning television should be free of commercials: I can support that, or a restriction on the number of food-oriented commercials. It is not enough to run a single good-food pitch in the midst of the glop, nor simply to urge parents to supervise. Why should parents be forced to *undo* damage, or to deny the medium to their children? Supercritic might disagree with my conclusions, but by the time he is old enough to stay awake through the programs, they'll have changed. Or Daddy will have the difficult task of telling him "no."

Reprinted with permission from *The National Observer,* p. 10 (8 November 1975). Copyright 1975 by Dow Jones & Company, Inc. All Rights Reserved.

Your Fare, Lady

RUSSELL BAKER

Russell Baker moves us—with his usual wit—from the kid-vid ghetto to "adult" television, encapsulating in a single sentence the awful truth about the "food being sold on the tube"—namely that "it has not been grown; it has been manufactured."

It seems to me you can't go more than five minutes with the TV set this year without seeing somebody eat something absolutely awful. Or somebody, usually a woman, getting ready to serve something to eat that is absolutely awful. I wonder if we have passed through some kind of cultural watershed here.

The big thing on television used to be headache. Every five minutes they would stop the entertainment, and on would come somebody with a headache, and then—bingo!—the headache would be miraculously cured. For 20 years at least, headache was the king of television.

I haven't clocked a typical evening on the tube this year, but my impression—and with television, impressions are all that count—my impression is that the preparation and eating of absolutely awful food is beating headache by at least 2 to 1. Not surprisingly, upset stomach and indigestion are also doing very well. My observations suggest that indigestion is neck and neck with headache while upset stomach is closing fast on hard-to-remove stains, in terms of time on tube.

I said that the food on television was absolutely awful, and that's not fair, of course, because I haven't eaten any of it, and don't plan to as long as I have the strength to resist force-feeding. The point is that the idea of this TV food—the concept—is absolutely awful. Food should be grown, but this food being sold on the tube has not been grown; it has been manufactured.

It is hard to understand the men who eat this food, because they are always smiling after the first mouthful, or nuzzling their wives after finishing the thing off. There is one mildly rebellious male who, upon being served factory-made chicken, asks whatever happened to real chicken.

He is quickly put in his place by chortling harridans who tell him the factory chicken is not only better than real chicken, but also much easier to cook. There are threatening overtones to this encounter which are reminiscent of Strindberg's man-woman hate scenes, but the male turns out to be a sniveler. He eats the phony chicken happily instead of throwing it at the television camera and announcing that he will get some real chicken and cook it himself.

What the feminists call sexism is superficially preserved in all these commercials, since they always cast the woman in the cook's role and make the husband the breadwinner home from his labor to play stern judge of the wife's cooking. This is only superficial, however. What is really going on here is something much trickier.

The point about this television food is that it requires no skill, little time and not much work to put it on the table. A typical teledrama, for instance, concerns two wives unboxing a spaghetti dinner. Both dinners come in boxes. Wife

One opens her box and finds nothing but spaghetti. She is in trouble because she will have to add meat. Not Wife Two. Her spaghetti dinner (the sponsor's, naturally) comes with meat boxed in. Everything in one box.

She nips off camera for a second and—presto! —reappears with a steaming spaghetti dinner with meat. Wife One looks surly and defeated, and with good reason, for she will now have to go to the food locker and open another box—of factory-made hamburger, perhaps. Wife Two had to open only one box to make dinner. Poor Wife One has suffered the drudgery of opening two.

So while the commercials seem to cast women in the cook's role, in fact they do not. How can the women be cooks when there is no cooking going on?

Most of what passes for cooking with this television food is nothing but opening, thawing and heating. The real message of the factory-food commercials is not that woman's place is in the kitchen. It is that if a woman has a benighted husband who believes such archaic clap-trap, she can fake the cooking effortlessly, thanks to factory-made food, have idle hours in which to do as she pleases, and then reduce the poor dolt to eye-rolling delight in her skill in opening a box.

Can any woman long be happy with such a man? Not likely.

These food commercials could bring back the headache.

Reprinted with permission from *The New York Times Magazine*, p. 6 (26 May 1974). Copyright 1975 by The New York Times Company.

International Advertisers Change Consumer Ways

RAMONA BECHTOS

Ramona Bechtos' piece from the international section of *Advertising Age* speaks for itself in a world where those she calls "emerging consumers" are often hungry. It is followed, on the next page, by an excerpt from a book called *Global Reach* by Richard Barnet and Ronald E. Müller. Is development really promoted they ask, by the blandishments of advertisers, coaxing both the destitute and the wealthy to become consumers?

NEW YORK, May 15—In this special International section, ADVERTISING AGE is putting the spotlight where it belongs—on the advertiser.

This issue is timed with the first international advertisers' conference held under the auspices of the International Advertising Assn. Sponsored by the Brazilian chapter of the IAA, it will take place in Rio de Janeiro May 22 and 23. Theme of the conference is "The contribution of advertising to developing countries and emerging consumers." It is, of course, an important focus because this is where the greatest percentage of growth can be expected.

Emerging nations undoubtedly can learn a great deal from the developed countries whose marketing and promotional structures have had a longer period to develop. No one would deny, however, that the developing economies have their special marketing needs and advertising focus.

The internationality of the world's consumers has been the subject of speeches and panel discussions for many years, with most marketing experts concurring that the similarities are greater than the differences. Human needs and wants are well nigh universal, with national differences more often than not merely a reflection of the level of the national economy.

Old taboos have been broken down in many areas, but some deep-rooted traditions show signs of never waning. It takes a keen marketer—at times with an assist from well formulated market research—to be able to tell the difference between the two categories.

For example, the German *frau* has long been proud of her baking skills, so who would have thought that she would succumb to the convenience of refrigerated dough for her beloved *apfel strudel?* Pillsbury of the U.S. and Gervais-Danone of France found her ready for it.

And who would have thought that the Japanese, who make an art out of everything from flower arranging to tea pouring to dining, would ever be found wolfing down an instant noodle dish from a Styrofoam cup? Nisshin of Japan has struck gold with such a product, and plans to expand it to the U.S., Brazil and beyond.

Examples of the influences of one country on another can be seen everywhere. When an Australian company sought a memorable name for its youth-oriented, unisex deodorant, it hit upon Uncle Sam and used an updated, kicky version of the symbolic American hero to propel the product through one of the most successful launches Downunder.

An Australian ice cream company, seeking a new product to boost its static sales, also found the answer on the other side of the world—in natural ice cream, made of all natural ingredients, from the U.S. And when a Canadian candy company wanted to sweeten its sales it did so by developing a totally different candy bar reminiscent of Danish pastry.

Perhaps discussions of such products as candy, ice cream and even deodorants seem a bit frivolous to societies whose immediate concern is to feed, house and educate its masses, but the basic marketing principles are often the same, whether one is selling a French perfume or a basic nutrient or even an idea....

Excerpted with permission from *Advertising Age,* 46 (20): 1+ (19 May 1975). Copyright 1975 by Crain Communications, Inc.

Engines of Development?

RICHARD J. BARNET and RONALD E. MÜLLER

The third great source of power of global corporations in poor countries is the control over ideology—the values that determine how people live.... Through TV, movie-house commercials, comic books, and magazine ads, foreign corporations unquestionably exert more continuing influence on the minds of the bottom half of the Mexican people, to take one example, than either the Mexican Government or the Mexican educational system. A small fraction of the Mexican population goes to school beyond the third grade. The officially admitted illiteracy rate is more than 27 percent. Contact with school is for the vast majority of the population fleeting, but exposure to TV and the transistor radio is lifelong....

Nor can government propaganda match the power of advertising. On some of the main thoroughfares of Mexico City, government slogans exhorting the population to cleanliness compete for attention with huge billboards advertising beer, cosmetics, smart clothes, and other symbols of the good life. These billboards, prepared with the latest techniques of modern advertising, offer Technicolor fantasies of luxury, love, and power that no message from the Department of Health, however uplifting, is likely to disturb.

Throughout the underdeveloped world, global corporations are thus successfully marketing the same dreams they have been selling in the industrialized world. Stimulating consumption in low-income countries and accommodating local tastes to globally distributed products is crucial to the development of an ever-expanding Global Shopping Center. The World Managers argue that they are cultivating tastes and educating for progress. Marketing the pleasures of becoming a "man of distinction" who knows and drinks good whiskey, of exercising power on the highway at the wheel of a new "Fury," or escaping to the South Seas via Pan Am offers the people of poor countries the prospect of "the good life" to which they can aspire. Telling poor people about products they have the money to buy right now, such as Coca-Cola and ITT's Twinkies (via its wholly owned subsidiary Wonder Bread), opens up new horizons. How, the World Managers argue, can the transfer of the consumption ideology, which had so much to do with the expansion of the U.S. economy, be bad for poor countries?

Whether the transfer of the marketplace ideology by global corporations is good or bad for development depends once again on what is meant by development. If the priority of development policy is to alleviate the most crushing problem of the underdeveloped world—mass poverty resulting from unemployment and inequality—then we must conclude that the transfer of the ideology of the global corporations to poor countries has had several disastrous impacts. First, despite Jacques Maisonrouge's claim that the global corporation is a great leveler and a great equalizer, corporate strategy actually reinforces the sharp class cleavages that exist in all poor countries. The principal targets of most global corporations are the enclaves of affluence within destitute societies. Peter Drucker, the father of the Global Shopping Center, points out that within the "vast mass of poverty that is India" there is "a sizeable modern economy, comprising 10 percent or more of the Indian population, or 50,000,000 people."...Obviously, expensive capital goods such as automobiles, luxuries such as fine watches and cameras, and costly services, such as a plane ride to New York, are available to only a tiny fraction of the population in underdeveloped countries, although in absolute numbers it represents a sizeable market. These items are frequently imports and exhaust scarce foreign exchange. The mobile minority, encouraged by advertising to adopt the eating, wearing, and traveling habits of the American upper middle class, live imported lives....

Quantitative evidence of the impact of advertising on the bottom 40 to 60 percent of the population in the underdeveloped world is meager. This is not the population that the advertising agencies are ordinarily paid by clients to canvass. There has been little research, and most of it is impressionistic. But what there is suggests that the "communications explosion" to which the World Managers often allude has not had the revolutionary impact that some feared in the 1950's, but rather the opposite. Evangelina Garcia, a specialist in "social communication" at the Central University of Venezuela and a consultant to McCann-Erickson, J. Walter Thompson, and other U.S.-based global advertising firms, says that the "most revealing and continually reconfirmed" finding of her studies on advertising is that the *marginales* (those who are barely hanging on) have "lost their perception of class differences." They think that there are, to be sure, rich and poor, she explained, "but that all have access to the same consumer goods" they hear about on the transistor or see on the TV. It is a matter of luck whether they have the money to buy them, and luck can change. Johnson's Wax conducted a survey of *marginales* and found that a common reaction in hovels with dirt floors was "I don't have a floor to wax, but I can buy the wax if I want to." Thus the byproduct of advertising campaigns is to give families without the bare necessities of life a spurious feeling of being middle class....

An important impact of imported advertising campaigns, Professor Garcia points out, is that "the values in the U.S. are reproduced in Venezuela, in relation to sex, love, prestige, race, etc." Today in Venezuela, she notes, "the housewife measures her happiness by whether she has a refrigerator...before a woman's happiness was to have children, depend on her husband, even to have goods but not to show them." Advertising, she concludes, creates a psychological dependence. One's sense of self-esteem is determined by what one buys. In effect, they are saying, "My security—my emotional security—depends upon what I consume." Advertising is popular among the very poor in Latin America. While a few intellectuals and nationalist politicians worry about the effects of scientific huckstering, most people appear to accept the rationale which the advertising agencies give for their activities. The advertiser is like a friend who tells you about all the wonderful things in the world that you didn't even know existed....

Global marketeers are not persuaded that there is anything wrong with spreading the thrill of consumption in poor countries. "The factory girl or the salesgirl in Lima or Bombay (or the Harlem ghetto)," says Peter Drucker, "wants a lipstick...There is no purchase that gives her as much true value for a few cents." The fact that she is in all probability malnourished and without a decent place to live does not mean that she is spending foolishly. Albert Stridsberg, an "international advertising specialist" writing in *Advertising Age*, says that we must rid ourselves of "the conventional range of ideas about what will minister to the poor man's physical needs. The psychological significance of his spending his money on a transistor radio may be more important then the physical benefit generated by spending the same money for basic foodstuffs." It is an interesting theory, especially when applied to a country like Peru where, it is estimated, a substantial number of all babies born begin life with serious, and possibly irreparable, brain damage due to malnutrition.

Creating and satisfying wants such as lipsticks and transistor radios while the basic necessities of life recede ever further perpetuates and compounds mass misery in poor countries. (In certain Peruvian villages a pathetic item is a piece of stone painted to look like a transistor radio. Peasants too poor to buy a real one carry it for status.) Global corporations have the enormous power to determine what does or does not give "psychological satisfaction." It is disingenuous to talk about the "dictates of the consumer" when the consumer is so thoroughly subject to the dictation of the modern technology of manipulation.

Evidence has been accumulating in the last few years that the diet of the bottom 40 to 60 percent of the world's population is actually getting worse. Alan Berg in his Brookings Institution study of world nutrition problems notes that whereas production of beef in Central America increased dramatically during the 1960's, the per capita consumption of meat in those countries either increased marginally or declined. In Costa Rica, to take the most extreme case, meat production increased 92 percent from the early 1960's to 1970 but per capita consumption went down 26 percent. The reason, Berg notes, is that the meat is "ending up not in Latin American stomachs but in franchised restaurant hamburgers in the United States..." There has been a per capita decline of production and consumption of milk in India. Since eggs cost anywhere from 40 to 70 cents a dozen in poor countries, they are prohibitive as a source of protein. (In 1969 the average American consumed 314 eggs; the average Indian 8.) The decline of real purchasing power of the world's poor and the flight of the "marginal" forces to the city means that more people are eating worse than ever before....

The deadly effects of the world hunger problem are obvious. In Brazil, children under five constitute less than one-fifth of the population but account for four-fifths of all deaths. According to Berg's study, malnutrition is the primary or contributing cause of death in 57 percent of all deaths in Latin America of one- to four-year-olds. The high infant mortality rate has a great deal to do with the high birth rate

characteristic of poor countries (and of poor families in rich countries). People produce more babies in hopes that some at least will survive. Berg estimates that about a billion persons in the world today suffer the effects of malnutrition. More than 300 million children suffer "grossly retarded physical growth" due to not getting enough to eat. According to the nutrition expert Myron Winick, "the evidence is becoming more and more weighty that malnutrition in infancy permanently affects the minds of the children who have been affected."...

The global corporations, it must be said, have compounded the world hunger problem in three ways. First, they have contributed to the concentration of income and the elimination of jobs. Second, through its increasing control of arable land in poor countries, agribusiness is complicating the problem of food distribution....

Finally, the companies' control of ideology through advertising has helped to change the dietary habits of the poor in unfortunate ways. Beginning in 1966, the major global food companies had begun research on low-cost protein foods, baby cereals, soft drinks, imitation milk, candies, snacks, soups, and noodles, and by 1968 a dozen such products were on the market. Berg questioned a number of food and pharmaceutical companies seeking to introduce such products in India and found that "corporate image was the most important general factor influencing their decision to become involved." While there was also a "strong thread of social responsibility" on the part of some executives, the fact that image is a prime motive means, he points out, that "corporate contributions to national nutrition are likely to be token."...

In his studies of changing dietary habits in rural Mexican villages, Joaquin Cravioto finds that the two products which peasants want and buy the moment they come into contact with the advertising message are white bread and soft drinks. Bread becomes a substitute for tortillas. Depending upon how enriched it is, there may be some gain in protein and vitamins, but a loss in calcium. But the most important impact of this shift in eating habits in poor villages is that it takes a much greater share of the virtually nonexistent family food budget. Coca-Cola, nutritionally speaking, is a way of consuming imported sugar at a high price. People like the taste, but its popularity, as Albert Stridsberg points out, is due to the advertising campaigns of the global giants. "It has long been known that in the poorest regions of Mexico," he notes with satisfaction, "where soft drinks play a functional role in the diet, it is the international brands—Coke and Pepsi—not local off-brands, which dominate. Likewise, a Palestinian refugee urchin, shining shoes in Beirut, saves his piastres for a real Coca-Cola, at twice the price of a local cola." The result is what the nutrition expert Jelliffe calls "commerciogenic malnutrition." It is not uncommon in Mexico, doctors who work in rural villages report, for a family to sell the few eggs and chickens it raises to buy Coke for the father while the children waste away for lack of protein.

The companies say they are not to blame if primitive people want to indulge their taste at the expense of their children and their own health. Whenever they try to sell food as being "good for you," executives claim, no one buys. But the reality is that companies are investing heavily in campaigns to sell nutritionally marginal food to economically marginal people. In Latin America, to take only one example of what Berg calls "antinutrition education" campaigns of the food companies, a cornstarch ad features a robust baby in order to give the false impression that this classic stomach filler of the poor is actually good for one. The villages and tribes of the world, Albert Stridsberg proclaims in *Advertising Age*, "are eager to become 'consumers.'" The problem, he says, "is to find products which can be priced within their financial reach and still pay for branded advertising support and return a reasonable profit." Company campaigns have succeeded in increasing consumption of white bread, confections, and soft drinks among the poorest people in the world by convincing them that status, convenience, and a sweet taste are more important than nutrition.

Global companies have used their great levers of power—finance capital, technology, organizational skills, and mass communications—to create a Global Shopping Center in which the hungry of the world are invited to buy expensive snacks and a Global Factory in which there are fewer and fewer jobs. The World Manager's vision of One World turns out in fact to be two distinct worlds—one featuring rising affluence for a small transnational middle class, and the other escalating misery for the great bulk of the human family....

Excerpted with permission from *Global Reach*, pp. 172-184 (Simon & Schuster, 1974). Copyright 1974 by Richard J. Barnet and Ronald E. Müller. Reprinted by permission of Simon & Schuster, a Division of Gulf & Western Corporation.

The Bottle Baby Scandal
Milking the Third World for All It's Worth

BARBARA GARSON

Among the new consumers are young mothers, many of whom abandon breast feeding to give their babies "modern" bottles. The role of advertising and other forms of promotion in what has been called the infant formula "scandal" has been widely debated. In this article from *Mother Jones*, Barbara Garson examines the motives of the contenders.

"In 1970, I visited a small town called Aliagua, in a very rural area of Luzon. . . . During my visit, an old friend of my family, who knew that I was a doctor, approached me and asked me to visit his newborn child, who was very ill. The baby was less than ten days old. He was burning with fever, dehydrated and suffering from severe diarrhea. I asked the mother how she had been feeding the baby and she replied that she was using Enfamil. She told me that this had been given to her on discharge from the hospital in Cabanatuan where she had delivered the child. The milk was given to her by a nurse who told her that her milk was 'inappropriate' for the baby."

So writes Dr. Jesus T. De La Paz, who practices obstetrics and gynecology in the Philippines. According to Dr. La Paz, 80 per cent of the sick infants in the pediatric ward at his country's San Pedro Hospital are bottle fed. Why?

Throughout the Third World, from Haiti to Venezuela to Nigeria to the Philippines, new mothers are leaving maternity wards with tins of powdered milk—free samples—supplied by American, Swiss and Japanese companies. In an attempt to do what's modern, what's best for their babies, they abandon breast feeding. And then, like the family in Aliagua, they try to reconstitute a powdered formula where they have no clean water, no suitable pot for sterilizing, insufficient fuel to boil their one bottle and nipple several times a day, and no refrigerator for the milk.

Above all, they do not have money to keep on buying enough formula. A laborer in Uganda would have to spend 33 per cent of the average daily wage to feed an infant on powdered milk. In Pakistan the figure is 40 per cent. In Haiti a secretary, a relatively well-paid worker, spends 25 per cent of her salary for substitute infant food. And so what happens is that poor mothers start to "stretch" the formula. In 1969 the National Food and Nutrition Survey of Barbados asked mothers of bottle-fed infants two to three months old how long a can of milk lasted. The can contains a four-day supply. But 82 per cent of the mothers said they made it last anywhere from five days to three weeks.

Some mothers who have run out of formula have been found mixing cornstarch with water to give the baby something that looked like milk. Others use cocoa, tea, or simply sugar water to stop the crying, at least temporarily. The British charity organization War on Want found a Nigerian mother feeding her baby water alone. She had seen the bottle and nipple pictured on a billboard and thought the manufactured items themselves provided the nourishment.

Unsterilized and diluted bottle formula exacerbates the two most common causes of infant sickness and death around the world: malnutrition and diarrhea. Actually, the two are "synergistic," as the doctors say: each makes the other worse. Underweight babies are prone to the infections that create diarrhea. And the baby with constant diarrhea receives less nutrition from what food it does get.

Since the late '60s, health officials in poor countries have been seeing these symptoms combined in a syndrome sometimes called Bottle Illness. In some hospitals in Africa these severely dehydrated babies are kept aside in beds labeled "Lactogen Syndrome" (Lactogen is the Nestlé Company's powdered formula). Dr. D. B. Jelliffe, a distinguished British pediatric nutritionist who now heads the UCLA School of Public Health's Division of Population, Family and International Health, has labeled the syndrome "commerciogenic malnutrition."

Whatever you call it, the syndrome involves no new diseases. The diarrhea results from the Third World's prevalent bacterial and amoebic infections, which can be contracted from drinking unboiled water. The malnutrition takes the form of marasmus (shown by the sunken eyes, prominent ribs, thin little arms and legs we've seen in the Bangladesh posters) and kwashiorkor (puffy face and feet, anemia and apathy).

What *is* new about "Bottle Illness" is the early onset of these poverty diseases in children. Ordinarily mother's milk, *even of an underfed woman,* will provide adequate nourishment for at least the early months. For a year to 18 months more it can sometimes provide a good protein supplement. Of course it is good for the mothers to eat well, but, unless the mother is virtually starving, the baby gets nourished.

Furthermore, mother's milk provides immunities against various diseases—something all the more important in countries with few public-health measures. No matter what water the mother drinks, the baby receives breast milk relatively free of the local infections. When poor people breast feed, malnutrition doesn't usually appear until well into the second year of life. Recently the Inter-American Investigation of Mortality in Childhood, conducted by the Pan American Health Organization, a branch of the World Health Organization, checked into the causes of some 35,000 deaths in 15 areas of the world, mostly in Latin America. The researchers found that because of the decline of breast feeding, childhood deaths from malnutrition now peak in the third and fourth months of life.

Of course death is only the extreme result. Milk companies would find little profit in distributing those free samples if every infant was going to die in two or three months. But one of the horrible aspects of this new form of malnutrition is that protein deficiency in the early months seems more likely to lead to permanent brain damage. We won't know the full effects of malnutrition that begins at birth until 15 or 20 years from now, for it had been relatively rare in the world until widespread bottle feeding came along.

For ghoulish family planners, let me stop to point out that bottle-baby deaths are not an effective population control. Rather, they tend to *increase* population. Study after study has shown that, regardless of the availability of birth control, people do not start having smaller families until they feel secure that their children will live to adulthood. When children die, people go on having big families in the hope that at least one or two children will survive. Furthermore, the decline of breast feeding may increase population, because there is some truth to the old wives' tale that you don't get pregnant while you're nursing. It's not foolproof birth control, but lactating mothers do have children spaced farther apart than bottle-feeding mothers.

"Foods You Can Trust"

The bottle baby problem really began in the late 1960s. By then it had become clear the U.S. birthrate was heading for an all-time low. Figures from Europe told the same story. Baby-oriented businesses throughout the overdeveloped world knew that they had to think of a strategy to cope with the baby bust.

Some companies diversified, but the big push went into finding new markets in the Third World. Ross Laboratories, for example, is the subsidiary of Abbott Labs, which manufactures Similac and Isomil. In 1969 the overseas portion of Ross' pediatric sales was 14.3 per cent; by 1973 it had risen to 22.2 per cent, amounting to $31.3 million. Following the same strategy, Bristol-Meyers (Enfamil and Olac), American Home Products' Wyeth division (SMA, S-26, Nursoy) and, biggest of all, the Swiss corporation Nestlé (Lactogen) expanded like mad. Throughout Asia, Africa and Latin America, the airwaves and the billboards began filling with slogans like "Right from the Start—the Foods You Can Trust."

Soon nutritionists began to object. After a series of meetings organized through the U.N., the companies agreed to modify their approach. Now their signs said things like: "The Next Best Thing to Mother's Milk." Their pamphlets spoke vaguely about the times when breast feeding is "inappropriate" or "unsuccessful." More important, in the last few years the milk companies have almost entirely dropped billboards and radio spots. They concentrate now on the most effective and direct approach to the new mother. The majority of the companies give out free samples, pamphlets, posters and contributions of equipment directly to hospitals; they give services to and sponsor conferences for the doctors and nurses. Thus, the

woman from Aliagua was given Enfamil by the nurse when she left the hospital. In some countries (Guatemala, for instance) "milk banks" connected with the hospitals sell a supply of formula to new mothers at cut rates, so it takes them a couple of weeks before they have to buy it on the open market and realize how expensive it really is.

But Nestlé, Bristol-Myers and some of the others don't stop with the hospitals. The milk companies now hire their own special "milk nurses." Dressed in nurse-like uniforms, they travel around in countries such as Jamaica or Malaysia visiting new mothers, providing gifts and advice, weighing the babies—and leaving infant formula samples. These "mothercraft personnel" or "milk nurses," incidentally, may or may not be medically trained. Indeed, the use of fully trained nurses as saleswomen is probably the more harmful practice, since it depletes a developing nation's small supply of medical personnel.

Dr. Roy E. Brown is a nutritionist and pediatrician, now at Mount Sinai medical school, who has practiced abroad for 11 years, including time in the Bangladesh refugee camps. (There, incidentally, he used a simple and successful technique to promote "relactation" among mothers who had previously ceased breast feeding.) He told me about a pediatric nurse he knew in Ethiopia in 1963:

"She was a beautiful woman who was not only an Ethiopian nurse but a nurse tutor. She had been to Sweden, where she got advanced training to teach other nurses. She was married and had one child of her own. She left the hospital when a milk company offered her three times what she was getting paid as a nurse.

"I saw her again in 1974. She had two children and was still employed by the milk company. I had become increasingly disturbed by what I had seen of bottle feeding around the world, and I tried to talk to her about it. She said she understood my point of view, but she wanted to make a good living. Her defense was that she did not advise people to stop breast feeding; she simply gave them information if they 'couldn't breast feed.' Besides, people were giving up breast feeding anyway, so at least she would supply them with a wholesome product and instructions."

Make Your Baby White

Mary Lee, a housewife in Malaysia, wrote this letter: "On 23rd August, 1976, I had an interview with a Bristol-Myers mothercraft nurse by the name of Mrs. Ho, who came to my house at my request. Mrs. Ho was wearing a white nurse's uniform and informed me she is a State Registered Nurse who trained here in University Hospital, Kuala Lumpur. On arrival Mrs. Ho presented me with a free sample tin of Enfamil powder infant formula without my asking for it. I told her I was thinking of weaning my baby from the breast, to which she said that Enfamil 'is just like breast milk.' She even pointed out on the sample tin the content 'choline,' which she assured me would make my baby's complexion beautiful and fair. In this community mothers feel it is very important to have fair skin...."

Mary Lee happens to be a doctor's wife. She was not particularly impressed by the white uniform, nor was she intimidated when the nurse worriedly weighed her baby. And she doesn't seem interested in making her baby more white with Enfamil. But what about a poor and unsophisticated woman?

Or what about a not-so-poor and -unsophisticated woman? During World War II, my mother, otherwise honest and patriotic, bought black market lamb chops. This was because her pediatrician prescribed an exact diet for each baby he treated. Four ounces of lamb chop, two ounces of cereal, three ounces of mashed banana. And this I was fed (and re-fed) despite the fact that I threw up three times a day for three years.

Before I was ready for the scraped lamb chops and mashed banana, I was bottle fed with a formula that entailed much measuring, sterilizing and breaking of bottles. Worst of all, the doctor set me on a four-hour feeding schedule.

My parents later told me how I cried stubbornly, sometimes for two and a half hours straight, while they sat in agony waiting for the scientifically determined moment when they could give me the bottle that would bring immediate satisfaction.

How could they do it? Why didn't they just pick me up and feed me the way their mothers had done? Well, my father's mother was dead and, besides, she had lost children while feeding the old way. And my mother's mother was an immigrant who spread newspaper on the floor after she washed it and kept live fish in the bathtub to make gefilte fish at Passover. I was going to get the best scientific chance in life.

And here's an even more sophisticated woman. When I was to deliver, I chose a hospital that allowed Lamaze and featured rooming-in. They brought me the baby after isolating her for 24 hours, and I nursed contentedly for a couple of days. Then the nurse said "The baby is not gaining any weight. Not an ounce after any feeding."

"But she's sucking," I insisted, "and she's not crying. Let me keep trying."

Then the doctor came in: "Not a single ounce."

I agreed reluctantly to let them start her on formula while I gave it a few more tries. But I knew the bottle would curtail the baby's sucking, and there wouldn't be too much hope after that.

While I was giving it that one more try, a woman who was cleaning the floor, with no white uniform, said to me: "That baby's not gettin' a thing."

"What do you mean?"

"Look," she said, pinching me roughly. "It's all clogged up." She showed me how to put a hot washcloth on my breast and squeeze hard. After an hour of hard work, milk started to flow. Apparently the 24-hour delay after the baby was born had caused the milk to "back up."

I should have nursed right away or started squeezing the milk out by hand. If it weren't for the cleaning lady, I, like the woman in Aliagua, would certainly have found that under modern conditions I was one of the many who "couldn't nurse."

The same thing happens in the Third World. There, too, people are being cut off from their past, moving away from their families. The Green Revolution (*Mother Jones,* August 1977) sends former subsistence farmers off the land and into the *favelas,* barrios, and shanty towns in the city. There, with modern medical help, many will find breast feeding "unsuccessful" or "inappropriate." Some can't nurse because they work or hope to work. Most, however, will choose more freely not to nurse. What would they do if the baby cried on the bus? Some don't want to be bothered. But most want to do what's best for their babies. They want to give their children the start that will help them out of the *favela* and into the modern world. Like buying an encyclopedia.

In the scantiest slum store they will find the powdered milk prominently displayed. (A chart in the February 1977 issue of the Brazilian trade journal *Modern Supermarket* shows that baby formulas have a profit margin of 72 per cent. This is three or four times higher than the profit margin for most other items.) On the labels of these products are pictures of plump, smiling children. And so, healthy mothers are feeding their babies watered-down imported milk in contaminated bottles in the hope we all share—to do the best by one's children.

The Nuns Go to Court

The bottle baby problem has not gone unnoticed. Activists have been fighting Nestlé in Europe for some time, and in the U.S. the Interfaith Center on Corporate Responsibility (ICCR)—connected with The National Council of Churches—has been publicizing the issue widely, especially to church groups. Therefore, when the Sisters of the Precious Blood, a Catholic teaching order based in Ohio, realized several years ago that they owned stock in Bristol-Myers, they quickly made the connection.

The Sisters tried first to speak to corporate executives about the problem. They found Bristol-Myers more difficult to deal with than the other milk companies, who were, if nothing else, at least willing to talk politely. Eventually, unable to get satisfaction, the sisters submitted a stockholders' resolution asking for information about Bristol-Meyers' sales policy abroad. In a proxy statement urging defeat of that resolution, the company said, among other things: "Infant formula products are neither intended, nor promoted, for private purchase where chronic poverty or ignorance could lead to product misuse or harmful effects."

Now it can in some cases be a violation of Securities and Exchange Commission (SEC) regulations to make misstatements in proxy material. After further frustrating dealings with Bristol-Meyers, the Sisters of the Precious Blood eventually filed a lawsuit against the company on these grounds. The strategy of the suit was to expose the lie. The Sisters attempted to show, first, that the company *did* promote its Enfamil formula to chronically poor people and, second, that the people who bought it were too poor or ignorant to use it safely.

As all TV viewers know, court testimony must always be based on firsthand knowledge. You can't submit statistical reports or get up and say "as everybody knows...." So, the Sisters and ICCR painstakingly collected testimony from 15 countries. There are affidavits that read something like: "I, Dr. So-and So, living in the town of Such-and Such, Venezuela, or Indonesia, or Guatemala, went to the following grocery stores in poor neighborhoods where I personally saw cans of Enfamil on sale." One exhibit was an Enfamil ad on the back page of the Barbados phone book, as personally observed by the witness, of course.

There are personal interviews, like these taken by Dr. Arthur L. Warner in Guatemala, where one in four slum mothers he talked to was bottle feeding:

"*Family B.* A young mother of two living in a shanty hillside settlement of Guatemala City decided to wean her baby at ten days, because a friend told her the milk was no good and too weak. She purchased Enfamil on the suggestion of a doctor in the public health 'well-baby' clinic. Her husband earns $3 a day (of which she spends about 75¢ for the infant's milk). They live without safe water and beside an open sewer. Their shack has many openings for flies. They have no refrigeration. She is illiterate. She must haul water...from a community spigot.

"Family C. A mother of three, living in a shanty development in Guatemala City, decided to wean her baby at two months because the child wasn't gaining fast enough and was sickly. A clinic nurse had suggested her milk had gone bad. [Local] water, generally considered contaminated since the earthquake...Fuel costs are high.... Boiling water costs the family up to $5 a month."

A doctor in Jamaica reviews the cases of 37 patients referred to the Tropical Metabolism Research Unit for severe malnutrition. "Twenty-five received infant formula. Five died."

And so the Sisters of the Precious Blood compiled thousands of pages. In one way their brief is an impressive document, and in another it is almost pathetic—this patient piecing together of minute firsthand accounts to show the world-wide workings of imperialism. To show what everyone knows.

In May of this year the case was dismissed, though the Sisters are appealing. The decision, by Federal Judge Milton Pollack, though a little difficult to read, appears to say:

The shareholders' resolution was only a request and wouldn't be binding on the board of directors even if it had passed. Therefore, it just doesn't matter. The court doesn't have to consider whether the proxy material contained a misstatement or whether the affidavits submitted by the Sisters are true, because no irreparable harm was done to any shareholder.

There is no law preventing corporations from doing irreparable harm to Third World babies.

Bottle on the Grave

Leah Margulies, small, lively and radical, heads the project on bottle feeding for the Interfaith Center on Corporate Responsibility. "I was hired with the general assignment to develop the relationships between multinational corporations and world hunger—agribusiness, cash cropping, you know. But it is very difficult to make it graphic that the world is starving, not because of drought, or floods, but because of economic dependency."

"So you decided to use the baby bottle case as an example?" I suggested.

"I didn't really decide. It grew up around us," Margulies said. "I did extensive research on multinationals in the early '70s. I was anxious to show the effects of the *normal* operations of capitalism, not the big scandals or fuck-ups. So I read *Fortune, Harvard Business Review, Forbes,* annual reports, speeches by corporate executives.

"And I developed my thoughts about economic dependency. The corporations operate in the Third World in a way that creates overall economic dependency as horrifying, impoverishing and unnatural as the dependency of a healthy mother on expensive powdered milk. The import of unnecessary powdered milk—forget Coca-Cola—now takes about one *billion* dollars a year from the Third World.

"But I tell you the truth, even after documenting the entire lawsuit—the facts, the figures, the affidavits—sometimes I still don't believe myself. I don't believe the world could be starving, that babies could be sick and dying just for a little profit.

"Like you remember the story about the graves in Zambia?"

I remembered it well. The film *Bottle Babies,* used widely by the church groups, ends with a shot of a child's grave near Lusaka, Zambia. The small grave is decorated with a crushed milk can and a little baby bottle. The narrator says, "Mothers put empty Nestlé's Lactogen cans and feeding bottles on their dead babies' graves, for they believe to the end that powdered milk and feeding bottles were the most valuable possessions their babies once had." I had wondered myself how to evaluate this dramatic detail. The film itself was apparently "re-enacted."

"Well, last week," Margulies continued, "I happened to see the film *Last Grave at Dimbaza*. The film is about apartheid, not about bottle feeding. No mention was made of that. But it shows the poverty and the horrible infant mortality. The film ends with a shot of those infant graves. My heart jumped. There—you could make it out if you knew what it was—there was that little can of powdered milk.

"But still, when you immerse yourself back in our U.S. reality once again, you don't believe it. For instance, the president of American Home Products is a kindly, charming man. I go in there with a room full of church people. We are all middle class. And this lovely gentleman says, 'Do you believe we would deliberately harm babies?'"

I questioned Margulies about the stockholders' approach. Did it make sense to ask corporations on their own to stop selling? Or to limit their market to the tiny number of Third World mothers (certainly under five per cent) who really can't nurse? She felt that the educational effect on the participating religious groups made it worthwhile. Also, the publicity can't hurt. And pressure here creates the climate for real regulation in the Third World. So far, though, the countries attempting to regulate milk companies are few. In Guinea-Bissau baby formula is available only by prescription. Papua New Guinea is cracking down on advertisements. In Jamaica, mothercraft personnel are forbidden to enter the hospitals, though it seems that some still do. And, in any case, they are active in all the slums. Malaysia and Guyana, among other countries, have launched national breast-feeding campaigns. But of course their resources are limited compared to milk company advertising budgets.

"I Have an Appointment"

Like Margulies, I, too, found myself suffering bouts of doubt. Infants crying from hunger when there is all the milk they need? Maybe this is just a radical "cause." Something blown up out of proportion.

I must check it out, I felt, someplace more neutral and scientific....

At the U.N. I spoke first to Dr. Jacob Schatan of the Protein Advisory Group. He is a mild, thin man, very reasonable sounding, but sad. He is Chilean.

"What is the scope of this bottle-feeding problem? Is it really so dangerous?"

"Everywhere there is a marked trend of decline in breast feeding." Dr. Schatan speaks in U.N. Reportese, though his gestures show concern. "It is a trend accompanying urbanization. I could not tell you the exact percentages for each country, but we can easily estimate the cost to the developing nations in the billions."

"Billions?" I asked. (He has an accent, and he mumbles.) "Billions with a *B?*"

"With a B."

"Do you think there could be legislation restricting the companies?"

"The Protein Advisory Group provides information from scientists to the U.N. system, not to countries. However, I would say you need legislation not in relation to sale, but legislation facilitating breast feeding for urban women. If a mother works eight hours, there should be a time and place to nurse at work. This is not done except in a few of the...uh..." (The pause is cautious, painful; finally, he gives up and uses the word.) "...socialist countries. And of course education. There must be an educational campaign."

Next I went to UNICEF, where I spoke to L.J. Tepley, senior nutritionist.

"How did the question of bottle-feeding first come to your attention?" I asked.

"And just how could I be concerned with children's nutrition without its coming to my attention?" (Tepley, a stocky American, is as bluff and direct as Schatan is cautious.)

"Is it really as dangerous as some think?" I asked.

"Does any of those papers..." (He pointed to a bundle of charts, reports and articles I had been collecting all week and was now spilling on his office floor. They were from the Columbia Medical School, Mount Sinai Hospital, the U.N., the Consumer's Union, the Brookings Institute, the ICCR, the milk companies themselves.) "Does *any* of them say bottle milk is *good* for poor people? Here." (He handed me an enormous envelope for all my papers.)

"We know the effects. They are awful. No one doubts it."

"Then why is it spreading?" I asked.

"The causes are two. Ignorance and money. Not necessarily in that order."

"What can be done?" I asked. "Can the milk companies be regulated?"

"I have to go," said Mr. Tepley. (I had dropped in on him unannounced around lunch time.) "I have an appointment."

And in New York...

A couple of years ago, the chief of the New York City Health and Hospitals Corporation announced proudly a money-saving contract with Ross Laboratories, the Abbott subsidiary that makes infant formula. Till then the city hospitals had been spending some $300,000 a year on Similac. But Ross was going to slash next year's price to less than $100,000, and in the third year of the contract the hospitals would be getting all the Similac they could use for free.

I decided to take a look around Lincoln Hospital in the Bronx. When I got to the maternity ward, it was feeding time. The sign in front of the swinging doors said, "No entry. Mothers with babies." While I waited, an orderly wheeled in a cart loaded with cases of Similac. Here they use the more expensive pre-mixed formula in individual disposable nursing bottles.

After a while I went down to the prenatal clinic. I asked the pregnant women, all black or Puerto Rican, whether they were going to breast feed or bottle feed. The answers were unanimous.

"What if I'm on the bus when the baby gets hungry?"

"If you're in the house with just your husband, okay. But if there are friends or family,

then you have to go into the other room."

"I eat a lot of junk. The baby would drain me."

"My milk wasn't good enough for my first one."

"What if you're out in the street? You can't just whip it out!"

In English, Spanish and sign language, the response was clear. Total repugnance at the idea of breast feeding.

I asked whether the nurses or doctors had said anything about breast feeding.

"They said Similac was just as good."

"They said you have to eat a certain diet, and I couldn't eat all those special vegetables."

"They give you pamphlets that say you should choose yourself."

The pamphlets handed out at the prenatal clinic are published by Carnation. The more detailed one, "You and Your Contented Baby," does indeed admit that "the breast-fed baby seems to have fewer digestive upsets than the bottle-fed baby." However, the seven-step instructions for breast feeding include language like "compress the nipple and the brown tissue horizontally," along with medical illustrations of areola and sinuses and indecipherable diagrams labeled "correct and incorrect positions for baby's jaw." This makes it all seem much more complicated than simply heating up a formula. Not to mention the fact that the picture of Carnation milk is in color and labeled "For over 35 years, millions of babies have thrived on Carnation Evaporated Milk formulas." A second, simpler pamphlet says nothing at all about the advantages of breast feeding.

Pamphlets notwithstanding, it is the official policy of the pre-natal clinic that breast feeding is best. The intake nurse told me that she is supposed to mention it to each mother. "But I know that they are going to say 'Echh, I can't do that.' And then there is a language barrier. I can give directions in Spanish, but I cannot talk about personal things. I do mention it, though, when I think they may be interested. And if one woman a week says 'Yes, I'd like to try,' then I feel very rewarded."

Back up in the maternity ward, the babies had

been put away. After an initial period of isolation, they are brought to the mothers every four hours, along with the bottles of Similac.

I stood with a group of new mothers in front of the nursery window talking about breast feeding, while we watched the nurse inside feed a newborn from a Similac bottle.

I asked the women if they knew what the formula would cost.

A couple said, "I have no idea." Some gave me a figure: "$5.50 a case," "$1.50 for the quart can of concentrate." One lady said, "I don't know what it will cost me because I don't know if they're giving mine Similac or Carnation." Apparently she was under the impression that she would have to continue to use whatever the hospital started the baby with.

But the majority of mothers said, "I won't have to pay for it because I'm on this program." The program was WIC (Women Infant Care), a federal program offering health care to mothers and well infants. One of the inducements to remain with the program is a monthly supply of baby products, including bottle formula.

"Will You Make a Profit?"

"I called Bristol-Myers," I said to Leah Margulies.

"Yeah?"

"And they put me on to Ed Simon in the P.R. office."

"Oh, yeah?"

"I asked him if any of your charges had affected their sales promotions abroad."

"What'd he say?"

"First, he said I was obviously prejudiced because the question implied that the charges were true. Second, he said, 'While not acknowledging any of the claims, it is safe to say we've made every attempt to strengthen our control over the sale of infant formula.'

"And then he started to read me all the clauses from their guidelines:

'Detailed information on infant formula . . . will be directed only to physicians and medical personnel. . . .

'Mothercraft nurses will perform in a manner comparable to government-sponsored public-health nurses, with their primary concern the assistance of mothers in the proper care and feeding of their infants, whether breast or formula fed. . . .'

"I was busy scribbling, trying to get it all down as fast as I could. Finally, I said, 'With all those restrictions, do you sell more or less Enfamil?'"

"What did he say?"

"He said they couldn't discuss information regarding the sale of specific products."

"One of the Sisters of Mercy made the same point during our meeting with Abbott in Chicago," said Margulies. "They were being very agreeable about modifying their sales techniques. 'Use of mass media will be dropped . . . no radio, billboards . . .

"Well, as we were about to leave, one of the Sisters said, 'Tell me, if you stop selling to people who are too poor to use the product safely, will you still make a profit?'

"There was absolute silence. It must have been a full minute.

"Finally one of the corporate executives picked it up and said:

"'That is the crux of the problem.'"

Barbara Garson is the author of "MacBird" and a book about routine work, now in paperback, *All the Livelong Day.*

Reprinted with permission from Barbara Garson and *Mother Jones,* pp. 33-34+ (December 1977).

Coke Tries to Widen Brazil Market

RAMONA BECHTOS

SAO PAULO—Not content to simply be the largest selling soft drink in Brazil and to hold a whopping 90% of the cola market, Coca-Cola is looking to boost its sales here by expanding the total consumption of soft drinks.

Per-capita annual consumption of soft drinks in Brazil is 95 bottles (of the 6½-oz. variety), according to Robert Cole, president of McCann-Erickson Publicidade, which acquired the Coke account in Brazil before getting it anywhere else. In an interview with *Advertising Age,* he said that Coke holds about a 32% share of all soft drink sales in Brazil, which in 1974 were 423,000,000 cases (with 24 bottles per case).

This puts Coke ahead of its big competitor, guarana, the generic name for a sweet-tasting refreshment which holds a 29% share of the soft drink market. (Guarana is now being sold in the U.S. and the United Kingdom on a small scale under the name Trop.)

The soft drink market in Brazil has a great potential for growth, Mr. Cole said. He noted that "in Rio de Janeiro and Bahia, when the temperature drops below 77°, the people pretty much stop drinking the stuff. So, there seems a tremendous market in promoting Coke off-season, as well as for in-home consumption." He feels that Brazilians must be encouraged to consume more soft drinks with meals eaten at home, where they drink mainly mineral water and some beer.

It also seems to some observers that all sodas would make gains if their manufacturers could persuade the people in this coffee-rich country to occasionally replace the seemingly ever-present black brew in every office with a soft drink.

Coke spends less than $2,000,000 annually in advertising, "an amazingly small budget here" for such a product, according to Francisco Gracioso, director-general of McCann/Brazil, and author of the book, "Homen do Marketing" ("Marketing Men").

Mr. Cole observed that Coke's budget is going up slowly, but added that the company is giving priority to using its capital for additional trucks and glass. There has been a shortage of bottles in Brazil, part of a general package scarcity.

For about four years, Coke's theme in Brazil has been *"Isso è que è"* ("This is it"), which is "our way of saying, 'It's the real thing'," noted Marcio Martins Moreira, creative director. He said that, meanwhile, Pepsi-Cola in Brazil has been working on a variation of the "Pepsi generation" theme, stating in essence that Pepsi gives you a "love" kind of feeling. . . .

Excerpted with permission from *Advertising Age,* 46(32): 3 (11 August 1975). Copyright 1975 by Crain Communications, Inc.

Din-Din

THOMAS WHITESIDE

In an oversaturated food market, what is there left to sell? Pet food. Thomas Whiteside's "Din-Din" first appeared in the *New Yorker* in November of 1976. The excerpt included here penetrates somewhat more deeply than earlier selections into the tactics of the food marketer, ever seeking new purchasers in an effort to achieve continued growth.

In a way comparable, perhaps, to that by which in reading the newspapers and watching the TV news I rather suddenly became aware of the word "Sunbelt" and the portent of the increasing population shift thereto, I have become aware lately in my television viewing of the prevalence of pet-food commercials on the home screen. Hardly before I realized what was happening, it seemed that I couldn't turn on my set without being confronted by pet-food ads. Now that I have become acutely conscious of the pet-food commercials on the air, it seems to me almost as though dogs and cats and their eating preferences are beginning to take over television, with human beings and human activities slowly falling back to a humbler place in the scheme of things.

In fact, if one concentrates on the content of the pet-food commercials it can easily appear that human beings are on the way out in the Darwinian sense, too. In the pet-food commercials, the pets are increasingly shown addressing the viewer directly on their own behalf and without human prompting. The animals are also shown talking together and engaging in all sorts of other behavior usually considered exclusively human. Thus, in one pet-food commercial a cat answers a ringing telephone by tipping the receiver off its cradle with a paw. A representative of the local supermarket is on the line, and the cat orders up dinner by saying "Meow" into the mouthpiece. The supermarket man recognizes immediately that the cat is ordering a cat food called Meow Mix. In a similar commercial, a cat is *singing* its order for Meow Mix:

> I want tuna,
> I want liver,
> I want chicken,
> Please deliver.

. . . As representations go, probably the most sophisticated inhabitant of the world of pet-food commercials is the cat Morris, which appears in the commercials for 9-Lives cat food. This cat is shown as being a choosy sort, especially in its eating preferences, and, through a human voice-over, is given to uttering its thoughts in a sort of interior monologue, mostly on the subject of cat food. The screen personality of Morris is one of advanced finickiness, displayed particularly in scenes in which the cat turns disdainfully away from the prospect of eating common cat food when its mistress (the audience sees only a pair of legs) cries coaxingly, "Din-din time!" The cat Morris also expresses its disdain of various attempts by its owner to entertain it—for example, by giving it an elaborate cat box—in a world-weary voice that I, for one, consider a bit fruity. In the commercials, Morris is stirred from boredom by an offer of 9-Lives, which it eats avidly, but after finishing the stuff the cat is shown as reverting to an attitude of languid archness. . . .

In pet-food commercials, the animal kingdom has made such inroads into the turf of human communication that not only have the pets assumed human capacities but human beings have been transmogrified into animal form. In a commercial for Gravy Train dog food, the scene is a kitchen. Two women are there, but they are wearing dog costumes and speak to each other through large dogs' heads. One of the two is a next-door neighbor who has just dropped in with a neighborly request. She exclaims, "Oh, Marge, Harry's boss is coming for dinner, and I ran out of food." The other dog-woman tells her neighbor not to worry. Helpfully, she produces a package of Gravy Train for the festive table. They discuss the meaty taste of Gravy Train. The scene then dissolves to the dinner party. All are sitting around the table dressed as dogs, Harry's boss included. Harry's boss is impressed by the dinner and, in a doggy voice, compliments the hostess: "Hmm! This Gravy Train is delicious crunchy dry!" And Harry, enthusiastically agreeing with his boss, declares through his dog's head that his own portion is "delicious with its gravy, too." Whatever the future of dog-costume dinner parties, all this reinforces one's vision of a general power shift to the Petbelt.

The advance of the prepared-pet-food industry in this country is certainly striking in economic terms. Fifteen years ago, the business was a relatively modest one; while canned dog and cat food was sold in the supermarkets, it wasn't accorded much space, and people often had to hunt around for it in obscure corners of the store. (In those primitive days, pets were getting by largely on table scraps and loving it.) By 1965, however, the amount of money Americans spent on commercially prepared pet food had risen to seven hundred million dollars. Since then, the business has grown to the point where people are spending two and a half billion dollars a year on this commodity.

Today, the sale of pet food has expanded so greatly that, instead of a few feet of shelf space, whole aisles of supermarkets are sometimes given over to the display of dog and cat food; in fact, the annual dollar volume of pet-food sales in the supermarkets has reached three times that of prepared baby food. Pet foods account for five per cent of all money spent in supermarkets on dry groceries. According to a survey by the A.C. Nielsen Company, the market-research organization, the average chain supermarket is devoting a hundred and eighty-two linear feet of shelf space to the display of pet food. Strolling down supermarket aisles, citizens look over and take their pick from a vast variety of products with names like Mighty Dog, Alpo, Kal Kan, Strongheart, Laddie Boy, Henny Pen, Jo-Bo, Chuck Wagon, Puss 'n Boots, Lovin' Spoonfuls, and Tender Vittles. In the course of a year, customers are buying, at an average price of thirty-two cents a pound, about seven and a quarter billion pounds of pet food. . . .

While available statistics may not quite serve to confirm one's strong individual impression—derived from all the pet-food commercials and the pet-food takeover in supermarkets—that a pet population explosion must be occurring in this country, there has unquestionably been in recent years a marked increase in the number of pets. Completely reliable statistics in this area are rather hard to come by, but according to current industry estimates there are now between fifty-seven and seventy million cats and dogs in this country—thirty-five to forty million dogs and twenty-two to thirty million cats. With the decline of the postwar baby boom, the increase in human population in this country has levelled off to about one per cent a year. But for some years the pet population appears to have been increasing at the rate of about three per cent a year, and it shows no sign at all of slackening off. The number of dogs in the United States now far exceeds the number of human beings in Canada, which is a mere twenty-three million.

If one compares the sales figures of the pet-food industry over the last decade with the population figures for pets, it seems that the increase in the consumption of pet food has been a lot greater than the increase in the number of pets consuming pet food. . . . It can probably be explained in part by various alterations in people's household habits in this country. For example, the traditional habit of feeding pets largely on scraps has been affected to some extent by people's habit of buying their meat in supermarkets rather than from local butchers. The family butchers would often supply them with all sorts of odds and ends for their pets. . . . But a great deal of the huge increase in the sale of pet food appears to be attributable to the strenuous promotional efforts of the pet-food manufacturers, whose television ads, with their shots of dogs, puppies, cats, and kittens in adorable action, not only have helped persuade pet owners to buy their products but may even have influenced many people to go out and buy pets so that they could dish out for them the pet food being advertised.

Never in the history of television, with its news coverage emphasizing wars, invasions, fires, bombs, and political chicanery, and its dramatic programs emphasizing shoot-'em-ups and missions impossible, has love been promoted so assiduously as in the pet-food commercials. . . .

In view of all the love and harmony that overflow the home screen and even soak into the names of the pet foods themselves (Lovin' Spoonfuls, Tender Vittles), one may visualize the promoters and actual producers of pet food as a genial and benign group—as eager to discuss and exult over their industry to outside inquirers as they are to depict their products on the airwaves. But this turns out not to be quite the reality, as I discovered recently when I approached a number of pet-food companies in hopes of having their officers discuss the pet-food business. In fact, I found those officers to be, collectively, a remarkably silent and secretive fraternity.

For example, attempts to obtain information from the officers of the huge Ralston Purina Company, of St. Louis, whose production accounts for thirty per cent of the country's entire annual pet-food business, were unavailing. . . . I found them—the promoters of the slogan "All you add is love"—most uncommunicative. It is possible that this air of Fortress Purina is the result of a certain amount of publicity which people in the pet-food industry could consider adverse—for example, various allegations in the press that some of the poor have been reduced to eating pet food as a regular part of their diet. . . .Suggestions have also appeared in the press from time to time that the enormous amount of pet food sold in this country represents a diversion of food energy into the mouths of pets when many millions of people are starving throughout the world. The pet-food manufacturers have undoubtedly preferred to ignore these suggestions, because countering them would necessitate dwelling upon the fact that most pet food is "not suitable," as they put it, for human consumption, and the manufacturers are extremely reluctant to go into details that might make their products seem rather less yummy than in the pet-food commercials. . . .

One of the companies I had approached, unavailingly, for information on the merchandising of pet food was Allen Products, with headquarters in Allentown, Pennsylvania. I had been particularly interested in talking to officials of Allen, because the company is the manufacturer of Alpo, a premium-priced canned dog food. Beginning in the mid-sixties and continuing until the economic recession took the edge off its competitive lead in its section of the business, Alpo was promoted into possibly the most spectacular success in the pet-food business. . . .

To advance the cause of Alpo, Allen Products greatly increased its advertising budget, especially for television, and instead of concentrating on spot advertising, as it previously had, it went heavily into network television advertising on a national basis. The claims made on national television implied that Alpo, at a higher price than the products of competitors, provided superior nutrition and was more appealing to dogs because it was an all-meat product, in contrast to brands that contained other ingredients, such as cereal. . . .

Alpo's competitors began making great efforts to promote the semi-moist brands of dog food—most of which contained a high proportion of soy meal or cereal as well as sugar—by attacking Alpo's grip on the market for high-priced dog food. General Foods, which put out a semi-moist dog food called Gaines-burgers, was advertising it as "the canned dog food without the can." The makers of other semi-moist products were promoting them with such slogans as "Dogs think it's meat, but it's more" and "More nourishing than the sirloin steak you'd eat yourself."

Alpo, striking back at the semi-moist-dog-food campaigns pretty much as Weightman had proposed, came up with a subsidiary slogan— "No sugar added." Its television ads also took to warning dog owners, in sincere and pointed fashion:

> Burger dog foods...can contain as much as twenty per cent sugar. There's also up to thirty-five per cent vegetable matter. How much real beef, or meat by-products are in a burger? Well, it would take at least ten burgers to equal the beef and meat by-products in one can of Alpo Beef.

. . . Certainly the huge Alpo promotion was not without problems that the competition might exploit. From the mid-sixties on, the Alpo promotional people had to contend with a growing set of "vulnerabilities," which included published reports on a number of veterinary studies of dog nutrition purporting to show that a diet made up exclusively of high-protein food— just what the Alpo ads on television were proclaiming as the ultimate in nutrition for dogs—might have adverse effects on the animals' health. One study claimed that digestive upsets and bone changes occurred in puppies that were fed diets consisting primarily of meat and meat by-products; moreover, such diets were said to exert ill effects on older dogs with liver and kidney problems. Another study concluded that there was no evidence to prove that animal protein was an essential constituent of a dog's diet at all. Ominously for the Alpo people, it looked as though such allegations were going

to result in some sort of action by the F.T.C. to put restrictions on the claims that pet-food companies could make about the benefits of all-meat dog food. . . . In any event, Ralston Purina had been systematically running down the worth of "all meat" canned dog food in television ads for its cereal-based Purina dry dog foods. . . .

It is perhaps germane, in contemplating the pet-food battlefield and the weaponry employed by the contending forces, that the Alpo people opposed their competitors not by modifying the comparatively high price of their products but by ordering up, at enormous cost, more and more television commercials to do the opposition in. The pet-food war was a war fought on television screens, and as the television campaigns to fight the competition grew ever more expensive, the competitors had to be even fewer and richer. This notion did not fail to strike the administrative-law judge in the Liggett & Myers-Perk Foods proceedings. "The record shows beyond any question," he wrote in his decision, "that entry [of competition] into most categories of dog food [merchandising] is largely determined by the ability to match the massive advertising expenditures of the industry's giants."

It was as though the advanced price of Alpo were itself a secret ingredient that added to its attractiveness to purchasers. . . .

With the unceasing advertising barrages on television, and with the emphasis on the virtues of high-priced dog food, it was as if price had become the touchstone not only of the quality of the product being offered but also of the quality of the purchasers—as if the social status of citizens could now be judged by the expensiveness of the dog food they bought. The merchandisers of the competing companies appear to have had few doubts about who was influencing the exercise of individual choice in matters of pet nutrition. A motivational-research study of the dog-food market that was prepared in 1972 for the Perk Foods division of Liggett & Myers puts the issue of consumer free will rather unsentimentally:

Advertising is usually down-graded by people as an effective element in their product and brand selections. They prefer to believe in the myths of their own autonomy in decision-making. . . . Advertising implies to an individual that peers value the same brand or product as he does. Therein, the individual is assured of the rightness of his choice. But such forms of advertising influence are not in the realm of the admissable.

No, indeed. Nevertheless, the pet-food manufacturers and advertisers have been eager to ascertain the outlook and social standing and buying habits of pet owners, and their precise attitudes toward their pets; and all the pet-food companies seem to have commissioned studies appraising these characteristics, sometimes in detail. In fact, the underlying tone of much of the pet-food advertising on the air undoubtedly reflects what the pet-food men conceive, through their market research, to be the spiritual and temporal tone of pet owners—particularly those with money to spend. A few such studies that I have been able to get my hands on make interesting reading, even if they are sometimes a bit complex, being peppered with terms like "ego-gratification," "surrogate child," "love object," "ambivalence," and "anthropomorphizing."

One of the first things I noticed in reading this literature is that, while pets are usually owned by families, the customer is usually referred to as "she." That is, the man of the house may buy the dog, but it's his wife who picks up the dog food at the supermarket. From the point of view of the pet-food people, "she" is an individual to be watched, and "her" motivations are to be analyzed, with care. Thus, "A Study of Attitudes Toward Pet Ownership," prepared on behalf of the Pet Food Institute, observes, under the subhead "Emotional Gratification," "It is interesting to note that it is primarily women who receive emotional support and satisfaction from their pets." A little farther on, the study goes into a few details. "There are many ways in which pets provide this kind of satisfaction," it says. "For example,

pets offer the opportunity to give and receive a totally involving kind of love, a kind which husbands or children often do not want or cannot tolerate." The study notes that animals do not "complain or recoil" from overattention or affection, "but rather, follow their owners around, are eager for bodily contact, and are even reported to stare at owners in a special way."

Later on, in an apparent reference to the man of the house, who, it is assumed, may be absent a good part of the time for one reason or another, the report asserts, "Pets mitigate guilt created by not being home with one's family." And it further notes:

> There were also signs that men use pets to relieve themselves of wives' overdependency or constant demands on their time. By having one or two pets to care for, the wives have more to do and also something else from whom affection can be given and received.

After such a characterization, the subhead of the section immediately following—"Pets fulfill perceptions of an ideal American home"—may seem a trifle flat. But things pick up again in a section headed "Pets provide a source of ego-gratification." The report explains that in addition to contributing to "feelings of successful family interactions," pets improve their owners' positive concept of themselves. Thus, "many women gain a tremendous sense of being 'good' when they take in strays." They "take pride in their pets doing special things," such as the way one of them "stalks his food," including birds. . . .The studies seem to agree that a household pet is increasingly regarded as (to use a phrase that occurs over and over in such documents) "a member of the family." In the family circle, as a document prepared for the Liggett & Myers-Perk Foods division emphasizes, *the dog occupies a key position with his own prerogatives and needs.*" It goes on to say, "An intricate form of communication is established in which humans watch for and anticipate the desires of the dog and in which he makes his feelings explicit."

The prevailing attitude of dog owners, as the

manufacturers of pet foods have undoubtedly been gratified to learn through these studies, is an interestingly indulgent one. The Liggett & Myers study puts the situation in this way:

> Many of the women [interviewed in the study] indulge their dog's behavior. He is allowed to behave in "human ways" in getting on furniture, in insisting that he "go with the family" and in his desires to go out on demand. Many are proud of their pet's idiosyncrasies.... The attitude is parallel to that seen in families with "permissive" atmospheres for children.... and opportunities for "self-expression" are many and are encouraged.

Thus, if the family dog one day turns up its nose at the grub put in front of it, the reaction of the owner, even if the owner understands that the meal is perfectly nutritious, is not to let the dog get good and hungry until it decides not to be so picky. "Few of these owners have tried to discipline the dog to eat recommended foods simply because they are supposed to be 'good for the pet,'" the Liggett study notes, and it also observes, "Those foods that the dog rejects or even eats reluctantly will not be repurchased." The report goes on to point out that when such instances of stubbornness occur "the owners seem to be secretly proud that their pets could not be coerced into eating something against [their] wishes."

Another motivational-research study prepared for Perk Foods in 1972, delves into possible sources of such secret pride, noting, "The factor of catering to a dog seems to indicate that some dog owners not only recognize their dogs as fussy and individualistic, but also cater to their dogs' behavior and preferences . . . to the extent of preparing special dishes . . . presumably in an effort to satisfy a dog's apparent tastes." The report ascribes such deference partly to "a personal projection of feelings about how a dog ought to feel . . . loved, wanted, and pampered." It is of little concern to owners that "dogs can readily learn to be fussy about what they eat so long as owners change dog foods . . . every time a dog refuses to eat." And why

are the owners so deferential to their dogs whims? "By ego projection, owners unconsciously want to teach their dogs to be and act like themselves." The Perk Foods research report explains that this level of ego projection involves a sense of satisfaction, if not pleasure, which the owner experiences in exerting control over the dog. Such control "extends to concern and regulation of a dog's nutrition, which, comparatively, is somewhat more intensely felt with respect to dogs than with respect to human members of the family." An interesting point, this—that while the children of the house may be subject to the slow nutritional rot of Cokes and other soft drinks and TV dinners, the dog of the house is the subject of the grownups' concern over healthy eating habits. The report goes on, "Some dog owners seem to create a state of dependency of their dogs 'good will' in their projection of personal feelings to a dog." It concludes:

> In effect, such owners condition a dog to be "a fussy eater," which in turn reinforces a belief that their dog is special, unusually discerning, and, in a general sense, superior.

... The 1971 marketing plan for Allen Products had already defined the Alpo target as people with incomes in excess of ten thousand dollars, and "primarily female heads of household"— that is, housewives who do the family supermarket shopping chores—"with emphasis upon the 35-49 age group." Pretty much the same group of women were the target of competing high-priced brands of canned dog food, and by the time the Alpo people and their competitors had had a fair whack at them with successive volleys of television commercials, they seemed determined not to skimp on their dogs' rations. In general, these women were estimated in market research to have a strong concern for pets and a pronounced desire—"often generated by guilt feelings," the 1972 Perk document noted—to include their pets as family members and to treat them in a permissive manner. And the Perk document pointed out, "More important for us is that they indulge the dog in terms of his food." The report went on, "The owners' 'ideal' is a dog food that is *very close to human food.* This satisfies the emotional needs of the owner and strengthens her belief that the animal is a family member." . . .

> Looking ahead, as consumer environments change . . . as people love their dogs more, placate and coddle them more and more, spend more money on them, vest their egos in their dogs, there is no reason why additional new product factors cannot be introduced to dog-food buyers.

The document went on to emphasize, "In view of a psychic transformation of dogs to quasi-human status in the home, there may well be further opportunities for developing product qualities and products that are analogous to human foods." Then, perhaps, a little more prosaically, it listed such product possibilities arising from the psychic transformation as "casseroles, meat loaf, chicken and dumplings, hot dogs, hash, and snacks." Farther along, it picked up the tone of things by adding to the canine-menu possibilities "canned meat balls *au jus* or canned burgers with bouillon sauce."

While the great meat war was being fought with television campaigns and in the supermarkets, the manufacturers of semi-moist and dry varieties of pet foods were, of course, increasingly active. They, too, were attempting to outdo one another in emphasizing the delectability of their offerings, sometimes to the point of causing them to rival, if not overshadow, in attractiveness the appearance of mere human rations. . . .Pet-food companies putting out brands of dog food stress, in glowing ads, the meaty hue of their products. It seems to matter little that this highly expensive effort is lost on the pets eating the food, since research shows that dogs are pretty much color blind. . . .

I learned in a talk with a Young & Rubicam account executive that the psychographic chart describes a "tremendous emotional range" of attitudes among owners, again with particular attention to women. "We rarely address our pet-food advertising to men," the Young & Rubicam man said. "Our chief prospects are women, since usually they are responsible not only for buying dog food but for the more onerous job of feeding the family dog. When you're selling human-food products, you can divide the mothers who are your prospects into 'suppliers' and 'providers.' Some mothers, the 'suppliers,' tend to feel they're doing their job if they keep the kitchen stocked and let others in the family help themselves. Other mothers *implant* themselves in the kitchen—they have a hand in everything that is put on the table. Pet owners tend to divide in pretty much the same way. Some sit back and wait for the dog to eat when he feels like it, and others are tremendously and utterly involved in what the dog eats and how he eats. You'd need a psychiatrist to explain the various relationships that exist! It's not an overstatement that many women would rather give up their husbands, or even their children, than their dog. The dogs are regarded as child surrogates. I've heard a woman say that when she walks in at night from the supermarket her husband might not even look up from his paper, or the children from the TV set, but the dog *always* acknowledges her coming back home. The way people feel about dogs is translated into buying habits. There's a psychological break between the buyers of dry dog food, who take a functional view of the dog, and the premium-canned-dog-food buyer—the indulgent feeder, the nothing's-too-good, emotionally motivated type. The moist-food user is somewhere in the middle."

The adman went on to speak of "the psychographic makeup of the customer" and her "emotional relationship" to various kinds of pet food. "To be talking in a canned-dog-food commercial about the nutritional makeup of the product would not answer that prospect's real needs," he said. "She wants a product that is going to be a *treat*—her dog is going to love her more if she buys that product." He continued, "Dry dog food—it's irrelevant to talk about dry dog food in emotional, indulgent terms. The owner is just interested in a healthy maintenance diet for the pet. Now, in selling a moist product you're dealing with people who want to give their dogs a palatable treat but find the inconvenience of opening canned dog food troublesome. A moist dog food offers the pet owner the rationalization of *treating* the dog yet at the same time indulging *herself.*"

Consequently, in advertising a moist dog food, the adman said, "the piece of reasoning you have to do is to calm the person's potential feeling of guilt." This potential feeling arises, it seems, from the customer's use of a "convenience" product—in this case, an easily opened and mess-free pouch. "What you have to say in your advertising, in effect, is that even though it's convenient, your dog will never know it," the account executive explained. In the advertising of convenience products (at least when they have been successfully launched in the market), there is a general understanding in the trade that there should be no mention of the actual labor saved. The Young & Rubicam man said, "It's a make-believe world, in which you never actually use the word 'convenience.'" In the case of the customer who will inevitably see commercials for Gaines-burgers, then "you address what is in the woman's mind, which is 'Will my husband get mad at me if I make use of this easy-to-open container instead of a can?'" He went on, "In a perfect world, you could tell that woman about the advantages of the soft-moist product—how simple it is to open up out of the cellophane pouch, how simple it is to throw the pouch away without her hands ever touching the pet food. But you don't. It's absurd, I admit—does the *dog* know whether it's convenient or not? Yet there's that little feeling of guilt to reckon with—that the woman feels she isn't doing the very best thing."

There are other areas, too, in which the admen apparently take care not to roil the psyches of the lady customers. Thus, while in dog-food commercials children are often to be seen playing with a dog ("People who feel compelled to demonstrate affection to a dog think the dog is content if the children are content with the dog—that's why you see them romping together in the commercials," the ad-man said), children are almost never seen in the commercials feeding a dog. "Our research shows that women pet owners resent commercials showing a man or children feeding a dog," the Y. & R. man said. "The women don't mind feeding the dog, but they resent other people being shown as doing the feeding. The attitude is that the man wants the advantages of the pet but not the work. A man might influence the purchase of a dog-food brand, but his decision is less important than the woman's." So in dog-food commercials it's nearly always the woman who is the ministering angel. In the world of pet-food merchandising, such perceptions of the susceptibilities of the women in the audience range far and wide, and provide a lot of work for the motivational researchers. A 1971 *Fortune* article on the economics of the pet-food industry quoted a market-research study of the Ralston Purina Chuck Wagon commercials (featuring a toy chuck wagon that scoots across the kitchen floor and disappears into a cabinet door under the sink) as analyzing audience reaction this way:

Wagons and cabinets are, symbolically, womblike enclosures. The perceived episode of a galloping horse under the woman's kitchen sink, getting into her cabinet, followed by the little dog that wants to be fed is a symbolic tale of impregnation. And for some homemakers the watching of this commercial is a means of recapturing unconscious fantasies about "having" a dog, or about "being" a baby dog that is always fed and happy.

On the other hand, a section of one research report for Liggett & Myers-Perk Foods dealing with the attitudes of owners toward dogs and their perception of their pets as family members notes, "There are indications that some... owners feel somewhat guilty about the fact that they did not really want a dog in the first place." It is obviously all very complicated.

Besides introducing realistic chromatic effects into their products, the pet-food companies have, of course, been going all out to emphasize the products' supremely tasty nature. People in the business claim that, in general, the tastier the pet food is supposed to be, the higher it is priced. However, the tastiness involved is heavily influenced by what owners consider tasty. . . .

Actually, there appears to be some question as to how well dogs, for example, can distinguish between the flavors of the many different animal parts contained in commercial dog food. Basically, it's just nourishment to them, and they can get by equally well on a total vegetable-cereal diet, although some animal amino acids are desirable as part of such a diet. However, if the owners of dogs can persuade themselves, or be persuaded, that one particular kind of prepared food or combination of ingredients is better for their pets than another, the dog's eating habits can become somewhat fixed on that particular food, much as the tastes of many children—with the help of incessant advertising campaigns for candies, prepared breakfast cereals, and soft drinks—can be fixed long into their adult life on foods containing large amounts of sugar. To the basic stuff of dry pet food the manufacturers add a spraying of fat and "palatability enhancers," as they are called, consisting of traces of such things as garlic and cheese—the very stuff of which fussy eaters can be made. The result has been a gourmet-pet-food race by the big companies in the business, with innumerable new gastronomic offerings being hawked, and "improved" versions being launched on the market. A commercial for a new Recipe product shows a dog sitting up and looking longingly at a cheeseburger sizzling away on an outdoor grill while an announcer explains, "If he sits up and says 'Please' for burgers and cheese, he's gonna love . . . new Recipe-brand Burger Dinner with cheese-flavored chunks." A commercial for

Gravy Train shows two dogs and a former problem: One ate Gravy Train, the other "something else." But the problem is no more—both pets are now on Gravy Train, because "Gravy Train made their gravy better tasting . . . beefy tasting, rich, thick, and so much darker than before." Gaines-burgers scrambled the situation further with the introduction of "new Gaines-burgers with real egg." A Gaines-burger TV commercial describes the egg as "one of nature's wonders," and promises, in addition to "the moist meaty taste dogs love," no less than "a quarter of a real egg in every burger." And commercials for Ken-L Ration Burger 'n Egg have escalated the egg race with "half an egg in every pouch. Three eggs in every six-pack." With menus like this being flung incessantly onto the home screens, is it any great wonder that some poor people who become hungry enough might succumb to eating pet food? . . .

However [the purchaser] may be viewing the great variety of choices and flavors of pet foods on the long stretches of shelves in the supermarkets, and however vast the trouble and money involved in replacing table scraps with gourmet offerings, the manufacturers see, above all, a highly profitable market that is advancing beyond its initial boom stage and is now in a stage of relative consolidation. At such a stage, the big gains to be exploited lie in the proliferation of brands and the seizure of particular shares of the existing market. Thus, all the delicious gravies and gourmet meals. A pet-food-company executive I spoke with not long ago remarked of the gourmet warfare currently being waged, "It's very much like the detergent business at the stage of competition where they had to come in with all the blue dots and the green dots."

Excerpted with permission from *The New Yorker*, 52:51-4+ (1 November 1976). Copyright 1976 by The New Yorker Magazine, Inc.

Pet Food Sales Up 8.4%; Growth Should Continue

JOHN C. MAXWELL JR.

The pet food industry put in a strong 8.4% gain in 1976.

This is one of the major growth areas of the food industry and trends indicate that there will be little let-up in the future. The pet population continues to grow at a faster rate than the general population. Pets serve not only as a child substitute, but also as protection as in the case of dogs.

Research indicates little reason to expect a change in this basic life style and, therefore, no change in the growth of this product group.

Ralston continues to be the real winner with a market share of 31.6%, up 0.8% in share from 1975. Carnation also shows good growth, with 11.5% of the market, an 0.4% increase in share from 1975 levels.

Pet food market shares

Annual retail sales ($ millions)

Product	Company	1975	1976	% change 1975-76
CANNED DOG FOOD				
Alpo	Liggett Group	$142.0	$145.0	+ 2.1
Ken-L Ration	Quaker Oats	90.0	90.0	—
Kal Kan	Mars Inc.	80.0	82.0	+ 2.5
Mighty Dog	Carnation	45.0	48.0	+ 6.6
Friskies	Carnation	26.5	46.0	+73.8
Recipe	Campbell	26.0	31.0	+19.2
Cycle	General Foods	—	24.0	—
Vets	Liggett Group	22.0	22.5	+ 2.3
Blue Mountain	Associated Products	20.0	21.0	+ 5.0
Skippy, Premium	National Can	16.7	20.7	+24.0
Skippy, Dr. Ross	National Can	19.0	19.0	—
Cadillac	U. S. Tobacco	18.0	19.0	+ 5.5
Rival	Associated Products	20.0	17.0	−15.0
Strongheart	Strongheart	14.0	15.6	+11.4
Twin Pet	Allied Food	6.0	6.0	—
Calo[1]	Borden	3.0	3.2	+ 6.6
Laddie Boy	National Can	3.5	3.0	−14.3
Hills	Riviana Foods	3.8	2.8	−26.3
Ideal[2]	Allied Food	2.7	2.5	− 7.4
Red Heart	Allied Food*	2.5	2.5	—
Dash	Armour	1.3	**	—
Henny Pen	Allied Food	1.1	1.1	—
Jobo	Allied Food	1.1	1.1	—
All others		77.8	57.0	−26.7
Total		$642.0	$680.0	+ 5.9

Product	Company	1975	1976	% change 1975-76
DRY DOG FOOD				
Dog Chow	Ralston Purina	280.0	302.0	+ 7.9
Chuck Wagon	Ralston Purina	96.0	96.0	—
Puppy Chow	Ralston Purina	76.0	92.0	+21.1
Gravy Train	General Foods	91.0	91.0	—
Friskies Dinner & Cubes	Carnation	60.0	60.0	—
High-Protein Dog Meal	Ralston Purina	47.0	55.0	+17.0
Gaines Meal	General Foods			
Jim Dandy Chunks & Ration	Jim Dandy	24.0	21.0	−12.5
		21.0	16.0	−23.8
Hunt Club Walter Kendall	Standard Brands	17.0	15.0	−11.8
Ken-L Ration Biskit & Meal	Quaker Oats	10.0	13.0	+30.0
Alamo Brand	Liggett Group	4.2	10.4	+147.6
Vets Nuggets	Liggett Group	12.0	10.0	−16.7
Field & Farm	Ralston Purina	—	6.0	—
Strongheart	Strongheart	3.5	4.0	+14.3
Purina Dinner Mix	Ralston Purina	—	3.5	
All others		119.3	135.1	+13.2
Total		$861.0	$930.0	+ 8.0
MOIST DOG FOOD				
Ken-L Ration Burgers	Quaker Oats	96.0	103.0	+ 7.4
Gaines Burgers	General Foods	90.0	85.0	− 5.6
Top Choice	General Foods	46.0	56.0	+21.7
Ken-L Ration Special Cuts	Quaker Oats	27.0	30.0	+11.1
Gaines Prime Variety	General Foods	16.0	16.0	—
Gaines Prime	General Foods	10.0	12.0	+20.0
All others		5.0	3.0	−40.0
Total		$290.0	$305.0	+ 5.2
WHOLE BISCUIT SNACK DOG FOOD				
Milk-Bone, Flavor Snacks	Nabisco	46.0	49.0	+ 6.5
Liv-A-Snaps, Beef-Snaps, Char-O-Snaps, Chik-N-Snaps	Liggett Group	5.5	6.0	+ 9.1
Say Cheese, People Crackers and Doggie Donuts	R. T. French's	5.0	5.0	—
Ken-L Ration Treats	Quaker Oats	3.5	4.7	+34.3
Gaines Biscuits & Bits	General Foods	3.0	2.5	−16.7
All others		16.5	17.8	+ 7.9
Total		$ 79.5	$ 85.0	+ 6.9

DRY CAT FOOD

Cat Chow	Ralston Purina ...	98.0	98.0	—
Friskies	Carnation	71.0	75.0	+ 5.6
Meow Mix	Ralston Purina ...	32.0	47.0	+46.9
Special Dinners ...	Ralston Purina ...	28.0	29.0	+ 3.6
Kitten Chow	Ralston Purina ...	1.0	5.0	+400.0
All others		10.5	16.0	+52.4
Total		$240.5	$270.0	+12.3

CANNED CAT FOOD

9 Lives	Heinz	90.0	113.0	+25.6
Friskies	Carnation	93.0	103.0	+10.8
Purina Variety Menu	Ralston Purina ...	50.0	50.0	—
Puss 'n Boots	Quaker Oats	40.0	38.0	− 5.0
Lovin' Spoonfuls ..	Ralston Purina ...	40.0	37.0	+ 7.5
Kal Kan	Mars Inc.	25.5	34.0	+33.3
Tabby	Lipton	23.0	23.0	—
Calo	Borden	4.5	3.4	−24.4
All others		100.0	98.6	− 1.4
Total		$466.0	$500.0	+ 7.3

MOIST CAT FOOD

Tender Vittles	Ralston Purina ...	67.0	77.0	+14.9
Whisker Lickins ...	Ralston Purina ...	2.0	18.0	+800.0
9 Lives Square Meal	Heinz	4.0	16.0	+300.0
Moist Meals	Quaker Oats	12.0	13.3	+10.8
Choice Morsels ...	Ralston Purina ...	6.0	—[3]	—
Tabby	Lipton	1.5	—[3]	—
All others		2.0	2.7	+35.0
Total		$ 94.5	$127.0	+34.4

*Through 1972 Red Heart marketed by John Morrell & Co. **Discontinued operations at end of 1976, amount sold in 1976 not meaningful. [1]Closed West Coast operation in 1975. [2]Ideal was bought by Allied Foods (Atlanta) on Feb. 1, 1976, from Wilson Co. [3]Discontinued.

Pet food sales
by type of product (estimated)
Annual retail sales ($ millions)

Type of pet food	1975	1976	% change 1975-76
Canned dog food	$ 642.0	$ 680.0	+ 5.9
Dry dog food	861.0	930.0	+ 8.0
Moist dog food	290.0	305.0	+ 5.2
Whole biscuit, snack dog food	79.5	85.0	+ 6.9
Total dog food	$1,872.5	$2,000.0	+ 6.8
Canned cat food	$ 466.0	$ 500.0	+ 7.3
Dry cat food	240.5	270.0	+12.3
Moist cat food	94.5	127.0	+34.4
Total cat food	$ 801.0	$ 897.0	+12.0
Total dog & cat food	$2,673.5	$2,897.0	+ 8.4

Source: Maxwell Associates. Earlier years' figures revised.

Reprinted with permission from *Advertising Age*, 48(7):44 (25 April 1977). Copyright 1977 by Crain Communications Inc.

When the Excuses Have to Stop

ERSKINE CHILDERS

In this article from *InterMedia,* the Director of the Information Division of the United Nations Development Program gives us a stranger's sudden glance at American television. He sees that our TV sets are selling more than dog food—even when it is only dog food they are advertising.

Learn from me the meaning of hunger and
    thirst.
When a man hungers, the waters guide what he
    eats. . .
And where can the root of what he eats be?
Where but in the world-food, Earth.

The Upanishads

The first really epochal issue of human society to confront broadcasting media since the 1939-1945 global war is at long last being exposed. Earth is in a gathering crisis of resource use-imbalance, and resource-depletion. It will reach everywhere, and affect everyone: it is going to demand adjustments by every segment and every instrument of Earth society. What adjustments will it demand of broadcasting and other organised communication media?

The traditional answer would probably be high-quality international and domestic 'coverage' and indeed this must be part of the response. But Earth's food, development and population crisis will demand very much more of broadcasting—the most potent and rapid technology for interdependence that humankind has yet devised. And here lies the extraordinary paradox: the broadcasting profession, with all its capacity for instantaneous global gathering of information, does not seem fully aware that, far from merely responding by

'coverage,' its concept of its very role in society may be shaken by this crisis.

For most of the broadcasting world, the concept of the role of electronic media in society is a cautiously, carefully timid one, surrounded by advisedly fragmented arguments about the power of the media:

One: Broadcasting acknowledges the power to bring every aspect of the human condition from any part of Earth into the ordinary home through news, analysis, and drama.

But, comes the cautious disclaimer, what the ordinary home *does* with this is not broadcasting's business or concern.

Two: Yet again, broadcasting has the power to teach.

But, comes the rider, this should be done in programmes expressly called Education (school or adult).

Three: Broadcasting has the power to sell products and influence people in their consumption habits.

But this has nothing to do with the programmes between the commercials. The two elements come together quite separately, from two separate sources of responsibility. It is a mere electronic and economic technicality that they converge into the same channel, on the same screen, before the same audiences (and in the same temporal message-stream).

'Politicians' (and social and political scientists), when face to face with broadcasting professionals, know that these careful riders to each proposition of media power are the broadcasters' main defences against political control. And along the lines of Ustinov's ambassadors, the broadcasters know that the politicians know that the broadcasters know, et cetera. In the rich part of Earth, this decorous intellectual and policy gavotte has continued now for many years, with only peripheral difficulties in most countries over things like the effect of TV Violence on Real Violence, or TV Sex, or smoking commercials, or party-political broadcasting time during election campaigns.

Most of the poorer countries originally professed the intention to invest in electronic media for far more explicitly purposive aims—development, education, nation-building. But much of the same pervasive western-libertarian ethos arrived with the shipments of hardware and the first generation of trained broadcasters. Since part of the doctrine has been that 'broadcasting finds its audience and grows accordingly,' and since its most easily found (and receiver-purchasing) audience was urban and middle/upper class, the reach and the idiom of this new instrumentality was until very recently heavily urban and middle/upper class. And since in the western world, broadcasting 'found its audiences' through across-the-board programming (news, entertainment, sports, features, and all) so the contents of training and the programming resources have been spread thin over this whole spectrum in most developing countries.

I remember, vividly, the afternoon in South Asia when even provincial townspeople in many Asian countries were able to see the first moonwalk, live by satellite link. That same day, with colleagues in government development ministries, I was wrestling with problems of communicating basic development innovations like grain protection and nutrition to villagers across distances of a few hundred miles. We knew that we had virtually no hope of using, for these development communication needs, the very same media that were on that day linking provincial towns with the Moon.

That night I stood looking up at that Moon, thinking of the millions of Asian children sleeping in active malnutrition beside parents who were not even aware of it, and of the thousands of rodents quietly gnawing into Asia's grain harvests, while the TV stations played out the last of the evening's locally dubbed Bonanza, FBI Story, and the newly competing Japanese equivalents. The moonwalk transmission was in *that* context something close to an incredible aberration. The western-originated assumptions about what broadcasting had to be used for seemed grotesquely irrelevant and wasteful.

The other evening, arriving in a rich northern country after six more years of largely broadcasting-starved rural development communication work in Asia, I spent an evening before a TV set. In that time-span, I watched a newscast of dead Asian children being unloaded from a truck for burial, and more dying of starvation—followed within minutes by a colourful commercial offering seventeen different tinned meals for rich-country cats. During the prime-time Thrillers and Shows which came next, I was urged to take up valuable options in protein-rich meat; a vitaminised skin cream; and protein-rich shampoo. A comedian made racist fun of a human being from an oil-producing country, prompting much aggressive laughter from the studio audience. I was offered more than 100 per cent of my daily nutrition needs if I consumed a particular brand of breakfast cereal; the next day I counted 38 distinct types of such food at the nearest supermarket (on a quick calculation, by the end of the evening I had been urged to consume in a day about four times more nutrients than my body actually needs).

The viewing continued with a grim documentary on famine and underdevelopment, followed by a panel discussion on whether development aid should be restricted to those nations 'most likely to survive and most worthy of help,' and in which some mentioned India's 'wasteful' sacred cows. This was followed by a commercial for dog foods with the dogs speaking like human beings. A major statesman was interviewed about possible military intervention in oil-producing countries. And my viewing ended for the night with almost frantic persuasion to buy an automobile with a large rebate check.

There are broadly two ways of reacting to this kind of single-evening record of TV experience. One would be to ask 'So what's new?'; and to add that the total evening surely reflected plenty of public-affairs 'coverage' of the gathering global crisis. The other would be to ask *what the total behavioural effect of these message-streams may have been on that rich country's audiences.* And here, of course, is where one enters upon dangerous ground, in the traditional view. Although all of us who have been professional broadcasters know perfectly well that every minute of programmed time does have behavioural effects, and that the progressive sequence of material must also have some combination of behavioural effects, these are not things to dwell upon too long. They provoke rejoiners that 'we're only responsible for our specific time-slot'; or 'we count upon the intelligence of the audience to derive balanced conclusions'; or 'you can't isolate broadcasting's effects from all other information and experience impacts.'

But are these traditional responses good enough, as our tiny space-ship whirls on its way into hunger and its new kind of tension? Again, someone will remark that all such questions about the media are inherently dangerous: 'Look, be very careful, that way lies 1984.' I submit that we have another kind of rendezvous in 1984—with the statistics of resource-imbalance and relative consumption which, on present trends, if not remedied, will produce in that very year a good grains deficit in the southern part of Earth on the order of 60 to 80 million tons. Combine this with the numbing, stop-the-world-I-want-to-get-off effect of 'good coverage' of hunger transmitted in the rich countries, mixed with a continued nightly riot of urgings to overconsumption; and in poorer countries the continued underuse of media for education and development; and one already has the outlines of History's verdict on Earth's media, their policyshapers, and their practitioners, by the end of the century.

The excuses have to stop. Broadcasters must surely review soon the power and the role of their instruments in a world where we know that:

- some 500 million people are, this day, actively malnourished;
- the annual expenditure on pet foods in just one rich country equals UNICEF's entire global budget;
- less than one-tenth of the grains fed to northern beef cattle (unnecessarily in terms of human protein needs) equals this year's global deficit in food-grains.

In a profession where we know that the electronic media, combined in sensitive programming with ground-level change agents (teachers, extensionists, etc.), could greatly accelerate rural development, every day of delay in reordering media-use priorities and communication systems in the southern part of the earth is a day lost towards—precisely—1984.

Media directors in many developing countries have recently become the first to challenge their share of traditional concepts. Large numbers among them now realise that their countries have not been using a potentially immensely powerful instrument where it was most needed in terms of their countries' human priorities.

But one government after another that has become determined to use technical media for programmed, behavioural-social objectives in education and development is now discovering that they are unprepared for the radically different software requirements of such media-use. For the engineers can indeed now provide a signal through a broadcast satellite, for example, in a mere couple of years. But new, especially trained and rurally sensitive software staff (who are not all going to be professional broadcasters, western-style, but selected teachers, extentionists, health educators, etc.) now have to be found to translate that signal capability into education and development innovation-diffusion; and new systems have to be devised linking all this for ground-level utilisation by change agents, who must also be trained and programmed.

In short, an adequate response to the challenge of hunger by broadcasting—with other media—in the lower-income countries may involve a sweeping re-examination of the very structures, locations, and types of programming authority that were set up largely under nominal western models. Some very dramatic options for investment and systems design might be required for many lower-income countries. For example, if once one postulates that electronic media investment should be designed and located on a top-priority basis to support rural development and food production, policy-makers may even decide that television, through a whole first (or new) stage of its growth, should be reserved for rural areas exclusively, leaving radio plus cinemas, etc., to serve the urban minority.

Such a picture may seem absolutely crazy to most broadcasters on first sight. But is this not only because we have all had a standard and notional model in our minds for decades—a model premised on non-purposive, non-social priorities?

A courageous review of the role of broadcasting in the rich countries in face of Earth's interdependence in resource-use would surely have to embrace studies on ways to modify the electronic promotion of unnecessary consumption. For example, a start could be made in extending the present health/medical supervision of the content of relevant commercials to include any content which promotes over-consumption of nutrients. Broadcasters themselves could undertake to provide a critically needed social service in sound nutrition education. This would itself put brakes on the present obvious over-consumption of nutrients in rich countries, much as has already been done as regards education about energy conservation.

Producers of current-affairs programmes dealing with hunger and poverty in the developing countries will undoubtedly need to ponder what Frances Moore Lappé had to say in a recent issue of *Harper's* magazine on 'Fantasies of Famine.' Writing of the visual images of wretchedness that have pounded upon Americans and others she said: 'Again and again our minds conjure up images of overwhelming numbers and unrelenting disaster.

'Journalists convey these images to us because they believe one picture is worth a thousand words. Indeed, by evoking a personal, emotional reaction they do engage us—for to focus on one hungry family in Africa is to tell the story of famine. Or is it?

'The opposite may be true; these photo-images may actually paralyse us into frustrated inaction. It can then require thousands of words to undo the intuitive but false conclusion of hopelessness drawn from a picture and replace it with the complex but real sense of the roots of hunger, a reality that can neither be photographed nor caricatured. How could a photograph capture the global system of production and use that operates to create scarcity?'

In short, openly taking into consideration the likely behavioural effects of programme-content will (with whatever initial shudders) be a prime need. Linked with it will be the need to develop, in broadcasting as in other media, the very highest degree of factually sound and expertly informed knowledge of the real roots of hunger and resource-use imbalance. Earth has never before confronted so immensely complex a set of economic, social, and infrastructural problems as are contained within the two simple words 'interdependence' and 'poverty.' If we are to come through this expanding crisis as one viable Earth Society we will need a standard of journalistic, investigatory, and presentation responsibility in broadcasting that amounts to taking the world through a crash education course in the resource-structures, resource-uses, and needed resource-management balances of our little spaceship.

New perspectives on the social responsibility of broadcasting in the crisis of interdependence should really emerge very easily from the very perspective of the technology. Next only to astronauts, broadcasters ought to be especially able to see our world whole, as one system, one society, one 'world-food—Earth.'

Reprinted with permission from *InterMedia*, journal of the International Institute of Communications, pp. 7-9 (March 1975).

Selling It!

"The mass media tell us continually to satisfy our emotional needs with material products— particularly those involving oral consumption of some kind. Our economy depends upon our willingness to turn to things rather than people for gratification—to symbols rather than our bodies. The gross national product will reach its highest point when a material object can be interpolated between every itch and its scratch."[1]

If consumption is—as the final reading in this volume suggests—as American as apple pie, there can be little doubt that what historian Daniel Boorstein has called "The American rhetoric" of advertising has helped to make it so.[2] There seems to be no end to the things Americans can learn to want; in our two-hundred years of nationhood we have criss-crossed the continent, finding needs to meet the nation's natural abundance, learning to waste when careful use slowed down the wheels of commerce. In that same 200 years, we have gone from expending a modest $200,000 a year to induce ourselves to buy, to an estimated 1976 advertising expenditure of three-and-a-half billion dollars—the price of stimulating prodigies of acquisition and consumption, of creating markets for everything from food, soap, and toothpaste, to toys and travel.

The readings in this section were chosen to raise some questions about the role of advertising in the complex of *food-related* problems we are examining. They were intended to raise those questions by letting advertising people speak for themselves about what it is they are *trying* to do with food, and by letting some of their critics comment about what seem to them to be the actual *effects* of advertising.

The first selection is one of my favorite pieces in the book. In it, the late sociologist Jules Henry, in a language as deliberately hyperbolic as that of the profession he elegantly excoriates, explores the relationship of advertising to American culture. Having identified a number of concepts underlying advertising's "philosophical system"—"pecuniary truth," "pecuniary psychology," "para-poetic hyperbole and the brain box," and "monetization"—he goes on to argue that the effect of advertising is not merely to sell products, but to promote the "most radical conception of *homo sapiens* that has ever been proposed." Because advertisers are interested in the consumer *only* as a consumer, they will use anything to sell, even treasured societal values which are thereby debased.

To a non-advertising person, the candor with which the ad industry discusses the economic benefits of social breakdown is sometimes almost disarming. In July of 1975, an *Advertising Age* front page story on changing markets happily reported the finding of a sociology professor that "the rising divorce rate and subsequent reformation of households probably indicates more of an increase of certain types of expenditures than if marriages were more stable. The experiences of Vietnam and Watergate," the report continued, "have turned idealism and interest in public service into cynicism and selfishness. For marketers, this probably means an increase of materialism among consumers."

---

[1]Philip Slater, *The Pursuit of Loneliness*, p. 83.
[2]*Advertising Age*, 19 April 1976.

Given such a "sales at any cost" philosophy, it was probably inevitable that Henry's discussion of the monetization of values, written in 1965, would in 1978 be outdated in a singularly painful way. J.F.K. fish stew was still "inappropriate" then; ten years later it was possible to find bicentennial toilet seats and Martin Luther King sides of beef.[3] At the same time food marketers were printing smiling faces on breakfast cereals (companionship for the child who eats alone?) and insinuating that squeezing a plastic pudding pouch was emotionally equivalent to hugging a loving friend. (I felt Jules Henry turning in his grave when my dairy—newly merged into a regional conglomerate— delivered my milk in a plastic-coated carton printed "LOVE from Dellwood.") It was this character- istic of advertising which led economist Richard Heilbroner to write that advertising was "...perhaps the most value-destroying activity of a business civilization."[4]

Yet it is sometimes argued that whatever the ultimate *effect* of advertising, its intentions are pure, that its real function is merely to make useful product information available to potential purchasers. It did, unquestionably, begin like that ("We have some fine spices newly arrived from the Indies...") but as historian Boorstein has pointed out in his review of two hundred years of American advertising,[5] "the main role of advertising in American civilization came increasingly to be that of persuading and appealing rather than that of educating and informing. By 1921, for instance, one of the more popular textbooks, Blanchard's *Essentials of Advertising,* began: 'Anything employed to influence people favorably is advertising. The mission of advertising is to persuade men and women to act in a way that will be of advantage to the advertiser.'"

So the issue is not whether advertising is informing or persuading. The issue is: is what is of advantage to the advertiser also of advantage to the advertisee?

In recent years, none among the professional persuaders has been so ardent, so imaginative or so spendthrift as the food advertisers. For where food is concerned, advertising has a special role. As was previously pointed out, in a country where population growth has slowed and activity levels have declined, the total value of food products consumed (and therefore food company growth) ought logically to stabilize or increase only slowly. Advertising has been mobilized to prevent that.

In 1976, the top food advertiser, General Foods Corporation, invested 275 million dollars, over 5 million dollars a week, convincing the American public to buy its products. In one year, between 1975 and 1976, General Mills *increased* its advertising budget by more than thirty-seven-and-a-half million dollars to a total of 131 million. And in the months of February, March and April alone, as the news story in this section reports, it spent an estimated two-million dollars promoting one product, Nature Valley granola bars—thus helping to complete the conversion of what had once been a "health food" cereal into one more highly sugared snack.

Television, especially network television, accounts for the majority of food company advertising, one-billion dollars of it in 1976. Over $150 million of the $275 million General Foods spent on advertising in 1976 was spent on network TV. Moreover, food and beverage advertising is the largest single product category on the tube, so that food advertisers are a powerful force determining network policy and programming. Thus products designed for oral consumption are among those most frequently promoted on our most persuasive and pervasive medium; and little that might seriously offend the producers of those products reaches the same audiences.

This barrage of advertising supports the proliferation of consumable products, which, as we have seen in the last chapter, has transformed the American food supply. Indeed, "...though not

---

[3]It is hard to know where to put "Billy Beer" in this context. Presidents' brothers don't appear, characteristically, to have been held in any special awe. One is tempted to say that Billy Carter knows this, that he is working a kind of double whammy, and that his beer may be successful on that basis alone. Certainly it's difficult to figure out what value might have been debased.

[4]Robert L. Heilbroner, *Business Civilization in Decline,* p. 113 (New York: W.W. Norton & Co., Inc., 1976).

[5]*Advertising Age* (19 April 1976).

generally recognized, the relationship between national advertising and supermarkets is a very close one, and it is unlikely that supermarkets could exist as we know them were it not for national advertising which encourages a high level of consumer demand...In a large supermarket...over 7,000 brands, varieties and sizes of items are available for purchase—of which 1500 (22%) were not there a year ago and 3500 (55%) were not there 10 years ago. The rate of new product influx means that every week...there are some 30 products that were not there the week before while almost as many products that were there a week ago are not there now."[6] Advertising, in short, creates a marketplace demand for food items which come and go with the speed of hula hoops. It promotes these products by any legal means available, to all the potential customers it can find.

Children are, as Henry points out, not exempt from this barrage. "What should businessmen do," he asks ironically, "sit in their offices and dream, while millions of product-ignorant children go uninstructed?" Against such an unthinkable eventuality, television advertising has proved a fabulous defense. For even preschool children, not yet able to comprehend the printed word, can be sold products by the twinkling tube; and what, after all, can better be sold to children than food and toys? Ultimately advertisers and networks together created a special marketplace for toddlers, Saturday and Sunday morning television—a dead-time for late-sleeping adults, an ideal time to hold an audience of early-up tots (who could be sold on "immediate gratification" products they would then pester their parents to buy).

By the end of the 1960's the potential effects of this advertising barrage had begun to generate concern in a number of places, among them the nation's capitol. There, in 1970, Washington consumerist Robert Choate gave some widely publicized testimony regarding the relative nutritional merits of breakfast cereals. Choate pointed out that of the many thousands of commercials a year beamed at children (the average child is variously estimated to see from 20,000 to 25,000 commercials a year), a very high proportion were for breakfast cereals that were both highly sugared and nutritionally poor compared to cereals advertised to adults.[7]

Choate's testimony, my own testimony reprinted here, and perhaps most effective of all, extensive efforts by a Boston-based consumer group called Action for Children's Television (ACT), have produced over the years a number of attempts to "regulate" advertising, especially food advertising, for the benefit of children. To date the only substantial accomplishments have been the elimination of vitamin advertising to children, and a significant reduction—from 16 minutes to 9½—in the total time devoted to commercials during each of the "children's hours."

Other suggestions aimed at making commercials more accurate, more information-packed, and "fairer," or at requiring stations to run messages promoting "good foods," have as yet had little effect—though the regulatory climate in Carter's Washington is encouraging. But as my article attempts to suggest, one difficulty with most efforts at improving the situation is that what is being dealt with is television—and young children. Children are highly susceptible, and below a certain age (which sometimes seems like around 35) people are not very logical thinkers. It is quite possible to give children completely accurate information (about the potential harm, for example, of consuming only highly sugared products) without dissuading them from eating those products. For television is persuasive in many implicit ways, just as food is chosen for other than logical reasons. With a barrage of television commercials, as I suggest in my testimony, you can go far beyond Jules Henry's "legally innocent prevarication" to the kinds of messages conveyed by a succession of ads for sweet products—e.g., that only sweet things taste good.

---

[6]"What Does Advertising Do for the Consumer?" National Business Council for Consumer Affairs Sub-Council on Advertising and Promotion (Washington, D.C.: Supt. of Documents, November, 1972).

[7]Robert B. Choate, "The Seduction of the Innocent," Testimony before the Subcommittee on the Consumer of the Committee on Commerce of the U.S. Senate, 23 July 1970 (Washington: U.S. Government Printing Office, 1970).

In fact, despite all the efforts at reform, the weekend morning landscape continues to look very much the same, as the John Corcorans' description of a morning of kid-vid in 1976 documents. With all those sugary cereals battling for space, not only on supermarket shelves, but in the kiddies' brain boxes, the overall message is still more than the sum of its parts—exposing its young audience to the risk of "audio-visual diabetes." Corcoran approvingly takes note of the emerging pro-nutrition message, but finds it totally outnumbered.

While cereals dominate the child market, a powerful brainbox battle is currently being waged by the fast-food marketers competing to lure the children to McDonalds or Burger King. In fact, as any regular observer of the TV food marketplace can observe, almost all the foods that appear in commercials are "fast." Why is that the case? Why is it that all food on the tube, as Russell Baker points out, "has not been grown" but manufactured?

Because television advertising is expensive, and only products with a high profit margin, products which have been highly processed, can afford to advertise on TV. There is considerably more profit in a Pringle which costs around $2.00 a pound and is immortal, than in a potato which costs a lot less and can rot; therefore it is clear that much more advertising money is available to support the sale of Pringles than to support the sale of potatoes.

The kind of creative thinking which moves products like Pringles off the shelves and into shopping carts is approvingly laid out once a year in a special Food issue of a very readable publication called *Madison Avenue Magazine*. We had originally hoped to include some excerpts here, for it is usually enlightening to those attuned to dismissing advertising as beneath serious consideration to tune into inter-advertiser talk of "positioning." (Is it an "adult" or an "all family" product? A "good tasting" or a "healthy" cereal?) The excerpt lost out, alas, in the permissions arena. Thus you are denied the opportunity to learn first hand that some agency executives now believe nutrition "sells" or to ponder the suggestion from one advertising man that "the natural cereals would be very smart to add vitamins; they would have a much better story to tell."[8]

Yet in an overstuffed United States, pushing non-nutritious foods, or tantalizing the customer into trying one more new product, may be looked on as only mildly anti-social acts. It is more difficult to look with tolerance on the effects of similarly directed advertising campaigns in less affluent societies. Bechtos' articles about international food advertising provide inadvertent confirmation for the selections they bracket. What is the effect of promoting the sale of luxury products to the rich minority in countries where the majority is poor? What is the effect of promoting the sale of non-nutritious food and drink to impoverished peoples whose nutrition will thereby be compromised? The Bechtos article proudly confirms the international effort to "change consumer ways," to break down "old taboos," promoting the sale of refrigerated strudel dough and instant noodles in styrofoam cups.

In the relative affluence of Europe and Japan such campaigns *may* have minimal nutritional implications. Even Pepsi's $2 billion three-month-long "Love" campaign, and Coke's push to displace mineral water and beer in Brazil, may appear relatively harmless. But the Barnet and Müller excerpt suggests that mass media campaigns by international corporations in developing countries may sometimes have much more ominous implications.

Markets, of course, must be found. Population growth in the U.S. has dropped off, and federally-financed food-supplement programs have helped bring "modern" infant formulas even to the poor at taxpayer expense. Ambitious marketers looked abroad, to the fabulous market provided by the exploding populations of the developing countries. Unfortunately, the penetration of those

[8]*Madison Avenue Magazine* (October 1976).

brain boxes, as Barbara Garson's piece on infant formula abuse recounts, has often had tragic consequences.

With Thomas Whiteside's "Din-Din," we appear to be moving from the tragic to the ridiculous. The excerpt was included here to remind us that in a rich country food consumption can *always* be made to increase, even in a society saturated with calories (and non-caloric products); when the child population declines, there are always animals to whom we can feed our surplusses.

The energy, creative talent and concern devoted to selling pet food—the charting of the psychographics of the pet owner—achieve a kind of stunning obscenity when they are viewed against the reality of the hungry world. Author/scientist C.P. Snow long ago warned us we risked having to watch the world starve on color TV; but he failed to warn us that the spectacle would be interrupted by pet food commercials.

"Din-Din" sets off the final selection, Erskine Childers' powerful "When the Excuses Have to Stop." Like Jules Henry, who began the chapter, Childers argues that these insistent messages are doing more than selling, they are changing our perception of the world, and are effectively obscuring the real food problem. Childers reminds us, quite appropriately, that we are in a worldwide crisis of resources, thus leading us back to where we began—and into the topic which will make up the remainder of this volume—the ecological cost of our food supply. One aspect of this cost, energy, will be addressed in the following chapter.

CHAPTER 5

Energy and Food – The Inter-Locking Crises

ENVIRONMENT NEWS

No. 9-1973

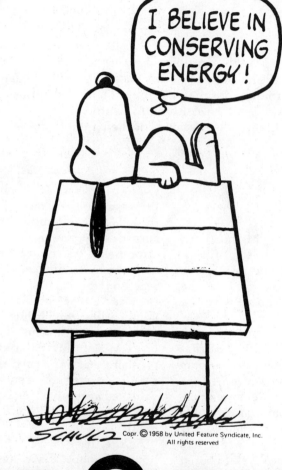

savenergy

U.S. ENVIRONMENTAL PROTECTION AGENCY

Note the fallacy in the government's own energy-saving pitch. The energy we need to save *is not our own.* Snoopy should be pushing a lawnmower, not relaxing!

Reprinted with premission from United Features Syndicate. Copyright 1958.

What Magic Wand?

T.M. BLAKE

"What Magic Wand?" provides us with an opening view of the energy crisis from the standpoint of what would once have been called a yeoman. T.M. Blake is an independent English farmer, for whom writing is clearly something more than a hobby. The *Soil Association*, the journal in which Blake's essay first appeared, is a kind of British equivalent of *Organic Gardening and Farming*; B.F. Schumacher of *Small is Beautiful* fame was president of the parent Soil Association until his death.

An Elemental Budget

1. A condition for survival.

The dark evenings of mid-winter in northern latitudes conjure up visions of fireside stories, ideas of fantasy and magic. Some mysterious domains have, in the past, belonged to the imagination. Today they are exposed with the brilliance of the fabulous picture-box. The Tele' transports us, like the magic carpet of the fairy-tale to exotic corners of the globe. Except that now a piece of magic called voltage has become much reduced. It is being starved of *energy*. Electric fires have been damped. Room temperatures fall from a comfortable warmth to a miserable chill. The image on the magic box shudders, vibrates and ripples as if a rock had dropped onto the surface of the crystal pool at which we gaze. So, almost before this story starts the pioneers of Western civilisation are faced with the idea that some magic elements of their Utopian technology are no longer magical. They are suddenly scarce: and the so capable vanguards of affluence may start to scramble for them.

This story is about the mushroom era. The era of runaway growth. The era during which mankind has so explosively increased his numbers, and during which a pioneering minority has lavishly increased its material standards of living. The era amounts to something less than two centuries. On the scale of the evolutionary time-span it is a mere few minutes. During those last 'few minutes' the human species has surged past equilibrium with its natural environment: an environment which comprises only the living and renewable resources of the seas and the earth's surface. In the past, for each and every species, population surges beyond natural equilibrium have been followed by a relentless consequence which has been decline or extinction. Indeed students of fossil history proclaim that more species have become extinct than have ever survived: and that some species vanished abruptly after a sudden surge of numbers beyond equilibrium with their environment.

Before these last 'few minutes' (or 'couple of hours' perhaps, if we count in the early Mediterranean civilisations), mankind grew in tune with Natural Order. Stemming from other sorts of life which appeared among the drifting chemicals of the primordial seas: building strange cells and molecules by primitive fermentations in an atmosphere without oxygen. Those first life-forms carried with them no prospect of continuity because the *energy* they needed for *growth* was borrowed from *non-renewable resources* which they depleted as they grew. So that any rapid self-propagated growth of that sort would, sooner or later, have used up its *capital assets* and destroyed the *condition* for its *survival*. Thus from the earliest moments of evolution primitive life-forms faced the same limiting factors which now face mankind. And since mankind has developed words for communication, the essence of that threat to first-life is perfectly portrayed with scientific accuracy by the same words and phrases that circumscribe our present dilemma: *capital, growth, energy, non-renewable assets* and many others.

But there is an important difference. When viewing evolutionary history we understand the intrinsic elemental *budget* of energy, substance and growth. We can illustrate it in the precise language of the Natural Laws which we have recently come to understand: with their undeviating rule-books which govern all the exchanges of substance and energy by which we live. Whereas in our present dilemma all those *capital* and *budgetry* terms are shrouded with the parasitical confusions of modern economics, they have become festooned with the verbiage of currencies and arbitrary monetary systems. We seem to have lost the ability to see the budget in elemental perspective. So, to help maintain that, all those words and phrases will, for now and in this story, retain their *capital* emphasis.

2. To render death complete.

Fortunately for us that earlier threat to first-life did not become critical. The pattern changed and the threat faded when the first green plants learned to harness the external *energy* of sunlight: using that energy to compound the carbon of the atmosphere with water. They learned how to split the hydrogen and the oxygen from the maverick molecule of water; and to use that hydrogen together with some other earth elements which water carries to build the new carbon/hydrogen and other molecules upon which most of today's living organisms depend. And while playing that trick performed another equally important by freeing the oxygen of the water as oxygen gas to the atmosphere; where some part of it converts to

ozone which has the convenient ability to absorb and screen ultra-violet radiation. That protective ozone shield against solar radiation was built up principally by early generations of green plants performing those magic tricks in wide proliferation. It enabled new life-forms to emerge from the protection of a water-shielded habitat, to evolve more complicated organisms leading to an outburst of plants and animals upon the earth's surface: and setting up with the ozone layer a sort of greenhouse effect which has raised the surface temperature above the level which could be sustained without it.

Thus to understand the conditions which encouraged the emergence of today's life-forms strikes a contemporary note when we consider our present efforts to tap the earth's store of nucleic energy: and while doing that protect ourselves from deadly radiation by enclosing the nucleii within a water-shielded habitat, thus applying in obverse an earlier trick of evolution. Truly there seems to be nothing new under our sun.

To appreciate the marvels of later patterns yet another trick needs to be illustrated. That during the long ages before the higher organisms were gradually evolved, the great proliferation of green plants discarded at the end of their growth vast residues of organic carbon compounds. And in due course, according to their nature and location, those residues became part of the planet's *capital resources: fossil fuels* in the forms of coal, gas, sulphur and oil. All of those *capital assets* were laid down once-for-all and once only. For mankind it was an era of fortunate provision.

But greater magic lay ahead. The pattern changed again. Some of the new life-forms upon the earth's surface developed a dominant role which they hold to this day. Massed microbial populations grew and sustained themselves upon the green plant residues: species upon species decomposing the organic residues, consuming each other, carrying through with decay, and recycling for future growth organic molecules, mineral elements, water and carbon-dioxide which had already served to grow and sustain previous generations of green plants. And while performing that function of returning dust to dust and rendering death complete, establishing also bit-by-bit a self-perpetuating life-cycle of growth and decay tuned to the rhythms of astronomical time-keeping: night and day, summer and winter. And because no beautiful consequence should be left unsung, building up in the process what man names the fertility of that thin smear upon the crust of the earth: the living topsoils which he has learned to use and abuse with his agriculture, industry and urbanisation. That superb pattern of the renewable life-cycle carried the higher organisms and mankind comfortably along until a 'few minutes' ago. Now it has become apparent that our species has soared past its equilibrium within that pattern. Some rethinking is necessary.

3. The Human Brain burns by the power of the Leaf.

Man has become unique upon the earth in developing an organic resource which progressively improves its capability and is also renewable. That resource, man's intellect, seems to hold the key which could forestall the inevitable consequences which have overtaken other species. The human brain has acquired the most advanced potential of any organic system that stemmed from the oxygenated atmosphere created by the green plants. Man is at this moment coming to understand in a general way that all living organisms, including himself, depend on many others for food and a tolerable environment. He is beginning to understand also that only the green plant has the magic to transduce external energy from space and convert it to chemical energy and substance which directly or indirectly he may put between his teeth to sustain himself. There is no other known transducer capable, like the green plant, of converting *energy* from space into biological *energy*. That provides the ultimate illustration of man's dependence upon his environment. The intellect boggles at the multitude and the scales of

the inter-dependencies from the infinitely large to the infinitely small. Indeed within each living organism and within each of its microscopic living cells, there exists system upon system: each to its own scale and each as complex as the outside environment. Thus the stream of blood cells carries more oxygen to the brain than to any other part of the body. And so the great nervous output of the brain which requires to burn all that oxygen to perform its function has become the unique specialisation which may save mankind from the consequences of unrestrained proliferation. Who could express that more perfectly than the American scientist and poet, Loren Eiseley? 'The human brain, so frail, so perishable, so full of inexhaustible dreams and hungers, burns by the power of the leaf.'

Perhaps *restraint* is a word that should also carry *capital* emphasis. Our present dilemma has to be seen in elemental perspective. There has to be a simple proposition which many people can understand. If that is possible to express in a sentence or two, it may be said that, having reached equilibrium with his Natural environment, man dug down through its crust to harvest some *limited resources* of a bygone age: *metals* and *fossil fuels* which were laid down when the planet was forming. By consuming such *capital* the human species has increased its numbers and standards of living far in excess of anything which may be sustained when that *capital* has been expended. Unless that is understood and acted upon by the exercise of *restraint* the runaway *growth* of homo-sapiens may come to be recorded in history as a temporary phenomenon. It may be said that the species opted for a short but exciting life.

Before the industrial age man learned to husband the fertility of that thin smear of earth, the cropping layer upon which he depends. He has made mistakes and is still making them, but with one or two notable exceptions fertility has been preserved. The industrial era however has been like a honeymoon in a bountiful territory where, as in most honeymoons, carefree expenditure of *capital* has seemed acceptable. Now the honeymoon can be seen to be at an end. So, like most honeymooners, the human species has to face up to living within a *budget*. An *elemental budget*. Unfortunately, as individuals know to their cost, it is difficult to break bad habits. After a century or more of profligate living off *capital* man's mind has become numbed about capital itself.

There is confusion about *capital energy* which is sustaining populations above their Natural equilibrium. There is confusion about energy for machines and work, and energy for people. Old (carbon fuels) and new (nucleic) forms of energy are equated together for the needs of industry and commerce. The needs of people for biological energy may be taken for granted and left out of the equation. That is serious because it illustrates that the dependence of today's intensive agriculture upon large inputs of combustible fuels is scarcely appreciated.

4. Man begins to die at birth.

There is confusion not only about *energy* as *capital*, but also about *entropy* which whittles away that *capital*. That is not surprising. Indeed about *entropy* there is significant confusion among scientists. Entropy, a combination of the two Greek words meaning work/transformation, is about the second law of thermodynamics. It is a universal law of Nature. It is an inescapable process. It is about deterioration and death. About running down. It embraces the inorganic physical world and the living organic world. Just everything is subject to entropy. Like gravity which pulls us down whether we like it or not, entropy makes sure that there is some loss of available energy with every exchange of substance in Nature. That is why the search for perpetual motion and eternal youth has always and will always fail to succeed. We know that a lump of coal contains energy in an organised form. We can burn it for heat or work. When it has burned, the energy is dispersed and run down. It has become dis-

organised and is no longer available. It has become what scientists name bound. Faced with that Natural law which is entropy, life-forms learned to strive against it. Rather than permit their living cells to wear out quickly with work, organisms devised the trick of constantly renewing their cells and living structure by drawing upon external energy for the biochemical changes.

The most important exception in all life to that method of struggling against run-down is that super-specialisation—the brain. If brain cells were constantly being renewed, it is improbable that the intellect of man—as it now is, would have evolved upon the planet. If the myriad brain cells were persistently undergoing replacement, they could not so well accumulate that organising capability which embraces memory, experience, wisdom, strategical planning and communication. In a rational universe surely that chanced-upon discrimination is almost magical. That we have acquired brains which burn oxygen at a rate out of all proportion to the rest of the body: with the result that over five or six decades we are able to build up an intellect with such a fantastic organising ability. So efficient has become that method of nourishing the brain, that the brain cells of a starving man will survive to the last while his body cells fade and run down.

The great lesson however is that everything whether it be the young tree which can split a rock or uproot a pavement, but eventually withers away; or the brain of an Einstein; everything is subject to the second law of thermodynamics. That is how man describes it in his rule-book. But it is Nature's law encompassing all of man's experience and knowledge and what he can only guess at. It fits even man's most recent ideas about the nature of the universe—a universe created by a cosmic explosion in a vacuum; expanding explosively: and later due to return to vacuum with implosive contraction. We ourselves are chemical substance. We need *energy* to sustain us. We depend upon green plants directly or indirectly. We perform exclusively within the laws of Nature. There is no cheating or dodging them. We have to submit to a discipline which gives nothing for nothing; and something only for its exact chemical equivalent, whether the currency of exchange be *energy* or *substance*. That is Nature's law of chemical equivalence. No matter by what method life-forms struggle against the laws of *entropy* and *equivalence*, the fight cannot succeed. An early part of Jain philosophy taught that man begins to die at birth. Seventy years ago T.H. Huxley wrote 'whether fungus or oak, worm or man, the living protoplasm is always dying; and, strange as the paradox may sound, could not live unless it died.'

5. *Decisions do not make resources.*

If we accept inescapable natural laws, we may be able to make better use of them when facing up to elemental budgeting. It is a challenge: and a challenge of that sort is more worthy of our unique intellects than indulging them with dreams of magic performances devised by man to evade the clauses in Nature's rule-book: or indulging them with dreams of magic wands and ideas about man's conquest of Nature as recently expressed by that respected and important man in view of all the world: the U.N. Secretary General, U Thant, who said: 'It is no longer resources that limit decisions. It is the decision that makes the resources. This is the fundamental revolutionary change, perhaps the most revolutionary that man has ever known.' Scientists, engineers, politicians, economists, nutritionists and all too many professionals settle for dreams built upon costs and returns in a financial world: dreams which may not be viable when equated to an elemental budget. Ideas to make dream deserts bloom: to make dream rain-forests of the tropics yield harvests like the soils of temperate latitudes: to win huge dream crops of a ten-fold increase in yield by the practice of large-scale hydroponics: to win untapped dream harvests of the green plant proteins of oceans: to win synthetic proteins from oils and wastes by ingenious schemes of

the laboratory. Those dreams and many like them shatter on the rocks of Equivalence and Entropy; and hydroponics upon the rock of pollution also.

It may be true that certain small and fortunately sited desert areas can be made productive with a regular massive input of *energy* from non-renewable *capital*. It is also true that on the larger scale desert areas cannot be made to produce in any sensible manner. Supposing for example 1,000 square miles of high desert is to grow wheat. In such a climate irrigating water equivalent to at least a 40 ins. rainfall will have to be found, pumped and circulated. That will require 4,000 tons of water for each acre in one year. It may have to come from seawater by distillation. To win 4,000 tons of water separated from its seawater salts demands an *energy* input which is something greater than the *energy* needed to heat 20,000 tons of cast-iron to its white-heat melting point. On a day-to-day basis that is about 50 tons of the *equivalent* for each acre each day: or for 1,000 square miles (each containing 640 acres) more than thirty million tons of white-hot iron-melting *energy equivalent* for each day of the year. All that is for water alone. It does not take into account enormous dressings of gypsum and other base elements needed to bring the surface smear towards a cropping soil: or the cultivations and fertiliser dressings needed to grow crops. And after that input of *capital energy* Calories won for no more than 3 or 4 million people each year in a world where the populations increase nearly ten times that number in the same period. On the contrary: rather than that idea put forward by the Secretary General of the United Nations Organisation, the most revolutionary change of the present century will be the understanding by man that he holds no magic wand. As Robert Ingersoll put it: 'In Nature there are neither rewards nor penalties—there are consequences.'

So, if there is one lesson to be learned from this story, it is that all magic stems from Natural Order, and that no magic which is not subject to Natural Order can stem from the human intellect. The lesson is taken from Nature that Loren Eiseley has so aptly named the Hidden Teacher. The lesson is there always whether it is observed or not. It has been by a number of intellects which have demonstrated the ability to relay it in simple words and stories which have moved people. Those who have understood and accepted the message seem to become naturally inspired with love and respect for the Hidden Teacher: so as positively to co-operate with Her systems and life-forms in every scale of the environment: beyond our own species and in other habitats: with our own species and within our special habitat: with our own living structures and the habitats those provide for their many internal micro-life systems to function. . . .

The lesson is always there. The implications of the lesson are the organisations of the individual intellects. Nothing can alter that. The pattern, design or whatever emerges points the answers to those vexing questions which disturb humanity. So, it is well to remember, that without the intellects there would be no questions. And always the intellects burn by the power of the leaf. Nothing can alter that. . . . If we wish to benefit from the lessons of the Hidden Teacher we have to seek a way towards changing attitudes. Towards conserving and sharing rather than grabbing and spending what is left of the world's resources. And towards the implications that go with it: such as, for many of us, doing with less foods and goods than we have been used to.

I believe one route above others should point the way to understanding. It is education for children of all ages. From primary school to dotage. In work and in leisure, and by all the media. And particularly for those with administrative authority in our complex society. Education about our universe, our planet, the patterns of Natural systems which make up our environment. About resources and food. About how much ENERGY is needed to boil a kettle; to make the kettle; to make a glass bottle to hold milk or a tin to hold food; to make a tractor; to cultivate land, sow crops, harvest and dry them; to process food, market and distribute it, cook it or freeze it. How much ENERGY is needed to raise and distribute water which is the first and most important food for all life: including the massed microbial populations of the soil. How much ENERGY is needed in agriculture to sustain the life-cycle turning over at a rate in excess of the natural capability of crop growth. How much coal is needed to make a ton of nitrogen; or to win a ton of coal from an automated coalface. How much ship's bunker fuel is needed to transport essential phosphates for our soils from Morocco or Florida. How much trawler's bunker fuel is needed to secure and deliver its catch. How vulgar animal and human energy may be sustained. About little calories in the laboratory and for machines; and big Calories to sustain people. How those who do not get enough big C's burn up the tissue protein of their own bodies to obtain them; and what that looks like—in pictures.

The elemental budget should permeate all education. We burn by the power of the leaf; and additionally by the power of any ENERGY we can find to boost the growth of the leaf. That is what matters above all else. It is the ultimate equation.

Reprinted with permission from *The Soil Association*, pp. 1-3 (April 1974).

The Entropy Law and the Economic Problem

NICHOLAS GEORGESCU-ROEGEN

Blake's poetic imagery is intended to seduce the reader into the more demanding prose of Nicholas Georgescu-Roegen, to whom we were introduced in Chapter 1; he here addresses us in person, explaining why conventional economics has failed to foresee our current food-resource, energy crisis—namely that it has cut itself off from the laws of nature.

II

...Some economists have alluded to the fact that man can neither create nor destroy matter or energy—a truth which follows from the principle of conservation of matter-energy, alias the first law of thermodynamics. Yet no one seems to have been struck by the question —so puzzling in the light of this law—"what then does the economic process do?" All that we find in the cardinal literature is an occasional remark that man can produce only utilities, a remark which actually accentuates the puzzle. How is it possible for man to produce something material, given the fact that he cannot produce either matter or energy?

To answer this question, let us consider the economic process as a whole and view it only from the purely physical viewpoint. What we must note first of all is that this process is a partial process which, like all partial processes, is circumscribed by a boundary across which matter and energy are exchanged with the rest of the material universe. The answer to the question of what this *material* process does is simple: it neither produces nor consumes matter-energy; it only absorbs matter-energy and throws it out continuously. This is what pure physics teaches us. However, economics—let us say it high and loud—is not pure physics, not even physics in some other form. We may trust that even the fiercest partisan of the position that natural resources have nothing to do with value will admit in the end that there is a difference between what goes into the economic process and what comes out of it. To be sure, this difference can be only qualitative.

An unorthodox economist—such as myself— would say that what goes into the economic process represents *valuable natural resources* and what is thrown out of it is *valueless waste*. But this qualitative difference is confirmed, albeit in different terms, by a particular (and peculiar) branch of physics known as thermodynamics. From the viewpoint of thermodynamics, matter-energy enters the economic process in a state of *low entropy* and comes out of it in a state of *high entropy*.[1]

---

[1] This distinction together with the fact that no one would exchange some natural resources for waste disposes of Marx's assertion that "no chemist has ever discovered exchange value in a pearl or a diamond." Karl Marx, *Capital*, I, 95.

To explain in detail what entropy means is not a simple task....

Energy exists in two qualitative states—*available* or *free* energy, over which man has almost complete command, and *unavailable* or *bound* energy, which man cannot possible use. The chemical energy contained in a piece of coal is free energy because man can transform it into heat or, if he wants, into mechanical work. But the fantastic amount of heat-energy contained in the waters of the seas, for example, is bound energy. Ships sail on top of this energy, but to do so they need the free energy of some fuel or of the wind.

When a piece of coal is burned, its chemical energy is neither decreased nor increased. But the initial free energy has become so dissipated in the form of heat, smoke and ashes that man can no longer use it. It has been degraded into bound energy. Free energy means energy that displays a differential level, as exemplified most simply by the difference of temperatures between the inside and the outside of a boiler. Bound energy is, on the contrary, chaotically dissipated energy. This difference may be expressed in yet another way. Free energy implies some ordered structure, comparable with that of a store in which all meat is on one counter, vegetables on another, and so on. Bound energy is energy dissipated in disorder, like the same store after being struck by a tornado. This is why entropy is also defined as a measure of disorder. It fits the fact that a copper sheet represents a lower entropy than the copper ore from which it was produced....

III

[Moreover] the elementary fact that heat moves by itself only from the hotter to the colder body acquired a place among the truths recognized by physics. Still more important was the consequent recognition of the additional truth that once the heat of a closed system has diffused itself so that the temperature has become uniform throughout the system, the movement of the heat cannot be reversed without external intervention. The ice cubes in a glass of water, once melted, will not form again by themselves. In general, the free heat-energy of a closed system continuously and irrevocably degrades itself into bound energy. The extension of this property from heat-energy to all other kinds of energy led to the second law of thermodynamics, alias the entropy law. This law states that the entropy (i.e., the amount of bound energy) of a closed system continuously increases or that the order of such a system steadily turns into disorder.

The reference to a closed system is crucial. Let us visualize a closed system, a room with an electric stove and a pail of water that has just been boiled. What the entropy law tells us is, first, that the heat of the boiled water will continuously dissipate into the system. Ultimately, the system will attain thermodynamic equilibrium—a state in which the temperature is uniform throughout (and all energy is bound)....

The law also tells us that once thermodynamic equilibrium is reached, the water will not start boiling by itself.[2] But, as everyone knows, we can make it boil again by turning on the stove. This does not mean, however, that we have defeated the entropy law. If the entropy of the room has been decreased as the result of the temperature differential created by boiling the water, it is only because some low entropy (free energy) was brought into the system from the outside. And if we include the

[2] This position calls for some technical elaboration. The opposition between the entropy law—with its unidirectional qualitative change—and mechanics—where everything can move either forward or backward while remaining self-identical—is accepted without reservation by every physicist and philosopher of science. However, the mechanistic dogma retained (as it still does) its grip on scientific activity even after physics recanted it. The result was that mechanics was soon brought into thermodynamics in the company of randomness. This is the strangest possible company, for randomness is the very antithesis of the deterministic nature of the laws of mechanics. To be sure, the new edifice (known as statistical mechanics) could not include mechanics under its roof and, at the same time, exclude reversibility. So, statistical mechanics must teach that a pail of water may start boiling by itself, a thought which is slipped under the rug by the argument that the miracle has not been observed because of its extremely small probability. This position has fostered the belief in the possibility of converting bound into free energy or, as P.W. Bridgman wittily put it, of bootlegging entropy. For a critique of the logical fallacies of statistical mechanics and the various attempts to patch them, see N. Georgescu-Roegen, *The Entropy Law and the Economic Process*, ch. VI.

electric plant in the system, the entropy of this new system must have decreased, as the entropy law states. This means that the decrease in the entropy of the room has been obtained only at the cost of a greater increase in entropy elsewhere.

Some writers, impressed by the fact that living organisms remain almost unchanged over short periods of time, have set forth the idea that life eludes the entropy law. Now, life may have properties that cannot be accounted for by the natural laws, but the mere thought that it may violate some law of matter (which is an entirely different thing) is sheer nonsense. The truth is that every living organism strives only to maintain its own entropy constant. To the extent to which it achieves this, it does so by sucking low entropy from the environment to compensate for the increase in entropy to which, like every material structure, the organism is continuously subject. But the entropy of the entire system—consisting of the organism and its environment—must increase. Actually, the entropy of a system must increase faster if life is present than if it is absent. The fact that any living organism fights the entropic degradation of its own material structure may be a characteristic property of life, not accountable by material laws, but it does not constitute a violation of these laws.

Practically all organisms live on low entropy in the form found immediately in the environment. Man is the most striking exception: he cooks most of his food and also transforms natural resources into mechanical work or into various objects of utility. Here again, we should not let ourselves be misled. The entropy of copper metal is lower than the entropy of the ore from which it was refined, but this does not mean that man's *economic* activity eludes the entropy law. The refining of the ore causes a more than compensating increase in the entropy of the surroundings. Economists are fond of saying that we cannot get something for nothing. The entropy law teaches us that the rule of biological life and, in man's case, of its economic continuation is far harsher. In entropy terms, the cost of any biological or economic enterprise is always greater than the product. In entropy terms, any such activity necessarily results in a deficit.

IV

The statement made earlier—that, from a purely physical viewpoint, the economic process only transforms valuable natural resources (low entropy) into waste (high entropy)—is thus completely vindicated....

Man's continuous tapping of natural resources is not an activity that makes no history. On the contrary, it is the most important long-run element of mankind's fate. It is because of the irrevocability of the entropic degradation of matter-energy that, for instance, the peoples from the Asian steppes, whose economy was based on sheep-raising, began their Great Migration over the entire European continent at the beginning of the first millennium. The same element—the pressure on natural resources—had, no doubt, a role in other migrations, including that from Europe to the New World. The fantastic efforts made for reaching the moon may also reflect some vaguely felt hope of obtaining access to additional sources of low entropy. It is also because of the particular scarcity of environmental low entropy that ever since the dawn of history man has continuously sought to invent means for sifting low entropy better. In most (though not in all) of man's inventions one can definitely see a progressively better economy of low entropy....

V

Economic thought has always been influenced by the economic issues of the day. It also has reflected—with some lag—the trend of ideas in the natural sciences. A salient illustration of this correlation is the very fact that, when economists began ignoring the natural environment in representing the economic process, the event reflected a turning point in the temper of the entire scholarly world. The unprecedented achievements of the Industrial Revolution so amazed everyone with what man might do with the aid of machines that the general attention became confined to the factory. The landslide of spectacular scientific discoveries triggered by the new technical facilities strengthened this general awe for the power of technology. It also induced the literati to overestimate and, ultimately, to oversell to their audiences the powers of science. Naturally, from such a pedestal one could not even conceive that there is any real obstacle inherent in the human condition.

The sober truth is different. Even the lifespan of the human species represents just a blink when compared with that of a galaxy. So, even with progress in space travel, mankind will remain confined to a speck of space. Man's biological nature sets other limitations as to what he can do. Too high or too low a temperature is incompatible with his existence. And so are many radiations. It is not only that he cannot reach up to the stars, but he cannot even reach down to an individual elementary particle, nay, to an individual atom.

Precisely because man has felt, however unsophisticatedly, that his life depends on scarce, irretrievable low entropy, man has all along nourished the hope that he may eventually discover a self-perpetuating force. The discovery of electricity enticed many to believe that the hope was actually fulfilled. Following the strange marriage of thermodynamics with mechanics, some began seriously thinking about schemes to unbind bound energy. The discovery of atomic energy spread another wave of sanguine hopes that, this time, we have truly gotten hold of a self-perpetuating power. The shortage of electricity which plagues New York and is gradually extending to other cities should suffice to sober us up. Both the nuclear theorists and the operators of atomic plants vouch that it all boils down to a problem of cost, which in the perspective of this paper means a problem of a balance sheet in entropy terms.

With natural scientists preaching that science can do away with all limitations felt by man and with the economists following suit in not relating the analysis of the economic process to the limitations of man's material environment, no wonder that no one realized that we cannot produce "better and bigger" refrigerators, automobiles, or jet planes, without producing also "better and bigger" waste. So, when everyone (in the countries with "better and bigger" industrial production) was, literally, hit in the face by pollution, scientists as well as economists were taken by surprise. But even now no one seems to see that the cause of all this is that we have failed to acknowledge the entropic nature of the economic process. A convincing proof is that the various authorities on pollution now try to sell us, on the one hand, the idea of machines and chemical reactions that produce no waste, and, on the other, salvation through a perpetual recycling of waste. There is no denial that, in principle at least, we can recycle even the gold dispersed in the sand of the seas just as we can recycle the boiling water in my earlier example. But in both cases we must use an additional amount of low entropy much greater than the decrease in the entropy of what is recycled. There is no free recycling just as there is no wasteless industry....

VI

The free energy to which man can have access comes from two distinct sources. The first source is a *stock*, the stock of free energy of the mineral deposits in the bowels of the earth. The second source is a *flow*, the flow of solar radiation intercepted by the earth. Several differences between these two sources should be well marked. Man has almost complete command over the terrestrial dowry; conceivably, we may use it all within a single year. But, for all practical purposes, man has no control over the flow of solar radiation. Neither can he use the flow of the future *now*. Another asymmetry between the two sources pertains to their specific roles. Only the terrestrial source provides us with the low entropy materials from which we manufacture our most important implements. On the other hand, solar radiation is the primary source of all life on earth, which begins with chlorophyll photosynthesis. Finally, the terrestrial stock is a paltry source in comparison with that of the sun. In all probability, the active life of the sun—during which the earth will receive a flow of solar energy of significant intensity—will last another five billion years. But hard to believe though it may be, the entire terrestrial stock could only yield a few days of sunlight....[3]

What has happened to man's entropic struggle over the last two hundred years is a telling story in this respect. On the one hand, thanks to the spectacular progress of science man has achieved an almost miraculous level of economic development. On the other hand, this development has forced man to push his tapping of terrestrial sources to a staggering degree (witness offshore oil-drilling). It has also sustained a population growth which has accentuated the struggle for food and, in some areas, brought this pressure to critical levels. The solution, advocated unanimously, is an increased mechanization of agriculture. But let us see what this solution means in terms of entropy.

In the first place, by eliminating the traditional partner of the farmer—the draft animal—the mechanization of agriculture allows the entire land area to be allocated to the production of food (and to fodder only to the extent of the need for meat). But the ultimate and the most important result is a shift of the low entropy input from the solar to the terrestrial source. The ox or the water buffalo—which derive their mechanical power from the solar radiation caught by chlorophyll photosynthesis—is replaced by the tractor—which is produced and operated with the aid of terrestrial low entropy. And the same goes for the shift from manure to artificial fertilizers. The upshot is that the mechanization of agriculture is a solution which, though inevitable in the present impasse, is antieconomical in the long run. Man's biological existence is made to depend in the future more and more upon the scarcer of the two sources of low entropy. There is also the risk that mecha-

nized agriculture may trap the human species in a cul-de-sac because of the possibility that some of the biological species involved in the other method of farming will be forced into extinction,...

VII

The upshot is clear. Every time we produce a Cadillac, we irrevocably destroy an amount of low entropy that could otherwise be used for producing a plow or a spade. In other words, every time we produce a Cadillac, we do it at the cost of decreasing the number of human lives in the future. Economic development through industrial abundance may be a blessing for us now and for those who will be able to enjoy it in the near future, but it is definitely against the interest of the human species as a whole, if its interest is to have a lifespan as long as is compatible with its dowry of low entropy. In this paradox of economic development we can see the price man has to pay for the unique privilege of being able to go beyond the biological limits in his struggle for life.

Biologists are fond of repeating that natural selection is a series of fantastic blunders since future conditions are not taken into account. The remark, which implies that man is wiser than nature and should take over her job, proves that man's vanity and the scholar's self-confidence will never know their limits. For the race of economic development that is the hallmark of modern civilization leaves no doubt about man's lack of foresight.... Once man expanded his biological powers by means of industrial artifacts, he became *ipso facto* not only dependent on a very scarce source of life support but also addicted to industrial luxuries. It is as if the human species were determined to have a short but exciting life. Let the less ambitious species have a long but uneventful existence....

---

[3] Four days, according to Eugene Ayres, "Power from the Sun," *Scientific American*, August 1950, p. 16. The situation is not changed even if we admit that the calculations might be in error by as much as one thousand times.

Excerpted with permission from *The Entropy Law and the Economic Problem*, Distinguished Series Lecture No. 1, University of Alabama, 1970. The lecture is reprinted in Dr. Georgescu-Roegen's *Energy and Economic Myths: Institutional and Analytical Economic Essays*, Pergamon Press, 1976.

The End of an Energy Orgy

KENNETH E. F. WATT

Just as Borgstrom reminded us that our present population/food crisis has a history, economist Kenneth Watt in this 1974 article from *Natural History* reminded his readers that the energy crisis of that season (and this) also have a history of several generations during which we have intoxicated ourselves with great gulps of energy. Much of the progress we have happily attributed to our ingenuity, hard work, and all-out superiority turns out to derive from the extraordinary energy-richness of our continent and its waters.

Americans have gobbled up sources of energy for centuries. Now we must learn to diet.

By next month, the United States, particularly the northeast, may be in danger of economic strangulation because of the fuel shortage. How could we be so ill-prepared? The answer is that we are the victims of a defective pattern of thinking that originated in a series of historical accidents in the nineteenth century. The ultimate consequence of this erroneous thinking was inevitable; the Arab export embargo merely hastened the arrival of a crisis that would have arrived by 1979 at the latest.

In the nineteenth century we consumed wood, whale oil, and buffalo at astonishingly high rates. This pattern of resource use had profound implications on our later development. By 1850, 92 percent of our energy came from wood, and Americans were consuming fuel wood at an annual rate equivalent to the burning of 7,091 pounds of coal per person. To put this into perspective, in 1969 the total consumption of energy in all forms; in pounds of coal equivalents, was only 6,993 pounds per capita in Switzerland, and 6,235 in Japan. Thus, by the mid-nineteenth century, and perhaps even earlier, the United States—by cutting down the trees that surrounded its population—had attained a level of energy consumption that two of the most technologically sophisticated nations on earth would not reach until about 120 years later.

Wood did not decline significantly as an important source of fuel until 1880. It was replaced by coal and some oil, which had been used for over two decades. Long before wood ran out, other sources of energy became available. This pattern was repeated three times: coal became important before wood ran out; oil became important before coal ran out; and gas became important before oil ran out.

Two other resources, now almost forgotten, led the United States early in its development to a very high level of resource exploitation. By 1847, we were using 313,000 barrels of whale oil per year, or about 0.014 barrels per person per year. This got the United States into early and heavy use of oil for lubrication and illumination and set the stage for heavy use of crude petroleum shortly thereafter. To indicate the magnitude of forward momentum in oil use, by 1928 the United States consumed 7.62 barrels of crude oil per person, while in the rest of the world, average per capita use in the same year was only 0.19 barrels.

The sperm whaling industry collapsed from

overexploitation in 1881, but by then crude oil in quantity was available to replace whale oil. As in the case of the shift from fuel wood to coal, the United States never got the chance to learn an important lesson: that the conversion from one energy economy to another takes a long time. Historically this country has taken from forty to sixty years to get a new source of energy to the point where it could supply 10 percent of the national energy needs.

We acquired a taste for meat early. By 1872 we were killing seven million buffalo a year. A meat-eating society requires more land per capita to produce food than a largely plant-eating society. This is because of the lower efficiency in solar energy use, which must pass through one extra trophic level in the food pyramid, from plants to herbivores, before it reaches man. A superabundance of buffalo, combined with a greater availability of space per capita relative to other countries, taught us to ignore land or food as critical limiting resources. The ultimate result has been that farmland has been cheap compared to the same land converted to urban purposes. Even in the last few decades the value of land used for farming has declined relative to the value of that same land used for urban purposes. The consequence has been a trend toward incredibly sprawling cities with no real urban center. Only in Canada and Australia have similar cities developed, and in those countries, too, the temporary superabundance of farmland has deceived the population into thinking it did not matter if cities grew by spreading out, rather than up. In countries where farmland is at a premium, the typical city building is seven or more stories. Indeed, in many old European cities, it is difficult to find a building less than seven stories high, and new buildings on the outskirts of cities are often ten to thirteen stories high.

Unconsciously, we learned several lessons from our experiences with resources in the last century; unfortunately, they were incorrect, the result of temporary situations in which we managed to get by because of extraordinary luck. One conclusion we reached was that resources are limitless, so there is no need to conserve them. This produced an economy characterized by low unit costs for resources relative to the cost of labor. Since there is no historical precedent for high resource prices, politicians today hesitate to permit prices to increase sharply in the interests of conservation. We were also taught that it doesn't matter if anything runs out, because there is always a substitute. This is one basis for the widespread and unshakable belief that atomic energy will arrive in the nick of time. Also important, because there was always a substitute ready in time, we have come to ignore the great importance of time itself as a critical limiting resource. Thus, we are unaware of the enormous time required to get new technologies working.

Our experiences in the nineteenth century led us as a nation to acquire excessive faith in "Yankee ingenuity." Because of our superabundance of resources, our ingenuity never encountered an insoluble problem. Thus, we overemphasize what we can accomplish, and naively believe that nuclear energy, solar energy, wind, or gravitational fields will produce another miracle for us....

We have deluded ourselves because of a set of historical accidents that were never perceived as unusual. Now we must quickly unlearn some erroneous lessons so that a future sequence of incidents such as the one that led to the Arab oil embargo will not catch us by surprise....

The time has come, in a sense, for America to grow up. For some two centuries we have lived luxuriously off the energy-rich land, like a spoiled child off wealthy parents. Now, crises are forcing us into a period of maturity, to an awareness of the consequences of high energy consumption. The development of this maturity could bring a style and richness of life that Americans have never known. But it will take all our Yankee ingenuity—and more—to reach such a golden age.

Excerpted with permission from *Natural History* magazine, 83: 16-18+ (February 1974). Copyright 1974 by The American Museum of Natural History.

The Energy Crisis: A Biological Vantage Point

BERND HEINRICH

Economists, like physicists and planners, tend to leave biology out of account. Here, an entomology professor suggests some of what we might have to fear should our Yankee ingenuity bring us unhumbled to the end of the petroleum era. Heinrich's article appeared first on the Op Ed page of the *New York Times* in November of 1973.

Berkeley, Calif.—One of the central themes in biology is the flow of energy through the ecosystem. Given the amount of this energy available to a species and data on birth and death rates, ecologists are able to make fairly accurate predictions of the species' population dynamics. As far as we know man is no exception.

As a population of squirrels which is outstripping its food resources and is forced to chew through tougher nuts in order to maintain itself, we are now similarly preoccupied with technology to obtain more energy. The squirrels can presumably not see beyond the immediate task. However, in order to avoid falling helplessly into the same cycles as the squirrels, we must examine the biological contexts of our actions even before we crack our "nut."

The energy used by living things on earth is derived from the thermonuclear fusion reactions occurring in the interior of the sun. Without this input of energy, life on earth would cease. Yet only a minute quantity of the sun's energy striking the earth is actually available to living things.

The energy from the sun that makes the clover grow, the horse run, and that powers our cars, is directly or indirectly due to photosynthesis, the chemical process revolving about one molecule—chlorophyll. The energy captured by the plants is passed on to the hervibores and then to the carnivores feeding on the herbivores. The lower end of this "food-chain" contains the largest total amounts of energy. The "bio-mass" with its available energy decreases further up the food chain. Depending on the size of the animals and their position in the food-chain, their numbers are limited accordingly.

Each species can multiply only until it reaches the "carrying capacity" of its environment—that is, until its food becomes a limiting factor for further growth and reproduction. An acre of woodland can only contain a limited number of rabbits. It cannot support a meat-eating wolf unless he also gets rabbits from elsewhere.

It has historically been similar with man. We are at the point where we must get our "rabbits" from elsewhere. Directly or indirectly, the availability of food and the organization of our society are related to energy. The hunting and gathering societies were operating near the top of the food-chain. They reached the carrying capacity of the environment at low absolute numbers because the energy available to them was extremely limited.

Man later learned to farm. Utilizing the energy near the bottom of the food-chain, where it was being captured from the sun, meant that less was used up by intermediaries and more was available to him. His numbers increased enormously. Next he learned to tap the stored energy of photosynthesis retained in the fossil fuels. This initiated the industrial revolution— and helped to create the population explosion. The concentration of large amounts of energy in one place allowed man for the first time to live outside some of the complex interrelationships with other organisms, at least in the direct sense.

Man presently has available, and is using, more energy than he or any other species has ever had before. Yet, we think we have not enough and we are clamoring for more, claiming that we are in an "energy crisis."

Man has faced limitations in the availability of energy many times before. In fact, it used to be a way of life, changed only temporarily when new supplies of energy were made available through new technology. He then had a temporary reprieve, until the population again increased. We now have increased to such numbers that, even by operating at the lower end of the food-chain and utilizing fossil fuels, energy is becoming a limiting factor to our comforts and to the carrying capacity of our environment.

The crisis is now real indeed, for our fossil fuels will eventually be depleted, and the large populations that now exist will be left with a small energy base. In order to broaden our energy base we are already bypassing the photosynthetic organisms as our ultimate energy source. We are utilizing hydroelectric and geothermal power. More recently we are harnessing nuclear power by utilizing Uranium 235 in nuclear fission reactors. However, Uranium 235 is relatively scarce and, like fossil fuels, may eventually be exhausted.

The "ultimate solution" to the energy crisis, as envisioned by some politicians, is the development of fusion reactors. Essentially this would involve harnessing the energy of reactions similar to those in the interior of the sun, the stars and the hydrogen bomb. Researchers in plasma physics, such as Dr. Francis F. Chen at U.C.L.A., think that such fusion reactors will be our energy source in the future. The energy produced by atomic fusion would be cheap. It is thought that there would be unlimited fuel for millions of years. Given enough demand for such a product, we cannot dismiss the possibility that the already successful work in many laboratories will eventually be fruitful. The immediate advantages are obvious. But as a biologist I ponder the long-term consequences.

An unlimited supply of energy has never been available to us or to any other species in the history of the earth. Its gradual release over the decades could, in an insidious way, be as devastating as that of the hydrogen bomb. Unlimited energy supplies, harnessed to our already sophisticated and expanding chemical technology, may make it possible to synthetically produce carbohydrates and proteins and bypass even the green plants as our ultimate source of food, or we might choose to build gigantic greenhouses for farms on the Poles.

We could build cities on the deserts, on the mountains and in the seas, on all of the lands that are presently fields and forests. It is possible that we could support a sustained population explosion for several hundred years and continue to multiply after there is "standing room only." The implications, yet unforeseen, are awesome.

The majority of animal species remaining now would certainly speedily vanish no matter how strict our conservation laws. But they would not be missed by the majority any more than the buffalo, the wolf, the prairie dog or the ferret are missed in New York City, or on the plains of Kansas, for that matter. Man is a cultural animal. The majority of mankind will be city dwellers. One cannot miss that which one does not know. Those who now savor the sights, sounds and smells of the wild creatures in their natural setting will be anachronisms. They will vanish like the American Indian from the plains and the Kalahari Bushman from the African veldt.

If we are cold or starving, we will be less inclined to save a forest or a prairie for visual or recreational pleasures or so that the prairie chicken may dance and the eagle may nest. We will not hesitate to plant corn. Most of us would not relish such options. However decisions made *one at a time* out of economic necessity will ultimately reduce our options to zero and result in irreversible changes. The more energy we harness and utilize without restraint, the more life forms will die out and the more irreversibly the world will be changed for those who will shortly follow us on *their* brief tour on earth.

The *long-term* solution to the "energy crisis" is obviously population control, rather than the deployment of new technology to provide more energy. The short-term solutions which we are so vigorously pursuing at the present time could create problems in the long run. Thinking in terms of decades may be short-sighted.

Assuming we do not want the envisioned scenario of the unlimited use of energy, what can we do to prevent it? For one thing, we could universally grant that the living space of other species must be given them as a right as fellow travelers on this our fragile lonely speck of cosmic dust. Secondly, since every person is a burden on nature's economy, perhaps those who procreate should be taxed heavily—and the proceeds given to those who do not. But such a policy can obviously work only in an educated well-fed society.

It has been said before that if we only react to circumstances we will assuredly become prisoners of them. The time has come to take a long-term look, to assess our options and to act before we are forced to react.

Reprinted with permission from *The New York Times*, Sect. 4: 15 (25 November 1973). Copyright 1973 by The New York Times Company.

Mechanization and the Division of Labor in Agriculture

MICHAEL PERELMAN

The realization that modern agriculture depended heavily on a fossil energy "subsidy" seemed to arise everywhere almost at once. In this relatively early paper, from the *American Journal of Agricultural Economics,* Michael Perelman points out the still startling fact that in energetic terms American agriculture is not efficient at all in comparison to what we have been taught to regard as much more "primitive" agricultural systems.

American agricultural technology is dependent upon an abundance of cheap energy. An energy crisis in the future or even a substantial rise in the price of energy will require that agriculture undergo a drastic reorganization. This paper investigates the nature and degree of agriculture's dependency on cheap energy with the hope that it will lead others to think about what an energy crisis would mean for agriculture.

"Cheap Energy" as a Source of Productivity

Until the harnessing of fossil fuels on the farm, most increases in the productivity of agricultural labor could be explained by increase in capital, labor, and land. With the advent of the tractor on the farm, productivity rose faster than capital [23]. In fact, productivity rose much faster than in industry [4, 6, 15].[1] Much of this increase in productivity can be attributed to increases in purchased farm inputs [19].

As late as 1920, more than 20 million horse-power was provided by horses and mules that had to be fed from the land [11, p. 21]. Not only was land freed by the coming of the tractor, labor was also freed because one man plowing with a tractor could do the work of several men plowing with mules. Replacement of human energy by mechanical power is shown in Table 1.

Another advantage of mechanization is related to the division of labor in agriculture. Earlier economists were not very optimistic about improvements in agricultural productivity since they believed that it depended upon the division of labor and that there was not much scope for improvement in the division of labor in the farm. This point was made twice by Adam Smith [22, pp. 6, 641] and was echoed by John Stuart Mill:

> Agriculture . . . is not susceptible of so great a division of occupations as many branches of manufacturers, because its different operations cannot possibly be simultaneous. One man cannot always be ploughing, another sowing,

---

[1] Farm productivity may now be leveling off. The USDA Index of Agricultural Productivity stood at 83 in 1955. During the next five years it rose to 96 and by 1965 had reached 101. Between 1965 and 1970 it fell to 99 [24, p. 464].

and another reaping. A workman who only practiced one agricultural operation would lie idle eleven months of the year. The same person may perform them all in succession, and have, in most climates, a considerable amount of unoccupied time. [20, pp. 131-132; see also 1]

Alfred Marshall also accepted the difficulty of the industrialization of agriculture which he said "cannot move fast in the direction of the methods of manufacturing" [18, p. 209].

But in fact, agriculture did move quite fast in the direction of manufacturing since the mechanization of agriculture meant that many jobs were transferred from the farm to the factory. For instance, the growing of hay for horses was replaced by the refining of petroleum for tractors. Workers displaced by the new machines migrated to the city where many of them were employed in producing machines and other nonfarm inputs for their comrades who remained on the farm. Between 1919 and the present, U.S. industries have employed almost 2 million man-years per annum in the production of goods and services used in American agriculture [9, p. 13].

Table 1. How mechanical power replaces human power

Year	Tractor Horsepower Millions	Cost of Operating and Maintaining Farm Capital Million Dollars	Man Hours of Farm Work on Crops Millions
1920	5		13,406
1950	93	5,640	6,922
1960	154	8,310	4,590
1969	204	11,500	3,431

Source: [25].

Energy Use in Agriculture

To show what high levels of energy consumption mean for agriculture, Fred Cottrell compared the energy budgets of Japanese and American farming [7]. He found comparable statistics for two rice farms—one in Japan and the other in Arkansas. Each had approximately the same yield per acre. In Japan an acre could be cultivated and harvested with about 90 man-days—equivalent to 90 horsepower hours. On the Arkansas farm, more than 1,000 horsepower hours of energy were used just to power the tractor and truck. Moreover, the nonresidential consumption of electrical energy exceeded 600 hp-hours. Cottrell did not even include the energy required to produce the tractors and equipment. On a national level, U.S. farmers burned about 7 billion gallons of motor fuel according to 1965 statistics [26].

The fertilizer industry consumes enormous amounts of energy. Current technology requires about 10^7 calories for each kilogram of nitrogen fertilizer produced commerically [8, p. 204]. In 1969 United States farms consumed about 7.5 million tons of nitrogen fertilizer which required about 2×10^{15} BTU's, which is equivalent in heat value to more than 1.5 billion gallons of gasoline of about 8 gallons for each American [24, p. 571]. But nitrogen fertilizer makes up only one fifth of our total commercial fertilizer supply [24, p. 570]. A. B. Makhijani [16] estimates that the overall average energy use in the fertilizer industry is a little less than 2×10^7 BTU's per ton of fertilizer. Since the total 1969 fertilizer usage was about 40 million tons, Makhijani's figures represent a total of about 8×10^{14} BTU's or a heat equivalent of more than 30 gallons of gasoline for every American.

Energy costs for the production of farm implements amount to 4 gallons of petroleum for every American, not counting the energy costs of supporting industries [17].

Electricity also contributes greatly to farm production. In 1970 U.S. farms consumed more than 50 trillion BTU's of electrical energy [13]. However, the production of one BTU of electrical energy requires 3.07 BTU's of fuel input [6, p. 8]. Thus farm electrical production actually represents more than 150 trillion BTU's or an equivalent of about 4 gallons of gasoline for every American, not counting the energy used by the supporting industries that supply that industry [17, p. 15].

The energy cost of the food processing sector is also significant. Makhijani estimates that this sector consumes about 10^{15} BTU's or an amount comparable to the consumption of energy by tractors [17, p. 12].

Much of the energy used in the distribution and processing of food should be charged to the organization of agricultural production that has minimized production costs through regional specialization. This specialization requires that food be transported longer distances and also that much food be processed to avoid spoilage in the often circuitous road from farmer to consumer. In 1971 $6 billion was spent for transporting food by rail and inter-city trucks [24, p. 545]. Brown and Pilz estimate that transporting food from farmer to consumer requires an unrealistically low figure of 1 billion gallons by assuming that all products move by rail in fully loaded cars with no empty back hauls.

Even the 1.8 billion gallons of fuel used for heating farm households are an important element of farm efficiency [26]. Previously, "cutting wood absorbed as much if not more time than any single task on the family farm" [12, pp. 37-38].

If efficiency is measured in terms of the conservation of energy, then American agriculture comes out very poorly. Harris [21, p. 262] estimated that Traditional Chinese wet rice agriculture at its best could produce 53.5 BTU's of energy for each BTU of human energy expended in farming it. But this energy came from people who burned rice in their bodies rather than fossil fuel. In the face of an energy crisis, the present system of agriculture could be irrational.

One method of getting a handle on the energy cost of agriculture would be to add the energy cost of operating tractors; the energy cost of producing electricity and farm implements; and the energy cost of the food processing industry. These activities require the

equivalent of about 110 gallons of gasoline for every American, or three times the amount of calories consumed at the table in spite of the energy costs excluded from this calculation.[2] For instance, farmers purchase products containing 360 million pounds of rubber, about 7 percent of total United States rubber production, and 6.5 million tons of steel in the form of trucks, farm machinery, and fences [5, p. 20]. Farms consume about one third as much steel as the automotive industry [5, p. 20].

For each unit of energy the wet rice farmer expends, he can get more than 50 in return; for each unit of fossil fuel energy we expend, farmers get one third in return. On the basis of this crude measure furnished by these two ratios, Chinese wet rice agriculture is more than 150 times as efficient as U.S. agriculture.

Conclusion

Agriculture uses more petroleum than any other single industry [5, p. 20]; yet agriculture is not the only user of energy in our society. In 1970 the United States consumed about 64,000 trillion BTU's of energy. The average American consumes the equivalent of about 2,000 gallons of gasoline per year; for instance, a typical American consumes the energy equivalent of about 10 gallons of gasoline annually just to watch a black and white television set [3, p. 7]. By that standard agriculture's consumption of 100 gallons of gasoline to feed one person does not seem extravagant. Besides, the U.S. uses more than 20 percent of its acreage for exports which feed citizens of other nations, and some of our crops are used for industrial purposes [24, p. 533].

The problem is that agriculture is supposed to be the *energy producing* sector of the economy.[3]

---

[2]The average American consumes about 3,000 kilocalories daily, or an average of 4,280,000 BTU's per annum. This amount contains as much heat as a little less than 34 gallons of gasoline. While some reviewers objected to a comparison between human energy and fossil fuel energy, the fact remains that agriculture appears to be a net energy drain.

[3]Some writers argue that crops have the potential of becoming a major energy source for the economy. Kramer *et al.* points out that corn silage grown as feed costs about $7.30/ton undelivered in 1971 and that the energy stored in this corn is equivalent to that of coal at $12/ton [14]. Of course the cost of corn silage "fuel" could be expected to rise as production increased to the point where the corn harvest could supply a sizeable fraction of our energy needs. Besides, fossil fuels are a much more concentrated form of energy which makes their transport simpler. However, as one writer has pointed out, much of the "decline of (harvested) materials before the onslaught of synthetic products in recent years is due to the enormous amount of scientific and technical research that has been carried out to ensure the fullest utilization of petroleum by-products. No comparable effort has been made for plant products..." [10, p. 51].

Harvested crops capture solar energy and store it as food or some other useful product. Yet the energy captured is small compared to the energy burned in the process. If the world is facing a future with rising energy prices, the highly mechanized technology currently used in the U.S. may be inappropriate.

References

[1] BREWSTER, JOHN M., "The Machine Process in Agriculture and Industry," *J. Farm Econ.* 32:69–81, Feb. 1950.

[2] BROWN, STEPHEN L., AND ULRICH L. PILZ, *U. S. Agriculture: Potential Vulnerabilities*, Stanford, Food Research Institute, Jan. 1969.

[3] BRUNE, W. D., JR., "The Economic Impact of Electric Power Development," paper presented at the National Engineers Week Symposium, Chico State College, Feb. 26, 1972, mimeo.

[4] CHANDLER, CLEVELAND A., "The Relative Contribution of Capital Intensity and Productivity to Changes in Output and Income in the United States Economy, Farm and Non-farm Sectors," *J. Farm Econ.* 44:335–348, May 1962.

[5] U. S. Congress, House of Representatives, Committee on Agriculture, *Food Costs—Farm Prices: A Compilation of Information Relating to Agriculture*, 92nd Cong., 1st sess., July 1, 1971.

[6] COMMONER, BARRY, AND MICHAEL CORR, "Power Consumption and Human Welfare in Industry, Commerce and the Home," to be published in *Electric Power Consumption and Human Welfare, The Social Consequences of the Environmental Effects of Electric Power Use*, eds. Howard Boksenbaum *et al.*, by the American Association for the Advancement of Science, Committee on Environmental Alterations.

[7] COTTRELL, FRED, *Energy and Society*, New York, McGraw-Hill Book Company, Inc., 1955.

[8] DELWICHE, C. C., "Nitrogen and Future Food Requirements," in *Research for the World Food Crisis, A Symposium Presented at the Dallas Meeting of the American Association for the Advancement of Science, December, 1968*, ed. Daniel G. Aldrich, Jr., Publication 92, Washington, D.C., American Association for the Advancement of Science, 1968.

[9] DOVRING, FOLKE, *The Productivity of Labor in Agricultural Production*, Illinois Agr. Exp. Sta. Bull. 726, Sept. 1967.

[10] FORTHOMME, P. A., "Can Rice Replace Petroleum," *Ceres* 1:50–51, Sept.–Oct. 1968.

[11] FOX, AUSTIN, *Demand for Farm Tractors in the United States*, USDA ERS Agr. Econ. Rep. 103, Nov. 1966.

[12] GATES, PAUL W., "Problems in Agricultural History, 1790–1840," *Agr. History* 46:33–58, Jan. 1972.

[13] HIRST, ERIC, National Science Foundation, Environmental Program, Oak Ridge National Laboratory, personal correspondence.

[14] KRAMER, MARC, THOMAS BAKER, AND ROBERT H. WILLIAMS, "Solar Energy," to be published in *Electric Power Consumption and Human Welfare, The Social Consequences of the Environmental Effects of Electric Power Use*, eds. Howard Boksenbaum *et al.*, by the American Association for the Advancement of Science, Committee on Environmental Alterations.

[15] LAVE, L. B., "Empirical Estimates of Technological Change in United States Agriculture," *J. Farm Econ.* 44:941–952, Nov. 1962.

[16] MAKHIJANI, A. B., personal communication.

[17] ——, AND A. J. LICHTENBERG, *An Assessment of Energy and Materials Utilization in the U.S.A.*, Electronics Research Laboratory Memorandum ERL-M310, University of California, Berkeley, Sept. 22, 1971.

[18] MARSHALL, ALFRED, *Principles of Economics*, 8th ed., London, Macmillan and Co., 1936.

[19] MEIBURG, CHARLES O., "Nonfarm Inputs as a Source of Agricultural Productivity," *Food Res. Inst. Studies* 3:297–321, Nov. 1962.

[20] MILL, JOHN STUART, *Principles of Political Economy*, ed. W. J. Ashley, London, Macmillan and Co., 1909.

[21] RAPPAPORT, ROY A., *Pigs for the Ancestors*, New Haven, Yale University Press, 1967, p. 262, referring to Marvin Harris, "Cultural Energy," unpublished.

[22] SMITH, ADAM, *An Inquiry into the Nature and Causes of the Wealth of Nations*, New York, Modern Library Cannan edition, 1937.

[23] TWEETEN, LUTHER G., AND FRED H. TYNER, "Toward an Optimal Rate of Technological Change," *J. Farm Econ.* 46:1075–1084, Dec. 1965.

[24] U. S. Department of Agriculture, *Agricultural Statistics, 1972*, Washington, 1972.

[25] ——, *Changes in Farm Production and Efficiency, A Summary Report, 1970*, Statis. Bull. 233, June 1970.

[26] ——, *Structure of Six Farm Input Industries*, 1968

Reprinted with permission from *American Journal of Agricultural Economics*, 55: 523-526 (August 1973). Copyright 1973 by the American Agricultural Economics Association.

Food Production and the Energy Crisis

DAVID PIMENTEL, L. E. HURD, A. C. BELLOTTI, M. J. FORSTER,
I. N. OKA, O. D. SHOLES, R. J. WHITMAN

"Food Production and the Energy Crisis," by David Pimentel and his associates at Cornell, excerpted here from *Science*, was a landmark in the analysis of the food/energy crisis. Painstakingly sorting out the energy inputs into a single crop, the authors documented the increasing energy intensiveness of U.S. agriculture, and raised questions about the world-wide implications of such a food-producing system in a time of growing shortages.

By 1975 the world population is expected to reach 4 billion humans *(1)*. As it continues to grow, there is increasing concern about ways to prevent wholesale starvation *(2)*. Concurrently, an energy crisis (due to shortages and high prices) is expected as finite reserves of fossil fuels are rapidly depleted *(3, 4)*. The energy crisis is expected to have a significant impact on food production technology in the United States and the "green revolution," because both systems of crop production depend upon large energy inputs.

Both the U.S. type of agriculture and the "green revolution" type of agriculture have been eminently successful in increasing crop yields through improved technology. The ratio of persons not on farms to each farm worker in the United States increased from 10 in 1930 to 48 persons in 1971 *(5, 6)*. This has led to great social change as numbers of unemployed, untrained farm laborers migrated to our cities *(7)*. In addition, the costs to the natural environment have been great, as is reflected in depleted soils, pollution, disruption of natural plant and animal populations, and natural resource shortages. One nonrenewable resource fast being depleted is fossil fuel—the most important element in the impressive yields and quality of agriculture in the United States. Energy is used in mechanized agricultural production for machinery, transport, irrigation, fertilizers, pesticides, and other management tools. Fossil fuel inputs have, in fact, become so integral and indispensable to modern agriculture that the anticipated energy crisis will have a significant impact upon food production in all parts of the world which have adopted or are adopting the Western system.

As agriculturalists, we feel that a careful analysis is needed to measure energy inputs in U.S. and green revolution style crop production techniques. Our approach is to select a single crop, corn (maize), which typifies the energy inputs for crops in general, and to make a detailed analysis of its production energy inputs. With the data on input and output for corn as a model, an examination is then made of

Table 1. Average energy inputs in corn production during different years (all figures per acre).

Inputs	1945	1950	1954	1959	1964	1970
Labor	23	18	17	14	11	9
Machinery (kcal $\times$ 10³)	180	250	300	350	420	420
Gasoline (gallons)	15	17	19	20	21	22
Nitrogen (pounds)	7	15	27	41	58	112
Phosphorus (pounds)	7	10	12	16	18	31
Potassium (pounds)	5	10	18	30	29	60
Seeds for planting (bushels)	0.17	0.20	0.25	0.30	0.33	0.33
Irrigation (kcal $\times$ 10³)	19	23	27	31	34	34
Insecticides (pounds)	0	0.10	0.30	0.70	1.00	1.00
Herbicides (pounds)	0	0.05	0.10	0.25	0.38	1.00
Drying (kcal $\times$ 10³)	10	30	60	100	120	120
Electricity (kcal $\times$ 10³)	32	54	100	140	203	310
Transportation (kcal $\times$ 10³)	20	30	45	60	70	70
Corn yields (bushel)	34	38	41	54	68	81

energy needs for a world food supply that depends on modern energy intensive agriculture....

Corn Production and Energy Inputs

To investigate the relationship of energy inputs to crop production, we selected corn for the following reasons. (i) Corn generally typifies the energy inputs in U.S. crop production for it is intermediate in energy inputs between the extremes of high energy-demand fruit production and low energy-demand tame hay and small grain production. (ii) Corn is one of the leading grain crops in the United States and the world. (iii) More data are available on corn than on other crops....

Corn yield per acre (1 acre = 0.405 hectare) in the United States has increased significantly from 1909 to 1971. During 1909, the corn yield averaged 26 bushels per acre, and during 1971 it averaged 87 bushels per acre. A sharp rise in production per acre started about 1950—a time when many changes, including the planting of hybrid corn, were taking place in corn culture. (17-19). The planting of hybrid corn probably accounts for 20 to 40 percent of the increased corn yields since the 1940's with energy resource inputs accounting for 60 to 80 percent (17, 20, 21). Hybrid corn and energy inputs

toward increased yields overlap because corn plants are often selected for characteristics that make the plant perform well under specific environmental conditions as, for example, with high fertilizer inputs. Without the appropriate genetic background, the corn plant will not respond to the fertilizer inputs and, of course, the corn plant cannot respond if fertilizer is absent.

While corn yields increased about 240 percent from 1945 to 1970, the labor input per acre decreased more than 60 percent (Table 1). Intense mechanization reduced the labor input and, in part, made possible the increased corn yield.

Machinery in agriculture has increased significantly during the past 20 years; the mean rate of horsepower per farm worker has increased from 10 in 1950 to 47 in 1971 (5). ... In our estimates we assumed that tractors and other machinery were used to farm 62 acres and assumed to function for 10 years (Table 1)....

For total U.S. corn production, fuel consumption for all machinery rose from an estimated 15 gallons per acre in 1945 to about 22 gallons per acre in 1970 (Table 1). Indeed, farming uses more petroleum than any other single industry (24).

The use of fertilizer in corn production has been rising steadily since 1945. An estimated 7 pounds (1 pound = 0.4 kilogram) of nitrogen, 7 pounds of phosphorus, and 5 pounds of potassium were applied per acre to the acres fertilized in 1945 (25). By 1970 the application of fertilizers had risen to 112 pounds of nitrogen, 31 pounds of phosphorus, and 60 pounds of potassium per acre (26). The increase in nitrogen alone has been about 16-fold.

Other inputs in corn production include seeds, irrigation, and pesticides (Table 1). The use of pesticides in corn has been increasing rapidly during the past 20 years and this parallels the general increase in pesticide use in the United States (27) (Table 1). About 41 percent of all herbicides and 17 percent of all insecticides used in agriculture are applied to corn (28).

Hybrid corn that is currently harvested has a higher moisture content because the newer varieties have growing seasons which extend further into the fall when drying conditions are poor (19). Moisture content above 13 percent (the maximum suitable for long-term storage) causes spoilage, and a drying process is used to reduce moisture (Table 1).

Agriculture consumed about 2.5 percent of all electricity produced (Table 1). The energy input for transportation is an important feature of modern intensive agriculture (Table 1). Machinery, pesticides, seeds, gasoline, and other supplies must be transported to the farm. Then the corn harvest must be transported to the place of use for animal feed or processing.

To gain an idea of the changes occurring over a period of time in corn production energy inputs, the years 1945, 1950, 1954, 1959, 1964, and 1970 were selected for a detailed analysis (Tables 1 and 2). Exact 5-year intervals were not selected because more complete data were available on these specific years than on others.

In 1970 about 2.9 million kcal was used by farmers to raise an acre of corn (equivalent to 80 gallons of gasoline) (Table 2). From 1945 to 1970, mean corn yields increased from about 34 bushels per acre to 81 bushels per acre (2.4-fold); however, mean energy inputs increased from 0.9 million kcal to 2.9 million kcal (3.1-fold) (Table 2). Hence, the yield in corn calories decreased from 3.7 kcal per one fuel kilocalorie input in 1945 to a yield of about 2.8 kcal from the period of 1954 to 1970, a 24 percent decrease.

The 2.9 million kcal input of fossil fuel represents a small portion of the energy input when compared with the solar energy input. During the growing season, about 2043 million kcal reaches a 1-acre cornfield; about 1.26 percent of this is converted into corn and about 0.4 percent in corn grain (at 100 bushels per acre) itself (29). The 1.26 percent represents

Table 2. Energy inputs (kilocalories) in corn production.

Input	1945	1950	1954	1959	1964	1970
Labor	12,500	9,800	9,300	7,600	6,000	4,900
Machinery	180,000	250,000	300,000	350,000	420,000	420,000
Gasoline	543,400	615,800	688,300	724,500	760,700	797,000
Nitrogen	58,800	126,000	226,800	344,400	487,200	940,800
Phosphorus	10,600	15,200	18,200	24,300	27,400	47,100
Potassium	5,200	10,500	50,400	60,400	68,000	68,000
Seeds for planting	34,000	40,400	18,900	36,500	30,400	63,000
Irrigation	19,000	23,000	27,000	31,000	34,000	34,000
Insecticides	0	1,100	3,300	7,700	11,000	11,000
Herbicides	0	600	1,100	2,800	4,200	11,000
Drying	10,000	30,000	60,000	100,000	120,000	120,000
Electricity	32,000	54,000	100,000	140,000	203,000	310,000
Transportation	20,000	30,000	45,000	60,000	70,000	70,000
Total inputs	925,500	1,206,400	1,548,300	1,889,200	2,241,900	2,896,800
Corn yield (output)	3,427,200	3,830,400	4,132,800	5,443,200	6,854,400	8,164,800
Kcal return/input kcal	3.70	3.18	2.67	2.88	3.06	2.82

about 26.6 million kcal. Hence, when solar energy input is included, man's 2.9-million-kcal fossil fuel input represents about 11 percent of the total energy input in corn production. The important point is that the supply of solar energy is unlimited in time, whereas fossil fuel supply is finite.

The trends in energy inputs and corn yields confirm several agricultural evaluations which conclude that the impressive agricultural production in the United States has been gained through large inputs of fossil energy *(8, 30)....*

World Food Supply

The shortages of food supplies in some nations *(2)* have prompted the United States to develop various international agricultural programs to aid in the "green revolution." Green revolution agricultural technology requires high energy inputs especially in fertilizers, pesticides, and hybrid seeds. Obviously, as energy shortages occur and costs increase, the success of the green revolution will be affected. For this reason, the problems of food production and energy demand on a worldwide basis are briefly examined.

In estimating the fuel energy needs to feed 4 billion humans, modern crop production technology similar to U.S. and green revolution agriculture is assumed. Energy data on U.S. corn will be used since it approximates average inputs and outputs in modern crop production. Our analysis indicated that about 2.9 million kilocalories of energy was used to raise an acre of corn in 1970—the equivalent of 80 gallons (2.5 barrels) of gasoline per acre (Table 2).

An estimated 330 million acres were planted in crops in 1970 (excluding cotton and tobacco) *(6, 51)*. With about 200 million people in the United States, this averages about 1.7 acres per capita; but since about 20 percent of our crops is exported, the estimated acreage is about 1.4 acres per capita. In terms of fuel per person for food, employing modern intensive agriculture, this is the equivalent of 112 gallons of gasoline per person (80 gallons per acre × 1.4 acres per

person = 112 gallons). Using U.S. agricultural technology to feed a world population of 4 billion on an average U.S. diet for 1 year would require the energy equivalent of 488 gallons of fuel.

...If petroleum were the only source of energy and if we used *all* petroleum reserves solely to feed the world population, the 415-billion-barrel reserve would last a mere 29 years [(415 billion barrels/448 billion gallons)/(31.5 gallons per barrel = 29 years)]....

Contrary to popular belief, U.S. food production costs are high *(54)*. Although only 16.6 percent of a person's total disposable mean income of $3595 in the United States was spent for food in 1970 *(5, 23)*, the percentage is small only because U.S. per capita earnings are high. ... The cost for 100 kcal of plant product is $38.

In India...the cost for 1000 plant kcal is about $10. Hence, the cost of producing 1000 plant kcal per day per year in India is significantly less than the $38 costs in the United States. This is in part due to the difference between nations in the plant crops used for food.

Conclusions

The principal raw material of modern U.S. agriculture is fossil fuel, whereas the labor input is relatively small (about 9 hours per crop acre). As agriculture is dependent upon fossil energy, crop production costs will also soar when fuel costs increase two- to fivefold. A return of 2.8 kcal of corn per 1 kcal of fuel input may then be uneconomical.

Green revolution agriculture also uses high energy crop production technology, especially with respect to fertilizers and pesticides. While one may not doubt the sincerity of the U.S. effort to share its agricultural technology so that the rest of the world can live and eat as it does, one must be realistic about the resources available to accomplish this mission. In the United States we are currently using an equivalent of 80 gallons of gasoline to produce an acre of corn. With fuel shortages and high prices to come, we wonder if many developing nations will be able to afford the technology of U.S. agriculture.

... To reduce energy inputs, green revolution and U.S. agriculture might employ such alternatives as rotations and green manures to reduce the high energy demand of chemical fertilizers and pesticides. U.S. agriculture might also reduce energy expenditures by substituting some manpower currently displaced by mech-

anization.

While no one knows for certain what changes will have to be made, we can be sure that when conventional energy resources become scarce and expensive, the impact on agriculture as an industry and a way of life will be significant. This analysis is but a preliminary investigation of a significant agricultural problem that deserves careful attention and greater study before the energy situation becomes more critical.

References and Notes

1. National Academy of Sciences, *Rapid Population Growth*, I–II (Johns Hopkins Press, Baltimore, 1971).
2. President's Science Advisory Committee, *Report of the Panel on the World Food Supply*, I–III (The White House, Washington, D.C., 1967).
3. A. L. Hammond, *Science* 177, 875 (1972).
4. P. H. Abelson, *ibid.* 178, 355 (1972).
5. U.S. Department of Agriculture, *Misc. Publ.* No. 1063 (1972).
6. ———, *Stat. Bull.* No. 233 (1972).
7. T. L. Smith, *International Labour Review* 102, 149 (1970).
8. L. Rocks and R. P. Runyon, *The Energy Crisis* (Crown, New York, 1972), pp. 12 and 131.
9. G. V. Day, *Futures* 4, 331 (1972).
10. M. Slesser, *Report to Program on Policies for Science and Technology in Developing Nations* (Univ. of Strathclyde, Glasgow, 1972).
11. E. Cook, *Sci. Amer.* 225, 135 (1971).
12. J. Darmstadter, P. D. Teitelbaum, J. G. Polach, *Energy in the World Economy* (Johns Hopkins Press, Baltimore, 1971).
13. P. E. Glaser, *Science* 162, 857 (1968).
14. K. L. Robinson, personal communication.
15. Food and Agriculture Organization of the United Nations, *Production Yearbook* 25, 35 (1972).
16. ———, *Monthly Bull. Agr. Econ. Stat.* No. 20 (1971).
17. C. V. Griliches, *Econometrica* 25, 501 (1957).
18. R. W. Allard, *Principles of Plant Breeding* (Wiley, New York, 1960), p. 265.
19. S. R. Aldrich and E. R. Leng, "Modern corn production," *Farm Quarterly* (1966), p. 296 and figure 150.
20. C. Grogan, personal communication.
21. H. L. Everett, personal communication.
22. U.S. Department of Agriculture, *Stat. Bull.* No. 344 (1964).
23. U.S. Department of Commerce, *Survey of Current Business* 52, table 10 (1972).
24. *Committee on Agriculture, House of Representatives* (92nd Congress, 1971), p. 20.
25. U.S. Department of Agriculture, *Changes in Farm Production and Efficiency* (Agricultural Research Service, Washington, D.C., 1954).
26. ———, *Fertilizer Situation* (Economics Research Service, FS-1, 1971).
27. ———, *The Pesticide Review 1970* (Agricultural Stabilization and Conservation Service, Washington, D.C., 1971).
28. ———, *Agricultural Economics Report* No. 179 (Economics Research Service, 1970).
29. E. N. Transeau, *Ohio J. Sci.* 26, 1 (1926).
30. P. Handler, *Biology and the Future of Man* (Oxford Univ. Press, New York, 1970), p. 462; H. T. Odum, *Environment, Power, and Society* (Wiley, New York, 1971), p. 115; R. A. Rappaport, *Sci. Amer.* 225, 117 (1971); G. Borgström, *Hungry Planet* (Macmillan, New York, 1972), p. 513; K. E. F. Watt, *Principles of Environmental Science* (McGraw-Hill, New York, 1973), p. 216.
31. D. Pimentel, H. Mooney, L. Stickel, *Panel Report for Environmental Protection Agency*, in preparation.
32. W. H. Johnson and B. J. Lamp, *Principles, Equipment, and Systems for Corn Harvesting* (Agricultural Consulting Associates, Inc., Wooster, 1966), p. 95.
33. F. B. Morrison, *Feeds and Feeding* (Morrison, Ithaca, N.Y., 1946), pp. 50 and 429.
34. E. J. Benne, C. R. Hoglund, E. D. Longnecker, R. L. Cook, *Mich. Agr. Exp. Sta. Cir. Bull.* No. 231 (1961); R. S. Dyal, *National Symposium on Poultry Industry Waste Management* (Nebraska Center for Continuing Education, Lincoln, 1963); R. C. Loehr and M. Asce, *J. San. Eng. Division* 2 (1969), p. 189; L. W. McEachron, P. J. Zwerman, C. D. Kearl, R. B. Musgrave, *Animal Waste Management* (College of Agriculture, Cornell University, Ithaca, N.Y., 1969), pp. 393–400; T. C. Surbrook, C. C. Sheppard, J. S. Boyd, H. C. Zindel, C. J. Flegal, *Proc. Int. Symp. Livestock Wastes* (American Society of Agricultural Engineers, St. Joseph, Mo., 1971), p. 193.
35. N. B. Andrews, *The Response of Crops and Soils to Fertilizers and Manures* (Mississippi State University, State College, ed. 2, 1954); R. I. Cook, *Soil Management for Conservation and Production* (Wiley, New York, 1962), pp. 46–61; S. L. Tisdale and W. L. Nelson, *Soil Fertility and Fertilizers* (Macmillan, New York, 1966).
36. R. E. Linton, *Cornell Ext. Bull.* No. 1195 (1968).
37. J. R. Miner, *Iowa Agr. Exp. Sta. Spec. Rep.* No. 67 (1971).
38. U.S. Department of Agriculture, *Crop Production* (Crop Report Board, Washington, D.C., 1970).
39. President's Science Advisory Committee, *Report of the Environmental Pollution Panel* (White House, Washington, D.C., 1965), p. 172.
40. C. J. Willard *Ohio Agr. Exp. Sta. Bull.* No. 405 (1927).

41. H. D. Tate and O. S. Bare, *Nebr. Agr. Exp. Sta. Bull.* No. 381 (1946); pp. 1–12; R. E. Hill, E. Hixon, M. H. Muma, *J. Econ. Entomol.* 41, 392 (1948); C. L. Metcalf, W. P. Flint, R. L. Metcalf, *Destructive and Useful Insects* (McGraw-Hill, New York, 1962), p. 510; E. E. Ortman and P. J. Fitzgerald, *Proc. Ann. Hybrid Corn Ind. Res. Conf.* 19, 38 (1964); R. E. Robinson, *Agron. J.* 58, 475 (1966).

42. L. C. Pearson, *Principles of Agronomy* (Reinhold, New York, 1967), pp. 73–84.

43. National Academy of Sciences, *Principles of Plant and Animal Pest Control* II, Publication 1597 (National Academy of Sciences, Washington, D.C., 1968), pp. 256–257.

44. H. B. Sprague, *N.J. Agr. Exp. Sta. Bull.* 609, 1 (1936).

45. R. D. Munson and J. P. Doll, *Advan. Agr.* 11, 133 (1959).

46. J. S. Drew and R. N. Van Arsdall, *Ill. Agr. Econ.* 6, 25 (1966); D. L. Armstrong, J. K. Leasure, M. R. Corbin, *Weed Sci.* 16, 369 (1968); F. W. Slife, personal communication.

47. R. J. Delroit and H. L. Ahlgren, *Crop Production* (Prentice-Hall, Englewood Cliffs, N.J., 1953), pp. 572–573); P. W. Michael, *Herbage Abst.* 39, 59 (1969).

48. G. F. Sprague, *Corn and Corn Improvement* (Academic Press, New York, 1955), pp. 643 and 663.

49. National Academy of Sciences, *National Research Council Publication* No. 1232 (National Academy of Sciences, Washington, D.C., 1964), pp. 77–89; *ibid.*, No. 1684 (1969), pp. 38–45.

50. D. D. Harpstead, *Sci. Amer.* 225, 34 (1971).

51. U.S. Department of Agriculture, *Agr. Econ. Rep.* No. 147 (1968).

52. H. Jiler, *Commodity Yearbook* (Commodity Research Bureau, Inc., New York, 1972), pp. 252–253.

53. National Academy of Sciences, *Resources and Man* (Freeman, San Francisco, 1969), p. 143.

54. G. Borgstrëm, *Principles of Food Science* (Macmillan, New York, 1968), vol. 2, p. 376.

55. U.S. Department of Agriculture, *Agricultural Statistics 1970* (Government Printing Office, Washington, D.C., 1970), pp. 28 and 430.

56. ———, *Fats and Oils Situation* (Economics Research Service, FOS-257, Washington, D.C., 1971).

57. G. R. Conway, *Environment, Resources, Pollution, and Society* (Sineurer Associates, Inc., Stamford, 1971), pp. 302–325; S. Pradhan, *World Sci. News* 8, 41 (1971).

58. J. N. Black, *Ann. Appl. Biol.* 67, 272 (1971).

59. U.S. Department of Agriculture, *Agricultural Statistics 1967* (Government Printing Office, Washington, D.C., 1967), pp. 34–35.

60. ———, *Crop Production, 1971 Annual Summary* (State Report Service, 1972).

61. ———, *Agr. Res. Ser. Stat. Bull.* No. 216 (1957).

62. ———, *Stat. Rep. Serv. Bull.* No. 408 (1967).

63. R. S. Berry and M. F. Fels, *The Production and Consumption of Automobiles. An Energy Analysis of the Manufacture, Discard, and Reuse of the Automobile and its Component Materials* (Univ. of Chicago, Chicago, 1973).

64. U.S. Department of Agriculture, *Bur. Agron. Econ. Bull.* No. FM 101 (1953).

65. U.S. Bureau of the Census, *Statistical Abstract of the U.S., 93rd Edition,* (Government Printing Office, Washington, D.C., 1972), pp. 600–601.

66. H. F. DeGraff and W. E. Washbon, *Agr. Econ.* No. 449 (1943).

67. U.S. Bureau of the Census, *Census of Agriculture 1964* II (1968), pp. 909-955.

68. E. O. Heady, H. C. Madsen, K. J. Nicol, S. H. Hargrove, *Report of the Center for Agriculture and Rural Development*, prepared at Iowa State University, for the National Water Commission (NTIS, Springfield, Va., 1972).

69. A. W. Epp, *Nebr. Exp. Sta. Bull.* No. 426 (1954).

70. T. S. Thorfinnson, M. Hunt, A. W. Epp, *Nebr. Exp. Sta. Bull.* No. 432 (1955).

71. *Corn Grower's Guide* (W. R. Grace and Co., Aurora, Ill., 1968), p. 113.

72. U.S. Bureau of the Census, *Statistical Abstract for the United States, 92nd Edition* (Government Printing Office, Washington, D.C., 1971), p. 496.

73. ———, *Statistical Abstract of the United States, 86th Edition* (Government Printing Office, Washington, D.C., 1965), p. 538.

74. U.S. Department of Commerce, *Census of Transportation*, III (3), (Government Printing Office, Washington, D.C., 1967), pp. 102–105.

75. Interstate Commerce Commission, *Freight Commodity Statistics, Class I Motor Carriers of Property in Intercity* (Government Printing Office, Washington, D.C., 1968), p. 97; ———, *Freight and Commodity Statistics Class I Railroads* (Government Printing Office, Washington, D.C., 1968); ———, *Transportation Statistics* I, V, VII (Government Printing Office, Washington, D.C., 1968).

76. U.S. Department of Transportation, *Highway Statistics* (Government Printing Office, Washington, D.C., 1970), p. 5.

77. *Handbook of Chemistry and Physics* (Chemical Rubber Company, Cleveland, 1972), Table D-230.

78. A. J. Payne and J. A. Canner, *Chem. Process Eng.* 50, 81 (1969).

79. G. Leach and M. Slesser, *Energy Equivalents of Network Inputs to Food Producing Processes* (Univ. of Strathclyde, Glasgow, 1973).

80. We thank the following specialists for reading an earlier draft of the manuscript and for their many helpful suggestions: Georg Borgström, Department of Food Science and Geography, Michigan State University; Harrison Brown, Foreign Secretary, National Academy of Sciences; Gordon Harrison, Ford Foundation; Gerald Leach, Science Policy Research Unit, University of Sussex; Roger Revelle, Center for Population Studies, Harvard University; Malcolm Slesser, Department of Pure and Applied Chemistry, University of Strathclyde; and, at Cornell University: R. C. Loehr, Department of Agricultural Engineering; W. R. Lynn and C. A. Shoemaker, Department of Environmental Engineering; K. L. Robinson, Department of Agricultural Economics; C. O. Grogan, Department of Plant Breeding; R. S. Morison, Program of Science, Technology and Society; N. C. Brady and W. K. Kennedy, Department of Agronomy; and L. C. Cole and S. A. Levin, Section of Ecology and Systematics. Any errors or omissions are the authors' responsibility. This study was supported in part by grants from the Ford Foundation and NSF (GZ 1371 and GB 19239).

Excerpted with permission from *Science*, 182: 443-449 (2 November 1973). Copyright 1973 by the American Association for the Advancement of Science.

The Uses of Power

BARRY COMMONER

In his book *The Closing Circle*, biologist Barry Commoner, Director of the St. Louis-based Center for the Biology of Natural Systems, analyzed our pollution crises as arising not from overpopulation but from our shift to "synthetic" instead of "natural" materials. Here, in an excerpt from his most recent book, *The Poverty of Power*, he sees the plight of the farmer as arising from much the same kind of shift. An agriculture no longer driven by solar energy can no longer provide a livelihood to farmers, he says, when our energy capital begins to run out.

For anyone, such as myself, who approaches it from the outside, agriculture in the United States presents a picture of enormous and apparently successful change. The storybook farm, with its menagerie of animals personally attended by the farmer and his family amid checkered fields of corn, oats, hay, and clover and a garden of fruits and vegetables, is long gone. Nearly all the horses have disappeared, their place before the plow taken by tractors, which—in a kind of parody of their predecessor's evolution—each year grow in size and power, many now riding on seven-foot wheels and carrying an air-conditioned cab. Most of the cattle have been banished to feed-lots—enormous pens where thousands of animals are fattened on truckloads of grain, tended more by bulldozers than by people. The chickens are no longer in the barnyard, scrambling about for food and laying eggs in nests of their own making: now they are congregated in long buildings, confined in rows of cages, their food and water delivered and their eggs and waste removed by endless belts.

Now the once-variegated fields are uniformly covered with a single crop. The corn no longer dries in the sun, but is harvested as moist grain which is fed into gas-burning drying ovens and trucked to feed companies—that supply the penned cattle and the caged chickens. Where once the animals' manure made the fields fertile, now it has become feed-lot waste. Instead, the crops are nourished by purchased chemicals. Other chemicals are used to kill weeds and insect pests, no longer kept in check by shifting crops from field to field.

The farm land, once a place where in almost every season some green leaf shimmered in the sun, is now more often bare ground, green for only a few summer months, when the single crop that is mandated by the market is rapidly grown, harvested, and turned into cash. And most of the people have left, no longer needed to tend the animals or to manage the seasonal variety of planting and harvesting. Those who remain are no longer preoccupied with daily decisions about how to mediate between the complex needs of their livestock and crops and the harsh demands of nature. Their decisions are now less numerous but much more portentous—whether to plant all of one crop or all of another, to take advantage of an expected market price; or whether to buy an expensive new machine or chemical, in the hope that it will increase their income sufficiently to cover the cost of the loan needed to pay the high purchase price.

All of these changes—most of them in the last thirty years—have been accompanied by spectacular improvements in agricultural production. Compared to 1950, in 1970 an acre of land planted to corn yielded three times as much grain; a broiler chicken gained nearly 50 percent more weight from its feed; a hen laid fifty more eggs per year (a 25-percent increase). In that time, farm output as a whole increased by 40 percent. And, as the proponents of the new agriculture are fond of reminding us, in 1950 each farm worker produced enough food for about 15 people and today the figure is well over 47 people per farm worker. If people have left the farm, it is because they are no longer needed there.

But there is also a major economic mystery here. Since the productivity of farm labor has increased nearly threefold and most of it is still supplied by farm families, we might expect them to be that much better off, economically, than they were. But they are not. Despite the huge increase in agricultural labor productivity and in total output, the real income of U.S. farms *decreased* from about $18 billion in 1950 to $13 billion in 1971. (These and the following figures are given in 1967 dollars to eliminate the effect of inflation.) Because the number of farms also decreased by 50 percent, the income per farm rose by 46 percent (from an average of about $3200 in 1950 to slightly under $4600 in 1971). However, this is much less than the average increase in the family income of *all* U.S. families in that period, 76 percent. Meanwhile, the total mortgage debt of U.S. farms rose from about $8 billion in 1950 to $24 billion in 1971.

These statistics tell us that the farm families which have accomplished the remarkable gains in agricultural production have not reaped most of the fruits of their labor. As a recent report of the National Academy of Sciences points out: "Agriculture as a major segment of the total economy has had to produce far more in order to earn as much; the terms of trade between agriculture and the rest of the economy have shifted against agriculture."

Who, then, *has* gained from increased agricultural production, if not the farmers?

My first clue to this puzzle came as I heard a lecture by Professor D. M. Woodruff, a distinguished and innovative agronomist at the University of Missouri. Professor Woodruff likes to begin his lectures by asking the question "What is the purpose of farming?" The usual answer, which is enshrined in every agronomy textbook, is: "To produce food and fiber"; but the answer that Professor Woodruff prefers is: "To capture solar energy."

This is a powerful insight. Once given this lead, it takes only a little reflection to realize that although only a minute fraction of the solar energy that reaches the earth is turned into useful work, nearly all of that energy is captured by agriculture and forestry. Agriculture is an energy-requiring process, and energy is the clue to the curious disappearance of the new wealth that farms have generated during the postwar gains in production....

Organic matter is the fuel that drives the great cycles of the ecosystem which support not only agriculture, but all life. Solar energy, trapped by the living plants, produces that fuel; Professor Woodruff is right.

The basic fact that agriculture is absolutely dependent on the energy contained in photosynthetically produced organic matter, and ultimately derived from the sun, has, of course, long been recognized in traditional farming practice. For example, one long-established principle was to maintain green crops on the ground for as much of the year as possible. This maximizes the capture of solar energy and the production of the organic matter that drives the soil cycles. Crops were grown in a yearly sequence, beginning with ones that green up early in the spring, through a summer crop, ending with one that remains green late into the fall.

The traditional scheme of combining animal and plant production on the same farm also recognizes the importance of organic matter for the soil cycle, energetically as well as in other ways. If the cycle is broken by growing a crop in one place and feeding it to animals in another, then their organic waste is not returned to the soil, but accumulates at the feed-lot. This practice converts manure from a useful carrier of solar energy and plant nutrients into a pollutant. Obviously, to maintain the integrity of the soil cycle, manure should be returned to the soil, where its nutrients can re-enter the biological cycle and its organic matter can provide the energy needed to drive it.

Crop rotations that include legumes are another good way to trap solar energy. The legumes' photosynthetic activity captures the energy needed to drive nitrogen fixation (by way of the organic products of photosynthesis) and thereby enriches the soil. Grasses seem to encourage the activity of nitrogen-fixing bacteria in the soil, perhaps by the organic matter sloughed off from their roots.

Given what we know about the natural cycles that maintain the fertility of the soil, and particularly their dependence upon energy, a system of agriculture that used solar energy efficiently would be based on a sequence of crops that are green for the longest possible yearly period, that are in a rotation which includes legumes, and that are mixed with animal production. This is, of course, the pattern of traditional agriculture. But this pattern has been largely destroyed by the post-war changes in agricultural production. By tracing the resultant effects on the farm's energy relations, and their economic consequences, we can find out where the added wealth produced by the new agriculture has gone.

In the U.S. Corn Belt, the common crop "rotation" is now usually corn-on-corn (corn planted in the same field year after year) or corn-on-soybeans, with the two crops planted in alternate years. This means that the soil is covered with energy-catching green leaves for only a short time each year. Corn matures in about ninety days and the leaves are full-sized and able to catch much sunlight for only perhaps half that time. And so, if only corn is grown, solar energy is trapped effectively for less than three months. For the rest of the year, the energy that the sun sheds on the land adds

nothing to the economy of the farm, or the nation. In the new agriculture, legume rotations have been drastically reduced; legume seed production declined 60 percent between 1959 and 1973. Even when soybeans are grown, they are usually on land that has been previously fertilized, so that nitrogen fixation (which is inhibited by nitrate in the soil) is rather inactive. And finally, with the animals raised in separate feed-lots, the only organic matter returned to the soil is the stalk residue of the crop....

Because of the shift from manure, legumes, and other organic fertilizers, the crop's nutrition is no longer provided by a biological cycle, driven by renewable, freely available solar energy; instead, by using inorganic fertilizer, it has become dependent on non-renewable, increasingly expensive fossil fuels.

Another example of this kind of shift in the energy dependence of the farm is the matter of drying grain. Corn, like most grains, is an enormously valuable food because it can be easily stored well past the harvest season. Grain resists decay because it is too dry to support the attack of bacteria and molds. In nature, corn readily dries on the stalk in the autumn sun, and in traditional agriculture the field-dried ears were harvested and stored, as such, in ventilated bins. But the familiar corn-crib is gone. In the late 1950s new harvesting machines appeared which stripped the still-moist grains from the ear, in the field. To be preserved, the grain had to be dried within a few days after harvest in large ovenlike machines fueled by propane. Once more an essential energy-requiring task was diverted from solar energy to fossil fuel.

Thus we must add to the conventional glowing picture of post-war agriculture a feature that is more subtle and less praiseworthy than the increased yields of corn and chickens: Particularly with respect to energy, the farm has become less self-reliant, more dependent on the outside economy. To maintain production, the farm must now rely on factories and refineries for more and more of the energy that is needed "to produce food and fiber." The farm's link to the sun has been weakened, replaced by a new and—as we shall see—dangerous liaison with industry.

The energy that the modern farm now imports from the industrial sector is delivered in diverse forms: as gasoline and diesel fuel (to run tractors and other machinery); as propane (to fuel grain driers); as electricity (to power milking machines, grain driers, and other stationary equipment); as fertilizers, insecticides, and herbicides, all chemicals that are synthesized in energy-demanding processes....

U.S. agriculture now consumes only about 4 percent of the total national energy budget. It would make little sense to cut down the agricultural uses of energy, however inefficient they are, in order to reduce the overall energy demand. Nor is there much logic in complaining that the farmer is "wasteful" because he makes less use of the sun than before. Solar energy is renewable, and, like the milk in the fable's miraculous self-filling pitcher, there is no way to waste it.

The real problem created by the shift to outside energy sources is economic (apart from the environmental problems due to fertilizer leaching into streams and lakes and the very serious toxic effects of insecticides and herbicides). This is evident in the farmer's balance sheets, as they are averaged out in standard U.S. Department of Agriculture (USDA) reports. And they tell us quite clearly where the increased wealth generated by the post-war development of "agribusiness" has gone.

In 1950 U.S. farms had a gross income of about $32.3 billion. Their expenses amounted to about $19.4 billion, yielding a net income of $12.9 billion. By 1970 gross income had increased to $57.9 billion (a 79-percent increase); but expenses had gone up even faster, to $41.1 billion (an increase of 112 percent), leaving a net income of $16.8 billion. With inflation taken into account, the net income of U.S. agriculture had actually *decreased* in that twenty-year period despite the introduction of the new technological marvels that have so greatly improved

agricultural production. Or, rather, because of them. The largest item in the farmers' rising costs is interest on loans and depreciation of machinery. These costs largely reflect the carrying charges of purchased material. These are the inputs brought into agriculture from the industrial sector, most of them—machinery, fertilizers, and chemicals—based on the intensive use of energy....

Part of the problem is not only that agriculture has been using more and more industrial goods, but that in some cases their use yields progressively less output. This is particularly true of nitrogen fertilizer. For example, in the United States the average amount of nitrogen fertilizer applied to corn annually has increased steadily. Between 1950 and 1959 the rate of nitrogen application increased by 26 pounds per acre and the average yield of corn increased by 16 bushels per acre (.62 bushels per pound of fertilizer). Between 1960 and 1970 the rate of nitrogen application further increased by 71 pounds per acre, but the yield by only 27 bushels per acre (.38 bushels per pound of fertilizer). In other words, the productivity of nitrogen fertilizer—the crop produced per pound of nitrogen applied—has been declining as the rate of application has increased. This reflects a basic biological fact: that there is a limit to the amount of growth that a plant can sustain, so that yields obtained for a given increment of nutrient element inevitably decline as more and more is supplied to the plant. There has been a similar decline in nitrogen productivity in U.S. agriculture as a whole: Between 1950 and 1970 the amount of nitrogen fertilizer used per unit of crop produced increased fivefold. In the same way, as insect pests become more resistant to the new pesticides, the amounts of these chemicals used have also risen faster than agricultural output. Such effects mean that the farmer gets progressively smaller returns in income from increased expenditures of this sort.

Thus, in economic terms, the great post-war change in agricultural production technology did a great deal more than simply increase output. It displaced farm labor with energy-dependent inputs: machines, power, and chemicals. As the amount of labor involved in farming went down, the amount of capital went up; the assets used in agriculture, per farm worker, rose from $9400 in 1950 to $53,500 in 1970. . . .

Here we can begin to see an explanation for the puzzling disappearance of the economic gains that one might expect farmers to receive from their additional production: Most of that wealth has been drained off by the industries—such as petrochemicals—that provide the new inputs, which substitute fossil-fuel energy for the solar energy on which agriculture has long depended.

By shifting its energy dependence from the sun to petrochemical companies, the U.S. farm has become linked to a multibillion-dollar industry which not only sells fuel to the farmer, but competes with him for it when it is in short supply. Propane is an illuminating example. The chief consumers of propane are farmers and the petrochemical industry, in which it is a major raw material for the production of plastics and synthetic fibers. In the 1973 energy crisis the industry cheerfully bid up the price of propane, so that farmers had trouble finding the propane they needed to dry their grain and then in some areas had to pay triple its former price. . . . Because they manufactured it themselves, for . . . petrochemical companies the high cost of propane was a purely bookkeeping transaction. . . .

Until the 1973 oil crisis this sort of economic vulnerability remained hidden. In the 1950s and 1960s, as the farmer became increasingly dependent on fuels and energy-intensive chemicals, their prices remained relatively low, in part because . . . the cost of the petroleum products from which they were manufactured remained constant, and even fell slightly (in uninflated dollars) between 1950 and 1973. As long as the price of fertilizer remained low, it did not really matter that its agricultural productivity was falling; it was still a worthwhile investment.

Then came the oil crisis of 1973, which . . .

was the signal for a sharp and escalating rise in the price of fuel. And with it the prices of energy-intensive products such as fertilizers and other agricultural chemicals increased drastically. Between 1970 and 1975 propane increased in price by 101 percent; nitrogen fertilizer by 253 percent; and pesticides by an average of 67 percent. In 1973 rising farm prices more than made up for the rising costs of fertilizer and other energy-intensive inputs, but these gains were lost by 1975. The process has left U.S. agriculture in a vulnerable economic position; if the selling price of farm commodities should fall, farmers will be hard pressed to meet the elevated prices of agricultural chemicals, and of fuel, that have been imposed on them by the energy and petrochemical corporations.

One can almost admire the enterprise and clever salesmanship of the petrochemical industry. Somehow it has managed to convince the farmer that he should give up the free solar energy that drives the natural cycles and, instead, buy the needed energy—in the form of fertilizer and fuel—from the petrochemical industry. Not content with that commercial coup, these industrial giants have completed their conquest of the farmer by going into competition with what the farm produces. They have introduced into the market a series of competing synthetics: synthetic fiber, which competes with cotton and wool; detergents, which compete with soap made of natural oils and fat; plastics, which compete with wood; and pesticides that compete with birds and ladybugs, which used to be free.

The giant corporations have made a colony out of rural America. Like Standard Oil forcing its product on old China, U.S. industry has molded the nation's farms into a convenient market and a weakened competitor. In both cases the economic weapon was energy.

All this suggests that if the modern farmer could find some way to reverse the direction of this technological "progress" and to reduce the use of energy-intensive inputs such as fertilizers and pesticides, he might suffer little or no loss in net income, the reduced gross income compensated by a comparable decrease in costs. Strangely enough, at least a few farmers in the Corn Belt have managed to do just that.

Farmers are, after all, independent folk, and despite the conventional wisdom as expounded by the USDA and most agricultural-research institutions, some farmers have remained skeptical of the value of the intensive use of chemicals. Some are concerned over the environmental effects of fertilizers and pesticides; some fear that exposure to pesticides is unhealthy; some have a moral commitment to maintaining the natural fertility of the soil. For one or more of these reasons, a few farmers (no one really knows how many) operating commercial farms on which they rely for their livelihood have given up the use of inorganic fertilizers and chemical pesticides, becoming, in effect, "organic" farmers. (The idea of "organic" farming or gardening, stripped of overzealous exaggerations and unsupported claims, has a firm scientific foundation. From what has already been said, it should be clear that the maintenance of organic matter in the soil cycle is a good indication of the system's natural fertility. There is also good reason to believe that organic substances which do not naturally occur in living things—such as synthetic pesticides—are likely to risk biological harm, so that excluding these substances from agriculture wherever possible also has a scientific justification.)

The existence of these farms creates the opportunity to test the validity of the conventional wisdom that the success of current agricultural practice—its level of production and economic returns to the farmer—would be impossible without the intensive use of inorganic fertilizers and synthetic pesticides. The position has been forcefully laid down by Secretary of Agriculture Earl Butz:

> Without the modern input of chemicals, of pesticides, of antibiotics, of herbicides, we simply couldn't do the job. Before we go back to an organic agriculture in this country somebody must decide which 50 million Americans we are going to let starve or go hungry.

Having located a number of such "organic farms," the Center for the Biology of Natural Systems was able to set up a simple way to test the validity of Mr. Butz's dictum: It compared these farms with neighboring conventional ones.

A research group headed by Dr. William Lockeretz studied sixteen commercial-sized organic farms that use neither inorganic fertilizer (other than phosphate rock) nor chemical pesticides, and sixteen conventional farms similar in size, location, and soil properties that used these inputs. Both categories of farms were combined crop-livestock operations; they raised about the same types of crops—corn, soybeans, wheat, and oats—except that the conventional farms raised relatively more corn. Both used about the same amounts and types of machinery (including grain driers).

The group analyzed the production of these farms for the 1974 season. The market value of the crops produced by the conventional farms was an average of $179 per acre, while the average value for the organic farm was $165 per acre. However, the operating costs of the conventional farms averaged $47 per acre, and those of the organic farms $31 per acre (the difference is largely due to the cost of the nitrogen fertilizer and pesticides used by the conventional farmers). As a result, the net income per acre of crop for the two types of farms is essentially the same: $134 per acre for organic farms and $132 per acre for conventional ones (this is not a statistically significant difference). The yields of different crops obtained by the two groups of farms are about equal, except for a small excess (12 percent) of corn yields on conventional farms as compared with organic farms.

The organic farms used only 6800 BTU of energy to produce a dollar of output, while the conventional farms used 18,400 BTU. Thus, organic farms appear to yield about the same economic returns as the conventional ones, but do so by using about one-third as much energy. In the terms of the farmer quoted earlier, they have managed to make as much money, without handling so much of it.

These observations, being based on only one year's results, must be regarded as tentative. As the study continues and we learn more about how the conventional and organic farms compare in their production, costs, and income, it will be possible to evaluate measures that might restore farming to a more thrifty use of energy, without undue loss in production. We hope to learn how to help the farmers find their way back to the sun.

Excerpted with permission from *The Poverty of Power*, pp. 159-175 (Random House, Inc. and Jonathon Cape, Ltd., 1976). Copyright 1976 by Barry Commoner.

Energy Use in the U.S. Food System

JOHN S. STEINHART and CAROL E. STEINHART

Chapter 3, "Whatever Happened to Food," examined the economic thrust that lay behind the endless diversification of the American food supply, and tallied some of the human costs involved. Here Drs. John and Carol Steinhart, a geologist and a biologist by training, examine another cost: what is the energy investment in our "modern" food supply? What does it cost energetically to eat a diet of Corny Snaps, Twinkies and Pringles instead of corn, wheat and potatoes?

In a modern industrial society, only a tiny fraction of the population is in frequent contact with the soil, and an even smaller fraction of the population raises food on the soil. The proportion of the population engaged in farming halved between 1920 and 1950 and then halved again by 1962. Now it has almost halved again, and more than half of these remaining farmers hold other jobs off the farm (1)....

Energy inputs to farming have increased enormously during the past 50 years (3), and the apparent decrease in farm labor is offset in part by the growth of support industries for the farmer. With these changes on the farm have come a variety of other changes in the U.S. food system, many of which are now deeply embedded in the fabric of daily life. In the past 50 years, canned, frozen, and other processed foods have become the principal items of our diet. At present, the food processing industry is the fourth largest energy consumer of the Standard Industrial Classification groupings (4). The extent of transportation engaged in the food system has grown apace, and the prolifera-

tion of appliances in both numbers and complexity still continues in homes, institutions, and stores. Hardly any food is eaten as it comes from the fields. Even farmers purchase most of their food from markets in town.

Present energy supply problems make this growth of energy use in the food system worth investigating. It is our purpose in this article to do so....

What we would like to know is: How does our present food supply system compare, in energy measures, with those of other societies and with our own past? Perhaps then we can estimate the value of energy flow measures as an adjunct to, but different from, economic measures.

Energy in the U.S. Food System

A typical breakfast includes orange juice from Florida by way of the Minute Maid factory, bacon from a midwestern meat packer, cereal from Nebraska and General Mills, eggs and milk from not *too* far away, and coffee from Colombia. All of these things are available at

Table 1. Energy use in the United States food system. All values are multiplied by 10^{12} kcal.

Component	1940	1947	1950	1954	1958	1960	1964	1968	1970	References
On farm										
Fuel (direct use)	70.0	136.0	158.0	172.8	179.0	188.0	213.9	226.0	232.0	(13-15)
Electricity	0.7	32.0	32.9	40.0	44.0	46.1	50.0	57.3	63.8	(14, 16)
Fertilizer	12.4	19.5	24.0	30.6	32.2	41.0	60.0	87.0	94.0	(14, 17)
Agricultural steel	1.6	2.0	2.7	2.5	2.0	1.7	2.5	2.4	2.0	(14, 18)
Farm machinery	9.0	34.7	30.0	29.5	50.2	52.0	60.0	75.0	80.0	(14, 19)
Tractors	12.8	25.0	30.8	23.6	16.4	11.8	20.0	20.5	19.3	(20)
Irrigation	18.0	22.8	25.0	29.6	32.5	33.3	34.1	34.8	35.0	(21)
Subtotal	124.5	272.0	303.4	328.6	356.3	373.9	440.5	503.0	526.1	
Processing industry										
Food processing industry	147.0	177.5	192.0	211.5	212.6	224.0	249.0	295.0	308.0	(13, 14, 22)
Food processing machinery	0.7	5.7	5.0	4.9	4.9	5.0	6.0	6.0	6.0	(23)
Paper packaging	8.5	14.8	17.0	20.0	26.0	28.0	31.0	35.7	38.0	(24)
Glass containers	14.0	25.7	26.0	27.0	30.2	31.0	34.0	41.9	47.0	(25)
Steel cans and aluminum	38.0	55.8	62.0	73.7	85.4	86.0	91.0	112.2	122.0	(26)
Transport (fuel)	49.6	86.1	102.0	122.3	140.2	153.3	184.0	226.6	246.9	(27)
Trucks and trailors (manufacture)	28.0	42.0	49.5	47.0	43.0	44.2	61.0	70.2	74.0	(28)
Subtotal	285.8	407.6	453.5	506.4	542.3	571.5	656.0	787.6	841.9	
Commercial and home										
Commercial refrigeration and cooking	121.0	141.0	150.0	161.0	176.0	186.2	209.0	241.0	263.0	(13, 29)
Refrigeration machinery (home and commercial)	10.0	24.0	25.0	27.5	29.4	32.0	40.0	56.0	61.0	(14, 30)
Home refrigeration and cooking	144.2	184.0	202.3	228.0	257.0	276.6	345.0	433.9	480.0	(13, 29)
Subtotal	275.2	349.0	377.3	416.5	462.4	494.8	594.0	730.9	804.0	
Grand total	685.5	1028.6	1134.2	1251.5	1361.0	1440.2	1690.5	2021.5	2172.0	

the local supermarket (several miles each way in a 300-horsepower automobile), stored in a refrigerator-freezer, and cooked on an instant-on stove.

The present food system in the United States is complex, and the attempt to analyze it in terms of energy use will introduce complexities and questions far more perplexing than the same analysis carried out on simpler societies. Such an analysis is worthwhile, however, if only to find out where we stand. We have a food system, and most people get enough to eat from it. If, in addition, one considers the food supply problems present and future in societies where a smaller fraction of the people get enough to eat, then our experience with an industrialized food system is even more important. There is simply no gainsaying that many nations of the world are presently attempting to acquire industrialized food systems of their own.

Food in the United States is expensive by world standards. In 1970 the average annual per capita expenditure for food was about $600 (3). This amount is larger than the per capita gross domestic product of more than 30 nations of the world which contain the majority of the world's people and a vast majority of those who are underfed. Even if we consider the diet of a poor resident of India, the annual cost of his food at U.S. prices would be about $200—more than twice his annual income (3)....

Seven categories of energy use on the farm are considered here. The amounts of energy used are shown in Table 1....

Little food makes its way directly from field and farm to the table. The vast complex of processing, packaging, and transport has been grouped together in a second major subdivision of the food system. The seven categories of the processing industry are listed in Table 1....

After the processing of food there is further energy expenditure. Transportation enters the picture again, and some fraction of the energy used for transportation should be assigned here. But there are also the distributors, wholesalers, and retailers, whose freezers, refrigerators, and very establishments are an integral part of the food system. There are also the restaurants, schools, universities, prisons, and a host of other institutions engaged in the procurement, preparation, storage, and supply of food. We have chosen to examine only three categories: the energy required for refrigeration and cooking, and for the manufacture of the heating and refrigeration equipment (Table 1). We have made no attempt to include the energy used in trips to the store or restaurant. Garbage disposal has also been omitted, although it is a persistent and growing feature of our food system; 12 percent of the nation's trucks are engaged in the activity of waste disposal *(1)*, of which a substantial part is re-

lated to food. If there is any lingering doubt that these activities—both the ones included and the ones left out—are an essential feature of our present food system, one need only ask what would happen if everyone should attempt to get on without a refrigerator or freezer or stove? Certainly the food system would change.

Table 1 and the related references summarize the numerical values for energy use in the U.S. food system, from 1940 to 1970. As for many activities in the past few decades, the story is one of continuing increase. The totals are displayed in Fig. 1 along with the energy value of the food consumed by the public. The food values were obtained by multiplying the daily caloric intake by the population. The differences in caloric intake per capita over this 30-year period are small *(1)*, and the curve is primarily an indication of the increase in population in this period.

... The values for energy use in the food system from Table 1 account for 12.8 percent of the total U.S. energy use in 1970.

Performance of an Industrialized Food System

The difficulty with history as a guide for the future or even the present lies not so much in the fact that conditions change—we are continually reminded of that fact—but that history is only one experiment of the many that might have occurred. The U.S. food system developed as it did for a variety of reasons, many of them not understood. We would do well to examine some of the dimensions of this development before attempting to theorize about how it might have been different, or how parts of this food system can be transplanted elsewhere.

Energy and Food Production

Figure 2 displays features of our food system not easily seen from economic data. The curve shown has no theoretical basis but is suggested by the data as a smoothed recounting of our own history of increasing food production. It is, however, similar to most growth curves and

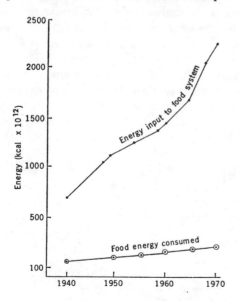

Fig. 1. Energy use in the food system, 1940 through 1970, compared to the caloric content of food consumed.

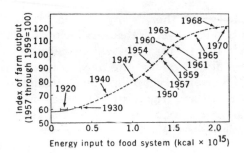

Fig. 2. Farm output as a function of energy input to the U.S. food system, 1920 through 1970.

suggests that, to the extent that the increasing energy subsidies to the food system have increased food production, we are near the end of an era. Like the logistic growth curve, there is an exponential phase which lasted from 1920 or earlier until 1950 or 1955. Since then, the increments in production have been smaller despite the continuing growth in energy use. It is likely that further increases in food production from increasing energy inputs will be harder and harder to come by. Of course, a major change in the food system could change things, but the argument advanced by the technological optimist is that we can always get more if we have enough energy, and that no other major changes are required. Our own history—the only one we have to examine—does not support that view.

Energy and Labor in the Food System

One farmer now feeds 50 people, and the common expectation is that the labor input to farming will continue to decrease in the future. Behind this expectation is the assumption that the continued application of technology—and energy—to farming will substitute for labor. Figure 3 shows this historic decline in labor as a function of the energy supplied to the food system, again the familiar S-shaped curve. What it implies is that increasing the energy input to the food system is unlikely to bring further reduction in farm labor unless some other, major change is made.

The food system that has grown in this period has provided much employment that did not exist 20, 30, or 40 years ago. Perhaps even the idea of a reduction of labor input is a myth when the food system is viewed as a whole, instead of from the point of view of the farm worker only. When discussing inputs to the farm, Pimentel et al. (3) cite an estimate of two farm support workers for each person actually on the farm. To this must be added employment in food-processing industries, in food wholesaling and retailing, as well as in a variety of manufacturing enterprises that support the food system. Yesterday's farmer is today's canner, tractor mechanic, and fast food carhop. The process of change has been painful to many ordinary people. The rural poor, who could not quite compete in the growing industrialization of farming, migrated to the cities. Eventually they found other employment, but one must ask if the change was worthwhile. The answer to that question cannot be provided by energy analysis anymore than by economic data, because it raises fundamental questions about how individuals would prefer to spend their lives. But if there is a stark choice between long hours as a farmer or shorter hours on the assembly line of a meatpacking plant, it seems clear that the choice would not be universally in favor of the meat-packing plant. Thomas Jefferson dreamed of a nation of independent small farmers. It was a good dream, but society

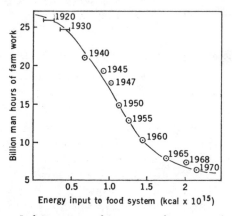

Fig. 3. Labor use on farms as a function of energy use in the food system.

did not develop in that way. Nor can we turn back the clock to recover his dream. But, in planning and preparing for our future, we had better look honestly at our collective history, and then each of us should closely examine his dreams.

The Energy Subsidy to the Food System

The data in Fig. 1 can be combined to show the energy subsidy provided to the food system for the recent past. We take as a measure of the food supplied the caloric content of the food actually consumed. This is not the only measure of the food supplied, as the condition of many protein-poor peoples of the world clearly shows. Nevertheless, the comparison between caloric input and output is a convenient way to compare our present situation with the past, and to compare our food system with others. Figure 4 shows the history of the U.S. food system in terms of the number of calories of energy supplied to produce 1 calorie of food for actual consumption. It is interesting and possibly threatening to note that there is no real suggestion that this curve is leveling off. We appear to be increasing the energy input even more. Fragmentary data for 1972 suggest that the increase continued unabated. A graph like Fig. 4 could approach zero. A natural ecosystem has no fuel input at all, and those primitive people who live by hunting and gathering have only the energy of their own work to count as input....

Some Energy Implications for the World Food Supply

The food supply system of the United States is complex and interwoven into a highly industrialized economy. We have tried to analyze this system on account of its implications for future energy use. But the world is short of food. A few years ago it was widely predicted that the world would suffer widespread famine in the 1970's. The adoption of new high-yield varieties of rice, wheat, and other grains has caused some experts to predict that the threat of these expected famines can now be averted, perhaps

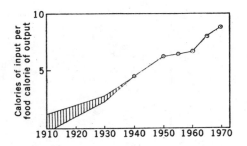

Fig. 4. Energy subsidy to the food system needed to obtain 1 food calorie.

indefinitely. Yet, despite increases in grain production in some areas, the world still seems to be headed toward famine. The adoption of these new varieties of grain—dubbed hopefully the "green revolution"—is an attempt to export a part of the energy-intensive food system of the highly industrialized countries to nonindustrialized countries. It is an experiment, because, although the whole food system is not being transplanted to new areas, a small part of it is. The green revolution requires a great deal of energy. Many of the new varieties of grain require irrigation where traditional crops did not, and almost all the new crops require extensive fertilization....

We know that our food system works (albeit with some difficulties and warnings for the future). But we cannot know what will happen if we take a piece of that system and transplant it to a poor country, without our industrial base of supply, transport system, processing industry, appliances for home storage, and preparation, and, most important of all, a level of industrialization that permits higher costs for food....

Where Next to Look for Food?

Our examination in the foregoing pages of the U.S. food system, the limitations on the manipulation of ecosystems and their components, and the risks of the green revolution as a solution to the world food supply problem suggests a bleak prospect for the future. This complex of problems should not be under-

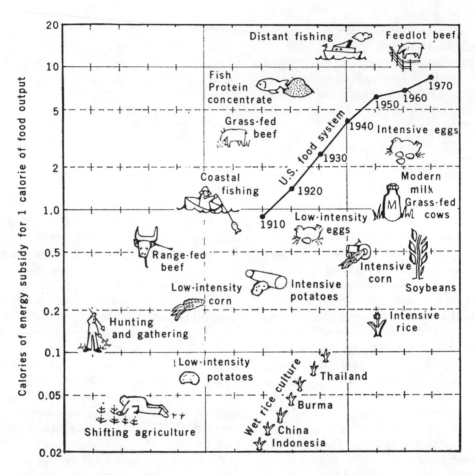

Fig. 5. Energy subsidies for various food crops. The energy history of the U.S. food system is shown for comparison.

estimated, but there are possible ways of avoiding disaster and of mitigating the severest difficulties. These suggestions are not very dramatic and may be difficult of common acceptance.

Figure 5 shows the ratio of the energy subsidy to the energy output for a number of widely used foods in a variety of times and cultures. For comparison, the overall pattern for the U.S. food system is shown, but the comparison is only approximate because, for most of the specific crops, the energy input ends at the farm. As has been pointed out, it is a long way from the farm to the table in industrialized societies. Several things are immediately apparent and coincide with expectations. High-protein foods such as milk, eggs, and

especially meat, have a far poorer energy return than plant foods. Because protein is essential for human diets and the amino acid balance necessary for good nutrition is not found in most of the cereal grains, we cannot take the step of abandoning meat sources altogether. Figure 5 does show how unlikely it is that increased fishing or fish protein concentrate will solve the world's food problems. Even if we leave aside the question of whether the fish are available—a point on which expert opinions differ somewhat—it would be hard to imagine, with rising energy prices, that fish protein concentrate will be anything more than a by-product of the fishing industry, because it requires more than twice the energy of production of grass-fed beef or eggs *(9)*. Distant fishing is still less likely to solve food problems. On the other hand, coastal fishing is relatively low in energy cost. Unfortunately, without the benefit of scholarly analysis fisherman and housewives have long known this, and coastal fisheries are threatened with overfishing as well as pollution.

The position of soybeans in Fig. 5 may be crucial. Soybeans possess the best amino acid balance and protein content of any widely grown crop. This has long been known to the Japanese who have made soybeans a staple of their diet. Are there other plants, possibly better suited for local climates, that have adequate proportions of amino acids in their proteins? There are about 80,000 edible species of plants, of which only about 50 are actively cultivated on a large scale (and 90 percent of the world's crops come from only 12 species). We may yet be able to find species that can contribute to the world's food supply.

The message of Fig. 5 is simple. In "primitive" cultures, 5 to 50 food calories were obtained for each calorie of energy invested. Some highly civilized cultures have done as well and occasionally better. In sharp contrast, industrialized food systems require 5 to 10 calories of fuel to obtain 1 food calorie. We must pay attention to this difference—especially if energy costs increase. If some of the energy subsidy for food production could be supplied by on-site, renewable sources—primarily sun and wind—we might be able to continue an energy-intensive food system. Otherwise, the choices appear to be either less energy-intensive food production or famine for many areas of the world.

Energy Reduction in Agriculture

It is possible to reduce the energy required for agriculture and the food system. A series of thoughtful proposals by Pimentel and his associates *(3)* deserves wide attention. Many of these proposals would help ameliorate environmental problems, and any reductions in energy use would provide a direct reduction in the pollutants due to fuel consumption as well as more time to solve our energy supply problems.

First, we should make more use of natural manures. The United States has a pollution problem from runoff from animal feedlots, even with the application of large amounts of manufactured fertilizer to fields. More than 10^6 kcal per acre (4×10^5 kcal per hectare) could be saved by substituting manure for manufactured fertilizer *(3)* (and, as a side benefit, the soil's condition would be improved). Extensive expansion in the use of natural manure will require decentralization of feedlot operations so that manure is generated closer to the point of application. Decentralization might increase feedlot costs, but, as energy prices rise, feedlot operations will rapidly become more expensive in any case. Although the use of manures can help reduce energy use, there is far too little to replace all commercial fertilizers at present *(10)*. Crop rotation is less widely practiced than it was even 20 years ago. Increased use of crop rotation or interplanting winter cover crops of legumes (which fix nitrogen as a green manure) would save 1.5×10^6 kcal per acre by comparison with the use of commercial fertilizer.

Second, weed and pest control could be accomplished at a much smaller cost in energy. A 10 percent saving in energy in weed control could be obtained by the use of the rotary hoe twice in cultivation instead of herbicide application (again with pollution abatement as a side benefit). Biologic pest control—that is, the use of sterile males, introduced predators, and the like—requires only a tiny fraction of the energy of pesticide manufacture and application. A change to a policy of "treat when and where necessary" pesticide application would bring a 35 to 50 percent reduction in pesticide use. Hand application of pesticides requires more labor than machine or aircraft application, but the energy for application is reduced from 18,000 to 300 kcal per acre *(3)*. Changed cosmetic standards, which in no way affect the taste or the edibility of foodstuffs, could also bring about a substantial reduction in pesticide use.

Third, plant breeders might pay more attention to hardiness, disease and pest resistance, reduced moisture content (to end the wasteful use of natural gas in drying crops), reduced water requirements, and increased protein content, even if it should mean some reduction in overall yield. In the longer run, plants not now widely cultivated might receive some serious attention and breeding efforts. It seems unlikely that the crops that have been most useful in temperate climates will be the most suitable ones for the tropics where a large portion of the undernourished peoples of the world now live.

A dramatic suggestion, to abandon chemical farming altogether, has been made by Chapman (11). His analysis shows that, were chemical farming to be ended, there would be much reduced yields per acre, so that most land in the soil bank would need to be put back into farming. Nevertheless, output would fall only 5 percent and prices for farm products would increase 16 percent. Most dramatically, farm income would rise 25 percent, and nearly all subsidy programs would end. A similar set of propositions treated with linear programming techniques at Iowa State University resulted in an essentially similar set of conclusions (12).

The direct use of solar energy farms, a return to wind power (modern windmills are now in use in Australia), and the production of methane from manure are all possibilities. These methods require some engineering to become economically attractive, but it should be emphasized that these technologies are now better understood than the technology of breeder reactors. If energy prices rise, these methods of energy generation would be attractive alternatives, even at their present costs of implementation.

Energy Reduction in the U.S. Food System

Beyond the farm, but still far from the table, more energy savings could be introduced. The most effective way to reduce the large energy requirements of food processing would be a change in eating habits toward less highly processed foods. The current aversion of young people to spongy, additive-laden white bread, hydrogenated peanut butter, and some other processed foods could presage such a change if it is more than just a fad... recycling of metal containers and wider use of returnable bottles could reduce this large item of energy use.

The trend toward the use of trucks in food transport, to the virtual exclusion of trains, should be reversed. . . .

Finally, we may have to ask whether the ever-larger frostless refrigerators are needed, and whether the host of kitchen appliances really means less work or only the same amount of work to a different standard.

Store delivery routes, even by truck, would require only a fraction of the energy used by autos for food shopping. Rapid transit, giving some attention to the problems with shoppers with parcels, would be even more energy-efficient. . . .

Energy, Prices, and Hunger

If energy prices rise, as they have already begun to do, the rise in the price of food in societies with industrialized agriculture can be expected to be even larger than the energy price increases. Slesser, in examining the case for England, suggests that a quadrupling of energy prices in the next 40 years would bring about a sixfold increase in food prices (9). Even small increases in energy costs may make it profitable to increase labor input to food production. Such a reversal of a 50-year trend toward energy-intensive agriculture would present environmental benefits as a bonus. . . .

Food is basically a net product of an ecosystem, however simplified. Food production starts with a natural material, however modified later. Injections of energy (and even brains) will carry us only so far. If the population cannot adjust its wants to the world in which it lives, there is little hope of solving the food problem for mankind. In that case the food shortage will solve our population problem.

References and Notes

1. *Statistical Abstract of the United States* (Government Printing Office, Washington, D.C., various annual editions).
2. *Historical Statistics of the United States* (Government Printing Office, Washington, D.C., 1960).
3. D. Pimentel, L. E. Hurd, A. C. Bellotti, M. J. Forster, I. N. Oka, O. D. Scholes, R. J. Whitman, *Science* **182**, 443 (1973).
4. A description of the system may be found in: *Patterns of Energy Consumption in the United States* (report prepared for the Office of Science and Technology, Executive Office of the President, by Stanford Research Institute, Stanford, California, Jan. 1972), appendix C. The three groupings larger than food processing are: primary metals, chemicals, and petroleum refining.
5. N. Georgescu-Roegen, *The Entropy Law and the Economic Process* (Harvard Univ. Press, Cambridge, 1971), p. 301.
6. *Patterns of Energy Consumption in the United States* (report prepared for the Office of Science and Technology, Executive Office of the President, by Stanford Research Institute, Stanford, Calif., Jan. 1972).
7. R. A. Rice, *Technol. Rev.* **75**, 32 (Jan. 1972).
8. Federal Highway Administration, Nationwide Personal Transportation Study Report No. 1 (1971) [as reported in Energy Research and Development, hearings before the Congressional Committee on Science and Astronautics, May 1972, p. 151].
9. M. Slesser, *Ecologist* **3** (No. 6), 216 (1973).
10. J. F. Gerber, personal communication (we are indebted to Dr. Gerber for pointing out that manures, even if used fully, will not provide all the needed agricultural fertilizers).
11. D. Chapman, *Environment (St. Louis)* **15** (No. 2), 12 (1973).
12. L. U. Mayer and S. H. Hargrove [*CAED Rep. No. 38* (1972)] as quoted in Slesser (*9*).
13. We have converted all figures for the use of electricity to fuel input values, using the average efficiency values for power plants given by C. M. Summers [*Sci. Am.* **224** (No. 3), 148 (1971)]. Self-generated electricity was converted to fuel inputs at an efficiency of 25 percent after 1945 and 20 percent before that year.
14. Purchased material in this analysis was converted to energy of manufacture according to the following values derived from the literature or calculated. In doubtful cases we have made what we believe to be conservative estimates: steel (including fabricated and castings), 1.7×10^7 kcal/ton (1.9×10^4 kcal/kg); aluminum (including castings and forgings), 6.0×10^7 kcal/ton; copper and brass (alloys, millings, castings, and forgings), 1.7×10^6 kcal/ton; paper, 5.5×10^6 kcal/ton; plastics, 1.25×10^6 kcal/ton; coal, 6.6×10^6 kcal/ton; oil and gasoline, 1.5×10^6 kcal/barrel (9.5×10^3 kcal/liter); natural gas, 0.26×10^3 kcal/cubic foot (9.2×10^3 kcal/m³); petroleum wax, 2.2×10^6 kcal/ton; gasoline and diesel engines, 3.4×10^6 kcal/engine; electric motors over 1 horsepower, 45×10^3 kcal/motor; ammonia, 2.7×10^7 kcal/ton; ammonia compounds, 2.2×10^6 kcal/ton; sulfuric acid and sulfur, 3×10^6 kcal/ton; sodium carbonate, 4×10^6 kcal/ton; and other inorganic chemicals, 2.2×10^6 kcal/ton.
15. Direct fuel use on farms: Expenditures for petroleum and other fuels consumed on farms were obtained from *Statistical Abstracts* (*1*)

and the *Census of Agriculture* (Bureau of the Census, Government Printing Office, Washington, D.C., various recent editions) data. A special survey of fuel use on farms in the 1964 *Census of Agriculture* was used for that year and to determine the mix of fuel products used. By comparing expenditures for fuel in 1964 with actual fuel use, the apparent unit price for this fuel mix was calculated. Using actual retail prices and price indices from *Statistical Abstracts* and the ratio of the actual prices paid to the retail prices in 1964, we derived the fuel quantities used in other years. Changes in the fuel mix used (primarily the recent trend toward more diesel tractors) may understate the energy in this category slightly in the years since 1964 and overstate it slightly in years before 1964. S. H. Schurr and B. C. Netschert [*Energy in the American Economy, 1850–1975* (Johns Hopkins Press, Baltimore, 1960), p. 774], for example, using different methods, estimate a figure 10 percent less for 1955 than that given here. On the other hand, some retail fuel purchases appear to be omitted from all these data for all years. M. J. Perelman [*Environment (St. Louis)* **14** (No. 8), 10 (1972)] from different data, calculates 270×10^{12} kcal of energy usage for tractors alone.
16. Electricity use on farms: Data on monthly usage on farms were obtained from the "Report of the Administrator, Rural Electrification Administration" (U.S. Department of Agriculture, Government Printing Office, Washington, D.C., various annual editions). Totals were calculated from the annual farm usage multiplied by the number of farms multiplied by the fraction electrified. Some nonagricultural uses are included which may overstate the totals slightly for the years before 1955. Nevertheless, the totals are on the conservative side. A survey of on-farm electricity usage published by the Holt Investment Corporation, New York, 18 May 1973, reports values for per farm usage 30 to 40 percent higher than those used here, suggesting that the totals may be much too small. The discrepancy is probably the result of the fact that the largest farm users are included in the business and commercial categories (and excluded from the U.S. Department of Agriculture tabulations used).
17. Fertilizer: Direct fuel use by fertilizer manufacturers was added to the energy required for the manufacture of raw materials purchased as inputs for fertilizer manufacture. There is allowance for the following: ammonia and related compounds, phosphatic compounds, phosphoric acid, muriate of potash, sulfuric acid, and sulfur. We made no allowance for other inputs (of which phosphate rock, potash, and "fillers" are the largest), packaging, or capital equipment. Source: *Census of Manufactures* (Government Printing Office, Washington, D.C., various recent editions).
18. Agricultural steel: Source, *Statistical Abstracts* for various years (*1*). Converted to energy values according to (*14*).
19. Farm machinery (except tractors): Source, *Census of Manufactures*. Totals include direct energy use and the energy used in the manufacture of steel, aluminum, copper, brass, alloys, and engines converted according to (*14*).
20. Tractors: numbers of new tractors were de-

rived from *Statistical Abstracts* and the *Census of Agriculture* data. Direct data on energy and materials use for farm tractor manufacture was collected in the *Census of Manufactures* data for 1954 and 1947 (in later years these data were merged with other data). For 1954 and 1947 energy consumption was calculated in the same way as for farm machinery. For more recent years a figure of 2.65×10^6 kcal per tractor horsepower calculated as the energy of manufacture from 1954 data (the 1954 energy of tractor manufacture, 23.6×10^{12} kcal, divided by sales of 315,000 units divided by 28.7 average tractor horsepower in 1954). This figure was used to calculate energy use in tractor manufacture in more recent years to take some account of the continuing increase in tractor size and power. It probably slightly understates the energy in tractor manufacture in more recent years.

21. Irrigation energy: Values are derived from the acres irrigated from *Statistical Abstracts* for various years; converted to energy use at 10^6 kcal per acre irrigated. This is an intermediate value of two cited by Pimentel *et al.* (*3*).

22. Food processing industry: Source, *Census of Manufacturers*; direct fuel inputs only. No account taken for raw materials other than agricultural products, except for those items (packaging and processing machinery) accounted for in separate categories.

23. Food processing machinery: Source, *Census of Manufactures* for various years. Items included are the same as for farm machinery [see (*13*)].

24. Paper packaging: Source, *Census of Manufactures* for various years. In addition to direct energy use by the industry, energy values were calculated for purchased paper, plastics, and petroleum wax, according to (*14*). Proportions of paper products having direct food usage were obtained from *Containers and Packaging* (U.S. Department of Commerce, Washington, D.C., various recent editions). [The values given include only proportional values from Standard Industrial Classifications 2651 (half), 2653 (half), 2654 (all).]

25. Glass containers: Source, *Census of Manufactures* for various years. Direct energy use and sodium carbonate [converted according to (*14*)] were the only inputs considered. Proportions of containers assignable to food are from *Containers and Packaging*. Understatement of totals may be more than 20 percent in this category.

26. Steel and aluminum cans: Source, *Census of Manufactures* for various years. Direct energy use and energy used in the manufacture of steel and aluminum inputs were included. The proportion of cans used for food has been nearly constant at 82 percent of total production (*Containers and Packaging*).

27. Transportation fuel usage: Trucks only are included in the totals given. After subtracting trucks used solely for personal transport (all of which are small trucks), 45 percent of all remaining trucks and 38 percent of trucks larger than pickup and panel trucks were engaged in hauling food or agricultural products, or both, in 1967. These proportions were assumed to hold for earlier years as well. Comparison with ICC analyses of class I motor carrier cargos suggests that this is a reasonable assumption. The total fuel usage for trucks was apportioned according to these

values. Direct calculations from average mileage per truck and average number of miles per gallon of gasoline produces agreement to within ± 10 percent for 1967, 1963, and 1955. There is some possible duplication with the direct fuel use on farms, but it cannot be more than 20 percent considering on-farm truck inventories. On the other hand, inclusion of transport by rail, water, air, and energy involved in the transport of fertilizer, machinery, packaging, and other inputs of transportation energy could raise these figures by 30 to 40 percent if ICC commodity proportions apply to all transportation. Sources: *Census of Transportation* (Government Printing Office, Washington, D.C., 1963, 1967); *Statistical Abstracts* (*1*); *Freight Commodity Statistics of Class I Motor Carriers* (Interstate Commerce Commission, Government Printing Office, Washington, D.C., various annual editions).

28. Trucks and trailers: Using truck sales numbers and the proportions of trucks engaged in food and agriculture obtained in (*27*) above, we calculated the energy values at 75×10^6 kcal per trucks for manufacturing and delivery energy [A. B. Makhijani and A. J. Lichtenberg, *Univ. Calif. Berkeley Mem. No. ERL-M310* (revised) (1971)]. The results were checked against the *Census of Manufactures* data for 1967, 1963, 1958, and 1939 by proportioning motor vehicles categories between automobiles and trucks. These checks suggest that our estimates are too small by a small amount. Trailer manufacture was estimated by the proportional dollar value to truck sales (7 percent). Since a larger fraction of aluminum is used in trailers than in trucks, these energy amounts are also probably a little conservative. Automobiles and trucks used for personal transport in the food system are omitted. Totals here are probably significant, but we know of no way to estimate them at present. Sources: *Statistical Abstracts, Census of Manufactures*, and *Census of Transportation* for various years.

29. Commercial and home refrigeration and cooking: Data from 1960 through 1968 (1970 extrapolated) from *Patterns of Energy Consumption in the United States* (*6*). For earlier years sales and inventory in-use data for stoves and refrigerators were compiled by fuel and converted to energy from average annual use figures from the Edison Electric Institute [*Statistical Year Book* (Edison Electric Institute, New York, various annual editions] and American Gas Association values [*Gas Facts and Yearbook* (American Gas Association, Inc., Arlington, Virginia, various annual editions] for various years.

30. Refrigeration machinery: Source, *Census of Manufactures*. Direct energy use was included and also energy involved in the manufacture of steel, aluminum, copper, and brass. A few items produced under this SIC category for some years perhaps should be excluded for years prior to 1958, but other inputs, notably electric motors, compressors, and other purchased materials should be included.

31. There are many studies of energy budgets in primitive societies. See, for example, H. T. Odum [*Environment, Power, and Society* (Wiley, Interscience, New York, 1970)] and R. A. Rappaport [*Sci. Am.* **224** (No. 3), 104 (1971)]. The remaining values of energy subsidies in Fig. 5 were calculated from data presented by Slesser (*9*), Table 1.

32. This article is modified from C. E. Steinhart and J. S. Steinhart, *Energy: Sources, Use, and Role in Human Affairs* (Duxbury Press, North Scituate, Mass., in press) (used with permission). Some of this research was supported by the U.S. Geological Survey, Department of the Interior, under grant No. 14-08-0001-G-63. Contribution 18 of the Marine Studies Center, University of Wisconsin–Madison. Since this article was completed, the analysis of energy use in the food system of E. Hirst has come to our attention ["Energy Use for Food in the United States," *ONRL-NSF-EP-57* (Oct. 1973)]. Using different methods, he assigns 12 percent of total energy use to the food system for 1963. This compares with our result of about 13 percent in 1964.

Excerpted with permission from *Science*, 184:307-316 (19 April 1974). Adapted from a chapter in *Energy: Sources, Use, and Role in Human Affairs*, Carol E. Steinhart and John S. Steinhart, Duxbury Press, North Scituate, Massachusetts, 1974.

Scarce Natural Gas Used to Lacquer Cans

If it's worth wearing a sweater so you can continue to drink beer, is it worth doing so in order to drink it from a throw-away can?

The Joseph Schlitz Brewing Company and the Miller Brewing Company are both building huge new breweries in Syracuse, New York. Both are planning to build can plants adjunct to the breweries already under construction.

The two breweries are asking for a combined annual total of 187 million cubic feet of natural gas for the can plants, for a lacquer-drying process on beer cans. This amount of gas would be enough to provide heat, hot water and cooking for more than 1,000 single family homes in the Syracuse area for an entire year!

The 1971 Public Service Commission (PSC) rulings, predating the breweries requests, placed restrictions on utilities for the attachment of any new customers. The PSC ruling also requires existing industrial gas customers to provide an alternate fuel system if their needs exceed 12,000 mcf annually.

Niagara Mohawk Power Corp. has already denied requests of at least 20 local firms because of the PSC ruling. These rulings were based on Federal Power Commission orders limiting the sale of natural gas by Consolidated Gas Supply Corp. of West Virginia, which supplies gas to Niagara Mohawk Power Corp. in Syracuse.

Tremendous pressure is being put on N.Y. State Governor Hugh Carey, Congressmen and Senators, as well as local officials and industrial leaders, to get the PSC ruling rescinded even though it would mean reducing allocations of existing gas service to commercial and then residential users. The Syracuse Herald Journal quotes Greater Syracuse Chamber of Commerce and Energy Task Force official Frank Lion as advocating spreading the increased cost of alternate fuel and shortages, across existing business *and residential* users.

The breweries are threatening to seek a new location for their can plants if they don't receive the gas allotment they desire, indicating 170 to 200 jobs would go with it. These are presently non-existing jobs.

Reprinted with permission from *Environment Action Bulletin*, 6(3):2 (8 February 1975).

The Other Energy Crisis: Firewood

ERIK P. ECKHOLM

What is the *minimum* energy, other than that directly required for body fuel, that a contemporary human needs for survival? Erik Eckholm of Worldwatch Institute answers that question in this paper on firewood. Survival requires, at a minimum, enough fuel to cook one's daily food. Eckholm points out that in many parts of the world that minimum is becoming harder and harder to acquire. The article excerpted here was printed in *The Ecologist*.

Dwindling reserves of petroleum and artful tampering with its distribution are the stuff of which headlines are made. Yet for more than a third of the world's people, the real energy crisis is a daily scramble to find the wood they need to cook dinner. Their search for wood, once a simple chore and now, as forests recede, a day's labour in some places, has been strangely neglected by diplomats, economists, and the media. But the firewood crisis will be making news—one way or another—for the rest of the century.

While chemists devise ever more sophisticated uses for wood, including cellophane and rayon, at least half of all the timber cut in the world still fulfils its original role for humans— as fuel for cooking and, in some colder mountain regions, a source of warmth. Nine-tenths of the people in most poor countries today depend on firewood as their chief source of fuel. And all too often, the growth in human population is outpacing the growth of new trees—not surprising when the average user burns as much as a ton of firewood a year.[1] The results are soaring wood prices, a growing drain on incomes and physical energies in order to satisfy basic fuel needs, a costly diversion of animal manures for cooking food rather than producing it, and an ecologically disastrous spread of treeless landscapes. . . .

An Economic Burden

The costs of firewood and charcoal are climbing throughout most of Asia, Africa, and Latin America. Those who can, pay the price, and thus must forego consumption of other essential goods. Wood is simply accepted as one of the major expenses of living. In Niamey, Niger, deep in the drought-plagued Sahel in West Africa, the average manual labourer's family now spends nearly one-fourth of its income on firewood. In Ouagadougou, Upper Volta, the portion is 20-30 per cent.[2] Those who can't pay so much may send their children, or hike themselves, out into the surrounding countryside to forage—if enough trees are within a reasonable walking distance. Otherwise, they may scrounge about the town for twigs, garbage, or anything burnable.

It is not in the cities but in the rural villages that most people in the affected countries live, and where most firewood is burned. The rural, landless poor in parts of India and Pakistan are now facing a new squeeze on their meagre incomes. Until now they have generally been able to gather wood for free among the trees scattered through farmlands, but as wood prices in the towns rise, landlords naturally see an advantage in carting available timber into the nearest town to sell rather than giving it to nearby labourers. While this commercialisation of firewood raises the hope that entrepreneurs will see an advantage in planting trees to develop a sustainable, labour-intensive business, so far a depletion of woodlands has been the more common result. *And the rural poor, with little or no cash to spare, are in deep trouble in either case. . . .*

Ecological Consequences

Because those directly suffering its consequences are mostly illiterate, and wood shortages lack the photogenic visibility of famine, the firewood crisis has not provoked much world attention. And in a way there is little point in calling this a world problem, for fuel-wood scarcity, unlike oil scarcity, is always localised in its apparent dimensions. Economics seldom permit fuel wood to be carried or trucked more than a few hundred miles from where it grows, let alone the many thousands of miles traversed by the modern barrel of oil. To say that firewood is scarce in Mali or Nepal is of no immediate consequence to the Boy Scout building a campfire in Pennsylvania, whereas his parents have already learned that decisions in Saudi Arabia can keep the family car in the garage.

Unfortunately, however, the consequences of firewood scarcity are seldom limited to the economic burden placed on the poor of a particular locality. The accelerating degradation of woodlands throughout Africa, Asia, and Latin America, caused in part by fuel gathering, lies at the heart of what will likely be the most profound ecological challenge of the late twentieth century. On a global basis, an ecological threat to human well-being far more insidious and intractable than the industrial pollution of our air and water—which has pre-empted thinking on environmental quality—is the undermining of the productivity of the land itself through soil erosion, increasingly severe flooding, creeping deserts, and declining soil fertility. All these problems are accentuated by deforestation, which is spreading as lands are cleared for agriculture and as rising populations continue their search for firewood. Rainwater falling on tree-covered land tends to soak into the ground rather than rush off; erosion and flooding are thus reduced, and more water seeps into valuable underground pools and spring sources.

The Dust Bowl years in the Great Plains of the thirties taught Americans the perils of devegetating a region prone to droughts. . . .

Dangerous Substitutes

In the Indian subcontinent, the most pernicious result of firewood scarcity is probably not the destruction of tree cover itself, but the alternative to which a good share of the people in India, Pakistan, and Bangladesh have been forced. A visitor to almost any village in the subcontinent is greeted by omnipresent pyramids of handmoulded dung patties drying in the sun. In many areas these dung cakes have been the only source of fuel for generations, but now, by necessity their use is spreading further. Between 300 and 400 million tons of wet dung—which shrinks to 60 to 80 million tons when dried—is annually burned for fuel in India alone, robbing farmland of badly needed nutrients and organic matter. The plant nutrients wasted annually in this fashion in India equal more than a third of the country's chemical fertilizer use. Looking only at this direct economic cost, it is easy to see why the country's National Commission on Agriculture recently declared that "the use of cow dung as a source of noncommercial fuel is virtually a crime.". . .

Even more important than the loss of agricultural nutrients is the damage done to soil structure and quality through the failure to return manures to the fields. Organic materials—humus and soil organisms which live in it—play an essential role in preserving the soil structure and fertility needed for productive farming. Organic matter holds the soil in place when rain falls and wind blows, and reduces the wasteful, polluting runoff of chemical nutrients where they are applied, thus increasing the efficiency of their use. These considerations apply especially to the soils in tropical regions where most dung is now burned, because tropical topsoils are usually thin and, once exposed to the harsh treatment of the burning sun and torrential monsoon rains, are exceptionally prone to erosion, and to losing their structure and fertility.

Peasants in the uplands of South Korea have found another, equally destructive way to cope with the timber shortage. A United Nations forestry team visiting the country in the late 1960s found not only live tree-branches, shrubs, seedlings, and grasses being cut for fuel; many hillsides were raked clean of all leaves, litter, and burnable materials. Raking in this fashion, to meet needs for home fuel and farm compost, robs the soil of both a protective cover and organic matter, and the practice was cited by the U.N. experts as "one of the principal causes of soil erosion in Korea."...

Firewood scarcity, then, is intimately linked to the food problem facing many countries in two ways. Deforestation and the diversion of manures as fuel are sabotaging the land's ability to produce food. Meanwhile, as an Indian official put it, "Even if we somehow grow enough food for our people in the year 2000, how in the world will they cook it?"

A Renewable Resource

The firewood crisis is in some ways more, and in others less, intractable than the energy crisis of the industrialised world. Resource scarcity can usually be attacked from either end, through the conservation of demand or the expansion of supply. The world contraction in demand for oil in 1974 and early 1975, for example, helped to ease temporarily the conditions of shortage.

But the firewood needs of the developing countries cannot be massively reduced in this fashion. The energy system of the truly poor contains no easily trimmable fat such as four to five-thousand-pound private automobiles represent. Furthermore, a global recession does little to dampen the demand for firewood as it temporarily has in the case of oil. The unfortunate truth is that the amount of wood burned in a particular country is almost completely determined by the number of people who need to use it. In the absence of suitable alternative energy sources, future firewood needs in these countries will be determined largely by population growth....

Fortunately trees, unlike oil, are a renewable resource when properly managed. The logical immediate response to the firewood shortage, one that will have many incidental ecological benefits, is to plant more trees in plantations, on farms, along roads, in shelter belts, and on unused land throughout the rural areas of the poor countries. For many regions, fast-growing tree varieties are available that can be culled for firewood inside of a decade.

The concept is simple, but its implementation is not. Governments in nearly all the wood-short countries have had tree-planting programmes for some time—for several decades in some cases. National forestry departments in particular have often been aware of the need to boost the supply of wood products and the need to preserve forests for a habitable environment. But several problems have plagued these programmes from the beginning.

One is the sheer magnitude of the need for wood, and the scale of the growth in demand. Population growth, which surprised many with its acceleration in the post-war era, has swallowed the moderate tree-planting efforts of many countries, rendering their impact almost negligible. Wood-producing programmes will have to be undertaken on a far greater scale than most governments presently conceive if a real dent is to be made in the problem.

The problem of scale is closely linked to a

second major obstacle to meeting this crisis: the perennial question of political priorities and decision-making time-frames. What with elections to win, wars to fight, dams to build, and hungry mouths to feed, it is hard for any politician to concentrate funds and attention on a problem so diffuse and seemingly long-term in nature. Some ecologists in the poor countries have been warning their governments for decades about the dangers of deforestation and fuel shortages, but tree-planting programmes don't win elections....

Even when the political will is there and the funds are allocated, implementing a large-scale reforestation campaign is an unexpectedly complex, and difficult process. Planting millions of trees and successfully nurturing them to maturity is not a technical, clearly boundaried task like building a dam or a chemical fertilizer plant. Tree-planting projects almost always become deeply enmeshed in the political, cultural, and administrative tangles of a rural locality; they touch upon, and are influenced by, the daily living habits of many people, and they frequently end in failure.

Most of the regions with too few trees also have too many cattle, sheep, and goats. Where rangelands are badly overgrazed, the leaves of a young sapling present an appetising temptation to a foraging animal. Even if he keeps careful control of his own livestock, a herdsman may reason that if his animals don't eat the leaves, someone else's will....

In country after country, the same lesson has been learned: tree-planting programmes are most successful when a majority of the local community is deeply involved in planning and implementation, and clearly perceives its self-interest in success. Central or state governments can provide stimulus, technical advice, and financial assistance, but unless community members clearly understand why lands to which they have traditionally had free access for grazing and wood-gathering are being demarcated into a plantation, they are apt to view the project with suspicion or even hostility. With wider community participation, on the other hand, the control of grazing patterns can be built into the programme from the beginning, and a motivated community will protect its own project and provide labour at little or no cost....

Alternative Fuels

Whatever the success of tree-planting projects, the wider substitution of other energy sources where wood is now being used would, if feasible, contribute greatly to a solution of the firewood problem. A shift from wood-burning stoves to those running on natural gas, coal, or electricity has indeed been the dominant global trend in the last century and a half. As recently as 1850, wood met 91 per cent of the fuel needs of the United States, but today in the economically advanced countries, scarcely any but the intentionally rustic, and scattered poor in the mountains, chop wood by necessity anymore. In the poor countries, too, the proportion of wood users is falling gradually, especially in the cities, which are usually partly electrified, and where even residents with little income may cook their food with bottled gas or kerosene. Someone extrapolating trends of the first seven decades of this century might well have expected the continued spread of kerosene and natural gas use at a fairly brisk pace in the cities and into rural areas, eventually rendering firewood nearly obsolete.

Events of the last two years, of course, have abruptly altered energy-use trends and prospects everywhere. The most widely overlooked impact of the fivefold increase in oil prices, an impact drowned out by the economic distress caused for oil-importing countries, is the fact that what had been the most feasible substitute for firewood, kerosene, has now been pulled even farther out of reach of the world's poor than it already was. The hopes of foresters and ecologists for a rapid reduction of pressures on receding woodlands through a stepped-up shift to kerosene withered overnight in December, 1973, when OPEC announced its new oil prices. In fact, the dwindling of world petroleum reserves and the depletion of woodlands reinforce each other; climbing firewood prices encourage more people to use petroleum-based products for fuel, while soaring oil prices make this shift less feasible, adding to the pressure on forests.

Fossil fuels are not the only alternative energy source being contemplated, and over the long term many of those using firewood, like everyone else, will have to turn in other directions. Nothing, for example, would be better than a dirt-cheap device for cooking dinner in the evening with solar energy collected earlier in the day. But actually developing such a stove and introducing it to hundreds of millions of the world's most tradition-bound and penniless families is another story. While some solar cookers are already available, the cost of a family unit, at about $35-50, is prohibitive for many since, in the absence of suitable credit arrangements, the entire price must be available at once. Furthermore, no inexpensive means of storing heat for cloudy days and for evenings has yet been devised.[3]

Indian scientists have pioneered for decades with an ideal-sounding device that breaks down manures and other organic wastes into methane gas for cooking and a rich compost for the farm. Over eight thousand of these bio-gas plants, as they are called, are now being used in India. Without a substantial reduction in cost, however, they will only slowly infiltrate the hundreds of thousands of rural villages where the fuel problem is growing. Additionally, as the plants are adopted, those too poor to own cattle could be left worse off than ever, denied traditional access to dung but unable to afford bio-gas.[4] Still, it is scientific progress with relatively simple, small-scale devices like solar cookers and bio-gas plants that will likely provide the fuel source of the future in most poor countries....

Back to the Basics

Firewood scarcity and its attendant ecological hazards have brought the attitude of people toward trees into sharp focus. In his essay "Buddhist Economics," E.F. Schumacher praises the practical as well as esoteric wisdom in the Buddha's teaching that his followers should plant and nurse a tree every few years.[5] Unfortunately, this ethical heritage has been largely lost, even in the predominantly Buddhist societies of Southeast Asia. In fact, most societies today lack an ethic of environmental cooperation, an ethic not of conservation for its own sake, but of human survival amid ecological systems heading towards collapse.

This will have to change, and fast. The inexorable growth in the demand for firewood calls for tree-planting efforts on a scale more massive than most bureaucrats have ever even contemplated, much less planned for. The suicidal deforestation of Africa, Asia, and Latin America must somehow be slowed and reversed. Deteriorating ecological systems have a logic of their own; the damage often builds quietly and unseen for many years, until one day the system collapses with lethal vengeance. Ask anyone who lived in Oklahoma in 1934, or in Chad in 1975.

References

1. Keith Openshaw, 'Wood Fuels the Developing World,' *New Scientist*, Vol. 61, No. 883, 31 January 1974. See also FAO, *Wood, World Trends and Prospects*, Basic Study No. 16. Rome: 1967, for a brief overview of world fuel-wood trends.

2. J.C. Delwaulle, 'Desertification de l'Afrique au Sud du Sahara,' *Bois et Forets des Tropiques*, No. 149, Mai-Juin 1973, p. 14; and Victor D. DuBois, *The Drought in West Africa*. American Universities Field Staff, West African Series, Vol. XV, No. 1, 1974.

3. See interview with A. Moumoumi, 'Potentials for Solar Energy in the Sahel,' *Interaction* (Washington, D.C.), Vol. III, No. 10, July 1975; National Academy of Sciences, Offices of the Foreign Secretary, *Solar Energy in Developing Countries: Perspectives and Prospects*. Washington, D.C.: March 1972; Farrington Daniels, *Direct Use of the Sun's Energy*. New York: Ballantine Books, 1974 (originally published 1964); Denis S. Hayes, 'Solar Power in the Middle East,' *Science*, Vol. 188, No. 4195, 27 June 1975, p. 1261.

4. C.R. Prasad, K. Krishna Prasad, and A.K.N. Reddy, 'Bio-Gas Plants: Prospects, Problems and Tasks,' *Economic and Political Weekly*, (New Delhi), Vol. IX, Nos. 32-34, Special Number, August 1974;

and Arjun Makhijani with Alan Poole, *Energy and Agriculture in the Third World*. Cambridge, Mass: Ballinger Publishing Co., 1975, esp. Ch. 4.

5.   E. F. Schumacher, 'Buddhist Economics,' in *Small is Beautiful: Economics as if People Mattered*. New York: Harper and Row, 1973.

Excerpted with permission from Worldwatch Paper 1, from *Losing Ground: Environmental Stress and World Food Prospects*, W.W. Norton, 1976. Copyright by Worldwatch Institute, 1776 Massachusetts Avenue, N.W., Washington DC 20036

Strip Mining in the Corn Belt

JOHN C. DOYLE, Jr.

Firewood as a minimum; and as a maximum? What is the *most* energy per capita any society can make use of? As we choke down one electric appliance after another—now a hot dog griller, now a pizza warmer—it is a question we seem determined to answer. With our coal resources, as the energy companies keep reminding us, we have energy to burn. John Doyle's report from the Environmental Policy Institute, from which the following pages are excerpted, urges those responsible for energy policy to keep in mind our need for something to cook, as well as something to cook with.

The Illinois Department of Agriculture estimates that the state is losing farmland at the rate of 80,000 acres a year. During the 10 year period between 1966 and 1975, about 1 million acres of Illinois farmland were lost to all other forms of urban and rural land use. The Illinois South Project has recently estimated that between 5,000 and 6,000 acres of productive Illinois agricultural land is lost each year to strip mining,[43] and the rate is likely to increase in the future if nothing is done to encourage the coal industry to forgo mining strippable reserves in favor of deep minable reserves. At least 172,000 acres of land in 40 Illinois counties have already been disturbed by strip mining, with most of this land being "part of established farms before it was acquired for mining purposes."[44] However, only about 15% of all strippable coal in Illinois has been mined to date.

The U.S. Bureau of Mines has calculated that a mere 3.2 billion tons of strippable Illinois coal,

mined at 37 million tons a year, would last about 88 years.[45] An all-out effort to mine strippable resources in Illinois...could lead to many years of disturbance, if not protracted destruction, of the state's agricultural economy. The potential disruptive time frame for Illinois' agriculture, measured in years of strippable reserves at 70 million tons a year, is nearly 300 years.

There are 19.5 billion tons of strippable coal in Illinois spread over at least 2.5 million acres in 40 counties, and probably many thousands of additional acres in the remaining 11 counties that have strippable coal reserves.[46] It is the nature of strippable coal resources like those found in Illinois to be thin at the surface. The coal resource in Illinois is geologically like a big underground iceberg, the tip of which is only exposed for surface mining at various locations around the state. Strip mining coal in Illinois is literally only "scratching the surface" of the total coal resource there, the largest block of

---

[43] Telephone conversation with Mike Schechtman, Illinois South Project, Carterville, Illinois, April, 1976. See also Illinois Dept. of Mines & Minerals, *1974 Annual Coal, Oil and Gas Report*, Table D, "Mining Permit Lands—Summary of Land Uses During Preceeding Five-Year Period," p.33, (acreage permitted between 7/1/74-12/31/74)

[44] Harold D. Guither, "Illinois Lands Affected By Strip Mining," *Illinois Agricultural Economics*, July, 1974, pp. 13-14.

[45] Bureau of Mines, U.S. Department of the Interior, "Strippable Reserves of Bituminous Coal and Lignite in the United States," BOM Information Circular, IC 8531, 1971, p. 35.

[46] This does not approach the potential figure of agricultural acreage that could be disturbed and/or destroyed by strip mining, especially since indirect and off-site effects of stripping operations can make many additional acres nonproductive for either a temporary or prolonged period of time.

which—about 141 billion tons—is found in thick deep-minable seams.

Strippable Illinois coal then, being geographically spread around the state in relatively thin seams, but being enough of a reserve to put off deep-mining starts in favor of strip-mining starts, will encourage a pattern of surface mining that will have a bit-by-bit, piecemeal impact on the state's agricultural economy, wiping out the economic base of a farm community here and a farm community there, having a slow but certain impact on the overall agricultural economy of the state. Once a farm community is disrupted and its members are forced to seek other forms of employment, there will be little possibility of bringing farmers back to land with an uncertain productive future. Consider the plight of one family farmer in Cherokee County, Kansas, whose local agricultural community once included about 20 family farmsteads:

In the early 1930's a large coal mining company (Gulf Oil Co.'s Pittsburg & Midway) moved their electric shovels into our county and started strip mining coal. They have worked continuously since that time. One by one they bought neighboring farms and proceeded to turn them upside down getting the coal. At this time there are thousands of acres that have been stripped.

The farmers left the area to purchase land elsewhere to farm. This increased demand for land elsewhere, contributed to the inflated price of land to the point it is unrealistic from the investment angle, to the production capabilities and the tax assessment ratio.

Since our land had been in the family for many years, we chose not to sell it to be stripped. They surrounded us with spoil banks. The farms have disappeared due to the digging until they are miles apart. The exodus of these farmers has been so great that it has had a great impact on the economy of the entire county.

They left thousands and thousands of these spoil banks. With the farm economy as it is, I know that if one person were given all the acres laid waste by coal mining, one family could not make a living from it.

The surrounding land that wasn't stripped has been [so] deflated in value due to the environment that it also works a hardship on the few remaining residents.

Since the topsoil is buried up to sixty feet deep, it isn't possible to reclaim this land to a very productive state.... [47]

The same kind of methodical destruction of small, viable agricultural communities has already beset parts of such Illinois counties as Fulton, Knox, Perry and Williamson, and is now moving into Adams, Schuyler and other counties. In Illinois' case, the dimensions of the problem may be even more serious due to the fact that a few large coal companies are retaining the stripped-over agricultural lands for various reasons,[48] including speculation, while other coal interests are going into the business of agriculture for themselves, with subsidiaries like that of Amax's Meadowlark Farms, which now controls about 100,000 acres of land throughout the Midwest.[49]

Peabody Coal Company's description of its "family-unit" farm organization on company-owned land that it uses for "livestock share-leasing" after strip mining conjures up images of "company farms" or even outright feudalism—certainly not the kind of agriculture communities most American farmers are accustomed to:

...Company policy is to reorganize the land into individual family units for a cooperative venture in farming and livestock production

[47] Lloyd Grove, Farmer, Cherokee County, Columbus, Kansas, from letter to the Environmental Policy Center, April, 1976.
[48] "In recent years, the major coal companies have followed a policy of holding most of the lands after stripping is completed. Although the reasons for this policy are not fully known, the most probable are: (1) a desire to retrieve the costs incurred for reclamation; (2) the possible opportunity for large landholders to benefit from the long-term rise in land values; (3) the possibility of new technology making it feasible to take out deeper veins of coal below that already stripped; (4) the convenience of access to lands owned where travel and access may be necessary in mining operations still underway; (5) the profit opportunities from grazing and other productive uses when reclaimed land is properly managed along with unaffected land acquired at the time that stripped land was purchased." Guither, *op. cit.*, p. 17.
[49] Vicke Gowler, "Amax Coal tells of program to reclaim land after mining," *The Quincy Herald-Whig*, January, 1976.

commonly called "livestock share leasing." The reason for the family unit size is that this policy will serve the local community better by preserving and maintaining the social and economic structures of the area. The land and the families seem to integrate back into the agricultural structure of the various communities, thus promoting better relations in the surrounding area.

Having divided the area into farm units of an economic size that will insure a farm family a good income and an additional challenge to increase their income by combining their efforts along with good management, the next step is to put the physical unit into operation. Most areas require extensive fencing which is done with company labor or by contract to a local farmer as off-season work and sometimes the new tenant builds the fence and is reimbursed by the company. Many times, former farm steads, as well as the mine plant sites, can be incorporated into the new units' facilities. In the past, barns and houses have been moved to new locations when possible, taking advantage of ideal sites adjacent to the lakes formed by the mining operations. The lakes insure ample supply of water and provide an excellent family recreation area for the tenants and their friends.[50]

Peabody, and other coal companies in the Midwest, are moving into beef cow-calf operations on their stripped-over farm lands. Their agricultural preference for reclaiming these lands to some productive agricultural use after mining is all too clear:

> ...The most promising and extensive of (agricultural uses) mentioned in Peabody's utilization of mined land is the beef cow-calf herd. At the present time, cows on Peabody's reclaimed pastures number over 5,000 head, managed as direct operations (hired labor), 50-50 livestock

share leases and grazing leases. Of all types of utilization the beef cow herd has the most promise of being successful from both the standpoint of site adaption and demand for the product. The demand in this country as well as most of the world is exceeding the production of beef. Market specialists and economists agree there is a bright future for beef production, particularly cow-calf operations for the next ten years and possible more so in the future.[51]

The unsettling prospect of such developments is that they are changing the character of Illinois agriculture in subtle and not-so-subtle ways: shifting high-yield, row-crop agricultural land to much lower-yield grazing/calving operations.[52] This trend among coal companies with their "agricultural enterprises" on stripped-over croplands in the Midwest, while not a publicly-noticeable change at the moment, is one worth confronting, particularly since the most productive beef cow-calving areas in this nation are those open range lands in our Western and Great Plains states which have the rich and varied native grasses necessary for balanced grazing and proper weight gain.

Perhaps it is no coincidence then that there is a discernible corporate trend toward grazing and calving on stripped-over farmland in the Midwest, while at the same time, our very best grazing lands in the West are also being targeted for their strippable coal reserves. What this country could conceivably end up with, given Project Independence-size surface coal mining appetites and the technologies and government policies big enough and generous enough to feed them, is the complete destruction of our most valuable native grazing lands in the West (like alluvial valley floors), and a shift from row-crop cultivation to grazing/calving operations on considerable portions of our most productive

50 Tom Higgins, Peabody Coal Co., St. Louis, Mo., "The Planning And Economics of Mined-Land Use for Agricultural Purposes," Research and Applied Technology Symposium on Mined-Land Reclamation, March, 1973, Pittsburgh, Pa. p. 148.

51 *Ibid.*, p. 145.

52 It would be ludicrous to even suggest that a calving/grazing operation on reclaimed Illinois farmland would in any way be equal to the value of undisturbed row-crop agricultural land. It may be more valuable to the coal company in terms of easier reclamation and some financial return on grazing, but states and localities would pay dearly, since farmland in Illinois that changes from row-crop agriculture to pasture loses about half its assessed valuation. Moreover, economic returns that would have been realized from continuing row-crop economies will be felt as losses for many years.

lands in states like Illinois, leaving a distinct shortfall of high-capability cropland necessary for growing high-protein grains and beans.

The inevitable corporate/government "agricultural fix" that would emerge under such a scenario would be one that spends millions of dollars on fertilizer, irrigation projects, and agricultural technologies to get minimum yields from marginal and sub-marginal lands.

Such is the "drift" of our lust for energy at any price—a myopic non-policy that will allow high-capability agricultural lands to be strip mined for coal even though there are clearly other alternatives available; alternatives that could preserve our agricultural communities and agricultural economies in *all* regions of the country; alternatives as simple as deep-minable coal or as demanding of commitment as solar energy. In the face of a world that can produce 3 billion people in less time than it takes mother nature to create one inch of fertile topsoil, we had better start moving toward those alternatives with some considerable speed.

Excerpted with permission from the Environmental Policy Institute, Washington DC.

The following item is reprinted in its entirety as it appeared in the Newsletter of the National Agricultural Chemicals Association. Read it and smile...or weep.

Agriculture—the nation's largest industry needs about 15 percent of the total energy consumed in this country. In turn, this industry creates more than $200 billion worth of food and fiber each year. Besides providing for the food needs of some 215 million people in this country, a sizeable portion of this production ends up in export markets. As a result of this export trade in agricultural commodities some $22 to 23 billion is available to pay for much of the petroleum imports upon which the country is becoming increasingly more dependent.

Reprinted from *NAC Newsletter*, p.3 (12 August 1976).

Only About Half of Public Knows U.S. Has to Import Oil

Only a little more than half of the American public is aware that the United States must import oil to meet its energy needs, according to the latest Gallup Poll.

Thirty-three percent of 1,506 adults interviewed April 29 through May 1 in more than 300 communities indicated they believed the country was self-sufficient in oil while 15 percent said they would not venture a guess.

Of those who were aware of the need to import oil, the Gallup organization reported, about a third (9 percent of all adults) knew that the amount shipped into the United States last year was 42 percent.

In the poll, Gallup found that residents of the Northeast and Midwest were more aware of the need to import oil than were people living in the warmer climates of the South and West.

Gallup said that the poll indicated that those who were best informed on the oil situation appeared to be most receptive to the call from President Carter for energy conservation and sacrifice.

For example, the polling organization said, among those who believe that Mr. Carter's proposals call for too many sacrifices on the part of the public 41 percent think "we have enough oil in this country."

Responding to the question, "From what you have heard or read, do you think we produce enough oil in this country to meet our present energy needs or do we have to import some oil from other countries," 52 percent replied "must import," 33 percent replied "produce enough" and 15 percent said "don't know."

Reprinted from the *New York Times* (2 June 1977).

Energy and Food— The Interlocking Crises

In 1970, the Kaiser Aluminum & Chemical Corporation published the fourth in its ongoing "Markets of Change" series, a group of well-written, brilliantly produced special issues of *Kaiser News*. This one was entitled "Food: An Energy Exchange System." To read it was to come away convinced that the only kind of energy used to produce American food was solar. (And, alas, despite their professional concern with calories, nutritionists often fail to credit even the sun.)

Until very recently, most people have thought seriously only about the calories they might get out of eating food, not about the calories that have gone into producing it. Consequently, we have neglected to notice that during the last half century we ceased to eat "potatoes made of solar energy" and, in ecologist Howard Odum's memorable phrase, began to eat "potatoes partly made of oil."[1]

This section has been designed to remind us all 1) of the intimate relationship between our food and energy crises; 2) of the ways in which we have (temporarily?) overstepped the photosynthetic limits; and 3) of the dangers inherent in some of the trade-offs we may be tempted to make in our scramble to maintain our high levels of energy consumption. My students always find the energy readings hard. I always agree with them. They are hard—but important.

Poet William Blake once wrote that energy was "eternal delight." In this chapter's first selection, a more contemporary farmer named Blake reminds us all of the enduring truth of that poetic fact. Energy *is* the common coin of the elemental budget, its availability setting an ultimate limit to food, to life, to *all* growth—even to thought. Blake lays out the basics of energy conversion, rightly emphasizing the miraculousness of the primary step wherein the chlorophyll of green plants transduces light—uses incoming solar energy to convert air, water, and a few minerals into matter substantial enough to bite into.

Both farmer Blake and economist Georgescu-Roegen (in his essay on entropy and economics) emphasize the critical difference between energy *income*—our daily input of solar energy, and energy *capital*—that ancient solar energy transformed by pressure, time and luck into what we know as coal, oil, and gas.

As the excerpt from Kenneth Watt points out, it was a series of "historical accidents" that mistakenly led us to come to think of energy as abundant, and an energy-intensive meat-heavy diet as "natural," when, in fact they have traditionally been scarce and "unnatural." We are now dependent upon ancient fossilized pockets of sunlight which can be used only once. Yet we have been rashly exploiting them to increase our numbers and our standard of living "far in excess of anything which may be sustained when that *capital* has been expended."

Unfortunately, as ecologist Howard Odum has observed, economists who were all trained during a stage of rapid growth "don't even know there is such a thing as a steady state . . . even though most of man's million year history was close to steady state. Only the last two centuries have seen a burst

---

[1] Howard T. Odum, *Environment Power, and Society*, p. 115 (New York: Wiley Interscience, 1971).

of temporary growth because of temporary use of special energy supplies that accumulated over long periods of geologic time."[2]

In nature, Georgescu-Roegen reminds us, things run downhill; order "naturally" degenerates into disorder. Energy once used to do something—anything—is energy no longer available to do something else. Thus what is in conventional economic terms the "value added" by labor when copper ore is smelted into a piece of copper, is in energetic terms "value lost" from the sum total of usable energy on earth. For in all such transactions, part of a finite store of usable energy—coal, oil, gas, electricity—has been converted into unusable heat.

Analyses like those of Georgescu-Roegen have led a number of observers to propose that energy rather than money be used as the common value against which the cost of other energy (and other things) is measured. The critical term here is "net energy," being defined as "the amount of energy that remains for consumer use after the energy costs of finding, producing, upgrading and delivering the energy have been paid."[3] Huettner, whose definition that is, goes on to point out that the idea of using net energy analysis as a general economic measure "rests on the concept of energy as the ultimate limiting factor, since substitutes for other inputs can always be synthesized from it...." For example, if we run out of high grade ores, we can always turn to lower grade ores which require more energy for refining to useful metals. If we run out of fresh water, we can always desalinate sea water—with energy. If we run out of soil fertility we can, and do, synthesize fertilizer by fixing atmospheric nitrogen—using natural gas as a raw material. If we run out of sunlight for photosynthesis, we can always install giant electric lights. And, if we run out of land on which to grow food, we can always synthesize fats, proteins, carbohydrates and vitamins—and mine the minerals we need—but only at an energy cost.

Huettner goes on to point out that *in the long run*, resources other than energy will be constraining, so that from an economist's standpoint net energy analysis is no more perfect than money as a tool for measuring whether one is getting one's "money's worth" from various activities. While the economists argue, however, "optimizing the arrangement of the deck chairs on the Titanic" (in E.F. Schumacher's felicitous phrase), it is important not to lose sight of the fact that where *energy* is the desired *output*, net energy analysis is essential. If you are trying to produce energy, no process can end up being economical, in monetary or energetic terms, which uses up as much or more energy than it produces. For example, if nearly as much energy has to be put into extracting oil from shale as can be got out of the shale oil, it is obvious that shale would not be an "economical" source of energy.

This is why, as Peter Bunyard has written, the rising price of OPEC oil did not end up making it "economic" to go after energy sources that were harder to get. "What the economists appeared to have forgotten was that energy is not quite like any other resource, since it is the basic resource determining the production of every other substance...."[4] Thus "when OPEC oil went up in price, it did not mean, as was naively thought, that other less readily mined sources of energy would become economic; for those sources were as dependent upon OPEC oil for their production as was any other material. Hence, in the North Sea the cost of developing an oil field shot up to nearly double in less than one year." And in the U.S., as elsewhere, the cost of bringing an atomic plant into production became even more prohibitive.

Of course, net energy analysis might not be useful if we had an unlimited supply of energy—if fusion were practical and really "clean" (at the moment it is neither), or if solar energy were fully exploited. Under such circumstances, however, as the brief essay by Heinrich argues, and as a later

[2] Howard T. Odum, "Energy, Ecology and Economics," reprinted in *Mother Earth News* from Ambio, 1973
[3] David A. Huettner, "Net Energy Analysis: An Economic Assessment," *Science* 192: 102 (9 April 1976).
[4] Peter Bunyard, "The Future of Energy in Our Society," *Ecologist* 6 (3): 89 (March/April, 1976).

section will more fully illustrate, we would be at considerable biological risk from the activities such abundant energies would permit us to undertake (or continue).[5]

But what does all this have to do with food? Simply this: Where energy is concerned, food is (or ought to be) a commodity quite different from any other. An activity like smelting steel, for example, inevitably requires an investment of energy capital. Food, on the other hand, does not. For food—plants and the animals which eat the plants—can readily be made of solar energy alone [6]; and since solar energy represents a regular "income," food ought to be a net *producer* of energy, never a sink for energy capital.

The efficiency with which "primitive" agriculturists exploited this energy-storage capacity inherent in man/plant systems was first brought to popular attention through an article on "The Flow of Energy in an Agricultural Society," published by anthropologist Roy Rappaport in a special "Energy and Power" issue of *Scientific American*.[7] Using careful measurements of the human energy expended by a tribe of New Guinea Indians in all the activities necessary to produce their yearly food supply—clearing their forest land, building fences, cultivating and so on—Rappaport found that the Tsembaga Indians "received a reasonable short-term return on their investment. The ratio of yield to input was about 16.5 to one for the taro-yam gardens and about 15.9 to one for the sweet potato gardens." These primitive cultivators, in other words, got about 16 food calories out of their system for every calorie of energy they put into it.

When I first began using Rappaport's article in my classes, in 1971, I would ask the students to guess whether the U. S. agricultural system was more or less efficient than that of the Tsembaga. They, having been properly schooled, already knew American agriculture to be the world's most efficient. It was a trick question, of course, the correct answer to which depended on the meaning one gave to the word "efficient." That much-celebrated American efficiency—measured in yield per man hour—undergoes a curious reversal when energy is counted in the equation. As Michael Perelman's brief article points out, American agriculture, taken as a whole, has a negative net energy yield, requiring three calories in to get one calorie out.

Three months after Perelman's article appeared, David Pimentel and his associates at Cornell University published a detailed analysis of the energy inputs into the production of a single U. S. crop, corn. Noting the concurrence of the food crisis and the energy crisis, they predicted the likely impact of the latter upon the former, given the heavy dependence of "modern" crop production methods on large energy inputs. The included excerpt from their detailed analysis of the energy inputs into the production of a U. S. corn crop is, like other energy analyses, difficult, but important. Their figures show that the largest energy inputs into corn were represented by nitrogen fertilizer, gasoline and the machinery itself. Though little corn was irrigated, the energy costs of irrigation were very high. Their analysis permitted them to make suggestions (omitted from the excerpt reprinted here) for alterations of farming practice designed to cut down on its energy intensiveness. Many of their suggestions, which are summarized in the Steinharts' sequel, sound astonishingly like the practices some "organic" agriculturists have long recommended.

But the energy-saving changes Pimentel, *et al.* suggested usually involve the re-introduction of labor—and labor remains the most expensive input into farming—even at today's inflated energy prices. The question was, could a real farmer afford to make such a change? The answer, or the beginning of an answer, was not long in coming. In July, 1975, the Center for the Biology of Natural

[5] Note that Heinrich assumes energy produced by atomic fusion would be cheap. Benoit (Emile Benoit, "Must Growth Stop?" Pgs. 161 - 182 in: Pfaff, Martin. *Frontiers of Social Thought: Essays in Honor of Kenneth E. Boulding,* North Holland Publishing Co., 1976) among others has pointed out that it is the fuel—sea water—which is cheap. The plants to extract energy from it would be so complex as to make the probability of cheap energy remote.

[6] In fact, the energy they *contain* is *all* solar energy—potatoes are not really made partly out of oil. Oil, as Odum has shown, merely reduces the loss of solar energy to other parts of the system.

[7] Roy Rappaport, *Scientific American*, 224(3): 117+ (September 1971).

Systems in St. Louis, Missouri, published the results of "A Comparison of the Production, Economic Returns, and Energy Intensiveness of Corn Belt Farms That Do and Do Not Use Inorganic Fertilizers and Pesticides." The description of those results—reproduced in this volume from a book by Barry Commoner, Director of the Center—leads one to the conclusion that in the long run farmers can't afford *not to* retreat from their energy-dependence. Commoner's analysis of American agriculture, not dissimilar from that of Pimentel, asks a different question: not how much energy has been used (for he argues that the total *amount* is trivial), but what has happened to all the *profits* from farming?

Thus the circle, which began with economics and led to energy, leads back again to economics. For, as Commoner points out, if the purpose of farming is the capture of solar energy, then the increasing dependence of farmers on energy controlled by a petrochemical industry which is both the farmer's supplier and his competitor explains why, despite its rising "efficiency," farming has not become more profitable. If farming is not profitable, of course, farmers stop farming, and the only ones who can continue to farm are large corporations who may themselves control many of the energy-intensive inputs.

But the energy-intensiveness of agriculture is only a small part of the problem. Most food is not consumed at the farm gate. If our potatoes "partly made of oil" are turned into Pringles by the food industry, clearly they have become more oil-soaked in the process.

The article by Steinhart and Steinhart takes us off the farm. Much more energy is consumed in the transport, processing, storage and cooking of food than is consumed in its on-farm production. Indeed, "food processing and related industries" is the sixth ranking industrial group in terms of energy use, accounting for some 7% of all energy used in the U.S. The Steinharts' figures show that *total* energy use in the food system was 12.8% of the total U.S. energy use in 1970, a figure which is probably conservative (see pg. 309). Over-all, they calculate, the U.S. food system requires something on the order of ten calories of energy input to produce one calorie of energy output (even without counting the original input of solar energy).

(On their energy efficiency chart [Steinhart, Figure 5], it is worth noting the position of distant fishing, i.e., fishing far from one's *own* shore. Keep the illustration in mind when fishing for a tiny shrimp called krill is offered as a "solution" in subsequent reading. The energy cost of distant fishing was, of course, one reason why fish protein concentrate, just below it on the chart, did not turn out to be a useful "low-cost" food. It is also important to take note of the location of feedlot beef on the energy efficiency chart. While there have been a number of disagreements about the precise extent of calorie and protein loss as one moves up from eating grain to eating grain-fed beef, the relative position of such beef on the energy-efficiency chart, compared for example to intensive rice, or corn or even intensive eggs, is an example of the kinds of ecological data that are being used to argue in favor of our moving to a more vegetarian diet.)

Coming off our food energy high would not be easy, even if we decided it would be worthwhile. The individual consumer, finding it hard to make a direct connection between having a throw-away beer can and a cold house, (pg. 318) is likely to continue drinking beer from cans. But the issue may in fact be somewhat more serious than whether or not our houses (or our cars) run out of gas. Energy inputs into food, of which we are just becoming aware, range all the way from the irrigation needed to grow vegetables on the once-desert that is California, to the natural gas used to lacquer throw-away beer cans. What is the cost to the food supply of our ever continuing search for more energy?

Only recently has it been called to our attention that the *demand* for energy, at least partly for energy to produce and process food, has begun to *compete* with food production—both in countries called "developed" and in those designated as "developing." The two articles which close this section simply hint at the complexity of the food/energy relationship. In "Firewood: The Other Energy Crisis," Erik Eckholm poignantly documents the extent to which the struggle for a minimum supply of energy, for cooking and warmth, results in the world's poor destroying the trees and ultimately the topsoil on which their very lives depend. The answer, reforestation, is obvious, but difficult to achieve (as Eckholm points out) when pressures on the land to provide minimum sustenance are so great.

There is much less excuse for *our* apparent indifference to the potentially devastating effects of an all-out search for energy. "Strip Mining in the Corn Belt" documents the trend toward sacrificing the indefinitely replaceable potential energy of food for the one-time energy of coal. When Illinois passed a mining control act in 1962, requiring the disposal of all future refuse from mining activities, 10,000 acres of land were already covered with "gob piles," mountains of acidic waste from abandoned mines. Not only are the costs of reclaiming such land formidable, but there is little chance it can be restored to high levels of productivity. The search for hydroelectric power, and often the simple pork-barrel politics of Washington, frequently threaten to inundate productive farm lands behind large dams. The search for energy from shale may alter ground water patterns and dry up western ranch wells.

No one knows for sure how much energy we can safely continue to use to produce our food. No one knows for sure how much fossil fuel energy remains available off our own shores. No one can yet tell when man's diverse activities (including his massive release of CO_2 through the burning of fossil fuel) will produce major climatic alterations, with unknown effects on the food supply. No one knows for sure whether strip mining in the drier western coal lands would convert grazing land into "National Sacrifice Areas,"[8] *never* productive again (as a National Academy of Sciences report suggested).

What we do know is that the food and energy crises are part of a single crisis of resource allocation and use, so intimately intertwined that we can never again in our search for energy afford to ignore its potential cost in food production capability. Is the energy crisis contrived or real, Bruce Hannon has asked. [9] "The conservative approach is to believe that it is real and act accordingly. If the crisis is real, we shall be viewed by future generations as terribly wise; if the crisis is false, we shall have had an instructive relief from the dancing mirage of our manifest destiny."

The short excerpt which ends the section is from the newsletter of the National Agricultural Chemicals Association. It is included, like the Snoopy cartoon with which the section opened, to remind us all how easy it is to be illogical—about something like energy, which we have so long taken for granted. If we are using energy to grow and process the food which we then export to get the money to import energy, we had better be sure we are coming out ahead.

[8]Robert Gillette, "Western Coal: Does the Debate Follow Irreversible Commitment?" *Science* 182: 456-458 (2 November 1973).
[9]Bruce Hannon, "Energy Conservation and the Consumer," *Science* 189: 95-101 (11 July 1975).

CHAPTER 6

Earth, Air Fire and Water: Problems and Their Solutions

what the ants are saying

DON MARQUIS

dear boss i was talking with an ant
the other day
and he handed me a lot of
gossip which ants the world around
are chewing over among themselves

i pass it on to you
in the hope that you may relay it to other
human beings and hurt their feelings with it
no insect likes human beings
and if you think you can see why
the only reason i tolerate you is because
you seem less human to me than most of them
here is what the ants are saying

it wont be long now it wont be long
man is making deserts of the earth
it wont be long now
before man will have used it up
so that nothing but ants
and centipedes and scorpions
can find a living on it
man has oppressed us for a million years
but he goes on steadily
cutting the ground from under
his own feet making deserts deserts deserts

the ants remember
and have it all recorded
in our tribal lore
when gobi was a paradise
swarming with men and rich
in human prosperity
it is a desert now and the home
of scorpions ants and centipedes

what man calls civilization
always results in deserts
man is never on the square
he uses up the fat and greenery of the earth

each generation wastes a little more
of the future with greed and lust for riches

north africa was once a garden spot
and then came carthage and rome
and despoiled the storehouse
and now you have the sahara
sahara ants and centipedes

toltecs and aztecs was a mighty
civilization on this continent
but they robbed the soil and wasted nature
and now you have deserts scorpions ants and
    centipedes
and the deserts of the near east
followed egypt and babylon and assyria
and persia and rome and the turk
the ant is the inheritor of tamerlane
and the scorpion succeeds the caesars

america was once a paradise
of timberland and stream
but it is dying because of the greed
and money lust of a thousand little kings
who slashed the timber all to hell
and would not be controlled
and changed the climate
and stole the rainfall from posterity
and it wont be long now
it wont be long
till everything is desert
from the alleghenies to the rockies
the deserts are coming
the deserts are spreading
the springs and streams are drying up
one day the mississippi itself
will be a bed of sand
ants and scorpions and centipedes
shall inherit the earth

men talk of money and industry
of hard times and recoveries
of finance and economics
but the ants wait and the scorpions wait
for while men talk
they are making deserts all the time
getting the world ready for the conquering
drought and erosion and desert
because men cannot learn

rainfall passing off in flood and freshet
and carrying good soil with it

because there are no longer forests
to withhold the water in the
billion metriculations of the roots

it wont be long now it wont be long
till earth is barren as the moon
and sapless as a mumbled bone

dear boss i relay this information
without any fear that humanity
will take warning and reform

archy

Reprinted with permission from *Archy & Mehitabel* (Doubleday and Company, Inc., 1933).

The Compost Pit

JOAN GUSSOW

The earth *is* a globe; everything *is* connected to everything else. What I throw over my shoulder *will* come up over the horizon and hit me in the face; without a clean environment we *cannot* produce clean food. Simple truths, here simply stated in a piece first published in the CAN newsletter.

My family and I have a compost pit. Several years ago we began to compost not only the garden wastes, as we always had, but everything that would decay: brown paper bags (when we couldn't avoid them), paper towels (when we had to use them), plus all our vegetable peelings, egg shells, bones and other assorted kitchen scraps. One day I began to think about what went into the compost pit—all those orange rinds with their load of Citrus Red #2, all the fruit peelings with whatever pesticide residues they contained, all the heavy metals used in paper manufacture—anything I threw out was incorporated into that crumbly black compost I dug out and threw into the vegetable garden in the spring. Some of those "additives," I hoped, got broken down by bacteria into harmless forms. But some of them, I suspected, just sat there, waiting to be taken up by my tender spring lettuce and fed to my family.

It was probably just a fantasy—in any case I am still composting, though I did stop throwing in the brown paper bags (largely for superstitious reasons). And I did a lot of thinking about what it really means to say that we live in a closed system—different only in scale from my kitchen-compost-garden-kitchen cycle. What it really means is that once something is there, it's *there.* We can't throw it *away* because in the long run there isn't any "away." This is especially true for those manmade compounds which nature has made no provision for breaking down (a nylon fishing line once somehow got into our compost pit and keeps turning up—absolutely unchanged—every spring). What I am trying to say is that the "purity" and nutritional value of what we eat are defined by the purity and nutritional value of what is available to eat—and the soil it grows in and the air it breathes and the water it uses. We will lose the whole battle if we simply turn inward and contemplate our stomachs.

Reprinted with permission from *Consumer Action Now*, p. 4 (January 1972).

The Undermining of Food-Production Systems

ERIK ECKHOLM

Only in the affluent lands is chemical pollution the principal threat. Elsewhere men stress the ecosystem in less elaborate ways. This sobering assessment is the introduction to Erik Eckholm's important book, *Losing Ground*.

Coaxing enough food from the earth has traditionally been guided by a certain simple logic: plow more land, intensify labor, refine techniques, and the supply of food will grow commensurately. But this has been the logic of humans, not of nature, and today's newspaper headlines tell with increasing frequency a different, more puzzling story. Millions of individuals, and sometimes whole countries, are learning the hard way that more work doesn't necessarily mean more food—that it may mean fatally less.

A Somali nomad builds his herd to record size, but the grassland is overgrazed, his cattle grow thin, and sand dunes bury pastures. A farmer in northern Pakistan clears trees from a mountain slope to plant his wheat; soon after, fields downstream are devastated by severe floods. In Indonesia, a peasant burns away luxurious hillside vegetation to plant his seeds; below, rice production drops as soil washed down the mountain chokes irrigation canals.

Over the course of ten thousand years humans have successfully learned to exploit ecological systems for sustenance. Nature has been shaped and contorted to channel a higher than usual share of its energies into manufacturing the few products humans find useful. But while

ecological systems are supple, they can snap viciously when bent too far. The land's ability to serve human ends can be markedly, and sometimes permanently, sapped.

The international discussion of environmental quality has, like that of many other topics, been largely pre-empted by the rich industrial world. The term "environmental crisis" joined the lexicon of journalism and politics only within the last decade, in response to the visible spread of acrid air and poisoned waters. Even within the field of agriculture, concern for ecological damage usually focuses on the polluting impact of misused chemicals.

These problems are pressing enough, and deserve all the attention they have received and more. Yet in the world war to save a habitable environment, even the battles to purify the noxious clouds over Tokyo and Sao Paulo, and to restore life to Lake Erie, are but skirmishes compared to the uncontested routs being suffered in the hills of Nepal and Java, and on the rangelands of Chad and northwest India. A far deadlier annual toll, and perhaps an even greater threat to future human welfare, than that of the pollution of our air and water is that exacted by the undermining of the productivity of the land itself through accelerated soil erosion, creeping deserts, increased flooding, and declining soil fertility. Humans are—out of desperation, ignorance, shortsightedness, or greed—destroying the basis of their own livelihood as they violate the limits of natural systems....

The littered ruins and barren landscapes left by dozens of former civilizations remind us that humans have been undercutting their own welfare for thousands of years. What is new today is the awesome scale and dizzying speed with which environmental destruction is occurring in many parts of the world. The basic arithmetic of world population growth reveals that the relationship between human beings and the environment is now entering an historically unique age of widespread danger. Whatever the root causes of suicidal land treatment and rapid population growth—and the causes of both are numerous and complex—in nearly every instance the rise in human numbers is the immediate catalyst of deteriorating food production systems. The number of humans reached one billion about 1830, two or three million years after our emergence as a distinct species. The second billion was added in one hundred years, and the third billion in thirty years. One day in late 1975, just fifteen years later, world population reached four billion. At the present rate of growth, the fifth billion will come in thirteen years and the sixth in ten years after that.

Seldom does the imagination translate these inconceivable abstractions into the events on the ground that give them meaning: farmers forced onto mountain slopes so steep that crops and topsoil wash away within a year; peasants making charcoal out of forests that are essential for restraining flood waters and soil erosion; droughtprone pastures plowed up for grain despite the high odds that a lifeless dust bowl will ensue. In some respects, these are Malthusian phenomena with a twist. Exponentially growing populations not only confront a fixed supply of arable land, but sometimes they also cause its quality to diminish. However, a second addendum to Malthus' gloomy formulation is also crucial. Today the human species has the

knowledge of past mistakes, and the analytical and technical skills, to halt destructive trends and to provide an adequate diet for all using lands well-suited for agriculture. The mounting destruction of the earth's life-supporting capacity is not the product of a preordained, inescapable human predicament, nor does a reversal of the downward slide depend upon magical scientific breakthroughs. Political and economic factors, not scientific research, will determine whether or not the wisdom accumulating in our libraries will be put into practice....

Earlier in this century a number of analysts, concerned primarily with the threat of soil erosion, catalogued the ecological calamities impending if humans did not change their ways. Erosion was sometimes painted as the greatest single threat to the future of human civilization. In the 1930s, as the Great Plains heartland of North America wasted away into the Dust Bowl—one of the century's more dramatic environmental debacles—previous warnings achieved an air of prophecy.

Then, as the Great Plains were recovering from their human-caused infirmity, World War II created environmental disasters of a different type and scale, and was followed by an era of economic expansion such as the world had never before seen. World agriculture, too, entered an era of remarkable gains, with global grain output far outpacing population growth since the late forties. Headlong economic growth in the richer countries, and in small pockets of the poorer countries, has created new environmental challenges as the refuse of industrialism piles up, but earlier predictions that land degradation would be humanity's downfall seem to have been disproved by history.

Or have they? The continuing growth in world food output and the remarkable climb of the gross national product in most countries, rich and poor, over the last two decades mask some basic facts that add up to a different story. National income averages conceal the billion or more people locked in cycles of abject poverty, misery, and exploitation, many of whom live in worse conditions than their parents did. World, and even national, food output totals conceal the stagnant or deteriorating productivity of huge numbers of farmers in the poorer regions and countries. Such figures veil the half-billion people suffering chronic malnutrition in the best of years, and the hundreds of millions who join their lot when food prices soar, as they have in the mid-seventies. The statistics of progress ignore the swelling urban shanty-town filled with refugees from untenable rural situations. In short, the aggregate figures for growth, both of agriculture and economics, disregard the casualties and the cast-offs of the global development process....

Ecological degradation is to a great extent the *result* of the economic, social, and political inadequacies noted above; it is also, and with growing force, a principal *cause* of poverty. If the environmental balance is disturbed, and the ecosystem's capacity to meet human needs is crippled, the plight of those living directly off the land worsens, and recovery and development efforts—whatever their political and financial backing—become all the more difficult. The soft underbelly of global rural development efforts, environmental deterioration is an often neglected factor that severely undermines their effectiveness.

The glaring disregard of the ecological requisites of progress is at least partially attributable to the rigid compartmentalization of professions, both in the academic world and in governmental agencies. When reading the analyses of economists, foresters, engineers, agronomists, and ecologists, it is sometimes hard to believe that all are attempting to describe the same country. The actions of experts frequently show the same lack of mutual understanding and integration. Engineers build one dam after another, paying only modest heed to the farming practices and deforestation upstream that will, by influencing river silt loads, determine the dams' lifespan. Agricultural economists project regional food production far into the future using elaborate, computerized models, but without taking into account the deteriorating soil quality or the mounting frequency of floods that will undercut it. Water resource specialists sink wells on the desert fringes with no arrangement to control nearby herd sizes, thus ensuring overgrazing and the creation of new tracts of desert. Foresters who must plant and protect trees among the livestock and firewood gatherers of the rural peasantry receive excellent training in botany and silviculture, but none in rural sociology; their saplings are destroyed by cattle, goats, and firewood seekers within weeks after planting.

A failure to place agriculture in its ecological context has been apparent at even the highest levels of global policy-making. Nowhere were forests so much as mentioned in the dozens of resolutions directed to eliminating hunger passed by the Rome World Food Conference of November, 1974, despite the accelerating deforestation of Africa, Asia, and Latin America and its myriad effects on food production prospects. The editors of the United Nations magazine *Ceres* were not speculating idly when they wrote in early 1975: "It is no coincidence that the forests of all the countries with major crop failures in recent years due to droughts or floods—Bangladesh, Ethiopia, India, Pakistan, and the Sahel countries—had been razed to the ground."

Even without the impediment of professional or disciplinary blinders, recognizing and controlling the causes of environmental deterioration present special problems. Precise figures on ecological trends and their impact on agricultural systems are scarce. This does not make the trends any less real or menacing; it does suggest the exceptional difficulty of isolating and measuring these factors....

World fisheries present an instructive, readily measured example of what happens when too much is demanded of a food-producing ecosystem. In this case it is more often the rich than the poor who have neglected ecological reality and reaped the penalties. While the differences between farming the land and extracting food from the oceans are obvious, declining catches in numerous regional fisheries demonstrate clearly that greater effort and investment can bring not just diminishing returns but, as fish stocks are depleted by overfishing, *negative* returns. And in the early seventies, the sum of these local pressures produced a three-year sustained drop in the total *global* fish catch. We must now ask how many localized land regions have already experienced similar absolute declines in food output due to environmental degradation—and how many entire countries may be following suit, as some in central Africa apparently have already.

Rapid population growth, miserable social conditions, and environmental deterioration form the ultimate vicious circle.... The only alternative at this stage of human history is to simultaneously meet this quandary at every point along its circumference, in an all-out effort to turn the negative chain reactions into positive ones....

Excerpted with permission from *Losing Ground, Environmental Stress and World Food Prospects*, W.W. Norton & Company, Inc. Copyright 1976 by Worldwatch Institute.

The Revolution in American Agriculture

JULES B. BILLARD

It seems only yesterday that modern agriculture was promising to save us all. And it *was* only yesterday. These precious 700 words we were given permission to quote represent less than a page of what was a lavish, colorfully-illustrated 39-page article in the February, 1970 issue of the *National Geographic*. A tantalizing taste—enough, one hopes, to let the optimistic flavor come through.

In a single lifetime, United States agriculture has advanced more than in all the preceding millenniums of man's labor on the land. To witness this revolution firsthand, I traveled the length and breadth of the Nation.... In California I watched a factory-on-wheels move down celery rows—severing, trimming, washing, crating, doing the work of forty men....I handled tomatoes bred for machine harvesting in one of today's amazing developments in plant genetics. I learned about heating cables buried underground to warm the soil so asparagus can grow in December....

The revolution farmers have fashioned may even be a major weapon in the battle against one of the gravest problems facing the world: the population explosion....The spread of modern agriculture...can help us buy time against world famine while we press efforts to control the mounting population. As Dr. George W. Irving, Jr., research administrator of the U.S. Department of Agriculture put it: "Our agricultural revolution is setting up things so that other nations can telescope what we have done."

... [There is] an incredible parade of machines at work today on U. S. farms: acre-eaters that in an hour can plow a hundred times as much land as a farmer with a string of oxen. Self-propelled combines that permit a man to ride in an air-conditioned cab to harvest a crop of corn that used to take a crew of 80 hands.... Helicopters to spray cucumber fields. In all, such a host of devices that today U. S. farmers are investing eight times as much capital as they did thirty years ago....

This trend to bigness and specialization finds no sharper examples than in the Nation's poultry industry.... Julius Goldman's Egg City, 50 miles northwest of Los Angeles...has two million hens. Julius Goldman got into the egg business in 1951... "In those days a farmer might make only a dollar or so a year per bird," Mr. Goldman said. "Now he's lucky to make half that. To gain efficiency we had to expand." ...I saw what that expansion has required: A mill to produce the 250 tons of feed a day.... Two wells to supply a daily demand for 100,000 gallons of water. A packing plant that cleans, inspects and packages a million eggs a day. Block-long buildings, each housing 90,000

White Leghorns, cooped five birds to a 16 by 18 inch cage, and with row after row of cages suspended three feet above the floor. ... A little tractor came by, equipped with an arm that plowed through the droppings on the floor beneath the cages...120 *tons* a day....

I got a more jolting awakening when I roamed the feed lots of the Blair Cattle Company in Blair, Nebraska. "One cow produces as much waste as 16 humans," Harry J. Webb, the company's president said matter-of-factly. "With 20,000 animals in our pens, we have a problem equal to a city of 320,000 people. But we kept that in mind when we bought this place."... Now four miles of feed bunkers and concrete roadways to service them lace the one-time grain farm. A quarter-million-dollar feed mill rolls corn into tasty flakes and mixes a molasses-flavored ration that puts 2.7 pounds of weight on a steer every day....

What will farming of the future be like? Dr. Irving...summed up a few of its facets for me. "Agriculture will be highly specialized," he said. "Farms in one area will concentrate on growing oranges, those in another area tomatoes, in another potatoes.... Fields will be larger, with fewer trees, hedges and roadways. Machines will be bigger and more powerful and able to do more operations in fewer trips across the land.... They'll be automated, even radio controlled with closed circuit TV to let an operator sitting on a front porch monitor what is going on. It isn't difficult to visualize agricultural plots several miles long and a hundred feet wide. Equipment straddling the strip will roll on tracks or paved runways...without a wheel-touch compacting the soil in the cultivated areas.... Such things sound fantastic, but already they exist in pilot form or in the research stage."

Excerpted with permission from *National Geographic,* 137 (2): 117+ (February 1970).

Soil and Oil

CORNELIUS H. M. VAN BAVEL

Where has the revolution gone? Where are the farms of the future—treeless, shrubless, hedgeless? "Eroding," says this brief editorial from *Science.* Echoing the final refrain of the last chapter, van Bavel reminds us of another connection between energy and food. Not only are we stripmining our corn lands to *find* energy, but we are mining our topsoils to pay for it.

Americans are perhaps tired of being reminded that annual oil imports have risen to 400 million metric tons per year, equivalent to 16 quads of energy, and costing $36 billion. They do not hear as much about a counterflow of agricultural products, mostly grains and soybeans, that has increased to 100 million metric tons per year, valued at $23 billion. These farm products represent a relatively small investment of 0.5 quad of fossil energy for machines, fuel, and fertilizers.

Thus, in large measure, the bounty of our farms supports and extends the profligacy of our energy consumption. At first sight, this trade-off between solar energy trapped in plants and the energy in nonrenewable petroleum resources may appear to be a profitable long-term arrangement.

But can the current levels of productivity in the corn, wheat, and soybean heartlands be sustained? In 1971, it was estimated that in the North Central United States, 67 percent of all cropland needed conservation treatment. Since then, highly erosive and sloping soils have been placed in production of export crops, replacing forage crops.

The seriousness of the erosion problem is further indicated by a more recent analysis showing that unrestricted land use would result in a national soil loss figure of 20 metric tons per hectare per year, twice as high as the maximum tolerable rate, according to expert opinion. This could imply that for each ton of grain going to Europe or Japan, we export several tons of topsoil to the Gulf of Mexico!

Soil is a crucial element in the farm production equation. How shall we live, if both soil and oil are depleted? Perhaps we need a negative severance tax on sediment—that is, payments for keeping soil in place. This idea was basic to the national soil conservation policy that has succeeded in breaking the back of the erosion problem, but not in reducing it to a tolerable level.[1] Meanwhile, the programs implementing the policy have been allowed to wither over the past two decades.

Ironically, this neglect is in part attributable to the phenomenal success of another national policy of even longer standing, namely federal-state cooperation in the use of public funds for farm production research, development, and demonstration.

Historical trends suggest that soil losses are not necessarily caused by high yields: good conservation and high productivity are compatible. But it is equally clear that some soils are being mined. The implication is that the free-

---

[1]See L. J. Carter, *Science,* 22 April 1977, page 409.

dom to use any land for any purpose is to be tempered with a judgment as to how the private and the common enduring interests are best served.

Who is responsible for this? Soil conservation practices often appear not to be good business over the short haul. We should not depend on ethically inspired voluntarism any more than we can in other conservation issues. The stewardship challenge is one for the nation and its institutions, to be met through a voluntary partnership based on material interests. But a mere revival of the old system and adequate funding of existing programs will not be sufficient.

Farm operations can have a significant en-vironmental impact, and undue loss of soil is classified as a nonpoint pollution source. Granting blanket exemptions for farm operations or regimentation through permits and fines are nonsolutions. But much can be said for an amalgam of short-term risk sharing in the production and marketing of crops with long-term risk sharing in the conservation of soils, as long as participation is voluntary.

Such a policy may not be popular. But it is fair to ask whether protection against the vagaries of weather and markets should be extended without assured conservation of the soil resource. Without such a provision, our now profitable solar energy enterprise may well decline through a bad trade of soil for oil.

Reprinted with permission from *Science*, 197: 213 (15 July 1977). Copyright 1977 by the American Association for the Advancement of Science.

Soil Erosion: The Problem Persists Despite the Billions Spent on It

LUTHER J. CARTER

The "ultimate vicious circle" of which Eckholm speaks at the end of his essay in this chapter grows out of the need of desperate humans to grow food...and, as van Bavel suggests, out of the desire of hard-pressed American farmers to wrest the maximum profit from their land. Here Luther Carter, in a report for *Science* magazine, points out in more detail the reasons why and the extent to which we are heedlessly losing our precious and once abundant topsoil.

The dust storms that have swept part of the Great Plains in recent months have been for many people a surprising reminder of the 1930's, when such storms were so devastating as to drive thousands of people from their farmsteads. And, in truth, conditions of the kind that produced the "Dust Bowl" in the southern Great Plains 40 years ago have in some areas reasserted themselves ominously.

Yet, while drought, high winds, and blowing dust have brought severe hardship and even ruin to many farmers this year, the chief significance of the dust storms does not lie in their immediate effects, however distressing. Rather, the dust storms are especially significant as spectacular if redundant evidence that effective soil conservation of the kind necessary to sustain the agricultural productivity of the Great Plains and other farming regions over the long term simply has not been achieved.

Indeed, although nearly $15 billion has been spent on soil conservation since the mid-1930's, the erosion of croplands by wind and water (in most of the United States, erosion is caused chiefly by water) remains one of the biggest,

most pervasive environmental problems the nation faces. The problem's surprising persistence apparently can be attributed at least in part to the fact that, in the calculations of many farmers, the hope of maximizing short-term crop yields and profits has taken precedence over the longer term advantages of conserving the soil. For, even where the loss of topsoil has begun to reduce the land's natural fertility and productivity, the effect is often masked by the positive response to heavy applications of fertilizer and pesticides, which keep crop yields relatively high.

This complacency on the part of a large part of the farming community helps explain why, in all the public and political furor over environmental problems during the last decade, soil erosion has received so little attention. Yet water pollution can never be eliminated as a serious national problem until the flow of farm sediments into rivers and streams is drastically reduced.

In fairness to the farmer, his tendency to put short-term profits ahead of conservation is not simply a matter of greed, for he has been feeling the effects of inflation and sharply rising costs for tractor fuel, pesticides, labor, and equipment. Many farmers struggle under a growing indebtedness, and their need for increased returns is often very real. Nevertheless, a failure to reduce erosion to acceptable levels—or to where soil losses are not much greater than accretions—could lead sooner or later to a major decline in crop yields.[1]

Familiar Remedies

Soil specialists generally agree that erosion can be reduced to tolerable levels by long-familiar engineering and biological methods and practices. These include contour plowing; terracing; stripcropping (with strips of wheat or other grain crops that give little soil protection alternating with strips of grass or legumes); rotating crops to improve soil structure; leaving harvest residues or litter on the soil surface; converting marginal erosion-prone land from crop production to pasture; planting shelterbelts or windbreaks; and—of increasing importance—practicing "minimum tillage," or disturbing the soil as little as possible in planting operations and thereby leaving strips of sod between crop rows.

(According to estimates of the U.S. Department of Agriculture (USDA), if minimum tillage practices were extended to 80 percent of all U.S. croplands—as compared to the 10 percent covered at the end of 1974—this in itself would reduce soil erosion by 50 percent or more. The continuing spread of minimum tillage, which offers the further advantage of reducing labor costs and the loss of soil moisture, is said to be one of the few encouraging new developments with respect to soil conservation.)

The seriousness of the soil erosion problem was pointed out 2 years ago in a little-noticed report prepared for the Senate Committee on Agriculture and Forestry by the Council for Agricultural Science and Technology (CAST), which is made up of representatives of about a dozen professional groups having to do with soil science, animal husbandry, seed improvement, agricultural engineering, meteorology, and the like. The CAST report said, among other things, that "five problem conditions are evident which could trigger a dust bowl" in the Great Plains and perhaps a part of the Corn Belt if a sustained drought were to occur.

One was that Great Plains farmers were reported to be changing from wheat-fallow or wheat-sorghum-fallow rotations to continous planting of wheat in order to take advantage of high wheat prices, even though this was eliminating strip-cropping for wind erosion control. Also, by plowing with moldboard plows to bury the seed of downy bromegrass (a pest that reduces yields when wheat is grown continuously from year to year without rotation), many farmers were leaving the surface bare of harvest residues that help hold the soil in place.

The other conditions cited were the extensive leveling of fields (in some cases creating barren patches of erosion-prone sand) to permit the installation of the new wheeled irrigation systems that turn in a wide arc from a center pivot; the conversion of rangeland to grain production in response to high prices for grain and low prices for cattle, an unfavorable development from the standpoint of soil conservation because of the greater susceptibility of cropland to wind erosion; and the increasing practice in the Corn Belt of plowing cropland in the fall and turning under the stubble or harvest litter that would otherwise have helped protect the soil from winter and spring winds.

Addressing the soil erosion problem nationally, the CAST report said more than a third of all cropland was suffering soil losses too great to be sustained without a gradual, but ultimately disastrous, decline in productivity. It is generally accepted among soil scientists that even "deep soils" cannot sustain a loss of more than 5 tons an acre per year without hurting productivity. Such scientists therefore see real

---

[1]See the article "Land degradation: Effects on food and energy resources" by D. Pimentel *et al.* (*Science,* 8 October 1976). According to the authors, 4 billion tons of sediments are carried by surface runoff into waterways of the 48 contiguous states each year, and three-fourths of it comes from farmland. They estimate that another billion tons of soil is lost through wind erosion, with by far the greater part of this loss occurring in the West.

cause for alarm in the fact that erosion losses nationally have been variously estimated at about 9 or 12 tons an acre per year, and that, in extreme cases, losses of 60 tons or more are recorded. Under normal farming conditions— discounting erosion losses—new topsoil forms at a rate of about 1.5 tons an acre per year.

As noted in the CAST report, the Soil Conservation Service's most recent *Conservation Needs Inventory* (published in 1967), reported that farmers in 7 of the 12 Corn Belt states were doing a better job of protecting highly erodible cropland in 1958 than they were a decade later, and that, furthermore, only 36 percent of the some 472 million acres of cropland existing in 1967 had been adequately "treated against soil erosion through such practices as strip-cropping and terracing."

Program Failures

In February, the General Accounting Office (GAO) issued a report[2] that helps explain why past soil conservation efforts have not been more effective. Representatives from GAO visited a total of 283 farms, chosen at random, in the Corn Belt, the Great Plains, and the Pacific Northwest and found that 84 percent of them were losing more than 5 tons of soil an acre per year on those croplands for which measurements were made. Even more disturbing was the fact that there was no evidence that the soil losses were consistently smaller for the farmers who had been participating in USDA conservation programs than for those who had not. Losses for both groups were found to be "well above the maximum tolerable level."

The GAO said that USDA, which has been spending several hundred million dollars annually on various soil conservation programs, had not been actively seeking out those farmers most in need of help; that in the case of the farmers the department had helped, it had not done enough to encourage them to carry out their conservation plans effectively and over the long term; and that less than half of the money ... had been used for measures primarily oriented toward conserving the nation's topsoil and that most of it had gone for improving crop yields. The GAO said that because of this, Iowa—the first state to establish a cost-sharing program for soil conservation—had withdrawn from the ASCS program after only 1 year. The GAO indicated that Congress as well as USDA was responsible for this situation because recent appropriations measures had allowed farmers and the local soil conservation districts wide discretion as to which practices to follow.

A particular criticism which the GAO made of the Soil Conservation Service (SCS) was that its some 2750 district conservationists spend a substantial part of their time preparing elaborate conservation plans for individual farms which are seldom followed and soon become out of date. Less than half of the 119 farmer "cooperators" whom the GAO visited were using the plans the service had prepared for them.

Thomas Barlow, a member of the Washington staff of the Natural Resources Defense Council (NRDC), a private activist group, says that the fundamental weakness in the soil conservation programs is that they are not effectively linked to USDA programs to which farmers look for economic security, namely those that provide price supports, farm loans, crop insurance, and disaster relief....

Actually, there has been a linkage between farm price supports and conservation practices going as far back as 1935, the year that the SCS was created as a part of Franklin D. Roosevelt's New Deal. But during most of this 40-year period, the farm commodity markets have been plagued with surpluses, and it has been relatively easy to persuade farmers to withdraw substantial acreages from crop production and convert them to pasture, shelterbelts, or other uses consistent with soil conservation.

In more recent years, however, as farm sur-

[2]Entitled *To Protect Tomorrow's Food Supply, Soil Conservation Needs Priority Attention*, this document (CED-77-30) can be obtained from the General Accounting Office Distribution Section, Room 4522, 441 G. Street, NW, Washington, D.C. 20548 for $1 (the report is free for students, teachers, libraries, and nonprofit groups).

pluses have been eliminated with the growth of overseas markets, farmers have felt a strong incentive—both because of the rising commodity prices and (in many cases) their growing indebtedness—to put as much of their land into production as possible....

The Senate has already taken a major step in response to the soil erosion problem by passing the Land and Water Resources Conservation Act of 1977. This measure, now pending action in the House Committee on Agriculture, would require USDA to prepare an appraisal of land and water conservation problems—and an action program and statement of policy to go with it—by the end of 1979....

M. Rupert Cutler, USDA's new assistant secretary for conservation, research, and education, told *Science* that the most promising new approach to the soil conservation problem will be through section 208 of the Clean Water Act of 1972. Under this section, each state is required to submit to the Environmental Protection Agency (EPA), by 1 November 1978, an enforceable plan for abating pollution from all identifiable sources, including such "nonpoint" sources as farmland....

But a question that EPA and USDA have not yet seriously dealt with is what to do about those farmers—and there could be many—who prove unwilling to adopt essential soil conservation practices. Section 208 leaves it to the states to provide the sanctions needed to bring recalcitrants into line. Yet, while some 18 states have enacted sedimentation control laws, Joseph Krevac, EPA's branch chief for "nonpoint" water pollution sources, says that in all but two of these states—Pennsylvania and Iowa—erosion associated with farming activities has been exempted.

Congress may find that...the most readily available sanction for enforcing compliance with 208 plan objectives is to make the adoption of adequate soil conservation practices a condition for participation in USDA financial assistance programs. And, since Congress has required floodplain zoning and the floodproofing of buildings as a condition for federal flood insurance, one can certainly argue that it would make equally good sense to insist on soil conservation practices as a condition for future farm loans, crop insurance, disaster relief, and maybe price supports.

The very idea of such a thing may be upsetting to farm groups....

Secretary of Agriculture Bob Bergland acknowledges that the soil erosion problem is severe, and his office has a policy review of it now underway. "We are losing 15 tons of topsoil out of the mouth of the Mississippi River every second," he observed at his Senate confirmation hearing. "We know we cannot do that forever. And yet we have only begun to scratch the surface in our conservation activities."

If the Administration does take up the Barlow proposal, there will be some other circumstances that may work in its favor. One is that farmers and the senators and representatives who speak for them in the Congress may conclude that, to obtain passage this year of the kind of farm bill the agricultural community favors, they had better not get at cross-purposes with the Administration and the environmentalists on a major issue of land stewardship. Another is that, with the scenes of billowing clouds of dust blowing in the wind on the Great Plains still fresh in everyone's memory, the public will know that the past stewardship leaves plenty to be desired.

Excerpted with permission from *Science*, 196:409-411 (22 April 1977). Copyright 1977 by the American Association for the Advancement of Science.

Rain Induced Erosion and Its Prevention

T. F. SHAXSON

Like the wind of the Great Plains, the torrential rainfall of the tropics is an enemy of the farmer, a producer of erosion. Modern "clean cropping" encourages soil loss from both causes and, as the excerpt reproduced here points out, what have been called "organic" farming practices turn out to be soil- as well as energy-saving. Shaxson's article appeared first in the May/June issue of the *Soil Association* in 1975.

This article, written by a member engaged in conservation work in Malawi, is published with the permission of the Ministry of Agriculture and Natural Resources, Malawi. It will be of particular interest to overseas members.

1. Introduction

In many parts of the world where intensities of rainfall in excess of about one inch per hour are to be expected, much thought and effort is needed in the prevention and control of accelerated soil erosion and in the reclamation of eroded lands. For many, a picture of erosion effects is given by stark photographs of gullied land in the last stages of exhaustion. But as Elwell has put it, "The soil is removed so gradually, so continually, that it is like the wearing-out of a suit which goes on unnoticed until, one day, it is threadbare. What was once an object of admiration and pride is used less and less until it is finally discarded. So it is with soil." In other words, once the gullies begin to form, the most

significant damage has already occurred.

The nub of the problem posed by soil erosion is that *while* it is occurring, fertile topsoil particles are being removed from around the nutrient-absorbing surfaces of the plants' root hairs; *after* it has occurred the soil is in an impoverished state, providing a poorer medium for plant growth in the following season.

The measure of erosion's true effects would be better given by statements of quantity of lost plant production than by quantities of soil and water collected downstream. Unfortunately the former is much more difficult to measure than the latter.

In the face of rising world population and requirements for better standards of living we cannot afford to tolerate the insidious and widespread effects of erosion which limit plant production. In the past much reliance has been placed on mechanical measures to heal the worst scars of erosion and, hopefully, to prevent more occurring. The purpose of the following article is to show how scientific sensitivity to land and soil conditions assists effective prevention of erosion, and how biological and mechanical measures are interrelated in minimising damage by unavoidable run-off water.

2. *The erosion process*

When the rate of removal of topsoil exceeds the rate of soil formation, accelerated erosion occurs. This results from the interaction of the erosivity of the climate with the erodibility of the land in any particular place.

In Britain there is little erosion of this sort, not because some soils are not potentially erodible (witness the wind erosion in East Anglia) but because the maximum rainfall intensities in most places generally do not exceed one inch an hour—in other words, the erosivity of the rainfall aspect of climate is low.

In many parts of the world however rainfall intensities may reach 10-12 inches per hour for a quarter of an hour or so during storms. The more frequently such storms occur, and the higher the intensities, the more erosive is the rainfall.

In these conditions the primary effect of rainfall is to dislodge soil particles from their resting place, while the main effect of subsequent run-off water is to transport dislodged soil materials. In so doing run-off water may or may not also cut gullies.

On reaching a bare soil surface, big raindrops' energy is dissipated by dislodgement of soil particles, splashing of these into the air (as much as three feet vertically and six feet horizontally) and compaction of the soil surface by ramming finer particles into the interstices between the larger ones, creating a surface that is less and less permeable to rain-water as time goes on. Thus, on bare soil, a decreasing proportion of incident rainfall enters the soil, while an increasing amount collects on and begins to run over the surface.

It is important to note that, while this compaction effect is also produced by passage of animals' feet and of machinery, it can also be produced *by rainfall alone* in areas of high-inten-

sity storms. This explains why severe erosion can occur on lands where animals or machines seldom if ever pass.

The key to minimising soil dislodgement—the precursor of soil loss—is thus to break the force of large high-energy raindrops by interposing a permeable barrier above or on the otherwise bare soil surface, such as the leaves and stems of natural vegetation or planted crops, an organic or inorganic mulch, or even (as experiments have shown) such diverse materials as mosquito-gauze or hessian suspended a little way above the surface.

If the surface can be maintained in a permeable condition by preventing this serious effect of rainfall impact, the soil will absorb more of the water and in so doing the volume available for the transporting functions of run-off will be minimised.

Trouble can be expected both where the soil surface is bare because no crop cover has yet developed in the early part of the rainy season, and also where the cover already there has been thinned or depleted by excessive grazing or too-frequent fires.

Thus, in the first instance, close attention to providing a dense effective cover to the soil not only encourages better yields of plant material from each acre, but at the same time minimises risk of erosion.

3. *The significance of organic matter:*

Organic matter both above, on, and incorporated into the soil surface is of primary importance in prevention of erosion and run-off. Not only does material at the surface dissipate the force of heavy rainfall, but also supplies to soil micro-organisms the substrate for production of humic gums which markedly contribute—together with the mechanical effects of plant roots—to the stability of soil structural units. Soil structural units that are weak (for whatever reason) permit more easy dislodgement of soil particles, and slump more readily than strong units under high-intensity rainfall.

In such conditions mechanical cultivations, if used injudiciously, can break down otherwise stable structural units and enhance erosion hazard. However, cultivation does have a role to play in breaking up more or less impermeable crusts that may have formed as a result of rainfall action, complementary to any requirements for tillage *per se*.

Reprinted with permission from *The Soil Association*, pp. 5+ (May/June 1975).

In a recent Seminar of Shifting Cultivation held in Nigeria, loss of organic matter in tropical soils was singled out as the most important factor in rendering land more prone to erosion.

In this context, principles of organic farming and gardening take on an added vital significance, being one of the main lines of defence against erosion....

Threats to the Atmosphere

MICHAEL B. McELROY

For a number of years I had a file folder on air-pollution, despite the fact that I hadn't yet decided what air-pollution had to do with food. McElroy's article may initially have the same effect on the reader. Air pollution does have to do with food, as you will know when you finish this essay excerpted from the Harvard Magazine. Dr. McElroy is a professor of atmospheric sciences at Harvard.

Concern over preserving the ozone layer has raised alarming questions. Among them: Do our basic agricultural policies pose a greater threat to health than aerosol cans ever did?

Every generation has its own historically unique vision of the end of the world. Children of the early Sixties grew up certain that doomsday would be announced with a shower of nuclear fireballs. But in the Seventies, the bomb has dropped from public consciousness, and international attention has focused on a new threat to humanity: the spray can.

In the past year and a half, the possibility that chemicals used in aerosol sprays could destroy the earth's protective ozone layer has sparked heated debate. Spokesmen for the aerosol industry claim that their products are virtually harmless, while many people have begun to believe (equally irrationally) that total ozone depletion is imminent, that the sun's rays will soon fry us all. Ozone is clearly the issue of the day. Prophets of thermonuclear disaster have even begun to argue about the effect a full-scale nuclear war could be expected to have on levels of ozone worldwide....

The aspect of this problem that first caught the public's attention was the possibility that a drop in ozone levels—and the resultant increase in the amount of ultraviolet radiation reaching the surface of the earth—might cause skin cancer. Many forms of skin cancer are relatively innocuous and may be repaired by surgery: the link between these skin diseases and exposure to ultraviolet radiation in sunlight has been well established for quite some time. But very recently, new findings have begun to suggest that ultraviolet exposure may have much more serious medical consequences. Testimony presented to the U.S. Senate by Dr. Thomas Fitzpatrick, Edward Wigglesworth Professor of Dermatology at Harvard Medical School, cites convincing evidence that some of the more dangerous forms of skin cancer, particularly malignant melanoma, are also associated with solar ultraviolet radiation.

Malignant melanoma is a medical tragedy at least as fatal as breast cancer.... If malignant melanoma is already spreading in the population with generally greater exposure to sunlight, the additional effects of ozone destruction could be dangerous indeed.... This fact alone makes it imperative that we study the processes controlling levels of atmospheric ozone, and that we take steps to prevent the release of chemicals capable of destroying ozone in significant amounts....

Nitric oxide very effectively catalyzes the removal of atmospheric ozone. Less than one part per billion of the atmosphere consists of nitric oxide; yet this minute amount is sufficient to lower the level of ozone to half of what it would be were nitric oxide not present.

In 1970, nitric oxide's potential effect on atmospheric ozone levels came under intensive study, following the prediction that the supersonic aircraft then being developed might emit significant concentrations of nitric oxide into the stratosphere. Stratospheric pollution poses special problems. The stratosphere is much more stable than the lower atmosphere we are familiar with, the troposphere. Pollutants deposited in the troposphere are periodically removed from the atmosphere by rain; it is only the continuous release of industrial chemicals into the lower atmosphere that keeps air polluted at those altitudes. In the stratosphere, however, it does not rain. Gases emitted into the stratosphere may stay there for five or ten years before the slow turning over of the atmosphere may carry them down into the troposphere, where rain can cleanse the system. For this reason, one pollution source in the stratosphere is roughly equivalent to about three hundred pollution sources of similar magnitude in the lower atmosphere. Stratospheric sources of pollution like the SST, are thus intrinsically more hazardous to the general environment.

All of these factors were taken into account in 1970 to predict the effect that large fleets of supersonic aircraft would be likely to have on the atmosphere. It was estimated at that time that 500 Boeing SST's flying daily would cause a reduction in ozone of 3 to 5 percent. The best calculations available today, using methods that have been proven accurate in estimating present levels of ozone and nitric oxide, show that these figures were well founded and accurate....

[But] it soon became apparent that a potentially greater threat to the ozone layer came from a source that looked much more innocent and was in fact already an integral part of American life. This, of course, was the aerosol can.

About a year and a half ago, attention began to focus on the widely used industrial gases known as Freons. These... had been released into the atmosphere for several years through aerosol sprays and leaky refrigeration units. (Although spray cans have been the more widely publicized source of Freons, leaky refrigerators actually contribute about as much Freon to the atmosphere as do aerosol cans.) Freon is extraordinarily unreactive. One reason why it is such a useful industrial product is that it can be mixed with various chemicals in a spray can without reacting with them, serving only to push those chemicals out into the air in a fine spray when the nozzle is pressed. It was always assumed that, since Freon is so inert, it could not react with anything to cause any conceivable environmental problem.

In fact,... Freon breaks down in the atmosphere to release atoms of chlorine. Like nitric oxide, these chlorine atoms can catalyze the conversion of ozone to molecular oxygen.... Chlorine has essentially the same effect on ozone as nitric oxide does, except that it is an even more efficient catalyst of ozone's destruction.

The Freon problem is compounded greatly by the long time-lag between the release of the gas at the earth's surface and its eventual removal from the atmosphere. After Freon is released, it slowly makes its way about the protective ozone shield; when unfiltered sunlight hits it, Freon breaks down, releasing chlorine atoms. The average chlorine atom will convert a great many molecules of ozone to molecular oxygen before it finally forms hydrogen chloride (HC1) and is cycled back to the lower atmosphere, where it is removed by rain. Almost all of the Freon that has been used by human beings over the last forty years is still in the atmosphere at some point in this cycle.

The remarkable thing about the cycle, from an environmental point of view, is that it takes a very long time to reach an equilibrium state. If the use of Freon were stabilized immediately and we began to release the gas into the atmosphere at a constant rate, it would still take more than 200 years before the atmosphere started removing the chlorine at the same rate as it was going in....

By current predictions, an annual growth rate of 20 percent in Freon use would lead to a 15-percent decrease in the ozone layer by 1995. And even if Freon were completely banned at any point, it would take at least a century for ozone levels to return to normal.

When these calculations first appeared, they were met—not unexpectedly—with several objections from the Freon industry. It was said, first, that these mathematical models were just theoretical, and that we had no evidence that Freon ever even reached the stratosphere....

A second objection was that even if Freon did reach the stratosphere, there could be some benevolent chemical process that would take the chlorine atoms away and bind them up in a harmless form before they did any damage to ozone....

[But] all of the data collected over the past year are strong evidence for the validity of these predictive models.

If Freon really is destructive to the ozone layer, then there can be only two solutions to the problem: find a way to replenish ozone in the atmosphere, or drastically curtail the use of Freon.... With our present technology, the only reasonable course of action is to stop releasing Freon into the atmosphere as much as is possible.

Once the importance of this objective is recognized, it should not really be very difficult to accomplish....

Although Freon pollution may come under adequate control in the near future, the investigation of this problem has uncovered many other potential threats to the atmosphere that may be much more difficult to deal with. Concern about the environmental effect of Freon spawned a wide-ranging research effort to investigate atmospheric chemistry; this effort focused largely on the interaction of biological systems with the chemicals of the atmosphere. As a result of the work, it is now becoming apparent that such essential biological activities

as agricultural production may ultimately produce large amounts of nitric oxide, the same ozone-destroying compound released by the SST.

This disturbing fact first came to light through the study of the biological nitrogen cycle. Nitrogen is essential to life. It is a vital element in amino acids, proteins, all of the things we're made of.... Nature has solved the problem of how to convert nitrogen from the atmosphere into forms useful to life (a process known as nitrogen fixation) in quite a remarkable way.... Most of the fixation we see today appears to occur through a symbiotic relationship in which bacteria infect the root systems of leguminous plants, which supply the bacteria with a nutrient. The bacteria allow the plant to grow, and the plant feeds the bacteria in turn.

If there were not an opposing process to put the nitrogen back into the atmosphere, we would have a very serious problem on a geological time scale: with biological nitrogen fixation continuing at today's rate, all the nitrogen in the atmosphere would be exhausted in only 10 million years, a small fraction of the age of the earth. This is prevented by the biological process called denitrification, which puts nitrogen back into the air at about the same rate that it is taken out, and which is carried out on land by organisms that use nitrates in the soil. When oxygen gets low, these bacteria are unable to continue breathing oxygen and start breathing nitrate (NO_3) instead. In the process, they exhaust the gases nitrogen (N_2) and nitrous oxide, or "laughing gas," (N_2O) back into the atmosphere....

An increase in the amount of nitrous oxide coming out of the soil and forming nitric oxide could cause serious damage to the ozone layer. It has been estimated that a tenfold increase in present levels of nitrous oxide would effectively eliminate ozone from the point of view of terrestrial biology.

An increase in atmospheric N_2O is more than likely to occur as an inevitable and predictable result of present agricultural policies. Nitrous oxide is formed, along with molecular nitrogen, when soil bacteria consume nitrates instead of oxygen. If the amount of nitrate in the soil increases, then the bacterial output of nitrous oxide can be expected to increase as well. And over the past 25 years, the use of nitrate containing fertilizers has been expanding at a very rapid rate. In 1950, the total global amount of nitrogen fixed industrially and converted to nitrates for agricultural use was 1½ megatons (1.5 million metric tons). In 1974 the amount fixed was forty megatons. The World Food Conference has predicted a need for 400 megatons to be fixed annually by the turn of the century simply to feed people. The industry's prediction of what they will be able to deliver, using chemical plants now under construction, is 200 megatons per year, five times the present rate.

Of course, industrial-fertilizer production is not the only global source of nitrogen fixation. Biological organisms, such as the leguminous bacteria described earlier, fixed some 170 megatons of nitrogen in 1974. During that same year, another forty megatons was fixed in automobiles and stationary power sources. These sources of fixed nitrogen will probably not expand at the same rate as the industrial production of nitrate fertilizer. Nevertheless, the over-all rate of nitrogen fixation can certainly be expected to at least double by the year 2000.

If denitrification increases at the same rate as nitrogen fixation (remember that they are complementary processes that should theoretically balance), then denitrification, and the production of nitrous oxide, could also be expected to double shortly after the turn of the century. According to the best theoretical models, this would cause a reduction in ozone levels in the neighborhood of 20 percent. This is clearly a significant effect, and one that may be very difficult to prevent. It's one thing to ban Freon and the SST in the interest of preserving the ozone layer; it's quite a different matter to curtail food production.

At the same time that over-all rates of denitrification are growing, nitrous oxide is being increasingly produced as an exhaust gas of denitrification. Under typical conditions, only about 4 percent of the gas produced in denitrification is nitrous oxide; the rest is molecular nitrogen. The bacteria themselves seem to care very little whether their exhaust product is N_2 or N_2O; both gases are just waste products as far as the bacteria are concerned.

What biological factors control the production of these two gases? Denitrification occurs as part of the process of organic decay in water-clogged soil—the water keeps oxygen from reaching the bacteria, and they grow instead by using the nitrate available to them. One variable that seems to control the output of nitrous oxide is the acidity of this decay medium. The more acid the medium, the more nitrous oxide the bacteria will produce.

Since denitrification takes place in water-clogged soil, an increase in the acidity of rain could easily lead to a more acid decay medium and increased nitrous-oxide production. In fact, this already seems to be taking place. Data show that over the 1960s there was a gradual rise in the level of N_2O. At first, this appeared to be the fertilizer effect, but closer examination showed that the rise in N_2O was occurring too early to be due to the use of nitrate fertilizers. It seems possible that this increase in nitrous oxide might be due at least in part to a change in the acidity of rain, which we know has taken place dramatically in certain local environments. Rain may be increasing in acidity as a result of other types of atmospheric pollution, notably the burning of sulphur-rich fuels and the automobile's production of nitric acid. This is certainly sobering, for, much as these air pollutants have been studied, it would have been difficult if not impossible to predict that they might destroy ozone through this rather complicated and indirect process.

With continuing research, more and more aspects of the problem of preserving the ozone layer are becoming apparent....

We are still just beginning to appreciate the complexity of the interactions between industrial pollution, natural biological processes, and atmospheric chemistry. Through an interdisciplinary approach, it is finally becoming possible to examine all of these factors together, and to define more exactly the role played by biological and industrial products in the atmosphere.

The effect of industrial pollutants on the atmosphere is not determined by the absolute amounts of chemicals released, but by the extent to which these industrial products change an already existing atmospheric pattern. For this reason, much recent work has aimed at identifying and measuring the chemicals released into the atmosphere by *natural* sources....

One final, vital area that still has not been adequately researched is the question of the total biological impact of the destruction of stratospheric ozone. The implications for the incidence of skin cancer are well documented and have received much publicity, but there are other issues as well. A number of reports produced by the National Academy of Sciences have suggested that certain marine species may reduce their photosynthetic activity as the level of ultraviolet radiation reaching the ocean increases. Such a decrease in photosynthesis would have a profound effect throughout the food chain. There are also some very problematical data suggesting that growth of some crops may be inhibited by ultraviolet radiation. Overall, however, we really do not know what the biological effects of significantly decreased ozone levels would be, and that is perhaps the most disturbing aspect of the problem. Our ability to predict changes in ozone levels has now outstripped our ability to predict the effect of those changes on the total biospheric system. The study of that biological impact is now of primary importance.

In the last several years, concern over preserving the ozone layer—which seemed at first to be a rather simple environmental problem—has led almost accidentally to a whole new way of looking at our atmospheric environment. With our present appreciation of the complexity of the biosphere and its relationship to the atmosphere, it has become obvious that a very major need exists for a large research program to cross disciplinary lines that have never been adequately crossed in the past. Biology, physics, chemistry, and mathematics each have an essential role to play here, not to mention oceanography, medicine, and general environmental studies. A truly interdisciplinary study is absolutely necessary if our understanding of the atmoshere is to keep pace with our ability to destroy it.

Excerpted with permission from *Harvard Magazine*, 78 (6): 19-25 (February 1976).

Sahelian Drought: No Victory for Western Aid

NICHOLAS WADE

Freon, SST's, nitrogen fertilizers—all these are man-made assaults upon the environment and can, if they must, be curtailed. Drought, on the other hand, can be assumed to be unavoidable—an act of nature not of man. The two articles that follow examine that assumption. Nicholas Wade's "Sahelian Drought" examines the overall effects of recent technological interventions on the all too recent famine in the Sahel. Randall Baker, in an article from *The Ecologist*, examines in more detail the effect of colliding cultural assumptions.

The famine that struck the six Sahelian zone countries of West Africa last year is thought to have killed some 100,000 people and left 7 million others dependent on foreigners' food handouts. The same or worse may happen again this year. The essence of the tragedy is that the famine was caused not by dry weather or some putative climatic change but, primarily, by man himself. Could not Western skills, applied in time, have saved the primitive nomads and slash-and-burn farmers from destroying their own land? Western intervention in the Sahel, Western science and technology, and the best intentioned efforts of donor agencies and governments over the last several decades, have in fact made a principal contribution to the destruction.

"One of the basic factors in the situation is overpopulation, both human and bovine, brought about by the application of modern science," says a former Food and Agricultural Organization (FAO) sociologist. According to a recent in-house report on the Sahel prepared by the Agency for International Development (AID), "To a large extent the deterioration of the subsistence base is directly attributable to the fact that man's interventions in the delicately balanced ecological zones bordering desert areas have usually been narrowly conceived and poorly implemented." "Too many of our projects have been singularly unproductive and . . . we have tediously reintroduced projects which ought never to have been attempted in the first place," says Michael M. Horowitz, a State University of New York anthropologist who has studied the nomad peoples of Niger. And to quote the AID report again, "It must be recognized that assistance agencies have ignored the principles [of effective resource management], and the consequence of indiscriminate support has produced negative results or, on occasion, disaster."

The symptoms of distress in the Sahel are easier to perceive than the underlying causes of the disaster. The six countries concerned—Senegal, Mauritania, Mali, Upper Volta, Niger, and Chad—are former French colonies that stretch along the southern edge of the Sahara desert. The land is mostly semi-desert that enjoys only 4 months of rainfall a year. But the grasses are sufficient to support the herds of cattle tended by the nomads, and in the southern regions millet and sorghum are grown, together with cash crops such as peanuts and cotton. By 1970, just before the collapse, the fragile steppe and savannah ecology of the six countries was supporting some 24 million people and about the same number of animals. This burden amounted to roughly a third more people and twice as many animals as the land was carrying 40 years ago.

The agent of collapse was a drought—the third of such severity this century—which began in 1968 and cannot yet be said to have ended. The grasslands started turning to desert, the rivers dwindled to a trickle, and by 1972, the fifth year of the drought, people, cattle, and crops began to die. "Our country is already half desert and our arable lands left are extremely reduced," the director of Chad's water and forestry resources told the FAO. By last year, Lake Chad had in places receded 15 miles from its former shorelines and split into three smaller lakes. The ancient cultural center of Timbuktu, a port fed by an inlet of the Niger river, was completely cut off and boats lay in the caked mud of its harbor. The nomads, forced to sell the surviving cattle that afforded their only means of subsistence, were reduced to the status of aimless refugees in camps around the major cities. Probably 5 million cattle perished, the staple grain crops produced low harvests, and nearly a third of the population faced a severe food shortage which, but for a massive infusion of relief supplies from the United States and other donors, would have ended in widespread famine.

Drought has clearly been the precipitating cause of the ecological breakdown in the Sahel, but attempts to blame the desiccation of the land wholly on the dry weather, or a supposed southward movement of the Sahara desert, do not quite hold water. A global weather change may indeed have squeezed the Sahel's usual rain belts southward, as climatologists such as H. H. Lamb argue, or, as others believe, the drought may be no more than an extreme expression of the Sahel's notoriously variable climate. The Sahara desert may indeed appear to be advancing downward into the Sahel—at the rate of 30 miles a year, according to a widely quoted estimate (which works out at 18 feet per hour). But the primary cause of the desertification is man, and the desert in the Sahel is not so much a natural expansion of the Sahara but is being formed *in situ* under the impact of human activity. "The desertification is mancaused, exacerbated by many years of lower rainfall," says Edward C. Fei, head of AID's Special Task Force on Sahelian Planning. According to the French hydrologist Marcel Roche, "The phenomenon of desertification, if it exists at all, is perhaps due to the process of human and animal occupation, certainly not to climatic changes."

Perhaps the most graphic proof of man's part in the desertification of Sahel has come from a curiously shaped green pentagon discovered in a NASA satellite photograph by Norman H. MacLeod, an agronomist at American University, Washington, D.C. MacLeod found on a visit to the site of the pentagon that the difference between it and the surrounding desert was nothing more than a barbed-wire fence. Within was a 250,000-acre ranch, divided into five sectors with the cattle allowed to graze one sector a year. Although the ranch was started only 5 years ago, at the same time as the drought began, the simple protection afforded the land was enough to make the difference between pasture and desert.

The physical destruction of the Sahel was not an overnight process. Its beginning can be traced to the French colonization of the late 19th century, when the Sahelian peoples lost with their political power the control over their range and wells which was vital to the proper management of their resources.

The Sahel—a term derived from the Arabic word for border—was once one of the most important areas of Africa. In the middle ages it was the home of the legendary trading empires of Ghana, Mali, and Songhai.

The key to the Sahelian way of life was a remarkably efficient adaptation to the semi-desert environment. Although the nomads' life-style may seem enviably free to those who dwell in cities, there is nothing random about their migrations. The dry season finds them as far south as they can go without venturing within the range of the tsetse fly. Between the nomads and the sedentary farmers who also inhabit this area there is a symbiotic arrangement: The nomads' cattle graze the stubble of crops and at the same time manure the fields. In exchange for manure the nomads receive millet from the farmers. With the first rains, the grass springs up and the herds move northward. The rains also move north and the cattle follow behind in search of new grass. According to Lloyd Clyburn of AID, "The migration continues as long as the grass ahead looks greener than that at hand, until the northern edge of the Sahelian rain belt is reached. When that grass is eaten off, the return to the south begins. This time the cattle are grazing a crop of grass that grew up behind them on their way north, and they are drinking standing water remaining from the rainy season." Back in their dry-season range the cattle find a crop of mature grass that will carry them for 8 or 9 months to the next growing season.

The traditional migration routes followed by the herds, and the amount of time a herd of given size might spend at a particular well, were governed by rules worked out by tribal chiefs. In this way overpasturage was avoided. The timing of the movement of animals was carefully calculated so as to provide feed and water with the least danger from disease and conflict with other tribal groups.

By virtue of what one writer has called "the essential ecological rationality of the nomadic pastoral regime," the herders made probably the best possible use of the land. The settled part of the population, the farmers, had an equally capable understanding of their environment. They knew to let the land lie fallow for long periods—up to 20 years—before re-cropping, and they developed an extraordinary number of varieties of their main staples, millet and sorghum, each adapted to different growing seasons and situations. Within the limits of their environment and technology, the peoples of the Sahel have, over the past centuries, demonstrated what University of London anthropologist Nicholas David calls "an impressive record of innovation...which is quite at variance with the common negative criticism of the African as unduly conservative." In fact, when the Sahelian peoples have been conservative and resisted changes advocated by Western experts, it has often been with reason.

It would be absurd to blame the collapse of this intricate social and ecological system solely on Western interference, and yet rather few Western interventions in the Sahel, when considered over the long term, have worked in the inhabitants' favor. Those who have studied the farmers' and herders' traditional methods, says an FAO report on the Sahel, believe that the destructive practices that are now frequent are due to the cumulative effects of "over-population, deterioration of the climatic conditions and, above all, the impact of the Western economic and social system."

Western intervention has made itself felt in many ways, some inadvertent, some deliberate. Introduction of a cash economy had profound effects on the traditional system. The French colonial division of the Sahel into separate states has faced the nomad tribes with national governments which have tried to settle them, tax them, and reduce their freedom of movement by preventing passage across state boundaries. Curiously, however, it has been the West's deliberate attempts to do good that seem to have caused the most harm. The West in this case means the French, up until 1960, when the Sahelian countries were granted independence, and the French, Americans, and others thereafter. The French should probably not be held particularly to blame; they were only following conventional wisdom, and there is little reason to believe that other donor countries would have handled the situation very differently.

The salient impact is of course the increase in

human and animal population that followed the application of Western medicine. The people of the Sahel are increasing at a rate of 2.5 percent a year, one of the highest rates of population increase in the world. If the nomads could have been persuaded to kill more of their cattle for market, the animal population might have been kept within bounds. Not foreseen was the fact that cattle are the nomads' only means of saving, and it in fact, makes good sense—on an individual basis—for a nomad to keep as many cattle on the hoof as he can.

As a result herd numbers increased hand over fist in the decade following independence, aided by 7 years of unusually heavy rains. According to the FAO, the number of cattle grew from about 18 to 25 million between 1960 and 1971. The optimum number, according to the World Bank, is 15 million.

While the herders were overtaxing the pastures, the farmers were doing the same to the arable land. Population increase led to more and more people trying to farm the land. An even sharper pressure was the introduction by the French of cash crops to earn foreign exchange. With the best lands given up to the cultivation of cotton and peanuts, people had to bring the more marginal lands into use to grow their own food crops. In many cases these ecologically fragile zones could not take the strain of intensive agriculture. The usual process is that the fallow periods of 15 to 20 years are reduced to five or even one. Fertility declines, slowly at first, and then in a vicious spiral. Poor crops leave the soil exposed to sun and wind. The soil starts to lose its structure. The rain, when it falls, is not absorbed but runs off uselessly in gulleys. Desertification has begun. "Let us be under no illusion," President Leopold Sedar Senghor of Senegal told a symposium on the African drought held in London last year, "the process of desertification had been precipitated since the conquest of Senegal [by the French], since the introduction of growing peanuts without either fallow or crop rotation."

What cash crops have done for the Sahelian farmland, deep borehole wells have done for the pasture. A thousand feet or more beneath the Sahel lie vast reservoirs of water that can be tapped by deep wells. Thousands of these boreholes, costing up to $200,000 apiece, have been drilled across the Sahel by well-intentioned donors. The effect of the boreholes was simply to make pasture instead of water the limiting factor on cattle numbers, so that the inevitable population collapse, when it came, was all the more ferocious. "Few sights were more appalling at the height of the drought last summer," according to environmental writer Claire Sterling in a recent article in *The Atlantic*, "than the thousands upon thousands of dead and dying cows clustered around Sahelian boreholes. Indescribably emaciated, the dying would stagger away from the water with bloated bellies and struggle to fight free of the churned mud at the water's edge until they keeled over.... Enormous herds, converging upon the new boreholes from hundreds of miles away, so ravaged the surrounding land by trampling and overgrazing that each borehole quickly became the center of its own little desert forty or fifty miles square."

Overgrazing of the Sahelian pasturelands was a consequence of too many cattle having too little place to go. As the farmers spreading out from the towns took more land under cultivation, they tended to squeeze the nomads and their herds into a smaller strip of space. Moreover, the nomads' ability to manage their own resources was slowly slipping away. Government interference reduced their freedom of movement, and the boreholes threw into chaos the traditional system of pasture use based on agreements among tribal chieftains. With all the old safeguards in abeyance, the cattle numbers began to chew up the ecology across the whole face of the Sahel. First the perennial grasses went. These usually grow up to 6 feet tall and put down roots as deep. If the plant is heavily grazed, its roots make a shallower penetration and, in dry periods, may fail to strike water. The perennial grasses are replaced by coarse annual grasses, but these, under heavy grazing and trampling, give way to leguminous plants that dry up quickly and cannot hold the soil together. Pulverized by the cattles' hooves, the earth is eroded by the wind, and the finer particles collect and are washed by rains to the bottom of slopes where they dry out into an impermeable cement.

Desertification has been hastened by the heavy cutting of trees for firewood. Trees recycle nutrients from deep in the soil and hold the soil together. Slash-and-burn techniques—the only practical method available to the poor farmer for clearing land—are the cause of numerous fires which, according to a World Bank estimate, kill off 50 percent of the range grass each year.

Under these abuses, the Sahel by the end of the 1960's was gripped by a massive land sickness which left it without the resilience to resist the drought. A whole vast area which might with appropriate management have become a breadbasket providing beef for half of Africa instead became a basket case needing more than $100 million worth of imported food just to survive.

The future prospects for the Sahel and its people are not very bright. Sahelian governments and the various donors have not reached any kind of agreement on long-term strategy for rehabilitation. Some donors—AID excepted—are still digging boreholes. Most of the development projects now under consideration were drawn up before the drought struck and are based on the unlikely assumption that when the rains return everything can go on as before. (A recent meeting of American climatologists concluded that planners should assume drought conditions in 2 years out of every 3.)

Much of the development money for the Sahel will have to come from the United States and France, but there seems to be little coordination or exchange of ideas between the two countries. Nor is there any general agreement on how the Sahel can be restored to self-sufficiency. Optimists, such as William W. Seifert of MIT, who heads a $1 million long-term development study for AID, believe that the Sahel could support its present human population provided that cattle numbers were reduced by a half or more. Unfortunately, there is no way, short of a major social upheaval, that the nomads will consent to reduce their herds. Projects involving controlled grazing, such as in the Ekrafane ranch, are impractical because there is not enough land to go around. AID plans to open up the lands to the south of the Sahel by clearing them of tsetse fly, but this would benefit only 10 percent of the population. Others are not so hopeful. "I don't think there is much optimism that significant improvements can be expected in the short term. All you can do is try to increase their margin for survival and hope that something turns up," says an agricultural specialist conversant with both AID and MIT development plans.

"Neither the leverage of modern science and technology," concludes an in-house AID report on the Sahel, "nor the talents and resources of large numbers of individuals and institutions currently being applied to relevant problems has occasioned more than minor progress in combatting the natural resource problems and exploiting the undeveloped potential." Which is another way of saying that Western ideas for developing the Sahel have not proved to be a spectacular success. Its ecological fragility and the vagaries of its climate make the Sahel a special case. But there are many other areas in the world where unchecked populations are overloading environments of limited resilience. The Sahel may have come to grief so soon only because mistakes made there show up quickly. Other Western development strategies, such as the Green Revolution, are, one may hope, more soundly based in ecological and social realities. If not, the message of the Sahel is that the penalty for error is the same Malthusian check which it is the purpose of development to avoid, except that the crash is from a greater height.

Reprinted with permission from *Science*, 185: 234-237 (19 July 1974). Copyright 1974 by the American Association for the Advancement of Science.

Famine: the Cost of Development?

RANDALL BAKER

Over the last decade the severe hardships experienced by those communities living in the Monsoon areas or in semi-arid belts between the Desert and the Sown have forced an international interest in a zone which has been undergoing radical environmental deterioration. Several detailed and well documented studies[1] have been presented to account for the worsening situation in terms of climatic change, whatever its cause, and there now seems to be an impressive volume of evidence to substantiate the view that climatic change is a major contributory factor. On the other hand, the pace of destruction and the advance of increasingly desertic conditions outward from the Tropical High-Pressure zones, is frequently accelerated rather than retarded by the introduction of advanced technology. Whatever the overall climatic prospects for these marginal areas of production there seems little doubt that 'planning,' inappropriate technology and administrative weaknesses have undermined their resilience in withstanding drought and have seriously disrupted what was previously a long-term balance between Man and Environment. The implication of this is that, what-

ever long-term strategy emerges from the research into climatic parameters, the basic errors of environmental mismanagement must not be perpetuated. There is disturbing evidence that this may happen unless we recognise precisely what the problem is and what steps are necessary to make planning more appropriate to the total situation.

This paper will examine, briefly, what has happened in the past from the point of view of the participants. The first part describes the situation as perceived at the time by the colonial officers. In each section the evidence is the same and it is only the interpretation of the circumstances which varies; for that reason, the principal generalisations made by the colonial officers are in italics. It is these generalised conclusions, rather than what actually occurred, which account for much of the inappropriateness of many of the induced changes.

The second part of the paper will present a different interpretation of the same evidence, this time from the point of view of the pastoralist, and will highlight the causal processes arising from the confusion between the two interpretations, which encouraged desiccation. A

[1]See the accompanying paper by Prof. Campbell and also: Bryson, R. A., 1974, "Drought in Sahelia, who or what is to blame?", *Ecologist,* Vol. 3 No. 10, p. 336-371. Winstanley, D., 1973, "Recent rainfall trends in Africa, the Middle East and India", *Nature,* 243, p. 464-465 and; Winstanley, D., 1973, "Drought in the Sahel zones: severity, causes and prospects", a paper presented to the symposium on Drought in Africa, S.O.A.S., July, 1973.

final part considers the implications for the future and what remains to be done.

Some generalisations and their consequences

Drought, famine and starvation are the stuff of history in the Monsoon belts, so much so that several groups record their chronology relative to years of great loss, disaster or suffering. There is nothing new about droughts; Joseph saw Egypt stricken by "seven lean years" and gained prestige from his foresight in handling this calamity. In the marginal areas of cultivation and in semi-arid range-lands a small deficiency in an annual rainfall total or a variation in the timing of the onset and sequence of rainfall can have consequences far beyond those associated with such small changes in rainfall in humid regions. It is in these areas also that, as a general rule, variability (percentage deviation from the mean) is at its greatest.[2]

Early contact between colonial administrators and pastoral nomads very often followed the pattern I shall try to outline here. The casual colonial observer saw a community *wandering aimlessly with their herds in an eternal search for pasture,* often concentrated in a specific circuit of rangeland whilst considerable extents of the grassland nearby remained unoccupied, as for instance between the tribal groupings in Karamoja, N.E. Uganda.[3] At first it was thought necessary to limit this *needless movement* in order to tax the inhabitants, utilise their labour on public work schemes to establish the roads network, government buildings, etc., and to prevent hostility, especially across the new colonial boundaries. Attempts to commercialise the economy met with little success as the inhabitants did not respond *rationally* to market forces operating through the price mechanism offering only a few scrub animals from time to time and using price increases as an opportunity to reduce the number of animals put on sale.

Sooner or later in these climates a natural drought occurs and the administration is horrified by both stock and human losses: a problem Europe had conquered earlier through *superior technology.* It was evident that one of the overriding problems of the moment was to utilise this superior technology and eliminate the *problem of drought* by modern hydrological technique. These, after all, were being *proven* in similar semi-arid or extensive rangeland environments in Australia and the USA.[4] Wells were drilled, tanks excavated and so the droughts, previously manifested as a shortage of water, wreak less havoc than before. Appalling losses still result from diseases and here refinements in veterinary medicine were able to effect radical improvement in the survival rate. It was *encouraging to see the awakening of pastoralist interest in better management* and the herders adopted both innovations very rapidly with an almost immediate effect on herd size. A new problem however began to emerge and capture the attention of agricultural advisers during the 1930s and 1940s: soil erosion and a general *drying up* of the area leading in some regions to an advance of the desert.[5] The "reasons" for this seemed to be:

1. The area was undergoing a *period of desiccation based on climatic change,* illustrated by the increasingly xerophytic characteristics of the vegetation as time passes. In the Sahel there was the frightening prospect of the rangeland being *swallowed up by an advancing desert.*[6]

2. This trend could be countered only by reducing the number of animals, for the area was no longer able to support such large and rapidly increasing herds and flocks as a result of the *drying* up. Howev-

[2] It must be stressed that the aridity/variability relationship is pronounced only at the macro level and, in more local circumstances the situation may be reversed—see Gregory, S., 1969, "Rainfall Reliability", in Thomas and Whittington's: *Environment and Land Use in Africa* p. 57-82.

[3] Baker, P.R., 1968, "Environment and cattle marketing in Karamoja." Occasional paper no. 4, Geography Dept., Makerere University Coll., Kampala.

[4] It is salutory to recall that, at this time, some of the American dustbowls were being formed by severe overgrazing and mismanagement.

[5] In this light it is very instructive to follow the activities and findings of the Anglo-French Forestry Surveys in West Africa—see: Prothero, R.M., 1962, "Some observations on desiccation in north-west Nigeria", *Erdkunde,* 16, p. 112-119.

[6] Wilson, J., 1964, in Langdale-Brown I, et. al.: "The vegetation of Uganda", Government Printer, Entebbe, p. 89-92.

er, despite the *obvious necessity*, people, through their *sentimental attachment* to their cattle would not sell and, when offered a better price, showed their irrationality by offering fewer animals on the market. As conditions worsen their lack of even the *basic principles of scientific management* was revealed by an overwhelming desire to increase herd size and, after a drought, to sell nothing at all...and they would keep goats, the *most* destructive of all stock. Thus *they* accentuate the destruction and helped turn the area into a desert.

Drought now appears in a new guise as starvation, for now, a shortfall in precipitation caused heavy losses in the ever diminishing vegetation or a failure of annuals to appear. Perennials where, as in Karamoja they previously dominated, disappeared and the spectre of erosion encouraged by the exposure of the soil now haunted the corridors of the local administration. Raiding, the *local sport*, reached alarming proportions and the whole area became a "disturbed district," the security forces took over and nothing ever got any better. All that investment, technology and patience was wasted as a result of a *creeping desert* and an *ungrateful, destructive palaeotechnic* group of *wandering troublemakers*. They must be "sedentarised" *and taught to be useful citizens.*

An alternative interpretation

Over a long period before the coming of the colonial power the pastoral nomads had evolved, possibly by trial and error, a survival strategy which, given their level of technology, minimised the risks of failure and starvation in a very hazardous situation. The way of life that this strategy involved was by no means an ideal existence for its long term ecological balance was based on severe privation, death through famine, drought, disease and warfare. Large numbers of both the human community and their herds could expect to meet an early death

so that the overall population remained stable or grew, at best, only very slowly.

To keep risk down to a minimum a series of options was evolved by each community in relation to the range of environmental opportunities and based on an extraordinarily detailed knowledge of the type, distribution and value of natural grazing resources. The options were limited by technology but, accepting that, they represented superlative adaptations which modern game theory would be hard pressed to improve upon. The details of the strategies have been covered elsewhere but the point that needs to be made is that many of the outward characteristics of these strategies, perceived as symptoms of "backwardness," "savagery" or "perverseness" by the colonial administrators and their successors, have a very respectable interpretation in the context of staying alive in the face of considerable odds. Sadly, much of the anthropological work done during the colonial period failed to deal with the herds and flocks as survival mechanisms: that was "taken for granted" and attention was focused on the extra dimensions of livestock in pastoral society. Thus a vital field of information on the subsistence strategy was absent and planners either worked blind or assumed pastoralists would respond like the ranchers of Texas.

Initially, the controls on movement instituted by the colonial authorities often failed to recognise that the pattern of grazing and migration of pastoral nomads was designed to allow flexibility depending on the prevailing conditions.[7] In years of good rainfall, semi-nomads such as the Karamojong of Uganda may remain around the homestead in both wet and dry seasons. However, when conditions are drier, then communities may move out along one of several routes which have proven their value in the past: the exact path relating to the precise sequence of events up to the decision. In extreme conditions some communities move their flocks and herds on to resources maintained for just such exigencies: parts of the Western Plains

7 Johnson, D.L., 1969: "The nature of nomadism", Dept. of Geography Research Paper No. 118, University of Chicago.

or Eastern hills of Karamoja or the *hema* enclosures of the Bedouin of south-western Arabia for instance. This season by season variation in distribution of people accounts, in part, for a false interpretation of disorder, randomness and aimlessness. Interference with such movement naturally threatens the security of the group by spatially reducing the risk-minimising options and this also helps to explain why the seizure of "unoccupied" land did so much to engender the bitter wars which typified the early days of colonialism in pastoral areas. The annexation of the dry season reserves of the Masai of Kenya and their distribution to European ranchers or the settlement of Suk on reserves of the Karamojong provide good examples of such action. The colonists' early perception of these tribes as "aggressive and unreasonable" is better explained by their response to this theft of their land and the threat to their survival than by any mystical characteristics attributed to the tribe's outlook or attitudes.

Commercialisation

To the foreign masters of an expanding and increasingly urbanising territory the obvious attraction of the semi-arid areas was as a storehouse of cheap protein either for the domestic market (e.g. Karamoja to Buganda in Uganda) or for export to a neighbouring territory (e.g. Niger to Nigeria). Attempts at commercialising the pastoral economies proved frustrating and largely unsuccessful, principally because in a society where herds and flocks not only form the basis of survival, but also symbolise wealth and are the mainstay of social interchange there is almost no incentive to convert them into cash, goods or services. Retail penetration amongst a moving community such as the Bedouin is necessarily difficult because the retailer is tied to his shop whilst the pastoralist is mobile and the amount which may be bought is limited by the problem of transporting the purchases once acquired. If the pastoralists are forced to part with animals or kind, for instance, through the institution of taxes payable in cash then it will be those of least value which will go: the sick, the barren and the immature in time of drought or hardship. What the market wants and when it wants it are of limited consequences under these circumstances. Though higher prices during a demand peak elsewhere might produce a sudden surge of selling, the total number of animals sold over the year might fall as the limited requirements of the pastoralists may be realised by selling fewer head. In early days this type of "economic perversity" did much to encourage the view that the pastoralists were simply not pulling their weight in the development/modernisation stakes and were set against change.

The price of innovation

This critical misunderstanding really explains almost all that followed. The pastoralists live in a high risk situation, they have evolved a risk-minimising strategy proven over time and based on holding the maximum number of productive animals in the face of heavy losses. They never keep all the animals together but spread them over different grazing areas and keep a range of animals able to utilise various niches in the ecosystem. The price of an innovation may well be death for, if it fails, there is no reserve capacity. A reluctance to change is only natural under these circumstances, especially when the social implications of possessing animals are added to the function in survival.

However, any generalisations which suggest a universal refusal to change are patently false and some innovations have been widely and rapidly adopted—though not always with beneficial results in the long run.

In this light, the introduction of water resources based on deep drilling, and the diffusion of veterinary prophylaxis form a potential threat to the ecological balance of enormous proportions. Where such innovations reinforce the traditional survival strategy by reducing the death rate of stock and allowing larger herds to survive they have been taken up very rapidly, because larger herds are seen by the pastoralists as providing *greater security*. The critical factor is that they are taken up within the traditional strategy; to reinforce it and *not* to generate a marketable surplus. Most of the extra stock are retained and certainly none are farmed with the primary object of selling them for profit.

This is the origin of the spectacular overgrazing which can be seen to radiate from the boreholes where animals congregate in huge numbers, in the Sahel, the Sudan, Botswana and other African drylands. It is also a major factor in the advance of xerophytic vegetation, soil-erosion and desiccation, even in relatively humid areas such as Karamoja. Ironically, the response on the part of the pastoral communities in the face of such rapid and unprecedented change has been to retrench: in effect to protect the system that has traditionally protected them. They try to increase the size of their herds as an insurance against dry years which become more severe in their effects as the quality of the vegetation is reduced by overgrazing. This only makes over-grazing more severe still, so that the picture is not so much of retreat to better grasslands before an advancing desert as of pastoralists mistakenly opening the door and inviting the desert in. A study in the devastated area of Karamoja which the author made after the droughts of 1961 and 1965 shows only too clearly the tragic attempts of a bewildered people to increase herd size and maintain "security" on a vanishing resource base.[8] The pastoralists no more understand what is happening to them than we have understood how their traditional grazing systems worked. Now we find ourselves urging pastoral communities to reduce cattle numbers while they feel a greater than ever urgency to increase them, because they mistakenly perceive cattle, not a combination of cattle with

grass, as being the true resource.

The present position and implications for the future

There is little need to highlight the present ecological situation in the semi-arid areas, for that has been illustrated only too graphically by the Masai who lost 400,000 animals in 1961, and by reports of the drought affecting the 25,000,000 people in the Sahel over the last seven years. Recent estimates place the advance of the Sahelian desert frontier at as much as 100 kms between 1972 and 1973[9] and the loss of stock at around 80 per cent of the total predrought herds and flocks. Formerly nomadic communities have been beggared by the total loss of their stock and now live in humiliating poverty in the burgeoning *bidonviles* around Nouakchott, Agadez and the towns of the Soudan belt. The previous symbiosis between herder and cultivator in which cattle were moved into fields to graze the stubble and provide manure for the soil is collapsing as even greater numbers of pastoralists are driven out of the desiccated lands to the north. They no longer return northwards before the time of the planting season, but remain in inevitable conflict with their settled neighbours.

Although it seems callous to look for any beneficial aspect to the Sahel drought and so much suffering it is fair to say that the wholesale destruction of herds and flocks does provide a brief respite for pastures to recover and in which to plan to control herd numbers and re-establish ecological balance. As yet it is not possible to say with any certainty whether the cause of the drought is (i) an equator-ward shift in global pressure systems limiting the incursions of more humid monsoonal conditionals in the wet season; (ii) a shift in local pressure systems due to higher temperatures in the soil and lowest atmosphere following a reduction in vegetation; or (iii) a rapid spread of desert

[8] Baker, P.R., 1968: "Problems of the cattle trade in Karamoja", in Berger H. (ed): *Ostafrikanische Studien*, Nuremberg, p. 211-226.
[9] Such reports have to be treated very cautiously, see *The Guardian* 20.9.1973.

conditions because of the overgrazing of perennial grasses and their replacement by annuals which cover the ground for only a short part of the year and expose the land to desiccation by the sun in the dry season.

The answer, if it is ever clearly discerned, will probably incorporate all three elements. However, the relationship between environmental degradation, overstocking and the introduction of watering and disease control is indisputable. The immediate priority is that we *should not* look upon the end of the present drought as the end of the "problem" and then, when the next crisis comes, go back to the same type of technological "dyke-lugging" as before. If this is the outcome then the situation can only worsen.

Some optimists frequently ask, "But surely all this arises from the Colonial presence, false comparisons with the temperate mother-land and an arrogant disregard for traditional cultures? Things are different now that these countries have governments composed of people of local origin." Unfortunately, this is not true because the new elite which forms the government is often drawn from the settled agricultural portion of the population as in Tchad, Uganda and Mali and rarely contains people of the nomadic background. These governments show a disturbing faith in the automatic benefits of western technology: the President of Niger for example has called for a "Marshall plan" of recovery for the six drought-stricken nations, in which wells play a central part. He wants the international aid community to drill 2,500 wells across Niger, to an average depth of 900 feet—an enormously ambitious project that would cost upwards of £100,000,000[10]. At the same time there is a growing interest in damming the Senegal river at an estimated cost of another £30,000,000. Both these projects have been presented as simple "once and for all" solutions to the drought problem and the question of the multiplying effect of overgrazing that they may

produce seems hardly to have been considered. It is quite essential that a solution is found for, over most of the land area of the Sahelian states, there is no obvious alternative to extensive pastoralism nor is there any readily discernible alternative export. Each year some 700,000 animals are exported to the Urban markets of coastal West Africa providing half of Mali's export earnings and 65 per cent of those of Upper Volta.[11]

Since mismanagement is contributing substantially to the increasing desiccation of the semi-arid areas, what prospects are there on the one hand of slowing down or halting the impact of change or, on the other hand, of restoring a long term equilibrium? Ultimately the final decision on what happens must be made by the governments of the afflicted countries and so the "solution" has a powerful political dimension. An International Labour Organisation study[12] revealed that all the countries concerned were committed to a policy of encouraging settled agriculture or ranching even though movement is the basis of the pastoralist's strategy for survival, and no clear, viable alternative has been put forward. Again, many of the governments regard moving populations as a nuisance (cf. the gypsies in Britain), a security threat and an embarrassment to a modern image. Moreover, there exists what may be best termed an "administrative trap" which effectively prevents decision-makers from either perceiving or dealing with the situation in all its aspects simultaneously. Briefly, government departments are limited by their policies, fields of operation, budgetary constraints, so that, often the overall problem of ecological imbalance in pastoral communities is split up between six or more ministries each dealing with separate aspects such as water, veterinary services, marketing, communications, security, agriculture and so on. Frequently no one is responsible for considering *social* aims, objectives and constraints. If foreign ex-

[10] Ibid.

[11] Swift, J., *The Times* 4.9.1973.

[12] International Labour Organisation, 1968 "Technical meeting on the problems of nomadism in the Sahelian region of Africa" Ref. RTNS/R.1.

pertise is brought to bear then it is usually bound by the terms of reference of the responsible ministry and given almost no time—even if the desire is there—to study socio-cultural factors. Swift has remarked, "At the present time the largest UN project ever undertaken in Mali is getting under way to develop the whole of the country's livestock industry, but it contains no pasture specialists, no ecologists and a derisory amount of sociological expertise."[13] Additionally, the short-term political rewards to be derived from investment in a spectacular well sinking programme is likely to prove far more attractive to governments than vitally needed interdisciplinary research into planning. There is no long term in politics. Lastly there is, largely as a legacy of colonialism, a disregard of traditional technology which has the taint of "primitiveness" and is equated in many minds with savagery. This results in a tragic loss of centuries of expertise and knowledge.

Alternatives

It is clear that, for many, a return to pastoralism is likely to be difficult and destructive. A large scale return should be prevented at all costs, by developing other opportunities perhaps through irrigation near the great exotic rivers, or based on *nappes fosses* or retreating flood waters. A recent estimate places the irrigation potential of the Sahelian rivers at 1 million hectares. The only alternative is migration, which is now more difficult with numerous independent states warily protecting their own unemployment figures. There would seem to be very few alternative sources of employment within these economies except where minerals occur (copper in Botswana, uranium in Niger, iron in Mauretania). Work must begin in earnest on defining a methodology to build on the expertise and ecological adaptation of traditional nomadism. A mechanism must be found to preserve the traditional ecological balance, through researching into the attitudes of pastoralists and discovering possibilities for commercialism which could transfer security away from livestock. Eventually, if the social structures and attitudes can adapt, it may be possible to reintroduce practices of basic pasture management. In view of the limited range of economic opportunities in many of the stricken countries, the rising world demand for beef, the shortage of protein foodstuffs in the Third World and the centuries of traditional knowledge encapsulated in the pastoral societies, it seems little enough to ask that an attempt be made to build on a basis of understanding.

In conclusion it may be true that the present situation is partly due to long term fluctuations in the climate. But there is much which can and should be done to reduce the impact of these fluctuations and to prevent their disastrous results from being exaggerated and distributed over an even greater area than is absolutely necessary.

---

[13] Swift, J., *The Times* 4.9.1973.

Reprinted with permission from *The Ecologist* (Wadebridge, Cornwall, U.K.), 4 (5): 170-175 (June 1974).

...and Oceanic Fisheries

LESTER R. BROWN, PATRICIA L. MCGRATH AND BRUCE STOKES

Only a few years ago, the oceans were thought to hold the promise of unlimited bounty, if only we could learn to exploit their resources fully. The excerpt from the Worldwatch Paper #5 reprinted here gives a quick overview of some of the problems our optimism has generated.

The hope that man will be able to turn to the oceans to satisfy his food needs as population pressure on land-based food resources mounts is being shattered. Newspapers in Tokyo, London, and Lima tell daily of increasing competition in oceanic fisheries and growing conflict among countries over scarce supplies of fish. Overfishing is commonplace and pollution of the oceans worsens steadily.

The annual world fish catch of close to 70 million tons (liveweight) represents one of humanity's major sources of high quality protein, substantially exceeding the world slaughter of beef. From 1950 to 1970, the world fish catch more than tripled, from 21 to 70 million tons. This phenomenal 5 percent annual growth in the fish catch far exceeded world population growth, raising average fish consumption per person from eight kilograms in 1950 to 19 in 1970.

In the five years between 1965 and 1970 alone, the world fish catch increased by 18 million tons, or 35 percent. If that trend had continued, the 1975 catch would have been about 95 million tons. But between 1970 and 1973, this longstanding trend was reversed and the fish catch declined by nearly 5 million tons. While population continued to grow, the average per capita supply of fish declined 11 percent during this three-year span, triggering dramatic price rises. (See Figure.) The 1974 catch is estimated at 69 million metric tons, a million tons short of the 1970 catch.

As stocks of key commercial species wane, the time and capital expended to bring in the shrinking catch rises. Many marine biologists now feel that the global catch of table-grade fish is at or near the maximum sustainable level. Of the thirty or so leading species of commercial-grade fish, a number are now overfished: that is, stocks will not sustain even the current catch.

Without cooperative global management of oceanic fisheries and control of the swelling flow of pollutants, the catch could decline even further. The problem is not merely the possibility of diminishing returns on investment in additional fishing capacity, but also the prospect of negative returns. In many fisheries, additional investment in fishing fleets now contributes to overfishing and actually lowers the long-term catch.

Rich and poor countries alike will suffer if oceanic fisheries collapse. Population pressures on limited agricultural land long ago forced the Japanese to turn to the oceans for their animal protein, and to develop a fish and rice diet. As a result, annual per capita fish consumption in Japan now exceeds 70 pounds in edible weight, the highest of any major country. The Soviet Union, frustrated in its effort to expand live-

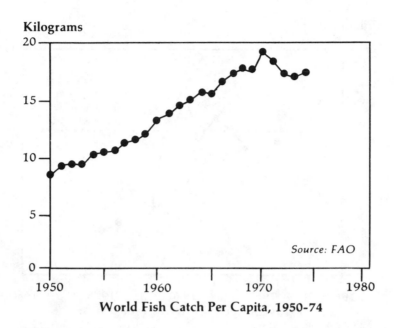

Kilograms

Source: FAO

World Fish Catch Per Capita, 1950-74

stock production, turned to the oceans for protein in a major way two decades ago.

More recently, low income countries with rapidly growing populations have also begun to look to the sea for protein. South Korea, India, Ecuador, and Peru now compete vigorously for a share of the catch in many fisheries, including the rich areas off their own coasts. Ecuador in particular has fined or confiscated many foreign vessels fishing within its 200-mile territorial limits.

Peru has been a leader in developing domestic fishing industries for badly needed foreign exchange. Beginning in the late fifties, its fishing industry underwent spectacular expansion. By the early sixties, Peru had emerged as the world's leading fishing nation, with its vast anchovy fishery accounting for one-fifth of the total world fish catch. For some years Peru has exported the bulk of the anchovy catch, supplying two-thirds of world fishmeal exports, a key protein source for poultry and livestock feeds in the industrialized countries.

In retrospect, it appears that the very heavy annual catches, ranging from 10-12 million tons in the late sixties and early seventies, exceeded

the regenerative capacity of the anchovy fishery. The combination of overfishing and a shift in ocean currents during 1972 and most of 1973 caused the anchovies to disappear from traditional offshore fishing areas. Clearly, future fishing efforts will have to remain safely within the estimated 9.5 million ton maximum sustainable yield, regardless of rising world demand. (See Figure.)

The Northwest Atlantic Fishery serves as another prime example of what happens when demand exceeds the regenerative capacity of commercially sought species. Its 350-year history makes it one of the world's oldest oceanic fisheries and perhaps a bellwether of other fisheries. The catch of this biologically rich region increased steadily until 1968, when it reached 4.6 million tons. Since then, the catch has fluctuated at lower levels, and it fell to 4.0 million tons in 1975, a 13 percent drop from the 1968 level. This decline occurred despite heavy investments aimed at expanding the fishing fleets of several countries.

Catches of cod, halibut, and herring peaked in 1968 but have all since dropped substantially, with declines ranging from about 40 percent for

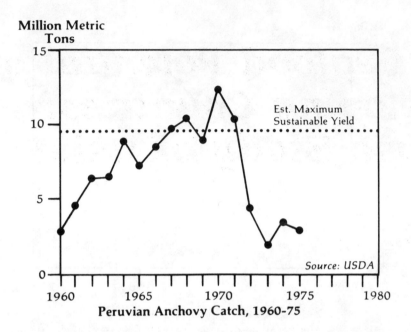

Million Metric Tons

Est. Maximum Sustainable Yield

Source: USDA

Peruvian Anchovy Catch, 1960-75

herring to over 90 percent for halibut. Since effort during this period never flagged, this decline very likely resulted from overfishing. As marine protein supplies lag behind the global growth in demand generated by expanding population and affluence, additional pressure will of necessity be shifted to land-based protein resources.

The years ahead will likely witness a continuously widening gap between population growth and the sustainable yield of oceanic fisheries. Should this occur, the impact on prices and nutrition will be felt everywhere. In an overpopulated and protein-hungry world, competition among countries for the limited and in some cases dwindling catch can only intensify.

Excerpted with permission from *Worldwatch Paper 5*. Copyright by Worldwatch Institute, 1775 Massachusetts Ave., N.W., Washington DC 20036.

The Seafood Potential of the Developing Countries: A Case Study of India

JAGADEESH REDDY

The following two papers consider the relationship between India and the ocean, suggesting on the one hand the potential of the ocean to provide food for a hungry nation, and, on the other, one of the ways not to go about it. The Reddy paper was first published in the *L.I.F.E.* (League for International Food Education) *Newsletter* in October of 1973; the Galtung paper first appeared in *Ceres* in the fall of 1974.

World Oceans and the Oceans of India

The ocean is not a forest nor is the fisherman a hunter who can drag a net in search of game. For this reason a diversified network of specialized scientific research institutions have been set up throughout the world to help the fisherman. A large number of research workers and industries all over the world are developing products out of the sea to meet the growing demand for food and to satisfy consumer requirements and taste. This field of exploration is virtually boundless—the global ocean which covers more than 70 percent of the earth planet now provides less than 2 percent of the world food supplies. Fishing is a widely developed industry providing employment to millions of people all over the world. Yet in many parts of the world, especially in India, fishing is still very primitive and very poorly exploited. India is surrounded by oceans on all three sides, namely the Arabian Sea, the Indian Ocean, and the Bay of Bengal. The coastline is about 5,000 Km. (3100 mi.). The fish resources of Indian oceans are among the richest but most poorly exploited in the world.

Indian Seafood Production

The fishery industry in India is still characterized by small coastal fishing vessels and traditional fishing methods. The present catch is made within a narrow belt about 15 miles from the shore to a depth about 30 fathoms (180 ft.). Harvesting is mostly by small indigenous fishing crafts such as catamarans, Teppa, sailing canoes, and many other nonmechanized country craft. These craft are primarily made by tying 4-6 rectangular logs shaped into a boat. They are dismantled after each day's operation and left on the dock until the next fishing day.

Small mechanized boats of 30-32 feet length are also used, mostly for shrimp fishing. At the present time there are only ten trawlers used for fishing operations.

The country's marine fish varieties are:

1) Major Pelagic (surface water) fishes, such as sardines, mackerel, tuna, anchovies, seer, and ribbon fish.
2) Midwater fishes, such as Bombay Duck, Silver Bellies, and Horse Mackerel.
3) Demersal (deep sea) fishes, such as perches, sciaenid, catfish, polynemids, flat fish, pomfrets, eels, sharks, skates, and rays.
4) Crustaceans, such as shrimp, lobster, and crabs; and
5) Molluscan resources, such as chank, oysters, mussels, clams, and squids.

Harvesting and Marketing

The fishing operations are on day-to-day bases. The country craft or the mechanized boats leave the shore about three in the morning and reach the fishing grounds by six. Harvesting lasts for 3-4 hours and then the boats need another three hours for the return journey. Nearly two-thirds of the time is spent travelling and only one-third in fishing. Even the mechanized boats do not have adequate facilities to stay overnight. The harvest is dumped on the dock (usually on the beach sand) and sold at auction. The fish are transported to market by head loads, cycles, buses, trucks, and railway. If the craft is family owned, the catch is marketed in the town by the ladies. The fish are occasionally sprinkled with water to keep them moist but are never iced even though marketing lasts for several hours.

Presently the catch consists mainly of Pelagic fishes (sardines and mackerel), crustaceans (shrimp and lobster), and frogs. Over 70 percent of the total fish catch is consumed fresh and only about 4 percent is canned and frozen; the world average is 28 percent fresh consumption and 23 percent canned and frozen. The major portion of the canned and frozen items is exported because of production costs and the attractive "price" offered by the foreign markets.

Consumption

According to FAO, the per capita consumption of fish and shellfish in India is 2.4 pounds per annum as compared to 86 pounds in Iceland and 71 pounds in Japan. In India the good quality shrimp, lobster tails, and frog legs are exported to curb the drain in foreign currency. Mollusks and many other gourmet seafoods are not harvested and not consumed in India because of local customs and conditions. In the coastal villages where fishing is the predominant occupation, the consumption of fish is greater than for any other source of animal protein. In big cities like Calcutta, fish is consumed on Sunday by low income households. The consumption of fish in the inland villages is limited to the few days a year when the ponds dry out. Then villagers are allowed to fish the ponds; at all other times fishing is prohibited. The inland medium-size towns very rarely get fish. The fish available in these markets are mostly fresh water fish which would spoil and lose characteristic good flavour by the time they reached the consumer.

At present India is producing about 1.8 million tons of fish and other seafood which is only 2.6 percent of the total world seafood supplies. In contrast, the geographically smaller countries, like Peru and Japan, are producing respectively over 15 and 14 percent of the world catch. According to many experts, the annual production can be increased by at least tenfold both by offshore and deep sea fishing (beyond 30 fathoms).

Inland Fisheries

The inland fisheries of India and their cultivation are over 2000 years old. The principal rivers including their tributaries and irrigation canals have a total length of about 87,000 miles and 4 million acres of cultivable waters. The cultivable brackish water is about 5 million acres. Only about 38 percent of these waters are being used for fish culture; the fish production is as low as 535 pounds per acre per year. This yield can be increased by another tenfold.

Seafood Exports from India

One of the most significant developments in Indian fisheries has been the unquestionable success of India's shrimp industry in moving dynamically into the major world markets. India is the second largest producer of shrimp, exceeded only by the United States. India has captured a major segment of the U.S. and Japanese markets. India is now the second-largest exporter of shrimp to the U.S. In 1951 India was not even listed in the U.S. shrimp import statistics. The quantity of marine products from India doubled between 1966 and 1972 and the value rose more than fourfold. In 1972 shrimp, frog legs, and lobster tails accounted for 86 percent in quantity and 93 percent in value of the seafood exports from India. Frozen shrimp was the largest commodity, accounting for 80 percent in quantity and about 88 percent in value.

Conclusion

In conclusion, India, with an estimated population of nearly 570 million people, is now going through a transition similar to the one in the 1966 drought. This year's drought is much worse than the previous one. Worldwide grain shortages and world political problems are among the major contributors to the widespread food shortage in India. People just want some food to eat—they are not concerned about its nutritional aspects. There are millions of people who want to eat fish but it is not available. The seafood industry in India is predominantly the shrimp industry which is primarily export oriented because of the high unit value realized by the fisherman and the processer. The government is encouraging and giving prime importance to this industry because of unsatisfactory trade balances with other countries. Using the present known technology of harvesting, processing, and marketing, India has tremendous resources that could be developed to increase its production and consumption by at least ten-fold. How soon we can achieve this and produce more food out of the sea must rest with government policies and priorities. Technologists can answer any necessary questions or can find a solution to any local problem.

Reprinted with permission from League for International Food Education *Newsletter*, pp. 1-3 (October 1973).

Technology and Dependence

JOHAN GALTUNG

*The internal logic of excessive modernization
in a fisheries project in Kerala*

As illustration of a general theoretical perspective and method of analysis that in our experience are applicable to very many development projects, we will use the Indo-Norwegian Fishery Development Project in Kerala, the southernmost state in India, or, more precisely, the effect of that project on the villages where it was initiated, Sakthikulangara and Puthentura, located between Cochin and Quilon towns on the Malabar Coast.[1] In no way is this an effort to present a complete evaluation of the project. Rather, it is an effort to elucidate what seems to the author to be the most salient features.

Initially, this project had only one important goal: to improve the living conditions for the poor along the coast, particularly for the very poor population of fishermen. Any measure of success should be in terms of increased standard of living in general and calorie-protein consumption in particular.

In order to analyse what happened with a view to emphasizing the salient features, let us turn to our very simple analytical tools.

Some major aspects of the principal economic activity of these villages, i.e., fishing, can be illustrated as in Figure 1. The point of departure, as in all economic cycles, is nature (n). This is the ocean washing the Malabar shores, and the producers (p) in the traditional cycle are the fishermen in their wooden canoes, and

further south in their catamarans, managing with age-old techniques to get some of the produce of the ocean into their boats. The gear is simple, the fishermen are plentiful, the catch is meagre, the economic productivity is low. But the catch is landed and marketed to the consumers, a considerable portion of whom are identical with the producers (self-consumption). These consumers give waste products back to nature. In the traditional cycle, one could hardly speak of much depletion (of fish), or of heavy pollution (by waste products)—low depletion and low pollution to a large extent being related to low efficiency.

Thus, it is probably correct to say that there was a certain ecological balance although the point should not be carried too far as it is romantic to assume that nature is in balance when it is untouched by man. But it is definitely true that the economic cycle was so limited, so small that there was little alienation. The fisherman was part of an economic cycle everybody could understand; everybody knew from where things came and where they went.

If we now turn to the cycle from a third perspective, that of exploitation, the picture is also well-known: an accumulation in the pockets of the fish merchants, little elsewhere. The fish merchants took risks, and they had and have complicated cycles of conversion where the monetary output may be only a minor fraction of the total. They also occupied key locations in the economic cycle, giving them considerable power.

Thus, the traditional cycle was characterized by three properties: ecological balance, limited

---

[1]See also Per Sandven, *The Indo-Norwegian Project in Kerala.* Oslo, 1959.

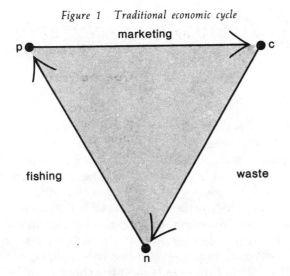

Figure 1   *Traditional economic cycle*

extension, uneven accumulation. A fourth and highly important feature was mentioned above: the cycle was low both in production (total output) and productivity; there was little catch, and very little catch per producer.

In other words, there was a motivation for doing something, and that motivation had two roots: get production up and exploitation down. However, in efforts to introduce a new economic cycle with increased production and decreased exploitation, other aspects were to a large extent ignored.

It is our basic tenet that it is wrong to analyse development projects component by component. There has to be some kind of total analysis, and there are many ways of doing this, whereby a more global impression of what took place can be developed. Thus, here is the formulation of this particular development project: an expansion of the economic cycle far beyond the level of the village, to the world level, as far as nature, producers and consumers are concerned. (See Figure 2).

Fishing still consists in harvesting nature, getting its produce; there are still producers, there are still consumers who consume the fish; and there is still waste. So far things can be said to be the same. The modern cycle is isomorphic

to the traditional cycle, the same elements can still be recognized; it is merely the famous economies of scale. But this is a rather superficial similarity, for not much more is similar.

Due to new methods of fishing, the harvesting of nature has been expanded. Thorough research has laid the basis for optimal ocean harvesting, indicating the need to go further out and deeper down. Nature (N), in short, can no longer be conceived of directly, but may be understood through the stories told by the new group of professionally trained fishermen on board the impressive, not only mechanized, but thoroughly modern steel and fibre-glass vessels, with electronic fish-finding devices.

Because of this, the producers (P) are no longer the traditional fishermen trained through imitation of the older generation, benefiting from the experience handed down by their ancestors.[2] For the pattern of modern fishing that was introduced is industrial fishing, whereby the fisherman is an industrial worker. As to the consumers: they are not the same as before either, and here comes what perhaps is the crux of the story. Briefly told, it may be said to have three phases, all of them part of this

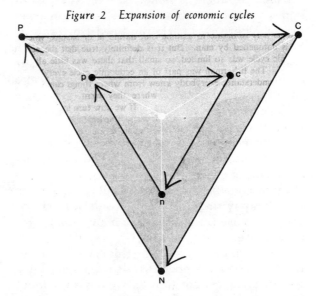

Figure 2   *Expansion of economic cycles*

[2]Arne Martin Klausen, "Technical Assistance and Social Conflict: A Case Study from the Indo-Norwegian Fishing Project in Kerala, South India." *Journal of Peace Research* 1964.

development project.

In the first phase, nature and producers are both expanded in the ways indicated. Fishing is less labour intensive, more capital and research intensive. It is done on an experimental basis, and much of the cost was borne by the Norwegian Government under the technical assistance agreement. One significant part of this agreement was the effort to introduce new methods of marketing, partly to make it more effective in order to expand the cycle, reaching consumers farther out, and partly to eliminate the middlemen, the fishmongers. One key element in connection with the expansion is the method of preservation. Beyond simple ice cooling, there are many alternative methods: the alternative chosen was deep-freezing of the catch duly sorted and prepared, and the preservation of the deep-frozen catch either in freezer, cold storage, or for shorter periods, in boxes with ice. Instead of the old bicycles transporting baskets of fish, insulated vans with considerable carrying capacity are introduced. Although the local fishermen of course could still fill their consumption needs and possibly more easily than before, the difficulty now was that the finished products became too expensive. Consumers were not obtainable at realistic market prices. There was certainly need (for protein) but not demand, articulated in the language a market economy will understand: the language of money. Before there was consumption at a very low level of technology; now there is a high level of technology, but still a very low level of consumption.

In the second phase, attempts were introduced to improve the situation. The choice was between using cheaper technology so as to produce cheaper consumer goods or finding consumers who can pay the price. The second method was the one chosen, and there are many reasons for that choice.

One obvious way of doing this is to try to cater to the upper and upper-middle classes of Indian society as target consumers. There is no doubt that they have the monetary power; the diffi-

culty is that they do not like fish, or at least did not consume much of it. Another difficulty lies in that the fish caught is not very elegant, that is, it is not fish with prestige or snob value.

Concentrating on elegant seafood

Efforts were then made to penetrate into the upper classes in Cochin and other places and demonstrate to the masses the farmer's willingness to buy and consume fish. The idea was that their life-styles could best be disseminated from the top to the bottom, through the laws of imitation. However, this was not a great success, neither at the top nor at the bottom nor in between. The consumption of fish did not greatly expand. And here it might perhaps be added that in a highly inegalitarian society like India, one cannot expect the top and the bottom of society to eat the same food. Food is stratified like people: in vertical societies food is also organized along a vertical axis. For food to be eaten by the well-to-do it cannot be too cheap; if, in addition, it should be eaten by the poor it certainly cannot be expensive. One might speculate that there could be a hierarchy of fish: that the top would eat salmon and the bottom herring, so to speak—but then it is not obvious that the bottom will feel inclined to eat herring just by watching and hearing about how the top enjoys salmon.

In short, a modernized technology existed producing a product for which there was insufficient demand to pay for the costs of the technology and in addition render a profit, small or big.

The solution came during the third phase: to concentrate on the part of the catch consisting of shrimps and lobsters. This is elegant seafood indeed, if not exactly fish; and prices are already high, partly due to scarcity and partly to demand. The contribution to the total price of modern technology would be smaller for lobster tails than for more humble fish, Indians and Japanese had started a small export industry during the 1940s based on frozen shrimps and lobsters. In the Indo-Norwegian project area, the local entrepreneurs saw the same opportunity, imitated the technology introduced by the Norwegians, and went in for the shrimps and lobsters. Needless to say, the price of these products was extremely far beyond what the very poor local population could pay, even to the extent that these products became abstract entities rather than concrete things available to the local population. But years had passed, and the goal was no longer local consumption.

The rise of the local entrepreneur

Expensive technology had now produced expensive goods; where were the customers willing to pay the price? The answer was very simple. In the rich countries, or more precisely in Japan and in the United States, both countries with enormous demand for seafood, and particularly for relatively cheap seafood produced in a country where labour costs are low. Old markets were expanded, new markets were found and the new consumers (C) were located far beyond the immediate horizon, indeed.

And thus, the cycle has been modernized not only in the sense that it has been expanded and integrated into the world economy in general, but also that all elements in the cycle are modern. What is caught is caught with the most modern technology, by modern fishermen, marketed with modern techniques to modern consumers. The cycle is of almost unlimited extension, reaching so far and so widely around the world that hardly anyone understands more than a tiny segment of it.

As for exploitation, the leading local entrepreneur in Sakthikulangara built his own ice factory with a capacity of 34 tons of ice, then bought 15 insulated vans and had an annual sales value of 30 million rupees (late 1969). His own profit was estimated at 4 million rupees: some of it was given back to the village in the form of a blue and white five-story temple, much of it invested in his own house, a palace protected by a high fence and guards with machine guns. Some other families also did well, extremely well by local standards. The GVP (gross village product) per caput no doubt increased steeply, making people talk not only about economic growth but even about little America. Social inequality, in short, rose tremendously, for most of the population continued as before, and those who were employed in the lobster and shrimp factories were very poorly paid, usually not even with a guaranteed daily income—they worked on an hour-to-hour basis, depending on incoming catch.

As to depletion and pollution: difficult to say. Since catch had been available for time immemorial with the traditional methods, it seems rather likely that highly capital- and research-intensive techniques would have a depleting effect. And there is little doubt as to the pollution: new smells, new types of wastes.

But there was production and productivity. More fish and other types of seafood were caught and killed than ever before in history, and certainly in more modern ways and by fewer people than ever before. The only difficulty with the whole operation was that the consumption of fish among those who needed this source of protein most did not go up. There are even indications that it went down.

Double-standard thinking

This story should not be seen merely as a case study relating to a particular area. It is far more general in its implications. However, to understand the implications, we must ask two questions. What are the factors contributing to the expansion of a cycle? Why is it that such an expanded cycle, although undoubtedly leading to increased production and productivity and to modernization, does not seem to improve the conditions lower down in society?

One very simple reason that a cycle tends to expand when a development project is undertaken is that it has to pass through new centres of administration, financing and research, and there are generally none located in the target area. Of course, there is the possibility of utilizing local administrative, finance and research potential. That could also have been done in this case, provided one had been aiming at a considably more modest goal of modernization. There was local leadership, some local capital (certainly not much), and some local expertise pointing in new directions. But this was not made use of since the whole assumption behind a technical assistance project is that the outsider—i.e., the Norwegians—would bring in modern technology. The whole idea of a technical assistance project, as it was conceived of in the 1950s and also today, is antithetical to utilization of local expertise. The local population can be used as consultants to pronounce themselves on details in the technology brought in from the outside. For the basic idea is the introduction of new technology. This is the *sine qua non* of the entire project: the new technology justifies the experts.

There is another factor, which was particularly relative to the level of thinking prevalent in the donor country, *in casu* Norway, some 20 years ago. One was firmly against double-standard thinking. What was good for Norwegians was also good for Indians because only the best was good enough. One should not have a rich man's technology and a poor man's technology. Development was to decrease the gap in the direction of the rich.

As a consequence of these two premises, the technology exported to the Kerala fishing villages had to be the most modern Norwegian technology at that time. If deep-freezing was the method considered the most developed in Norway in the 1950s, then extremely strong arguments would be needed to put alternative, less modern technologies on the political horizon. If these alternative technologies, such as drying, cold or warm smoking, were now considered outmoded or subdominant relative to the leading technology, they would not meet the bill.

Similar considerations apply to financing and research. The investment needed to modernize fisheries was of considerable magnitude and could not be obtained locally. It was obtained partly from Norway, partly from the central government, and since this meant that much capital was invested in a small area that was favoured by this input, it had to be defined as an experiment, not as a gift nor as a lasting venture. As a matter of fact, there was probably a limit to the amount of success one could have: a lasting total success would be a liability because of the injustice it would cause between the population of those villages and the surrounding millions. This was evidenced by the fact that some people tried to smuggle their family members and others into the area in order to benefit from the various types of services. An economic cycle that would share the benefits more evenly among recipients all over the state of Kerala, all over India and all over the world for that matter, would thus have something in favour of it—something alien to the project from a technological point of view but important from a political angle.

But more inportant than this was the fact that the project was administered by an Indo-Norwegian Standing Committee with regular meetings, usually in New Delhi. The meetings took place far above the heads of the local population, near to the corridors of power in Oslo and New Delhi, among men communicating in the English language, members of the same world culture, much more similar to each other than the Norwegian administrator/expert to the fisherman on a peripheral island in northern Norway. That this top-level communication process was easier for the Norwegians than communication with the minds behind the faces looking at them in the village area when they drove in or out of the Norwegian camp with its offices and living quarters, its tennis courts and gardens, faces pressed against the fences with expressionless eyes, goes without saying. Not only was the local language, *malayalam*, a very difficult one; the whole pattern of thinking, the cognitive styles, the local culture were incomprehensible to all except at a superficial tourist level, and to the very few who were particularly dedicated.

The Centre's gains

When it comes to research there is a similar picture. Modern technology is research intensive; traditional technology is labour extensive in the sense that its expertise is based on dozens, hundreds of generations of accumulated experience, filtered through complex communication processes and internalized (often implicitly rather than explicitly) in the local producer.

If development is to be based on modernization, it is almost unavoidable that economic cycles are spun in and out of the centres of research in addition to the centres of finance and administration. Very often research, finance and administration are found at the same place, in a private or public corporation.

The net result of all this is a new type of economic cycle that, perhaps, can be illustrated by Figure 3.

In this economic cycle the focus is on a division of labour between Centre and Periphery, with the Centre delivering research and technology (know-how and show-how), administration and capital, and the Periphery doing what is indicated in Figures 1 and 2, but in a modern way. What this division of labour means is that the tremendous experience

Figure 3 *A modern division-of-labour economic cycle*

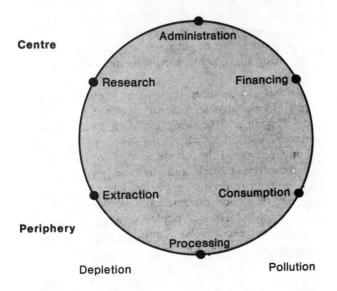

Figure 4   The centre-periphery export-import cycle

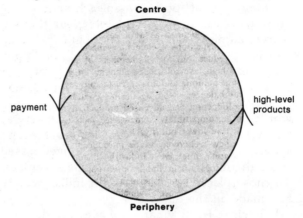

gained through trial and error, through doing the research, including the practical experiments, not only knowing the results, is given to the Centre; that the corresponding experience and control relating to administration and finance are also kept by the Centre; and that the Periphery receives solutions, decisions, and investment (loans/grants). The Centre grows with this process, develops an experience that can be used in other projects and in other parts of the world. The Periphery also gains something in principle: a modern technology is introduced, production and productivity go up. But then there are the negative sides to the equation.

First, a pattern of dependency is in all probability created. The Centre will continue doing research and stimulate a demand for the most recent technology. The Centre will also develop new administrative frameworks, for instance multilateral, international organizations, and stimulate a demand for participation in these organizations by offering information and decisions that high-level representatives of the Periphery country's own people have participated in formulating. This dependency pattern is relatively clear: only Periphery countries with very clear goals and strategies of their own will be able to resist. The strength of the Centre is always in part based on the weakness of the Periphery.

The Periphery may gain independence by defining a cut-off point. At an early stage of the project, it was made completely clear that research, administration and financing should go entirely over to Indian hands after some time. But these Indian hands were not located in Sakthikulangara/Puthentura, but in New Delhi, Bombay and Hyderabad/Bangalore, etc. In other words, for the local poor fishermen, there was probably scant comfort in knowing that the high spheres of the cycle to which he belonged passed through Indian rather than European centres. To those placed in the centre of Indian society this made all the difference.

It is clear from what we have said that the economic cycle induced by the Norwegian project was both alienating and exploitative: alienating because of its enormous extension, exploitative because the Centre gains so much more than the Periphery.

Who hears the malnourished?

But, it will immediately be objected, frozen shrimps and lobsters did not simply disappear; there was payment in return for them. Potentially, this payment might even be used to buy protein to be distributed to the masses in those villages. Needless to say, nothing of the sort happened, although the idea looks nice on paper. What happened instead is complicated to understand and even more complicated to demonstrate.

The payment in Figure 4 can be split into many components.

Obviously, a certain proportion will always go to (or be retained by) the Centre to pay for services, know-how (patents) administration and financing (servicing loans). A proportion goes into maintenance and modernization, also to the Centre, of the world, or of India. By Indian regulations, hard currency earning export industries may decide over a certain proportion of currency earned, provided it is used to cover this type of expenses. To some extent, this may be said to reinforce a dependency pattern since the exporter will probably be highly motivated to control how the money is put to use. But it must always be remembered that investment in increasingly modern machinery does not itself mean satisfaction of basic human needs.

Third, with export markets found in hard currency regions, chances are extremely high that the currency will be used to procure capital goods needed for industrialization and for military purposes elsewhere in the Indian subcontinent instead of being used to buy foodstuffs. Those who articulate the need for capital goods near the power centres speak with a considerably louder and more articulate voice than those who suffer from malnutrition in the backwaters of Kerala.

The fourth portion may be identified with profits. Of these profits, some may be kept abroad under a gentleman's agreement between the Indian exporter and the foreign importer, but the major part is probably taken home.

For an intermediate cycle

We would characterize this development project as a bad one, regardless of the facts that a modern technology has been transmitted to certain segments of the Indian structure and that fewer people make more catches in a more modern way than at any time before in Indian history. The purpose of a project of this kind must be to improve more human lives.

The question remains whether we can make use of this type of thinking to derive some ideas about alternative development strategies.

Development is defined as a process that leads to, as a minimum, the satisfaction of elementary needs (food, clothes, shelter, health, education) for all members of society, is compatible with a high level of local autonomy in goal-setting as well as instrumentation, and to a reasonable level of equity and ecological balance. Nothing of this contradicts the idea of increased production and increased productivity, but if there should be an incompatibility somewhere, then technical efficiency would have lower priority.

Thus the new technology to be introduced cannot be too research and capital intensive. Industrial fishing as it is conceived of today does not in and by itself constitute a solution to the problem of the poor fisherman. Hence the search for an intermediate economic cycle, which is a broader idea than the search for an intermediate technology, and it is very much doubted that one has to be an expert on fisheries in the modern sense in order to see some of the outlines of an intermediate cycle, including an intermediate technology.[3]

Any intermediate technology would have to be judged not only by its ability to satisfy the needs of the Periphery, but also to be directed by the Periphery. This in itself points in the direction of beach fishing rather than ocean fishing. On the other hand, if some simple type of mechanized craft is wanted, the intermediate economic cycle would at least have to be stretched in the direction of a factory capable of producing cheap and simple inboard or outboard motors. In a world that has not yet (with the exception of the People's Republic of China[4]) started asking fundamental questions about the total economic cycle, the factors taken into account in a cost-benefit analysis would be limited in number and scope. The idea of intermediate cycles would force one to ask whether it can be produced locally—meaning neither "village" nor "country" but something in between. That technology does not exist today, for which reason one might have to concede the necessity of involving industrialized centres outside the extended project area.

When it comes to the crucial point of preservation of the catch, it seems obvious that less capital-intensive methods have to be found. Drying and smoking are perhaps the two most obvious methods, but others also exist, such as more use of ice rather than freezing. It is surprising that so little was done to look into these possibilities, and that can probably best be explained by the built-in need to export modern technology. It is quite possible that such intermediate methods would have negative effects both in terms of depletion and pollution; trees might have to be cut excessively to produce the wood needed for the heat and smoke, and this would in itself lead to pollution But then it might be that other sources could have been found, such as solar energy.

A new direction for research

At this point it may be objected that research in this field is not very likely to take place in these villages; in fact, it will probably rather take place in the Centre. This may be true in our presently distorted world, but if the result is a technology that would make sunny districts in the Periphery autonomous where energy is concerned in a way that can neither be depleted nor lead to significant pollution, this would be a minor consideration. Again, that technology is not with us today, so what we are making here is the usual plea for a redirection of technological research.

We have tried to indicate a set of criteria for the steering and the evaluation of development projects, all of them within a framework of thinking defined by an analysis of the economic cycles being used by the project. The conclusions arrived at concerning this particular Indo-Norwegian project are far from positive. However, this is of minor significance in relation to the basic problem of designing and implementing different types of cycles with better ecological balance, less exploitation and less alienation. For although the modern cycles described above are still increasing in scope and number and depth, the awareness of their tremendous shortcomings seems to be mounting. And this article is one little contribution, however small, to the increase of that awareness.

[3] E. F. Schumacher, *Small in Beautiful,* Blond & Briggs, London 1973.

[4] Johan Galtung and Fumiko Nishimura, "Learning from the Chinese" (mimeo). Oslo, 1974.

Reprinted with permission from *Ceres,* the FAO Review on Agriculture and Development, pp. 45-50 (September/October 1974).

Should We Eat Krill?

BARRY BONDAR and P.J. BOBEY

If technology can move India from subsistence fishing to shrimp export, it can move the rich nations of the world from whaling to krilling. The following three pieces consider the prospects and pressures for the exploitation of this new ocean "resource."

The world's oceans are grossly over fished and as the traditional species become scarcer—new sources of marine food are being researched. Among the most recent to come under scrutiny are oceanic zooplankton or krill. *In this article two Canadian students examine the possible benefits to be derived from a large scale use of krill against the probable ecological cost resulting from such a radical interference with the oceans' ecosystems.*

Using recent technological improvements several governments are now on the way to creating a viable zooplankton harvesting process and it is time to look at both the benefits and the dangers of such an operation.

Perhaps the most important zooplankton type presently considered for harvest is commonly called "krill." Of the various worldwide species of krill which exist, only the Antarctic species, *Euphausia superba* has the qualities which make for economical harvesting. These include an adequate size for efficient capture, being plentiful and continually concentrated into swarms as well as having a good protein content.

The nutritive value of krill is high. On a dry matter basis, samples of *E. superba* were found to contain 24.6 percent lipid, 49 per cent protein, 2.5 per cent chitin and 9.8 per cent ash. The krill is also high in vitamins A and B as well as in essential amino acids like arginine, lysine, leucine and phenylalanine. Other substances such as potassium, iron, manganese and zinc are also present. Perhaps the most important factor in the economic harvesting of this form of krill is the fact that they aggregate into distinct lens-shaped swarms through-out every known phase of their life cycles.[5] It appears that crustaceans of various age classes differ fairly well in their size and generally do not mix,[6] which means that each swarm generally consists of only one specific age and size group. Since the *Euphausia surperba* has a life span of over four years, there are usually four types characterized by the length of the organisms within each unit. Although the patches vary in size from 0.5 by 1 metre up to 150 by 400 metres, the fact that this form of krill constantly swarms means that units of comparatively dense concentration can be harvested.

High costs

High costs are inevitable. In the first place there is the sheer distance that a fleet must travel in order to reach the Antarctic; ships must be equipped with some form of processing plant on board since spoilage is high within forty-eight hours, and much research must already have been done so that the fishermen can predict the location and swarming activities of the krill. Visual as well as hydro-acoustic observations are used in tracking down krill, which tend to be found in areas with circular water movements.[7] The main surface swarms are most commonly present in the area of the Scotia Sea where the Weddell Sea waters closely approach the warmer waters of the West Wind Drift. But there are a wide variety of environmental factors and intrinsic Euphausiid behavioural patterns which create unpredictable swarming patterns.

Generally, the largest catches are obtained during the day in the continental shelf regions by towing the net close to the bottom. During the night, the vertical migrations of the Euphausiid disperse the organisms throughout the vertical water column. Catches are also affected by temperature change. It has been observed that commercial concentrations of krill are often found where the temperature is close to 3.5°C.

Due to the unpredictability of the Euphausiid patches, new methods have been attempted to induce swarms of krill to concentrate in dense enough units for commercial harvesting. Stasenko (1967)[8] and Semenov (1969)[9] have indicated that *Euphausia superba* moves toward dim light regardless of the colour. Night fishing using large spotlights directed toward the water's surface can therefore locate and increase the density of surface swarms. Generally, side trawls, fish pumps or towed nets of varying sizes (depending upon what size range of krill is desired) are the main devices used for the collection of the krill.[10, 11]

Light lures may also be used in areas of weak surface currents by attaching lights to floating bouys thereby attracting dense swarms of Euphausiids. A scoop net can then be dropped around the swarm and closed beneath it. Initial experiments on the reactions of Euphausiids to electrical fishing methods are also being carried out.[11]

At present, several countries are involved in the experimental use of krill, although this is as yet on a limited basis. The U.S.S.R. has recently advanced a 10 per cent krill and 90 per cent cheese mixture to the consumer market under the brand name "Korall" and states that the product is selling well.[1] Furthermore, feeding trials of krill on young pigs by Soviet scientists have shown that the material can be used as a high quality animal feed.[10] In countries such as Canada and the United States where sea foods do not constitute a major part of the diet, krill would most likely be used as an additional source of animal feed. In addition, Euphausiids used for direct human consumption have long been collected on a small scale by Japanese fishermen and have been boiled, dried in the sun and mixed with rice to produce a rice cake known as "Tsukudani."[10] Other countries presently involved on a small scale include Norway and Canada where the krill captured is used as bait, food for trout or other "farmed" fish or as a pet food.[10] If technological considerations and problems can be solved, it appears that krill can form a viable commercially exploitable resource.

What we must now consider is the total amount of krill which can safely be removed from the Antarctic ecosystem. At present there is no reliable data on the productivity of the krill in the Antarctic, except for several rough estimates such as those made by J. A. Gulland (1970).[12] Based on a 10 per cent efficiency in energy transfer from the phytoplankton to the herbivorous krill, an annual production of some 500 million tons was calculated. A second estimate was based upon the standing crop biomass and a one year life span which resulted in a productivity of approximately 75 million tons. K. Radway Allen (1971)[13] later revalued this data to a level of 150 million tons taking into account the four year life span of *Euphausia superba*. As a result, only extremely crude values for both the productivity and the standing crop biomass can be obtained until extensive studies have been undertaken.

Since virtually nothing is known of the biotic or the abiotic factors controlling the abundance of the krill, it has been suggested by MacKintosh (1971)[14] and others that man should for the time being simply take over the role vacated by the greatly reduced baleen, sei, minke, and right whales in an attempt to utilise the expected surplus of krill. The surplus has been calculated to be not less than 30 million tons and may very well be more but no data is available to show that such an increase has actually occurred. It has further been pointed out that the reduction or removal of a consumer does not inevitably result in a surplus of the food.[14] Dr. B. Stonehouse has shown that it is unwise to assume that the removal of the whales has necessarily left a gap in the ecosystem that man can fill. Indeed, there may have been a compensating increase in the numbers of birds, crab eater seals, smaller minke whales, antarctic fish or squid populations to counteract the space left by reduced whale stocks. Later work by MacKintosh (1970)[15] has indicated that minke whales and crab eater seals do not appear to have increased greatly and that the excess krill, if any, could be being absorbed by fish or squid or by the carnivorous zooplankton which feeds on krill.

Recent studies have shown that the ability of krill to form vast concentrations in the pelagic waters of the Antarctic and its availability to the organisms which feed on it mark it as a principal link in the complex trophic interactions of the Antarctic.[16] Indeed, krill has been found in the stomachs of thirty-one fish species belonging to twelve families of Antarctic, Subantarctic and even migratory subtropical fish.[17] It also constitutes the main diet of such organisms as whalebone whales, crab eater seals, penguins and migratory birds. The *Euphausia superba,* therefore, is a critical link between the primary and the predatory levels of the Antarctic food chain.

The experience of whaling has shown that once an industry with huge capital investment has developed it is often too late to exercise effective control (indeed Dr. G.G.L. Bertram suggests that in the long term, the cheapest way of harvesting the krill may be to allow whales to recover and then to crop them again). At present the world has a totally inadequate legal frame-work governing the ownership of high sea resources such as fisheries. For this reason, immediate attempts must be made to set up international regulations to protect the highly dynamic Antarctic ecosystem, before exploitation begins.

All the facts lead us to the conclusion that no large scale harvesting of krill should be allowed until the ecological implications of such harvesting have been studied in depth and international treaties based on such studies have been agreed by every nation involved.

REFERENCES

1 *Commercial Fisheries Review* 31 (9) p.62, 1969
2 *Commercial Fisheries Review* 32 (1) p.79, 1970
3 Discussion "Utilization of Krill and Other Resources of the Southern Ocean by Man", *Antarctic Ecology* (Holdgate, M W editor) Volume 2 p.229 Academic Press, London, 1970
4 Discussion "Changes Consequent Upon the Reduction of Whale Stocks", *Antarctic Ecology,* Holdgate, M W (editor) Vol 2 p.227, Academic Press, London, 1970. *Biology* Vol 7, Academic Press, London, 1967
5 Sir F S Russell, Sir M Yonge (editors) *Advances in Marine Biology* Vol 7, Academic Press, London, p.156.
6 Makarov, R R, Naumov A G, and Shevtsov V V, The Biology and the Distribution of the Antarctic Krill, *Antarctic Ecology,* Vol 2, pages 173-176, Academic Press, London, 1970
7 Ivanov, B C, On the Biology of the Antarctic Krill (*Euphausia superba*), Marine Biology (Berlin), 7, p.340-345, 1970
8 Zenkovich, B A, "Whale and Plankton in Antarctic Waters" *Antarctic Ecology,* Academic Press, London 1970, p.83-185
9 Semenov, V N, Translation No 93, Fisheries Laboratory, Lowestoft, 1970
10 Parsons, T R, "Plankton as a Food Source", *Underwater Journal,* February 1972 p.30-36

11 Sir F S Russell, Sir M Yonge (editors) *Advances in Marine Biology*, Vol 7 Academic Press, London 1967

12 Gulland J A, "The Development of the Resources of the Antarctic Seas", *Antarctic Ecology*, Vol 2, Academic Press, London, p.217-223

13 Allen, K R, "Relations Between Production and Biomass" *J Fish. Res. Bd. Canada*, 28, p.1537-1581, 1971

14 MacKintosh, N A, "Whale and Krill in the Twentieth Century", *Antarctic Ecology*, Vol 2, Academic Press, London, p.196-221, 1970

15 MacKintosh, N A, "Whales and Krill in the Twentieth Century", Eng. National Institute of Oceanography Collected Reprints, 18 pages, 1970

16 Sir F S Russell, Sir M Yonge (editors) *Advances in Marine Biology*, Vol 7, Academic Press, London, p.177-181, 1970

17 Pernitin, Yu E, "Consumption of Krill by Antarctic Fishes", *Antarctic Ecology*, Vol 2, Academic Press, London, p.177-181, 1970

Reprinted with permission from *The Ecologist* (Wadebridge, Cornwall, U.K.), 4 (7): 265-266 (August 1974).

Food From the Sea

S. J. HOLT

Dear Sir,

The timely article by Bondar and Bobey ("Should we eat krill?" August 1974) appeared just before a "consultation of experts" convened by the Food and Agriculture Organization of the United Nations on that subject, at the time of a meeting of its inter-governmental Committee on Fisheries in October. Unfortunately participants were not, I think, aware of the article, nor were the important questions raised in it extensively discussed.

The Federal Republic of Germany should, by the way, now be added to the list of technologically advanced countries with programmes of research on krill with a view to harvesting. The main Russian product now is krill paste—to which there is, apparently, some "consumer resistance"—and the Japanese are marketing it as a form of frozen shrimp.

A more or less independent group of scientists, sponsored by the FAO Advisory Committee on Marine Resources Research and financed mainly by the United Nations Environment Programme, is now reviewing the estimates of the depleted whale resources used by the International Whaling Commission, and trying to evaluate the ecological relationships of the whales with their food supply and their competitors. It is true that existing data are tenuous; on the other hand it is clear that catch rates of krill would have to be very much higher than by present methods, not only for economic operation, but also to compete with the rate of catch that could eventually be taken with equivalent effort from restored whale stocks.

The need for a long-term programme of research on cetaceans, especially of the large whales, has now been internationally and officially recognised. During an "International Cetacean Decade" it will be necessary to monitor Antarctic whale populations independently of any continuing data from the drastically cutback whaling operations, and it has been suggested that specially chartered vessels might be used for this purpose, under the aegis of UNEP.

Yet, less biological oceanography is being done now in Antarctic waters—apart from basic studies near the ice edge by Antarctic expeditions, and the narrowly conceived krill exploration—than before. It seems reasonable to suggest that a large scale investigation of the Antarctic marine ecosystem should be launched as a combined operation. But why, some ask, should this be done by international organisations? Why not—even cooperatively—by the nations that are already interested in and able to mount such programmes? I have tried to show elsewhere why it should not be left entirely to them. Briefly it is because, even if the UN Conference on the Law of the Sea leads to agreement for a 200 mile wide Exclusive Economic Zone the living resources within which are under the jurisdiction of the coastal state, some of the "unconventional" resources such as squid, lantern fishes and krill will be beyond that zone. How much will be outside, and how much within, we cannot say, because we do not yet know the geographic distribution of the resources, and there are also large uncertainties as to the eventual frontiers of a hundred or more EEZ's and an international or "high seas" zone.

Further, since interested states have, under the Antarctic Treaty, until now held in abeyance their territorial claims on that Continent, the eventual status of the ocean area up to 200 miles offshore from it is anybody's guess. Ominously, some Parties to the Antarctic Treaty are now showing interest in the mineral resources of the continent itself—including huge reserves of offshore oil—and we cannot assume that the territorial claims will remain dormant.

So, observing that most of the nations now interested in krill are among those whose fleets depleted the whale stocks, and whose populations are not evidently short of protein, it seems in order to suggest that research and development on krill, and other biological resources of the Antarctic—including the whales —should be overseen by some organization responsible to the world community as a whole, including the developing nations whose people now consume neither whale products, nor krill, nor other items from one of the main marine resources in the Southern Hemisphere. The cooperation of the powerful nations, and of such specialised organisations as the IWC, will of course be desirable, even essential, but there seems to me to be an overwhelming case for a substantial international research operation in addition. To mount this the assistance of both UNEP and the World Bank and other funding organs of the UN system should be sought. To plan it, those *non*-governmental international organisations which have long been interested in Antarctic problems should

be involved: the Scientific Committee on Antarctic Research and the Scientific Committee on Oceanic Research (both parts of the International Council of Scientific Unions) and the International Union for the Conservation of Nature and Natural Resources. A useful lead has also been given by Unesco's Intergovernmental Oceanographic Commission, whose International Coordination Group for the Southern Ocean recently reported that it "shared a growing and world-wide concern regarding the impact of uncontrolled exploitation of krill, pelagic fish and other living resources..."

Meanwhile environmental interest groups should perhaps press, if not for a moratorium on krill harvesting, at least for the early establishment of a rather low international limit to the annual experimental harvest, pending better understanding of the situation. If, as seems possible, the International Sea-Bed Authority being negotiated by the UN Conference on the Law of the Sea, also has some responsibility for administering certain other aspects of the use of ocean space, it could be an appropriate body to implement such restraints, either directly or through an Agency such as FAO.

S.J. Holt.
Professor of International Ocean Affairs,
Royal University of Malta

Reprinted with permission from the author and *The Ecologist*, 5(2):70-71 (February 1975).

Antarctic Problems: Tiny Krill to Usher in New Resource Era

DEBORAH SHAPLEY

The 12 nations[1] that are signatories to the 1961 Antarctic Treaty, which dedicates their activities on that continent to scientific, peaceful ones, are moving toward a new treaty to manage Antarctica's living resources. These consist primarily of a species of 3-inch long crustacean found teeming in offshore waters, which also happens to be one of mankind's newest and richest sources of food.

The effort to achieve such a treaty, which has been urged by environmental groups for some time, has broad international significance. Other nations of the world have been eyeing Antarctica's resources—its presumed minerals such as iron and gold and its possible wealth of offshore oil and gas. But the resource most likely to be exploited soon is the krill (*Euphausia superba*). Krill abound in such huge swarms in surface waters that recently a West German ship, using a new technique likely to find wide application, is reported to have scooped up 8 to 12 tons in a single hour!

The sudden move by the Treaty nations signals a growing realization by the 12 governments, and by the scientist-diplomats who specialize in the arcane field of Antarctic policy, that, as one says: "People are realizing that Antarctica is a huge bank of resources that may have to be tapped, that it is something more than an oddity in the earth's crust."

J. H. Zumberge, chairman of the National Academy of Sciences' Polar Research Board, goes on to say, "The idea that Antarctica can be held forever as a scientific laboratory is losing ground." The group of 12 who have had Antarctica more or less to themselves for nearly 20 years, will recognize this new interest formally, soon, when they admit their 13th member, Poland, a nation frankly interested in krill fishing as well as in Antarctic research.

The Antarctic Treaty does not discuss resource exploitation, and thus does not expressly prohibit its signers—or anyone else—from exploiting the region's wealth. At present, any nation, exercising its high-seas freedoms, can fish for Antarctic krill. Likewise any nation could prospect for minerals or drill for offshore oil—although both would be highly impractical at this time. However, the Treaty does obligate its signers to conserve the continent's resources and protect its enviroment, and because of this obligation, the Treaty nations seek a new agreement on krill.

Therefore, at the recent meeting in London from 14 to 18 March, the Treaty powers moved to address the problem of managing the krill. The thinking among diplomats there, according to U.S. and Western sources, was that an agreement to manage the krill would be relatively easy to achieve. It could set a useful precedent for addressing the more difficult problem of oil,

[1]The 12 countries are Argentina, Australia, Belgium, Chile, France, Japan, New Zealand, Norway, Union of South Africa, Soviet Union, United States, and United Kingdom. Seven other nations have acceded to the treaty but have no say in deliberations. These are Brazil, Czechoslovakia, Denmark, East Germany, Netherlands, Poland, and Romania.

gas, and mineral exploitation. Such a treaty, some diplomats admit, could stave off the periodic rumblings at the turbulent, 120-nation law of the sea conference about including Antarctica's riches within its purview.

So it has fallen to the humble krill, which has gone almost unnoticed in the world's diet—let alone in international geopolitics—to become the vehicle for reconciling the 1961 Antarctic Treaty, whose clear aim is the preservation of Antarctica for scientific research, with the realities of a resource-hungry world.

Krill are tiny crustaceans barely capable of swimming, that drift in huge masses near the surface of Antarctic waters. They feed on phytoplankton; and, in turn, they are eaten by most higher life forms in the area, such as whales, seals, birds, fish, and others. Thus they are the cornerstone species of all Antarctic life.

Moreover, because decayed krill enrich Antarctica's coastal waters and continental shelves, they may be important to the spread of nutrients throughout the world's oceans by northward-flowing Antarctic bottom water currents.

But the most important fact about the krill is that they comprise a vast natural source of protein, and hence to many nations are a tantalizing new source of food. Gerard Bertrand of the Council on Environmental Quality says that a 70-million-ton annual harvest of krill would equal no less than the entire fish catch from the rest of the world's oceans. Yet today, well under 1 million tons are caught by the few nations that conduct "exploratory fishing" for krill: Japan, the Soviet Union, Taiwan, West Germany, and now, Poland. Only Japan and the Soviet Union market krill for human consumption, and in Japan, krill tempura is said to be tasty. But breakthroughs in the technology of krill fishing, largely by the West Germans, will make larger scale harvesting more practical, indeed, some say, inevitable. Says Bertrand: "The pressure will come. The world need for protein will require the utilization of krill."...

The details of a future treaty are not yet clear. Its initial objective, however, would be to set some limit on the amount of krill that could

be harvested, while gathering information to use as the basis of long-term management of the krill stocks. Estimates of how much can be harvested safely vary wildly—from 10 to 100 million metric tons; indeed no one knows the size of the total standing stock, which may be as much as 1 billion metric tons. Says CEQ's Bertrand, "Nobody knows how many krill there are. Less than 5 percent of the area has been sampled in a highly detailed way, and only in the last 2 years has anyone systematically tried making such samples."

Krill are primarily eaten by whales, but with the decline in the whale stocks in the last decade, some people have concluded that there must be a resulting "surplus" of krill that can be fished commercially. However, scientists and ecologists doubt that such a krill "surplus" even exists—and want to know more about the krill stocks before large-scale operations begin. The object of a treaty, therefore, would be to begin managing the resource before—rather than after—commercial fishing gets underway.

But the Antarctic Treaty powers are moving on the krill question not simply out of zeal for the environment. They have been under considerable political pressure to recognize the fact they, as well as other nations, want to exploit the krill and perhaps other, nonliving Antarctic resources. In today's international setting—for example at the law of the sea conference where the unclaimed seabeds are to be managed by 120 nations—the fact that 12 nations (principally of the developed world) can dominate this "oddity in the earth's crust" seems odd indeed....

A second pressure on the Antarctic Treaty nations is the fact that many nations, themselves included, are extending their own coastal fishing zones to 200 miles from shore. Seven of the 12 Treaty powers have territorial claims in Antarctica, which they maintain in principle, although the Treaty itself holds all such claims in abeyance.

When these nations extend their own fishing zones, they have a delicate choice: they can either also declare 200-mile exclusive fishing zones off the coasts of Antarctica, and thereby reassert their claims in violation of the treaty; or they can choose to *not* declare such a zone, implying that they are relinquishing their claims. A new international agreement on Antarctica's living resources will help these countries resolve this dilemma.

While under pressure to act on the resource question, the Treaty nations are anxious to avoid creating an image of themselves as a club that considers the continent its exclusive preserve. Thus, they want the krill treaty to include Taiwan, West Germany, and other non-treaty nations that plan to fish for krill in Antarctic waters. In addition, the group of 12 is getting ready to admit Poland probably within a year—and bracing itself for the fact that other resource-hungry nations may wish to follow....

Excerpted with permission from *Science*, 196:503-505 (29 April 1977). Copyright 1977 by the American Association for the Advancement of Science.

Genetic Improvement of Crop Foods

NORMAN BORLAUG

The observant reader will have noted by now that the most optimistic pieces in the book also tend to be the oldest. Here the father of the Green Revolution outlines its virtues and castigates its enemies.

Genetic engineering is making it possible for farmers in even depressed areas to produce more food of higher nutritional value to feed the world in the next three decades. The time thus bought may enable man to gain control of population growth—unless the Emotional Environmentalists succeed in turning back the clock on modern agriculture.

My talk is about the genetic manipulation or improvement of cereal grains. But first, I would like to make some comments on overall increases in food production in the last few years. I am referring to what has been commonly called by the press "The Green Revolution" in food production, especially in Asia.

It would perhaps be more apropos to speak about changes in production patterns in the Western Hemisphere. Nevertheless, I think that the two cases that I have selected will illustrate the magnitude of these changes more easily than if I tried to speak about progress in a great number of countries. In India and in Pakistan, we are dealing with 700 million people. Trying to tackle the complexities of expanding food production in this kind of situation is similar to the magnitude of the food production problems for all the Americas plus a good share of the population of Africa as well. Yet India and Pakistan, where the problem is greatest, are two relatively small countries. What has happened in these nations in the last four years? Take the case of wheat, for instance, considering only India for the moment. In 1965, which was a very favorable year, India's wheat output reached an all-time high of approximately 12 million metric tons. The most important fact is that this peak in wheat production was achieved largely by increasing yields per acre. This is very significant because there is very little additional land that can be brought under the plow. This increase in crops must be the pattern of attack for most of the densely populated countries of the world, which are already running out of arable land.

Hope Dawning

Beyond increased food production, what else does this portend? I have restricted these comments to wheat, but I have no doubt that in the next four years—if we have peace—there will be a similar expansion in the production of rice. Considerable progress has also been made in the production of maize, or corn, in the past four years. So, for the time being, we have made a significant increase in food production in this very densely populated part of the world. This enables us to buy a little time—one, two or three decades—if we continue to work at this problem from all angles and receive continued support from the governments concerned so that food production may stay ahead of population growth. After this period, I hope man will have regained his senses and adjusted his population growth—in order that the absolute essentials for a decent life may be available to all born into this world.

I think the stepped-up production of wheat is having a very significant impact on the total economy. I would like to emphasize that in a country such as India or Pakistan and in most of the Near East and Southeast Asia, a vast segment—80%—of the total population lives on the land, supported mostly by a subsistence agriculture, and has very little to sell. They actually live outside the economy of their country, but if there is a sudden increase in grain production from 12 to 23 million tons, many of these small farmers will participate in the economy. They now have something to sell—a state of affairs which never existed previously.

A whole series of changes is thus set in motion at the village level. The peasants buy things they never had before—simple machines, more fertilizer, more pumps, more motors and casings—and most of these products are made in India. They start buying consumer goods. If you are the head of the household, you might buy a Singer sewing machine in order to provide better clothes for the family, or a transistor radio. The latter allows the Government to broadcast educational programs to all backward villages that were hitherto completely isolated. Most important of all, hope has replaced despair. You can't use a yardstick to measure what hope means in terms of indirect benefits, but I am convinced that they are very substantial.

Mixed Blessing

There are certain disadvantages, however, of which we must be aware. The cereal grains are displacing some of the natural sources of protein on which millions of people in the near Middle East subsist. They are displacing such important protein crops as chick beans, pigeon peas, beans and lentils. This is a most undesirable development and must be corrected....

Genetic Engineering

Most people in the developing countries rely heavily upon cereals as their principal source of protein. We must take a look at the limitations of these cereal proteins. In the first place, none of them provide enough of one or more of the essential amino acids if they constitute a large part of the total dietary protein intake. Lysine, an essential amino acid, is of course lacking in all the major cereal grains. The second most limiting amino acid will vary with the different cereal grains. Nonetheless, we can start out with lysine. How can we do something about improving the nutrient value of our cereal proteins? There are three general approaches: (1) We can breed new varieties of grain with an improved balance of essential amino acids. This is a relatively new approach. It has been developed only in the last seven years. I call this "genetic engineering." (2) Using genetic engineering, we can develop varieties that are higher in total protein production by manipulation of genes. (3) We can develop improved cultural practices for any conventional variety, or better yet, for varieties that have built-in genetic improvements or an improved amino acid balance, increasing their production through such manipulations as proper application of chemical nitrogenous fertilizers—or growing cereals and certain legume crops in rotation. We can also increase the total percentage of proteins in this way.

These three avenues are open to us when we try to do something about the protein problem through the cultivation of plants. This genetic breeding—or genetic engineering or manipulation of genes—came into being as recently as 1964 with the discovery of the potential importance of the Opaque-2 gene in corn. I would like to point out that the Opaque-2 gene in corn, used as a genetic marker, was discovered and described in the 1920s by Jones and Singleton in Connecticut. But no consideration was given at the time to the significance of its other potentialities. Not until 1964, at Purdue University, did Nelson and Bates discover that the gene also produced higher than normal levels of lysine in Opaque-2 Corn. It turned out also to have much higher levels of tryptophan—lysine and tryptophan being the two most limiting amino acids in corn. Normal corn has about 2% lysine in the endosperm protein; the Opaque-2 corn has about 3.39% lysine in the endosperm protein. This is a very significant increase. It is not only evident from chemical analysis but the biological value likewise reflects it. When the growth rate of rats fed Opaque-2 corn was compared with their growth rate on normal corn, important differences were found. The same was true when weanling pigs were fed similar diets in which the main or only source of protein was either Opaque-2 corn or normal corn. They grew at a much more rapid rate. This work was done at Purdue and in Colombia.

The final "clincher" was the discovery that when children suffering from kwashiorkor were fed Opaque-2 maize by Dr. Pradillo and his group at the Zambali Medical School in Cali, Colombia, they responded beautifully.

Shortcomings Overcome

There were many shortcomings in the original Opaque-2 corn. First of all, this was a very poor corn for a basic type. If you are going to use these genes, you have to incorporate them into the background of a whole series of corn varieties or hybrids that are peculiarly adapted to a region. This takes time. It takes a whole series of crosses and backcrosses. You have to be able to follow this in segregating populations

so as not to lose this gene. As long as you are dealing with the original Opaque-2, it is self-evident because this is a soft endosperm or soft kernel type and you can spot this easily in the different kernels in an ear of corn, for example.

This kind of corn also has serious innate defects. Since the kernel is opaque, light is not transmitted through it as it is through a normal kernel such as may be seen in translucent hard endosperm corns. Also, these opaque kernels have low density. Therefore, the same number of kernels per ear will yield less—generally 8-10% or even as much as 14% less—grain. Offhand, this corn would therefore be completely unacceptable to the ordinary farmer, especially the small traditional farmer. Moreover, this soft kernel texture makes it vulnerable to damage by insects, both in storage and shortly before harvesting. Many of these kernels are also damaged by fungi before the ear matures. So there are considerable handicaps in trying to use these genes to improve the nutritional value of maize. Moreover, the kernels are much less attractive and have different milling characteristics and different dough-handling properties, all affecting their possible acceptance by the farmer.

What is the current status of developing varieties and hybrids that will be acceptable for commercial use in the case of Opaque-2 derivatives? Many varieties and hybrids are being converted to Opaque-2 types. The disadvantages I have mentioned have prevented their full acceptance in most cases up to now... None of these new varieties, however, has yet come into general use in largescale farming or in the area in which my organization is particularly interested , small subsistence-farming. . . .

Future Promising

. . .[But] particularly in the past year or two, hope has been growing that the Opaque-2 corn derivatives or hybrids will find large-scale acceptance. The reason for optimism is that there are now several known genes that will correct the softness of the kernel. Using these, you can maintain the high lysine and high tryptophan values of the original transfer from the Opaque-2 type....

Our group feel[s] there is a good chance that within two years large, commercial quantities of seed will become available that will not only have high nutritional value but will comprise a broad built-in adaptability to altitudes, temperatures and latitudes.... The prospects for accomplishing this very soon are excellent.

Cereal, Man-Made

What are the possibilities on other fronts, using other cereals? In 1967, a gene with a similar effect was found in barley. It has been called "hy-proly." This was found in an indigenous Ethiopian variety, a natural mutant. Swedish research workers... are incorporating it into improved barley varieties and aim to use it as a more efficient source of feed for producing animal proteins....

We have worked for six years on a man-made cereal which... is called "Triticale" from the Latin words *triticum* for wheat and *secale* for rye. Triticale is a cross between wheat and rye....

We became interested in the possibilities of using this wheat-rye combination as a prime source for protein in order to attack the world nutritional problem.... We have improved the architecture of the plant so that it will respond better to improved cultural practices and improved use of fertilizer, and we have thus increased the yield of grain. It is still not as high as in the case of our best-yielding wheat. But ...some of these lines have unusually good protein efficiency ratings: the full equivalent and perhaps considerably better than Opaque-2 corn!...

Triticale offers a new possibility. Here is an entirely man-made cereal. If we can overcome one defect that still remains—grain plumpness—then there is an excellent chance that this cereal can compete successfully with any of the other small-grain cereals such as wheat, barley and oats and can serve a very useful purpose in areas where small grains are the basic source of plant protein.

What about wheat and rice? They are the two most important grains. Up to now we haven't done too well with them as far as the change in amino acid patterns goes. We hope that progress will be made shortly by increasing the total levels of grain protein in both these crops. The genes are known, and some varieties have already been produced which will yield 1-2% more total grain protein than their progenitors. There is plenty of opportunity for further improvement while we continue our search for genes with better amino acid patterns. Genes have been found for both wheat and rice, but they have not been easy to use so far. More efficient ones may yet be discovered.

Two Dangers Lurking

To summarize: Considerable progress has been made in the last two years in expanding cereal grain production. But it is modest indeed compared to total needs. We must remember that, according to the Food and Agriculture Organization and also the World Health Organization, half of the world's people are still undernourished, badly nourished or malnourished. This is not a very pleasant picture!... There is no room for complacency because of the monster lurking in the wings—population growth!

There is another great danger lurking on the horizon that threatens our ability to expand food production: the emotional environmentalists, who are attacking on two different levels. On the food production front, they are using an organic gardening experiment, based largely on a few tomato plants grown in the backyard, to project ahead how to feed 3.7 billion people! It is questionable whether this experiment is a very good foundation upon which to make such calculations. When they are back home in their privileged nations (such as this one), they work on another front—trying to bring political pressure to bear to pass legislation outlawing the use of chemical fertilizers. If this should come to pass, we are all—sooner or later—doomed to starvation. On the pesticides front, there are these lobbies of emotional environmentalists...attempting to legislate against pesticides that are needed...to protect our food crops....

Last Biological Second

Nonetheless, I am very optimistic about the future of man. He has come a long way during the 2 million years since he stood up on his hind legs after he emerged—probably from the bush in East Africa....Man has indeed come a tremendous distance in this last "biological" second....

Excerpted with permission from *Nutrition Today* magazine, 7 (1): 20-21+ (January/February 1972). Copyright January/February 1972 by Nutrition Today, Inc., 101 Ridgely Avenue, Annapolis MD 21404

Miracle Seeds and Shattered Dreams in Java

RICHARD W. FRANKE

Java, hungry and overpopulated but with vast agricultural potential, would seem an obvious candidate for the kind of revolution Borlaug describes. In this article from *Natural History*, Richard Franke describes the outcome of the Javanese Green Revolution.

The Green Revolution may lead to larger harvests, but larger harvests do not always lead to full stomachs.

Culturally, politically, and economically, Java is Indonesia's most important island. It is also one of the world's richest agricultural regions. Streams, carrying an abundance of soil rich in nutrients, flow from the more than thirty active volcanoes along Java's central ridge. From time to time the volcanoes erupt, spewing out lava that eventually turns to fertile soil in the warm and humid valleys and on the coastal plains.

For hundreds of years Javanese farmers have ditched, terraced, plowed, planted and weeded this marvelous confluence of natural elements to produce the rice on which their lives depend. So rich is the soil, so dependable the water supply, so excellent the climate, that for centuries the population has increased, and the land has supported not only farmers and their families but also princely dynasties, courts, traders, armies, and eventually even the industrial development of Java's recent colonial rulers, the Dutch.

But the outcome of the island's history has not been a happy one for Java's peasants. By the turn of the twentieth century, the strains of population growth and the expropriation of rice lands by Dutch sugar interests had begun to produce the paradox so common in the underdeveloped world today—increased profits for the wealthy few and a declining standard of living for the mass of producers. Throughout the depression of the 1930s, the Japanese occupation during World War II, the war for independence from the Dutch in the 1940s, and to the present day, this decline has continued. It has brought the people of Java to the verge of famine and created ever worsening conditions for the vast majority of the island's 80 million inhabitants.

With an annual per capita income of less than $80 in 1969, Javanese peasants are among the poorest in the world. Nutritional standards are declining at an alarming rate. In 1960 the average Javanese consumed 1,946 calories per day, 200 short of United Nations minimum recommendations. By 1967 consumption had dropped to 1,730 calories. Protein intake is declining as well. Minimum adult recommendations call for 55 grams of protein per person daily. In 1960 the Javanese consumed 38.2; by 1967 this had fallen to an average of 33.4, meaning that millions of the poorest farmers and laborers subsist at even lower levels.

In Javanese villages and in the sprawling urban slums of the island's largest cities, the results of this undernourishment are obvious even to the casual observer. Children stare dully, unable to focus properly. Many persons have reddish hair and distended bellies, both signs of various stages of malnutrition. High rates of influenza, dysentery, tuberculosis, and more recently, outbreaks of cholera constantly plague a population physically too weak to resist disease. Cuts and burns heal with exasperating slowness, adding to the risk of infection. Even the body size of Javanese has been declining over the past fifty years, a result of the worsening diet. Java, it would seem, has received far too little help from the wealthy nations of the world.

Yet this island has been the object of one of the most elaborate food production schemes of the past two decades. Between 1967 and 1972 the government of Indonesia and its Western allies spent well over $100 million, mostly on Java, in an attempt to produce nationally 15.4 million tons of rice—the amount needed for self-sufficiency—by 1973. By the 1972 harvest, however, the program was clearly failing; the 12.2 million tons produced in that year were at least 2.1 million short of the need. With international food supplies at their lowest levels in years, the Indonesian government was able to purchase only 1.5 million tons abroad, leaving a 600,000 ton deficit, which in turn increased local rice prices by 30 percent in just a few months.

To make matters worse, the government has almost ignored soybean production, which has undergone an absolute decline, causing protein intake to drop even below the disastrous levels of 1967. In the countryside of Java and in the urban slums, this will mean a further decline in nutrition for an already badly undernourished people.

How has this tragedy come about? Why have all these millions in expenditures failed to stem

further impoverishment among the majority of Javanese? The answers lie in the blindness of development theorists to the social and political realities of Java and in the nature of aid programs from the wealthy nations—programs based on these faulty theories.

The program that was to have overcome the food shortage on Java is called the Green Revolution. The product of more than two decades of scientific research, the program is part of a broad and optimistic experiment occurring in several developing countries. Under the auspices of the Rockefeller Foundation, a seed research laboratory was established in Mexico City in 1944. Within several years, technicians had produced new varieties of corn and wheat with yield potentials far above those of local Mexican varieties.

By 1962 the Ford and Rockefeller Foundations united to establish the International Rice Research Institute at Los Banos, the Philippines, hoping the successes with wheat and corn could be duplicated with rice.

Sooner than expected, a genetic cross was achieved between a variety of rice from Indonesia and one from Taiwan. The result was a strain, IR-8, capable of doubling the yields of most local Asian rices. So profitable did the germ plasm from the new seeds seem that experts eagerly fostered their dissemination across the fields of southern Asia. By 1968, India, Pakistan, Thailand, the Philippines, Taiwan, South Vietnam, and Indonesia had begun large-scale planting of IR-8 and associated varieties of "miracle seeds."

With such a technological boon in hand, agricultural development planners began to revise their outlook on the development process. They now began to view as simpler, and more strictly economic, problems they had once seen as the results of psychological barriers, set up by "traditional" peasants unaccustomed to the idea of innovation, and institutional barriers, such as the outmoded labor and tenancy arrangements. If the new seeds could offer tremendous production increases at the level of the family farm, then perhaps all that was necessary to achieve their acceptance was the assurance that individual planters would earn a high rate of profit.

Such a position is represented in the highly influential study by Chicago economist Theodore Shultz, *Transforming Traditional Agriculture* (1964). In looking for ways to lower production costs to farmer-producers, thus increasing the profits from the farming enterprise, Schultz argues that if outside lending institutions can provide finance that will lower risk and if outside research and development organizations can pay for and even execute trials and experiments, then nothing should stand in the way of widespread acceptance of the new technology.

Economic planners were quick to take the cue from Schultz's proposals. During the 1960s, development programs and the discussions that surrounded them emphasized the construction of dams, irrigation works, harbors, markets, and roads. They advocated the provision of loans for fertilizer, pesticides, and above all, for new seeds.

With this new philosophy, the miracle of the Green Revolution should have been easily transmitted from the laboratory of the geneticist to become the major force for development in much of the impoverished world. Or so it seemed. The recent history of agricultural development programs on Java, however, reveals how poorly the theory and the seeds have fared.

Interest in agricultural development in Indonesia dates from the early 1950s. Reacting with a first flush of nationalism against the half-hearted agricultural extension system of the Dutch, the head of the national extension service proposed a way of intensifying contact between farmers and technicians. In each administrative unit, made up of about 15 villages, a five acre farming plot was set aside where both farmers and technicians could experiment with different planting and growing techniques. Practical and imaginative in its conception, the program failed primarily for lack of government funds.

By 1959 planners had fashioned a new program. This experiment, known as the "paddy center," consisted of large areas of almost 2,500 acres each, served by a central facility for credit, fertilizer, seed distribution, and education. The program began to show signs of failure by 1962-63, chiefly because rice produced in these centers had to be sold to the government, and the government kept its price lower than the open market price. Farmers resented the loans, while planners felt that they were too easily available and were undermining the farmers' "sense of responsibility."

As the government continued to introduce new but ineffectual programs, some Javanese farmers took the initiative for change into their own hands. Under pressure from a growing movement of peasant and workers' associations the government was forced to pass a series of land reform acts, beginning in 1960. Within months, however, the makeup of local land reform committees was so embroiled in politics that other kinds of agricultural programs were also likely to become engulfed. By 1964, tensions between landowners and the landless had become so great that violent confrontations were frequently reported from the countryside.

With the peasants becoming involved in politics, an elite group within Indonesia's upper-class university system made their own plans. In 1963 some idealistic students and teachers at the College of Agriculture of the University of Indonesia, noting that their history of service to farmers and food production was somewhat less than illustrious, came up with the idea of personally aiding the farmers. The students planned to go into the villages, live with the farmers, teach and learn from them, and take their experiences back to a following group of students who would do the same.

The first year of the program was a heady success. Starting out in an area not far from the university, twelve students lived in three villages, worked in the fields with the farmers, offered suggestions for improved cultivation techniques, listened to farmers' points of view, and interceded with local government and private institutions on the farmers' behalf as only elite students—and perhaps radical political organizations—would dare to do at the time. Per acre yields rose 50 percent over regular plots, from 1,984 to 2,866 pounds per acre (before processing), and this happened before the introduction of the miracle seeds from Los Banos.

With only their own ideas, enthusiasm, and dedication, Indonesian students and farmers were doing with locally bred improved seeds what experts and advisers from outside were later to claim required the services of aid organizations, private foundations, and multinational corporations.

By the next rainy season, enthusiastic administrators from the Department of Agriculture had taken over the program from the university. More than 400 senior students from nine different schools lived and worked with farmers in more than 200 villages, amounting to 27,000 acres of paddy land. Despite difficulties in supplying some villages on time and some decrease in talent and enthusiasm due to the program's rapid expansion, another kind of success was achieved.

Students won the confidence of farmers as the government had never done. The potential of their actions showed itself in one village where local officials had stolen fertilizer intended for the project. The students responded by sending a well-documented letter to the officials threatening that if the fertilizer was not made available to the farmers, copies of the letter would find their way to even higher officials. The fertilizer came.

As the program expanded, it did not just involve greater numbers of students and farmers and larger amounts of land. Peasant leagues and radical political movements were growing in east and central Java, and the new program to increase rice production became entangled in the web of Indonesian politics. What the students at Indonesia's top agricultural college were discovering in their first few seasons with the farmers, Indonesia's Communist party had begun to learn and teach years earlier.

In 1953 the party had called for its workers to live in the villages and study the social and economic conditions there, working at the same time to win the confidence of smallholders and farm laborers. The program's slogan was "three togethers": eat together, live together, work together; and organize to help small farmers and farm laborers overcome their fear of action. By these methods the party hoped to surmount what it considered the major obstacle to Indonesia's economic development—social and political control by a powerful ruling group.

At the same time the party was giving the farmers technological advice. In addition to attacking the powerful bureaucracy as "feudal remnants" and "imperialist forces," radical leaders urged farmers to adopt the "five principles": plow deeply, plant closely, use more fertilizer, improve seedlings, and improve irrigation.

The Communist party and student activists came to regard technology and strong political organizations for the poor as joint necessities in any attempt to bring about a more efficient use of resources on Java, both natural and human. Unlike most Western theorists, they rejected a simplified view of technology alone as the means to greater food production.

Javanese politics gave them precious little time, however, to test their theory. In September, 1965, as 1,200 students were starting the program for the rainy season, the long-smoldering struggle between landowner and landless, between Moslem storekeeper—religious official and Javanese Buddhist-Hindu farmer, between the Indonesian army and the Communist party, finally broke out into the open and ripped apart the fragile coalition that Indonesia's first president, Dr. Sukarno, had vainly tried to patch together. The army won.

During much of the rainy season of 1965-66 Indonesian society was embroiled in a protracted slaughter of known or suspected Communists. On Java alone, between 200,000 and one million persons were killed and radical peasant and workers' organizations destroyed. Little was done that year to increase the production of food.

By the dry season of 1966, the slaughter had come to an end in most areas. Despite the enormous social dislocations, the government expanded the area planted in rice from 27,000 to 415,000 acres, and this occurred in the first dry season that had ever been made a target of the rice production increase idea.

Dry season planting, however, was not the only innovation. At the invitation of the new military regime, American and West European advisors, most of whom had been thrown out of the country in 1963-64, now returned in large numbers to help put together a new development effort in Indonesia. In June, 1967, the government contracted with CIBA (Chemical Industries of Basel, Switzerland) to have this giant multinational corporation provide the technical apparatus for an experimental project to increase rice production in a small area in south Sulawesi (Celebes), to the northeast of Java.

Although no evaluation of the project was made, contracting with Western corporations continued at a rapid pace. By the rainy season of 1969-70, the West German companies Hoechst and A.H.T., the Japanese Mitsubishi, and a new, unknown company called Coopa were also offering the new agricultural technology, which for the first time included the miracle seeds from Los Banos. Together these companies provided fertilizer, miracle seeds, pesticides, and management advice for 2,470,000 acres, more than 20 percent of the entire wet-rice land of Indonesia.

Even from the start this massive program ran into difficulties. The new pesticides, untried on Indonesian fields, killed not only the harmful rice stem borer and various grasshoppers, as they were intended to do, but also the fish in the irrigation canals, an important source of protein in the peasant diet. One critic of the program asserted privately that one of the German companies was spraying onto the fields and into the canals the very chemical that had previously killed millions of fish in the Rhine, but the government never investigated this charge. Above and beyond all the stories and

complaints, one fact was evident: farmers were not repaying the loans they had been granted.

Complaints continued. Students reported that in many areas the packages of fertilizers, seeds, and pesticides were not arriving. Then the latter part of 1969, just about the middle of the 1969-70 planting season, the nature of Coopa, the mysterious corporation, became clear. Reporters for *Indonesia Raya*, a major muckracking newspaper in Jakarta, discovered a company letter dated in Vaduz, Liechtenstein, on the same day as the day of its arrival in Indonesia. Company officials had claimed registration was in Italy, but this was only part of the problem for, as the paper reasoned, "even the most modern airplane in the world cannot carry a letter from Liechtenstein to Indonesia in less than one day." When further evidence came in, the only question remaining was which generals secretly owned the company? At a cost of more than 150 million rupiahs (equal to $400,000 at the time), Coopa failed to deliver the technology for which it had contracted, and when evidence began to link the company's operations with members of President Suharto's personal staff, the President announced that the entire affair would be handled out of court. The development planners' idyllic rate of profit seemed to have become highly elusive.

Scandal ridden as it was, the total program of multinational corporation agriculture rolled on into the dry season of 1970 before the real reaction came. Continuing reports of unsatisfactory harvests were added to stories of inefficiency and corruption. Even in the best agricultural area, harvests had fallen off from 2½ tons per acre in 1965 to 2 tons per acre in 1968-69; in many regions crops were almost entirely lost because pesticides and fertilizers never arrived. Some government offices reported harvests of as little as from 220 to 882 pounds per acre, and a major famine occurred on the north coast of Java involving 100,000 persons.

Various international lending institutions, including foreign embassies, commissioned private studies of the program, and all agreed that no matter how perfect it looked on paper, something was not working. That that "something" was intimately related to the destruction of peasant and student political power and the rise of a bureaucratic military state was apparently outside the realm of development theory. The example of the students who once forced the government to deliver fertilizer was lost in the midst of theories that saw political action from below as insignificant, perhaps even threatening, in comparison to the power of technology.

Since the program was failing, something new had to be tried. By the rainy season of 1970-71, American and Indonesian planners launched a new program, incorporating many features of the pre-1965 experiments. First, interest rates on farmer loans were reduced from 3 to 1 percent. Secondly, the program was not packaged: a farmer could choose his own fertilizer and pesticide dosages without endangering his chance of getting seeds or a preharvest cost-of-living loan. Aerial spraying of pesticides, a major source of farmer opposition to the foreign companies' program, was discontinued altogether. Finally, to insure that the rate of profit would not be disturbed by price instability, the United States provided surplus rice that could be alternately injected into, or withdrawn from, regional markets. Farmers, it was hoped, would finally begin to see a profit from their harvests. The new plan, however, was doomed to failure by factors at the village level.

Like the national society of which they are a part, Javanese villages are highly stratified, with access to production resources distributed most unequally among different groups. A village along the north coastal plain of central Java illustrates this problem well. Excellent soil, good irrigation, nearby transportation, milling facilities, markets, and a long history of farmer acquaintance with new technology through their experience with the sugar factories should have made this a perfect place for a Green Revolution success story. Most farmers, however, cultivate plots of less than one acre, too small to support their families. They are forced,

therefore, to supplement their farming with outside jobs. Since not enough jobs are available, many of the farming households ought to go bankrupt, but they do not. In the village a group of large landowners, government officers, and town employees command capital for the small farmers. The capital takes the form of loans against the future labor of poor farmers, a form of debt-bondage in which the farmers must give up their option for outside jobs and be permanently on call to their patrons.

The mechanism is simple. During the pre-harvest period, small-holder families may run out of cash or food. If unable to find work outside the village agricultural economy, they are forced to attach themselves to a wealthy family by asking for a loan. Since they have nothing to offer in repayment—their next harvest will be no more effective in bringing them even a minimum of subsistence (much less a surplus) than was the last—they become permanently indebted, accepting a 30 to 50 percent cut under the market wage for farm labor and giving up the opportunity for future labor arrangements outside the village.

In such a situation, miracle seeds might seem highly beneficial. In addition to improving everyone's production of food, raising the standard of living, releasing the central government from its dependence on food imports, and lowering food prices, the productivity increases of from 50 to 100 percent on local farming plots of smallholders might eventually offer them the opportunity to reassert their independence from the lenders. That, however, is just the problem.

The wealthier families have clearly perceived the danger of too much technical progress of this sort, and during the rainy season of 1970-71 and the dry season of 1971, they used various means of preventing the smallholders from gaining access to the loans or to the technology. In some cases meetings to publicize government loans were never called, but notice of bank loans was passed along lines of kinship and neighborhood, thus kept within the circles of the village elite. In some cases subtle hints were delivered to small farmers; not much is needed to convince a family on the brink of starvation that they are better off with the security of the wealthy patron than striking out on their own even if the chances of success seem to be high. Failure to a family farm is not quite like bankruptcy for a modern business; there are no courts to handle starvation proceedings.

By the end of the dry season in September, 1971, the new technology was being utilized only on about 40 percent of the available paddy land, representing only 20 percent of the 151 households in the village. Poor families were totally absent from the list of participants. For them the promise of economic development meant only an increase in the wealth and lending potential of their patrons, and an opportunity for more of their class compatriots to fall into permanent debt and servitude.

In other parts of Java, the relationship between the social classes has deteriorated beyond the increased debt-labor bondage. In south-central Java, wealthy households are using the increased productivity of their fields to actually buy up paddy land from poorer families, driving the latter into the already jobless urban areas. In west Java, a region where landholding differences are even more extreme, some wealthy farmers have even begun buying Japanese-made rice-field tractors and home milling facilities, thus pushing an even greater number of landless and smallholding households out of the remnants of the rural labor market. The very possibility of technological success is creating a human disaster. For the poor, the Green Revolution in Java offers only the choice between servitude and homelessness.

What will the development theorists say about all this? Their answer lies in their actions: the programs continue as before with no substantial changes. The technology advocates, the rate-of-profit theorists, the military dictators, and the large landowners are attempting to produce enough food for the people of Java. They are failing. Their optimistic plans and programs have created only increased human suffering and promise more of the same. Perhaps solutions will come, not from the development experts, but from the small farmers and landless laborers of Java.

Reprinted with permission from *Natural History* magazine, 83 (4): 10-12+ (January 1974). Copyright 1974 by the American Museum of Natural History.

Farming the Edge of the Andes

STEPHEN B. BRUSH

Sophisticated is, a term we reserve for urban citizens of "advanced" cultured, not for farmers following traditional subsistence agriculture. Stephen Brush's article from *Natural History* reminds us that the wisdom of the old may be needed to compensate for the hazards of the new.

Despite assurances of bountiful harvests through the use of Green Revolution technology, some Peruvians wisely follow centuries-old planting strategies.

High in the Peruvian Andes before planting time, peasants sort over their collections of seed potatoes, selecting out of a possible fifty varieties those types that will be suitable for particular fields. In spite of low productivity, the many varieties of one plant and the way they are planted assure the peasant that he will not starve if drought, flood, or disease destroys part of his crop. These traditional patterns allow him to farm with minimum dependency on far-flung trade networks that are often liable to economic and political vagaries.

In contrast to the diversity of peasant fields, the advanced agriculture of industrialized nations strives toward the high production of one crop through extensive genetic experimentation and soil fertilization. Peasants in many parts of the world are being induced to abandon their traditional agriculture and to adopt the results of the newer technology. Within the last

decade, pressure for this change has increased with the breeding of high yielding varieties of maize, wheat, and rice, and with the profitability of transferring technology from Western to third world nations. Rapid population growth, the costs of importing food, and the rural exodus to cities have pressed the urgency of this change. The admirable goal of this effort—known as the Green Revolution—is the provisioning of an increasingly hungry world with food. But as this revolution proceeds, lessons that could be learned from traditional peasant agricultural systems are mostly ignored.

In the Peruvian Andes, where traditional agriculture predominates, peasants deal with one of the steepest environmental gradients in the world. Single mountain slopes, often spanning several thousands of feet in altitude, embody numerous ecological zones where there are differences in temperature, rainfall, exposure, slope, drainage, and soil composition. Altitude and exposure determine the different plant communities that grow in these zones.

The agriculture of both peasant societies and great civilizations such as the Inca Empire has been based on a finely tuned understanding of the ecosystems that span the Andes from the dry Pacific coast to the dense jungles of the eastern foothills. This sensitivity persists into the present.

Uchucmarca is one village whose survival has depended on a close adherence to steep valley ecosystems. Located in northern Peru near the Marañón River, a principal tributary of the Amazon River, the village is situated at an altitude of 9,950 feet, halfway up a forty-mile-long valley that covers more than 10,000 feet in altitude. The valley's climates are as diverse as those along a line from Texas to Alaska.

Slightly more than one thousand people live in Uchucmarca and another thousand live in smaller hamlets and homesteads scattered throughout the valley. Like many other isolated villages on the eastern slopes of the Andes, Uchucmarca is connected to the outside world by steep mountain trails passable only by foot and on horseback. The nearest road is six hours away and a twelve-hour journey is required to reach the nearest market center with such amenities as electricity.

Uchucmarca's self-sufficiency comes from the wide variety of crops produced in the valley's six ecological zones. Although the zones blend into each other, their different altitudes produce a gradient of environments. The lowest zone, between 4,200 and 4,900 feet, is a narrow alluvial basin between steep, dry hills studded with columnar cacti and thorny trees. Lying well within the rain shadow of the eastern cordillera, this area receives no appreciable rain, and the zone's principal crops—sugar cane, coca, manioc, chili peppers, and fruits—must be irrigated.

Above this zone, the *kichwa fuerte* zone runs up to 6,200 feet. In this area the valley widens and increased rainfall allows a dense scrub forest. Although precipitation is still too sparse and irregular to support extensive cultivation, some families venture to grow wheat and maize here. For most people, the important product of the *kichwa fuerte* is firewood, a resource rapidly being depleted.

The major grain-producing zone, the *kichwa*, climbs from 6,200 to 8,200 feet in the wide,

middle valley below grass-covered hills. Uchucmarca's farmers believe this area contains the valley's optimal agricultural land, with warm days, frost-free nights, and a regular annual rainfall of about twenty inches. During July and August, almost the entire village population decamps for this area to spend a month or two enjoying the mild climate and harvest festivals.

Above 8,200 feet the valley narrows again as the *templado* zone begins. As its name implies, this is a temperate area situated between the warm, drier zones in the lower valley and the cool, moist ones above. Steep slopes covered with low bushes and trees preclude extensive cultivation. But on more level ground, a wide variety of crops such as maize, wheat, barley, lentils, and field peas are grown.

Uchucmarca is located at the lower end of the next zone, the *jalka*. Lying between 9,900 and 12,000 feet, this zone is the center of the cultivation of potatoes and other tuberous crops. Potatoes are the bread of the Andean people. No meal is satisfactory without them, and hunger is defined by their absence. The origins of Andean civilization may be traced in part to agriculture in the *jalka*. In this valley, both modern and pre-Columbian populations expended more labor on more land for these crops than for any other. Temperatures are cool here, and frosts are common during the clear nights of the short dry season between May and September.

Above this zone, the *jalka fuerte* zone ascends to almost 15,000 feet. Here, above the limits of crop cultivation, rolling pastures of bunchgrass, sedge, and Andean tundra are swept by cold winds and are often covered by clouds that tumble down from the eastern Andean cordillera—a line of craggy rock outcrops and cliffs where condors nest. Llama and alpaca have long since disappeared from these pastures, although their prehistoric abundance is evident in the ruins. Now, cattle, sheep, horses, mules, and pigs graze here, representing the most important source of cash to the villagers.

The Uchucmarcan economy includes subsistence strategies designed to provide access to these ecological zones and their products for each individual household. Although no person has absolute ownership of any parcel of land—a right held exclusively by the village—individual households are granted virtually permanent rights through inheritance or by the village council.

Like most peasants in Latin America, the Uchucmarquinos present an image of egalitarian poverty. Most families, however, are fairly well off in that they have enough food for the table. The daily fare is simple: wheat cakes of stoneground whole wheat flour, parched and roasted maize, beans or peas, roasted barley flour, mutton soup, a few pieces of dried beef or mutton, and quantities of steamed potatoes.

An average family of four persons cultivates about five acres of land that are spread among small plots in various parts of the valley. Using only simple tools—a short-handled hoe, a pick, and a shovel—and with only oxen to supply power, agriculture is arduous and time consuming. Hiking to and from cultivated plots may occupy several hours per day. My research reveals that the average farmer spends almost 60 percent of his work time tending his fields and herds.

Most households attempt to obtain rights to as many parcels in as many zones as possible. Shortages of land and labor, however, prevent most households from achieving self-sufficiency. These shortages are compensated for by a set of alternative stratagems, such as reciprocal labor exchange, hiring laborers who are paid in crops as well as in cash, barter between households specializing in one crop, and a system of sharecropping that exchanges land for labor. Every household in the village employs each of these stratagems to some degree.

To insure a full larder, households try to grow six or seven different crops in different parts of the valley. Another guarantee is to plant the same crop in several fields. A single household may thus have three or four potato fields in the *jalka*, as well as fields planted in

wheat, barley, maize, and field peas in two or three of the lower zones. The peasants may also diversify crops in one field: maize, squash, and beans, for example, are always planted together because these different crops utilize different soil nutrients. This tactic may balance the failure of one crop with success in another if a family does not cultivate numerous plots.

Another way to reduce the risk of food shortage is to plant numerous varieties of one crop, especially potatoes, in a single field. There are more than 2,000 named potato varieties in Peru; in Uchucmarca alone, the peasants can identify some 50 varieties. The potato is indigenous to the Andes, and the area harbors a tremendous gene pool, both wild and domesticated. In the Andes, continuous cross-pollination between domesticated and wild potato varieties frequently creates new strains.

This large number of potato types provides some measure of security for the average Andean peasant. Agricultural success in Uchucmarca is fraught with danger: from earthquakes, landslides, hail storms, and sudden frosts, as well as damage by insects and disease. Saints, such as San Isidro, who watch over the fields and who are favored with candles, prayers, and fiestas do not guarantee success. Although all families depend on different crops as well as on their kinsmen and neighbors, their final safeguard against hunger is their ability to grow enough potatoes.

In most traditional communities, a first line of defense against crop destruction is maintenance of as wide a genetic base as possible and selection of different types more resistant to frost, blights, and insects. But no single variety of potato is able to withstand all of these, and none has total resistance to any single pest. By growing many varieties, however, the peasant reduces the risk of hunger if one field or variety is attacked by a particular pest.

In Uchucmarca, a common practice is to plant fast-growing varieties during the drier part of the year; this avoids late blight, which increases during the months of heavy rain. Another practice is the cultivation of certain frost-resistant varieties in flat, bottom areas of the high valley where frost, but not late blight, is common. Other varieties are cultivated on hillsides where late blight, but not frost, is common.

A third stratagem used by Uchucmarcan peasants to assure a potato harvest is to cultivate fields for only one to three years before returning them to a long fallow of eight or more years. Farmers usually sow potatoes in the first year and other Andean tubers—oca (*Oxalis tuberosa*), mashua (*Tropaeolum tuberosum*), and ullucu (*Ullucus tuberosum*)—for one or two subsequent years. The long fallow period lowers subsistence risk in two ways: by reducing the amount of erosion and soil loss and by killing disease vectors such as nematodes and fungi, which remain in the soil and depend on continued potato plantings to survive.

A final means of reducing crop destruction is the bordering of fields with hedgerows of living plants such as sauco bush and agave. Ostensibly maintained to keep out destructive livestock, the roots of the plants retard soil loss due to wind and water erosion and create quasi terraces. Soil loss is also reduced by plowing and cultivation, which tends to build up soil behind the hedgerow, slightly leveling the field on steep slopes. Hedgerows also provide refuges for wild varieties of domesticated plants as well as for insects, which pollinate, and birds, which prey upon pests. Despite criticism leveled at hedgerows for the space they require, they are one of man's most important agricultural inventions.

In spite of the success of isolated villages in meeting their food requirements, Peru faces annual food deficits and must import food. Agricultural production has not grown as rapidly as the population. To meet this dilemma, the Peruvian government and international development agencies initiated a program in 1974 to develop high-yielding potato varieties and to promote advanced agricultural technology based on the extensive use of chemicals. This effort, centered at the International Potato Research Center outside of Lima, is modeled on research programs for maize and wheat in Mexico and for rice in the Philippines. Although a miracle-variety potato may never be produced, several new strains have been developed that are capable of substantially higher yields than the traditional ones. These new varieties may increase yields by two or three times those of traditional varieties, lifting production from roughly three to eight or nine tons per acre. Along with agrochemical technology, these varieties have been introduced to several areas of Peru.

Uchucmarca and other villages along the eastern slopes of the Andes, however, have not adopted these new varieties or the new technology. Peasants say that the new strains are tasteless and of a watery consistency. Traditional varieties, especially the favorite floury-textured ones, tend to be higher in protein and have better protein quality than the improved strains. Crude protein of the native types averages roughly 2.48 percent versus 2.07 percent for the new types. Protein equivalency ratios—a measure of protein quality—indicate that some of the native varieties are more than 50 percent higher in quality than the most commonly planted "improved" variety. Also the new strains require heavy fertilization, while the traditional varieties do not. Good tasting potatoes, by the Andean standards, are incompatible with heavily fertilized fields.

Another deterrent is that the seeds of the new varieties and the technology they require are far too expensive for peasants: fertilizer, fungicides, and insecticides alone cost about sixty dollars per acre. There are no public or private loans available in the valley, and the present scale of potato production by an individual household does not now justify the long and expensive journey needed to search for credit. Uchucmarcan peasants are accustomed to producing potatoes with little or no cash expenditure. The average annual cash investment per plot is less than two dollars, the cost of hiring a team of oxen for two or three days. Outside labor, if needed, is traditionally paid for in the crop itself.

The general adoption of the new varieties would eliminate the rich gene pool of indigenous varieties and force the farmer onto an ecological high wire where the narrowly based genetic crop may fall prey to a recently evolved disease. Examples of such disasters are plentiful: the 1970 corn blight in the United States, coffee blights in Brazil, and the Irish potato famine of 1845. Further reduction in the gene pool of indigenous varieties may severely limit the ability to respond to such genetic dangers.

The developers of new high-yielding varieties are aware of this danger and have countered it by creating germ-plasm banks such as the U.S. Department of Agriculture station at Fort Collins, Colorado, where seed varieties of one crop are frozen or tubers are kept in cold storage. Such methods are satisfactory, provided the seeds and tubers remain viable under such conditions and the machinery for keeping them does not fail. Recognizing that neither of these provisions is certain, Hugh Iltis, a botanist at the University of Wisconsin, has proposed maintaining selected "genetic landscapes," that is, setting aside regions where specific crops would be off limits to agricultural technology. Such a proposal would avoid accidents, such as power failures, and allow the natural process of cross-pollination between wild and domesticated species. Iltis recommends the establishment of an international potato diversity preserve in the Lake Titicaca basin of Peru and Bolivia.

Like the native potato fields, the economies of traditional villages are relatively stable, but low-yielding, systems. The adoption of new, high-yielding crop varieties and agrochemical technology depends on restructuring traditional cultural and economic patterns. But Keith Griffin, an economist at Oxford University, notes that the credit and rural assistance that supports the Green Revolution is often biased away from the peasant in favor of large commercial producers. Francine Frankel, an economist at the University of Pennsylvania, has observed the effects of this bias in India, where the living standards of the poorest peasants have deteriorated in some areas and where the Green Revolution has undermined traditional peasant relationships. If these services and subsidies fail, the peasant may have no alternative but to join the exodus to cities.

The passing of traditional cultures under the guise of modernization results in a world made the poorer. This passing may be inevitable. What is not inevitable, however, is the loss of these cultures' insights and resources, so essential for the future of our hungry planet.

Reprinted with permission from *Natural History*, 86 (5): 32+ (May 1977). Copyright 1977 by The American Museum of Natural History.

The Greening of the Green Revolution

ROBERT RODALE

Robert Rodale, editor of *Organic Gardening and Farming* from which this article is taken, is most assuredly one of those "emotional environmentalists" Borlaug feared would blunt the Green Revolution—if indeed he is not something worse. Rodale, however, offers a surprising insight on how energetic, economic, and environmental concerns may live in harmony with progress.

Natural food-producing methods are starting to look good again—all over the world.

I first saw the Green Revolution in action when I was in India, about a year ago. Many farmers there were growing the high-yielding types of rice created by the International Rice Research Institute in the Philippines. Those strains of so-called "miracle rice" yield two or three times as much as traditional rice plants. To get that added yield, fields need more fertilizer, have to be irrigated more efficiently, and farmers also have to spray more with pesticides to protect their investment in fertilizer and water "inputs."

What did the Indian rice farmers think of that situation? Most that I talked to were happy. The energy crisis had already escalated their fertilizer costs, but if they could get irrigation water, they were getting good yields and were making more money than they used to.

The Green Revolution has been a very controversial feature of the world food scene, though. The new plants and advanced growing methods have had side effects. Farmers in very poor countries have been converted by the Green Revolution into buyers of chemical fertilizers and pesticides on a rather large scale. They have been made vulnerable to the rapidly rising costs of those products. The varied native strains of wheat, rice, corn and other plants have been made obsolete—replaced by a handful of super plants. While those new plants produce well for a time, they become vulnerable to epidemics of plant disease. Theoretically, at least, a new strain of a plant virus or other disease could sweep across all of southern Asia, attacking the same plants everywhere. Before the Green Revolution, such plagues were limited because each province or village grew slightly different kinds of plants.

There have been many other criticisms of the Green Revolution. All have stemmed from the fact that the Green Revolution has been an effort to transplant to developing countries an agricultural system that has been developed to suit the needs of America, the richest and most advanced farming country in the world. Our farms are usually large, with few workers. Farms in less affluent countries tend to be very small, and often have a surplus of labor. U.S. farmers have the money or the credit to buy large machines and to finance crop storage. In Green Revolution countries, many farmers are desperately poor. All kinds of other differences in situation stem from those conditions. In the face of those truths, does it make sense to try to superimpose the American system on places like India, Mexico, Thailand and similar countries?

Those questions were in my mind when I visited the International Rice Research Institute last February. Located at Los Banos, a couple of hours' drive south of Manila, IRRI (pronounced like Lake Erie) is the second oldest of the nine international institutes that are centers of Green Revolution technology. And since rice is the basic food of about a third of the world's people, IRRI is probably the most important. Founded in 1962 with Rockefeller Foundation money, IRRI now gets much help from other foundations and especially from the U.S. government and the governments of Asian countries. Its current budget is about $10 million a year.

The drive to IRRI takes you first through an opulent suburb of Manila, then past modern factories spotted along a seven-mile stretch of four-lane turnpike. Back on the two-lane road, you begin to get the real feel of the Philippines. The land is tropical, but not the thick jungle that I had imagined—at least in the lowland areas. Banana trees grow wild. The towns are crowded with simple wooden houses, usually two stories. Roadside stands sell steamed corn on the cob, melons, fruit, and novelties catering to the Philippine peoples' desire to ride in decorated cars. I'll always regret not stopping to buy one fringed car curtain lettered with the words "God Bless Our Trip."

At Los Banos, the road to IRRI leads through the campus of the University of the Philippines. Most impressive! It's like the Ivy League, but with palm trees. The IRRI installation is at the far end of the campus, located on 80 hectares (about 198 acres) acquired in the late 1950s.

The architectural atmosphere here aims for the international modern style—ceramic panel walls, large glass windows, and air-conditioning. Even in February, the heat builds up during the day. "Wait until the April rainy season," my guide said. "Then it really gets hot."

From the beginning, IRRI has tried to do things in a first-class way. Robert F. Chandler, Jr., the original director, was a stickler for perfection. One staffer told me how he fussed until even the memo forms were printed just right. Chandler is now semi-retired and lives in Massachusetts. The current director, Nyle C. Brady, is one of the great names of U.S. agricultural science. His book *The Nature and Properties of Soils* is a classic text, known and used by hundreds of thousands of ag students. Before coming to IRRI, he was Director of Science and Education for the U.S. Department of Agriculture.

There is a happy atmosphere among the people at IRRI. A visitor gets smiles and pleasant greetings from almost everyone. And I saw quickly that IRRI people were being pleasant and friendly to one another. They all were busy, yet I heard no complaining and detected none of the professional jealousy that seethes beneath the surface of almost all research institutions. I did meet one grouchy scientist, but he admitted right off that he was a grouch and advised me to take what he said with a grain of salt.

Many of the people I met spoke of contentment with their work. What pleased them most was the spirit of international cooperation and the lack of commercial secrecy and competition. Dr. W. Ronnie Coffman, a senior plant breeder, told me that at IRRI he could get his hands on any strains of rice he wanted. "Back in the U.S.," he commented, "much of the crop germ plasm is in the hands of companies working on their own special strains. A breeder can work with only part of what's available." Several scientists told me that they preferred to spend their whole careers at the international institutes, where they could get the cooperation needed to do good work.

Finally—Rice Without Pesticides

When IRRI was formed, farmers throughout Asia were growing types of rice that had long, weak stems and wide, droopy leaves. Fertilizing produced heavy heads, which made the plants lodge, or fall over. The grain would then get wet, or be eaten by rats. Yield was low.

IRRI scientists saw the opportunity to produce semidwarf strains of rice, which would have strong, stiff stems. Within a few years of the founding of the institute, they did just that. Their new rice strains not only could stand up well when fertilized, but also had narrow, erect leaves which allowed more sunlight to penetrate the leaf canopy. That increased photosynthesis, in effect making the rice plant into a more efficient collector of solar energy.

The most famous of these early improved strains was IR8, the first "miracle rice." When handled according to IRRI directions, IR8 and some of the other early strains yielded three to five times as much grain as traditional varieties. The Green Revolution in rice farming was given its first push forward by that plant.

Then the bad reviews started coming in. IR8 didn't taste as good as the old rice. Its grains tended to fall apart and get mushy during cooking. Insects and disease attacked the plants. Many farmers weren't able to supply the fertilizer, pesticides or extra irrigation water needed to get large yields. Big farmers had more success with the new rice strains than the poorer farmers, creating social problems. The "miracle" got a black eye.

The troubles with IR8 were not entirely unexpected. "They knew IR8 had weaknesses when it was introduced," Dr. Brady told me. "But those early rice strains gave us a breathing spell. They were trying to keep food production ahead of population growth. IR8 showed what could be done."

IRRI has learned from its mistakes and is aiming its efforts in very practical directions. "Today we work more in the real world—not in the world of experiment stations and rice farmers," Dr. Brady continued. Helping the small farmer is the watchword. Small farmers, after all, are what Asia has by the millions. If they are displaced from the land, there will be no room for them in the already jam-packed cities.

Dr. Brady told me that the current IRRI thrust is to create rice plants that need fewer inputs. Built-in tolerance to pest attack is being given very high priority in the development of new rice strains. Ability to withstand floods and droughts is also an important goal of the plant breeders. The need for fertilizers is being reduced by the design of new methods for placing nutrients as close as possible to the root zone, where they won't wash away and where the plants can reach them easily. Much research is going into the development of total cropping systems, blending the new plants, improved small machines, and all other ideas for improving production into a total package. Almost all the research on these cropping systems is done on farmers' fields, instead of on experiment station plots. Scientists find quickly what problems the small farmers have, and can try to solve them. The farmers themselves are deeply involved in the process of creating new cropping systems.

IRRI's biggest recent breakthrough was revealed to me by Dr. Coffman, a quiet talking Kentuckian. "We now have a rice that is so resistant to insects that it can be grown without the use of any pesticides," he said. "It's IR36, and will be released this fall. We've tested it at seven different places in the Philippines."

I stopped taking notes and looked him in the eye. "Tell me that again," I asked.

Ronnie Coffman leaned back in his chair and gave me a short lecture on rice insects and the problems of pesticide use. "The majority of Asian farmers can't afford pesticides," he began. "Not only that, but some of the worst insect pests can't be controlled by poisons. The brown plant hopper is one. The brown plant hopper not only causes hopper burn, but it transmits grassy stunt virus. Tungro, the worst virus disease of rice, is transmitted by the green leaf hopper."

"If you spray to try to control these insects,

you're talking about five different pesticide applications," he said. "That's quite expensive. The Japanese and Taiwanese have emphasized the chemical approach to rice insects, because they can afford it. But they're finding that chemicals really don't do the job. Actually, the poverty of the farmers we are working with may be a stroke of good fortune. It's forced us to develop resistant plants, which really are a solution."

"What do the chemical companies think about your work?" I asked.

"We have those fellows worried," Dr. Coffman said. "They turn white when we bring them in here and show them rice plants resistant to darn near anything. You name the rice problem today, and we have a variety that's resistant to it."

My next question was whether insect and disease resistance like that could be bred into crop plants grown in the U.S.

"Theoretically, it's possible," Dr. Coffman explained to me. "But from a practical point of view it would be very difficult. There's so much secrecy in plant breeding in the U.S. You don't have access to all the germ plasm the way we do here. There'd be too much frustration."

Had we talked longer, we might have mused about how the pesticide approach is ingrained into the thinking of most American farmers. They are comfortable with the idea of trying to kill bugs. Most farmers in the U.S. just don't realize that it's possible to create plants that can stand up to almost any kind of insect attack. A massive research effort would be needed to do that, but it is possible.

An Interest In Organics

On my last day at IRRI, I spent a final half hour with director Lyle Brady. We talked mostly about the history of IRRI, and its changing mission. Finally, I asked him what he thought of organic farming.

"I think it's good," he said. "I went to China last year and saw how they use every bit of organic matter," he continued. "The Chinese system of recycling is fantastic. I wish the same principles could be used in the Philippines and elsewhere. It's a sound practice—no question of it."

"Back in the days when nitrogen fertilizer was cheap," Dr. Brady continued, "we used to use 150 kilograms per hectare (133 pounds per acre) without worrying. But the price of fertilizer now is forcing us to use techniques that will let us grow more food with fewer inputs. It makes me sick when I see rice straw being burned—the common practice throughout Asia. They haven't yet learned how to make compost."

After returning home, I mailed Dr. Brady a copy of Dr. F.H. King's book *Farmers of 40 Centuries*, which describes in great detail the Chinese farmer's passion for saving and using organic matter. Dr. King was a high research official in the U.S. Department of Agriculture in the late 1800s, who spent several years in the Orient observing farming methods. I can think of no book that tells more convincingly the need for organic practices in Asia than does *Farmers of 40 Centuries* In a letter of thanks for sending the book, Dr. Brady commented that "The messages contained therein are not only interesting, but of vital importance."

Clearly, the Green Revolution I saw being created now by the International Rice Research Institute is quite a different thing than the Green Revolution I had read about. Many of the mistakes of the past have been corrected. new work is definitely headed toward making the life of small farmers easier. There are important organic directions to the work being done, though it is not a plan for organic farming the way we think of it here. But in the Philippines and much of Asia, the Green Revolution is getting greener.

Reprinted with permission from *Organic Gardening and Farming*, 23 (7): 34-40 (July 1976).

Toward a Dynamic Balance of Man and Nature

R. F. DASMANN

Ecologist Raymond Dasmann gave this address to a conference sponsored by the International Union for the Conservation of Nature at Kinshasa in September, 1975. It was one of those pieces I came across (reprinted in *The Ecologist*) at a time when the "morning's war" in *my* mind had moved me once again toward fear. Though I understood immediately that I was a biosphere person, and hence part of the problem, Dasmann's insights made me hopeful then—as they do now.

I doubt that many people here have an easy feeling about the future of mankind, or our ability to protect and maintain the networks of plant and animal life upon which the human future ultimately depends. Nor do I believe it likely that many of us believe that the hope for the future lies in more research, or in some new technological fix for the human dilemma. The research already done has produced truths which are generally ignored: We are reaching the end of technological fixes, each of which gives rise to new, and often more severe problems. It is time to get back to looking at the land, water, and life on which our future depends, and the way in which people interact with these elements.

Our attitudes toward the future of mankind and the human environment vary considerably with our point of view. Those of us in international organizations are likely to assume a globalist viewpoint. To a globalist, environmental and human problems often appear to be without solution, or their solution involves such massive inputs of money, energy, raw materials, education, and so forth, that any effort seems puny. But only a few environmental problems are really global in nature—and even they usually have solutions which can be applied rather easily at the local level. For example, if we are really threatening the stability of the ozone layer by using aerosol spray cans, it is a simple matter to give them up. They add virtually nothing to the quality of living for any individual, and those who manufacture them can make just as much money doing something else. Similarly, nobody is going to be much affected if the SST never flies again. The future of whales is a global problem, but its solution involves only a change in attitude of comparatively few people in a few countries—and some redeployment of economic effort.

Most conservation problems exist on particular pieces of ground, occupied or cared for by a particular group of people. Attempts to solve them at a global, or even national level often strike far from the mark, because they fail to take into account the attitudes or motivations of the people concerned. At the United Nations conferences in Bucharest and Rome we were presented with a global view of population and food problems. Globally it appears virtually catastrophic that a world population of 4 billion people is continuing to increase in the face of declining reserves of energy and minerals, and world food reserves that can be wiped out by the vagaries of weather and climate. Globally it appears vital that population growth be brought to a halt, quickly, by whatever means are feasible. This attitude seems either absurd or malevolent to somebody in Zambia or Zaire, where land and resources are relatively vast in relation to the numbers of people, although it may appear totally realistic to a person in Barbados or Bangladesh. It is also apparent to those who think about it that the addition of one person in the United States, which consumes inordinate amounts of energy and materials per capita, is far more likely to bring the world closer to crisis, than the addition of 20 new people in Tanzania. Similarly, food problems viewed globally are solved by massive transfers of wheat or rice from one place to another, and the establishment of world food banks. But the long-term solution to such problems probably lies in making each local community, each province and state, relatively self-sufficient in food—or at least capable of quickly attaining self-sufficiency if this be required. A Bengali who is dependent upon the uncertainties of weather in Kansas for his day-to-day survival is in a perilous condition indeed.

During the past few decades people have been encouraged to look to their nation's capital, or worse yet, to the United Nations, for solutions to problems that had always been considered, in the past, to be local affairs. But the tendency to depend upon the national government for decisions on the management of local resources inevitably creates delay, confusion, and often ends up with the wrong solution for each local community through trying to reach the right solution for all. *Thus providing water for a nation's population—as viewed from the top, can mean the need to build giant dams and canal systems, costing hundreds of millions of dollars, and taking many years. At the local level providing water may mean only*

developing some roof-top collectors, storage tanks, and giving some attention to the management of vegetation on the local hills and valleys. It might take a little money, some labour, and a few months of effort to improve the situation. But who will make that local effort if the responsibility lies with the government, and particularly if the government is likely to over-ride such a local initiative? Similarly, the *provision of electricity, viewed from the top, may seem to require the installation of a massive high-risk nuclear plant, and an environmentally disruptive national grid of power lines. It could also mean, at the local level, the installation of a windmill, or a small stream diversion through an axial flow generator.*

It is true that the simple local solution does not appear to work for the people in big cities. But there are questions we need ask about that also. Why are people crowding into big cities? Would it not make more sense to provide for them to move back to areas where they can look after themselves? Why do we build cities in such a way that their inhabitants are forced to become helpless dependents on agencies they cannot control? Since we must rebuild most cities anyway, why not build them to encourage in each neighbourhood the greatest degree of self-reliance, local initiative, and self-sufficiency?

If we attempt to conserve nature at a national level, we pass a great number of protective laws and hire people to enforce them. Decisions on protection, management, and administration are made by experts in the capital. Agencies come into existence with administrators who rarely have time to visit the field. We know the results, they are all around us. For each new protective law, we develop new specialists in the circumvention of that law, greater in number than the law enforcement agents. For each area in a national park or reserve, a larger area outside is degraded or made less productive. Or so it has seemed to go.

In some earlier papers I have promoted the idea that *human societies can be divided into two categories, with some in transition from one to the other. These are ecosystem people and biosphere people.*

Ecosystem people are those who depend almost entirely upon a local ecosystem, or a few closely related ecosystems. Virtually all of the foods they eat, or the materials they use, come from that ecosystem—although there will be some limited trade with other ecosystem groups. Because of their total dependence on a local system, developed usually over many generations, they live in balance with it. Without this balance they would destroy it, and cease to exist, since no other resources are available. The balance is assured by religious belief and social custom—everything is geared to the rhythms of nature—to phases of the moon, changes of seasons, flowering and fruiting of plants, movements and reproduction of animals. Such people have an intricate knowledge of their environment—the uses of plants for food, fibre, medicine. Every species, every thing, in their environment has some meaning or significance. Recent studies have shown that most such people did not live impoverished lives. Instead they tended to have adequate food, good health, abundant leisure—many of the features of the good life that others today strive for and rarely achieve. Once everybody on earth was in this category. Now only a few so-called "primitive" peoples, living more or less in isolation, survive.

Biosphere people are those who can draw on the resources of many ecosystems, or the entire biosphere, through networks of trade and communication. Their dependence on any one ecosystem is partial, since they can rely on others if any one fails. Drawing as they do on planetary resources they can bring great amounts of energy and materials to bear on any one ecosystem—they can devastate it, degrade it, totally destroy it and then move on. All of those who are now tied in to the global network of technological society are biosphere people. They are the people who preach conservation, but often do not practise it.

If we were to enquire when nature conservation in Africa was most effective, the answer would be "long before the words 'nature conservation' were ever spoken." Nature conservation prevailed in Africa in the days before the

agents of the biosphere societies first appeared—in other words before European technological society put in its appearance. In those days everybody lived in what we now call national parks and scarcely any species of animal or plant could be called threatened. Now the global conservationists and national administrators of the biosphere culture try desperately to protect species and to establish national parks in places where ecosystem people once lived. Effective conservation is at its lowest ebb. This is called progress. In the old Africa there were decision makers in the villages. Their decisions seemed to favour conservation. Now we try to influence national planners in the capital to achieve nature conservation. But the village decision maker still decides whether or not he will kill the last leopard in his stretch of country. Something is out of balance. Can the balance be restored?

We have lived too long with the idea that there is merit in bigness—an economy of scale that is important to efficiency. We suffer from the delusion that international or national organizations are best equipped to solve all conservation and development problems. It is a delusion. Aid poured in from the top with the idea that it will filter down and benefit poor people seldom filters very far. The filters are too fine, and scarcely anything drips through. Bigness creates dependency. Economies of scale lead to sociologies of economic helplessness. This should be increasingly obvious. The British economist E. F. Schumacher has written a book entitled *Small is Beautiful* and subtitled *Economics as if people mattered*. It should be required reading for decision makers, large or small. I think it is time we should be talking about "Development as if people mattered." We might then begin to build a system from the ground up that was ecologically sustainable, that would continue to provide for humanity for all time to come.

Marc Dourojeanni has pointed out the trifling amount of tropical rainforest that has actually been included in effective national parks or equivalent reserves—less than 2 per cent—probably not 1 per cent if we were to include only those reserves that really functioned in the way that they should. He has further noted that in Peru, if plans go through, we may see 10 per cent of the rainforest protected. In other words, at the culmination of an impressive national conservation effort, 90 per cent of the tropical rainforest is still left available for forms of use that will certainly create major modifications if not destroy it completely. If this does happen, what will be the fate of the islands of rainforest left in national parks. Will they be secure? It seems unlikely. Our host country, Zaire, has an impressive array of national parks. Those listed in the UN list cover over 7 million hectares. *But nobody can really believe that conservation can be effective if we have 10 per cent or less of the country in protected areas and the rest of the country is wide open to exploitation.* To be meaningful we must begin to restore conditions in which conservation will be a way of life for most people, where it will be a partner in development activities, where agriculturally productive land and natural areas are interspersed and the village forest is as important as the village field. In other words we need to restore some of the old partnership with nature that once existed throughout Africa. In the old days the partnership existed without people being aware of it. Now, with more people, we need a more conscious partnership. Some so-called "primitive" groups of people today still have it. We could all learn from them.

It is not suggested that any people be forced to live without the real benefits that technological advancement can bring: education, medical care, communications, transportation efficiency, and so on. It does mean, however, separating the gold from the dross—accepting the benefits while rejecting the energy and material wastage, the unnecessary consumption of scarce materials, all of the useless activities and societal patterns that end up with alienation of people and environmental impoverishment. What we really need is "conservation as if people mattered" and "development as if nature mattered."

To get there from here I believe we must aim at selective decentralization. Authority to solve local problems should always be held at the local level. Development should be localized, at a human scale, and intended to solve human problems. This has been stressed in the paper by Omo-Fadaka, and I will not repeat it. Nothing should be done by the province that can be done better by the village. Nothing should be referred to the nation that can be solved by the province. Those most likely to be directly affected by development decisions should have the most active role in reaching those decisions. No development decision should be made without full exploration of its effects upon human society and the natural environment. This does not mean that the local, the small scale, should prevail in all activities. Transportation networks need national coordination. Copper mines, smelters, refineries will require massive inputs of energy and labour—they can't be supplied by a few wind generators. Equally, however, one does not need a gigawatt power plant to meet the energy needs of farms and villages. In fact supplying energy needs in such a way inevitably creates the feeling of alienation and dependence that results when one has no understanding or control over one's means for survival.

It is particularly worthwhile to consider the speeches and discussions of the energy session of this meeting, where Odum, Leach and Omo-Fadaka presented their papers. If we take this together with other recent statements, such as that of the IUCN energy task force—we see that the energy panaceas that were being advanced with confidence a decade ago are likely to be a lethal problem in themselves and no solution to any existing problem. Any nation that pursues the nuclear energy alternative not only increases the existing rate of fossil fuel depletion, but further opens the path to nuclear war, nuclear blackmail and sabotage, the high risk of nuclear-power-plant accident, and finally the impossible task of finding a secure means for disposal of nuclear wastes. *The nation that adopts the nuclear option helps to endanger the future of life on earth and almost guarantees the growing restrictions of human freedom imposed by the need for increasing security measures. Furthermore, it is no answer to the energy problem, but may mitigate against finding long-term solutions.*

To those nations that wish to pursue the technological development alternative, apparently offered by the past behaviour of such countries as the United States, the answer is that there is *no way* such a pathway can lead to long-term economic development. The energy and materials wasting economy of the United States should be an example to the rest of the world of what *not* to do. *There is no possibility that it can go on for very much longer, without impoverishing the world.* All of the evidence from energy analysis, materials analysis—or most particularly from the increasing alienation of people from identification with government policy and practice show that present trends cannot and will not continue. Any country that hopes to follow this example is following a path to nowhere, from which the United States must find some way back.

The development pathways that hold promise are those that make most intelligent use of locally available renewable or inexhaustible energy resources—those based on the sun and the derivatives of solar power wind, vegetation, wastes, hydropower and the like. Using these and basing development on local, conservation-oriented land-use practices, building from indigenous knowledge and skills each nation can find a way for improving the lot of its people—not just for a decade or two, but for the foreseeable future. Somehow the political decision makers at high levels of government and the economists who advise them must be made conscious of the need to find ecologically sustainable ways of life. That these in turn will be oriented toward nature conservation is inevitable. Unfortunately, I know no way short of serious catastrophe to persuade many national decision makers of the need to shift away from short-term solutions. Politicians live for the short term. So I can only suggest that the local decision makers, the people themselves, hang on to whatever they can of their traditional ways and build slowly on them to achieve economic development at their own pace, and on their own terms. Faced with the arrogance and recklessness of governments of nation states, who prefer the glamour of jousting with one another in the international arenas of power to solving the problems in their own domains—this is not much hope. But it is all there is to offer for most of the world, when political leaders prefer fighter planes to manure spreaders.

Thus far I have not mentioned the word "life style" although I have been talking about the problem. However, if important decisions for the future must be made by individuals in their local communities—then the attitudes and ways of life of each individual become important. It is no use preaching pacifism if you work in a munitions factory. Is there any point in preaching conservation if you live in a style that wastes energy and materials and places excessive demands upon the world's living resources? Most of us, I fear, have grown up with the idea that conservation was the responsibility of governments, and that the duty of conservationists was to persuade governments to do the right thing. The idea that the first duty of a conservationist was to practise a conservation life-style only really became obvious when the ecological truth became known that the population crisis, the energy crisis and all other crises were interlinked and related to how each of us lived from day to day. In the 1960s a generation of young people grew up in the United States and in some other countries who began to accuse their elders of hypocrisy—because they preached peace while they waged war, and talked ecology while working for organisations that exploited the environment. Many of those I know simply refuse to work for agencies or companies that wage war, exploit the environment or threaten the future of the planet. They would rather go hungry. Often they do go hungry, but most can find non-exploitative ways of life.

I personally believe that conservation organisations and agencies have a particular responsibility to practise a conservation-oriented way of life. I do not want to point any fingers—but it would be interesting to know how many gallons of jet fuel were burned, how many trees were cut down, how many kilowatts of electricity burned to bring us all together here in Kinshasa? It would be interesting to know also whether we have influenced any decision makers as a result?

Reprinted with permission from Dr. R.F. Dasmann. A talk presented to the technical session of the IUCN General Assembly, Kinshasa, Zaire, 1975.

Earth, Air, Fire and Water: Solutions and Their Problems

In going over the materials I had collected as potentially useful for this book, I came across an article first published in the *Ladies Home Journal* for September, 1915. It was entitled "You Will Think This A Dream," and its author was Charles P. Steinmetz, long-time chief engineer of the General Electric Company. His theme was the wonders that electricity would produce, and his predictions were astonishingly correct: electricity would regulate temperatures automatically, keeping us warm in winter and cool in summer; electricity would be used for cooking, and much cooking would be done right at the table; electricity would bring us concerts in the home, synchronized motion pictures and "talking machines"—and the elimination of noisy, space-consuming trolleys.

Steinmetz made only one serious error. He did not foresee that these benefits would have their costs; he forgot to ask about the side effects. "Cities," he wrote in 1915, "will become sanitary—no dirt, dust or smoke will be possible. The streets will be beautifully clean. There will be no reason for dust or dirt... The atmosphere will be perfectly clear... with clean pure air we shall be able to raise evergreen pine trees in the city, and it is healthful to have pine trees where you live... [electricity] will be very cheap and it will not pay to install meters and have them read..."[1]

Poor Steinmetz should not be faulted for sharing his generation's technological optimism—for his innocence about the possibility that out of our continued progress toward a life of total ease, some unexpected side effects might arise. We, the inheritors of the dreams Steinmetz proffered, are only now, and with painful slowness, learning to look gift horses in the mouth.

Yet where food is concerned, necessity tends to make optimists of us all. So there are still some who argue that here at least we have no option but to damn the torpedoes; in the face of inexorable population growth there are still those who urge an all-out assault on nature with fertilizers, pesticides, herbicides, irrigation, hybrid seeds and the rest—to force Mother Nature into prodigies of production. Yet, increasingly, as Mother Nature fights back—salting up irrigated lands, changing her rainfall patterns, building pesticide resistance into those of her creatures we define as pests—there is a growing awareness of the need to take natural systems into account.

Here is a paragraph from the introduction to a 1975 report from the National Academy of Sciences' *Enhancement of Food Production for the United States*:

> "Research strategy of the past, in line with the admonition of Jonathan Swift in *Gulliver's Travels* was to grow two ears of corn where one grew before. Enhancement of productivity should still rank first among research priorities, but there are now other important—and not always complementary—objectives. *Increased production must now be sought with the lowest possible inputs of non-renewable resources of land, water, energy and fertilizer, and with achievable minimum environmental impacts.*" (pg. 5, ital. J.G.)

This chapter is about some of the environmental limitations on food production.

---

[1] *Equilibrium*, 2:2 (July 1974).

Plants, it has been said, are made of earth, air, fire and water. The last chapter was about fire. This chapter is about earth, air, water, human inventiveness and some of the other inputs man has used to make the earth bring forth food to support him. It is about the fourth law of ecology, which says, "There is no such thing as a free lunch," and about the first law, which says, "everything is connected to everything else." It is about "solutions" which do not take connectedness into account, and about the problems those solutions create even if—indeed especially if—one or another input to production appears, as it did to Steinmetz, unlimited.

The opening piece in this chapter—an excerpt from a somewhat longer essay printed in *CAN* in 1972, describes in personal primer terms the concept of interconnectedness in a closed system, which is the basis of the understanding that you can never do only one thing. In the much more sobering assessment which follows, Eckholm calls our attention to the world-wide devastation in our life-support systems being wrought by the frantic attempts of poor and hungry men to wring a living from the earth.

As the reader will have observed, the remainder of the chapter has been organized somewhat differently from the other chapters—as suits the implication of its topic. It is non-linear, sometimes apparently disconnected, and inevitably incomplete. Yet it is really of a piece. Even though the readings themselves deal with a variety of discrete topics, they are, as will become clearer, not really disconnected. It is the primary message of this chapter that they *cannot* be disconnected—that in the natural world any input is, inevitably, connected to any other, and that this web of interconnections is *always* more extensive and more complex than we can at first (or perhaps ever) imagine beforehand. Hence we must always intervene in natural systems tactfully and watchfully.

A story is sometimes told of a South Sea island plagued with mosquitoes to which Western health personnel came bearing mosquito sprays. Sometime after their beneficent intervention the roofs of all the houses fell down. As it turned out the mosquitoes had been the usual diet of lizards who lived in the roofs of the houses. When the lizards ate the insecticide-filled mosquitoes, they died and were eaten by the village cats. And the cats died. And since the cats had been keeping the rats out of the grass roofs of the huts, the rats ate the roof supports and the roofs fell down. One could, of course, impregnate the roof supports with rat poison, or import rat-proof steel eye beams—technological solutions which might keep the roofs up and might, in their turn, create other unanticipated fallouts.

The question is, what is the appropriate response to such a problem? Schumacher considers that question, in relation to a similar story, in his piece called "An Economist's Look at Farming."[2] "Some years ago in Canada," he writes, "the Newfoundland fishermen had changed over to Japanese fishing-nets of artificial fibre. The advantages were marvellous. These nets would never rot and they never needed to be dried; they were immensely strong, and they were held in place by bouys which were also of plastic and had similar advantages. This made life easier for the fishermen: it was, if you like, 'progress.'

"But since the fishermen's life is what it is, nets sometimes get lost at sea, and inevitably the old type of net would soon rot away and end up as nothing. But these new indestructible nets did not. What happened was that any number of fish got caught in them, lost their buoyancy when dead and dragged the nets down to the ocean floor with their weight. There the dead fish rotted and drifted away in scraps or were eaten, until the net with its small buoys had regained enough buoyancy to rise to the surface and start the process over again. It's a process that continues, and since it is practically impossible to find these nets there's no reason why it shouldn't go on almost for ever. 'Progress,' in this particular version, has generated a fully automatic fish-destroying process. . .

---

[2] E. F. Schumacher, "An Economist's Look at Farming," *Soil Association*, (November/December, 1974).

"It is very revealing, "Schumacher goes on, "to see the different ways in which different people respond to this story. There are some whom I have elsewhere called 'people of the forward stampede': they immediately come forward with a technological answer, a little electronic bleeper built into those buoys so that the nets can be found and recovered. And there are others—I have called them the 'homecomers'—whose instinct is to think in more biological terms, and to propose either a return to natural fibres or else a development of biodegradable fibres for use in those Newfoundland nets."

Now both these stories, the one about the grass roofs and the one about the fishing nets, are stories with morals. They emphasize the fact that natural systems have their own internal logic and that our foolish notion that we can simply over-ride that logic in order to provide comfort for our species is false. Though it is a fact that we often lose sight of, humankind depends wholly on growing plants as the primary producers of foodstuffs (and oxygen). It is not true, as our supermarkets insinuate, that we depend on the beneficence of General Foods or Kelloggs. Once we have firmly in mind our dependence on plants in nature (and not in White Plains or Battle Creek), we can begin to understand how important it is to look critically at all the things which interfere with the growth of plants—and to examine ways in which a variety of our consumption "needs" apparently unrelated to eating, have begun to compete with food plants and the inputs required to produce them.

In the last chapter we considered the contest between stripminers and corn farmers. Another example, well publicized several years ago, was the competition for fertilizer nutrients between crop lands in India and lawns, golf courses and cemeteries of suburban United States. Or consider the implications of the disappearance, under those same suburban amenities, of prime farmland in peri-urban areas, or the prolific use of water potentially needed for agriculture to produce lawnscapes in our southwestern deserts.

In any undertaking such as agriculture, where a number of factors must work together for the overall success of the enterprise, the abundance of the supply of all other inputs is immaterial when any *one* becomes limiting. What factor will finally become limiting in American agriculture? Will we, as some have argued, run out of phosphate, that mineral nutrient more intimately associated with the spark of life than nitrogen? Is it light itself? Will we so cloud our solar window with the effluents from our overdeveloped society as to reduce the inflow of light, thus hindering photosynthesis itself and the plant growth it generates? Or is it topsoil, a resource present in its greatest abundance before the advent of man, at the end of the 350 million years of growth and decay of plant and animal life.

There are those who believe we will do ourselves in with toxic chemicals; that we will so pollute the food supply—advertently with inadequately tested "additives," and inadvertently with the "accidental" introduction into the food producing environment of substances designed for other purposes—that we shall slowly but inevitably wipe out our own species. The Japanese, whose industrialization has been more heedless even than ours (partly because it has been so geographically confined), have produced the terrifying Minimata disease by dumping mercury-containing wastes into a food-producing lagoon. Italy has destroyed the agricultural potential of a Lombardy countryside by the accidental release of a deadly chemical-plant toxin; and Jacques Cousteau has announced that he will no longer dive in the Mediterranean because it is too polluted (confirming a long-held personal suspicion that mussels pulled from the harbor in Naples were the original source of the admonition, "See Naples and die").

Here in the United States we have polluted an entire state, Michigan, with what may have been a single bag of fire retardant (mistakenly substituted for a bag of feed supplement) mixed in with livestock rations. The initial fall-out from that contamination included destruction of 23,000 cattle, 5000 pigs and sheep, 1½ million chickens, 2600 pounds of butter, 340,000 pounds of dry milk products, 1500 cases of canned eveporated milk, 18,000 pounds of cheese, about 5 million eggs, and

865 tons of feed.[3] Meanwhile we talk of using chemicals to *increase* the total supply of food. So alarming has this toxic environment become to some observers that at least one consumer writer has argued that we are going to have to turn to "pure" synthetic foods in the coming generations because "we have so fouled our environment with industrial chemicals that most nature-created food is unfit to eat."[4] Unfortunately such an anthropocentric solution ignores a number of other critical biological roles our food plants play—how, for example, do we propose to produce oxygen?

But although pollution is a critical problem, there is nothing in this set of readings about its potentially devastating effects on our food supply. There is also nothing here on weather (unless one counts the articles on the Sahelian drought—a work of man as well as of nature), even though climatologists appear to agree on the fact that our weather (and hence our crop yields) will at the least become more unpredictable than they have been over the last decades.

Such incompleteness of coverage in this chapter is as inevitable as the inter-connectedness which produces it. For if everything is indeed connected to everything else, then only a discussion of "everything" would be complete. Here we have another answer to the question raised in Chapter 3: is our technological food supply part of the solution to world hunger, part of the problem, or neither? For if everything is connected, then advertising is connected to air quality just as Pringles are connected to energy use—and pet food to world hunger. If advertising fans our desires for things (and it does), and if production of these things (disposable bottles, aerosol cans, second homes, plastic bags, green lawns, white laundry) begins to use up pieces of the world important in food production (energy, ozone, open land, petro-chemicals, phosphate rock), then excessive demand for *anything* may have an impact on our food producing capacity. And if our food supply is itself not only unnecessarily using up resources, but is cutting us off from an awareness of what we are doing to our food producing environment, then clearly our food supply is part of the ecological problem, is part of the interconnected web of causes and effects that will ultimately determine the sustainability of human life on earth.

So the first and over-riding message of this chapter is that things are always more complex than we think; and there are always more factors involved than we are likely, at least at first, to consider. The second message, which arises naturally from the first, is that the notion of unlimitedness in anything is a snare and a delusion.

We have seen in the last chapter that energy has become a major factor in agriculture both here and abroad. But there are still optimists who refuse to see energy as limiting—ever. True, they say, fission energy seems less promising than it once did. So too, if energy costs involved in extracting the energy are counted, do petrochemicals derived from shale and the Athebaska Tar Sands. And limits to water availability appear to have dampened some of the optimism about on-site conversion of poor quality strippable Western coal. But perhaps we shall find a way to control fusion, or (more likely) perhaps we will find a way to capture economically the energy of the sun.

But even if we escape the limits energy imposes, we will still not have escaped the limits put on us by the fact that we are part of a complex biologically-controlled flow of energy and materials, which we interrupt at our peril. "Human intrusions on the natural order," Denis Hayes has written, "are often bungling and at times catastrophic. With endless cheap energy at our command there will be those who wish to turn Siberia into a vacation resort, to melt the polar icecaps to bring fresh water to the Saharan Desert, to construct cities on the ocean floor, and to shrink the average work week to twenty or ten or perhaps zero hours. To fear such undertakings is not so much to love Siberia the way it is as to quake at the unanticipated consequences of such enormous changes."[5]

[3] *FDA Consumer* (February 1977).

[4] Carper, "The Case for Food Chemicals," *Newsweek* (7 March 1977).

[5] Hayes, Worldwatch Paper #4—"Energy: The Case for Conservation."

Given such encompassing understandings, the readings tend to speak for themselves. When I put this chapter together, the appropriate "solution" with which to begin seemed obvious—Jules Billard's agricultural optimism classic from the *National Geographic* of February, 1970. Unfortunately I was given permission to quote no more than a tantalizing 700 words. Yet even those brief excerpts manage to give, I believe, the tone of an article that never ceases to amaze, reminding one ever more forcibly as the years go by of the awe and innocence with which most of us once viewed the wonders of "progress."

In 1970 Billard was delighted with the discovery that farmers were heavy users of electricity, for "niceties" like radiant-heated pig pens; in the aftermath of the energy crisis his discovery jolts us into an instant realization of how things have changed. In less than a decade we have become much less sanguine than he about the unquestioned virtues of pesticides. "New pesticides and safer ways of using them pop [sic!] from the laboratories," he wrote ecstatically. We are also less pleased about the prospect of farmers turning crop lands into profitable recreation areas.

When one (or a dozen) bags of fire retardant can contaminate a state, concentrations of animals like those of "Egg City" or the Blair Cattle Company feed lots are more alarming than awe-inspiring. Billard's picture of the agriculture of the future—fields unmarred by trees, hedges, and roadways—is unnerving in the face of swirling clouds of dust (unchecked by hedgerows), part of our dwindling topsoil. It is frightening to think of those fields "several miles long and a hundred feet wide" hit by a new version of the corn blight or attacked by a pesticide-resistant chewing insect. The characteristic of the agricultural system Billard describes is terrifying vulnerability—the inevitable characteristic of an over-simplified ecosystem.

And so, earth. The first discrete topic in the chapter is topsoil, the *sine qua non* of any sustained agricultural system. The two articles included here are from *Science* and are recent, as is widespread serious concern about topsoil loss. Van Bavel's editorial begins by pointing out another food/energy trade off: in order to pay for our imported oil we are putting back into production poor sloping lands which are subject to severe erosion and ultimate total loss of productivity. Luther Carter reviews recent concern about the problem, and recent attempts to do something about it.

Our general indifference to erosion appears to arise at least partly from our growing urbanization. We don't *live* on farms any more. We had a drought recently more severe than that of the dust bowl era; but most Americans didn't even know about it—TV's city-oriented weather persons are always hoping for a "nice" day. Because we do not know where our food comes from, we cannot be roused to protect the systems on which it depends.

T. F. Shaxson's brief excerpt points out that organic matter in the soil is a major factor in erosion reduction. Since this is a chapter on connections, it is worth keeping the soil-preserving role of crop residues in mind when it is proposed, as it has been, that we "solve" the energy crisis by collecting such residues to burn as fuel.

Though the rediscovery of the problem of erosion is relatively recent, destruction of the topsoil that supports him has been the mark of civilized man. As Carter and Dale point out in their book *Topsoil and Civilization*, the only areas of the globe which have supported civilizations over long periods of time are those in which moderate rainfall and a relatively flat terrain prevented the washing away of topsoil. In other cultures, less well endowed by nature, erosion eventually destroyed the fertility base on which the civilization was built—on which, in point of fact, all civilizations were built.

Yet as Carter and Dale point out in a last chapter entitled, "Can the U.S. Survive," "the odds very much favor a continuing steady decline in the basic stock of topsoil in the United States. When the topsoil is gone," they continue, "and there may be only a few inches now to work with, one will be lucky to get back the seed if he plants it . . . The crop output may be shored up, maintained and even increased for a time by various scientific tricks of the trade, and this is what is deceiving the country as to the true situation." These tricks of the trade, it should be noted, almost always require large energy inputs, high nitrogen fertilization, repeated use of pesticides and herbicides, and irrigation. Everything *is* circular.

It is hard to realize how dependent plants are on air. We put them in soil, feed them with fertilizers, and water them. Yet without air they cannot survive, and without what they do to air (removing carbon dioxide and replacing oxygen), neither can we. We had a small scare several years ago, related to a report that we were running out of oxygen. We had hardly recovered from that alarm before we were hit by a somewhat less comprehensible threat, that we were running out of ozone. This time more research didn't make the problem go away. Indeed, as Professor McElroy's article reprinted here from the *Harvard Magazine* makes clear, our initial concern over SSTs and even spray cans begins to seem trivial compared with the threat that we may be destroying the ozone layer by our efforts to increase food production. He suggests that increased nitric oxide in the atmosphere (a by-product of nitrate-containing fertilizers used in increasing amounts to boost agricultural output) may be destroying the ozone layer which protects us from too much ultra-violet light.

Moreover, the release of ozone-damaging nitrogen compounds may be further increased when soils are exposed to acid rain. The acidity of rain appears to have been increasing markedly, especially over the northeastern United States over the last decades,[6] as a consequence of the increased introduction of sulfur dioxide into the atmosphere. The additional sulfur dioxide appears to result from the increased use of clean natural gas instead of "dirty" coal, and from the use of taller smokestacks fitted with precipitators to remove particulates from smoke. (In other words, as a consequence of measures aimed at pollution control!) Increasing use of fossil fuels will tend inevitably to increase sulfur emissions, thus increasing rain acidity. And while the overall effects of acid rain are not known, it probably reduces plant growth, leaches nutrients from both plants and soils, causes high levels of fish mortality among valuable food fish, and otherwise reduces the productivity of both our lands and our waters.

Yet while ozone is decreasing in the upper atmosphere, there is evidence that, down below elevated ozone levels caused by man's activities are causing marked reductions in crop yields, and (even more importantly) in nitrogen fixation in plants (thus requiring the use of more nitrogen fertilizers). In 1976 the EPA reported that ozone "even at a concentration within national air quality standards" produced a 40% reduction in plants' ability to convert gaseous nitrogen into usable form.[7] Other pollutants such as cadmium—a pollutant generated by, among other things, coal-fired power plants and the rock used to produce phosphate fertilizers—also reduced the conversion of nitrogen into fixed (usable) form.

And because *everything* is connected, soil erosion itself affects the air—dust blowing off eroding cropland is believed to have the potential for triggering global climate changes, including the alteration of rainfall patterns so as to produce more drought and dust-producing soil erosion. And that particular insight brings us to the Sahel, and two articles which deal with the interaction between land and water and climate and progress. Wade's piece suggests the vulnerability of the Sahelian ecosystem. The Baker article suggests the collision of value systems. Both underscore the message that we must be cautious in "doing good," lest we inadvertently do bad.

So much for earth and air (and fire). The water here is salty, though it could as well be fresh. Only a few years ago, the oceans were thought to hold the promise of unlimited bounty if only we could learn to exploit their resources fully. The excerpt from the Worldwatch Paper #5 reprinted here

[6] *Science* (14 June 1974).

[7] *Environmental News* (4 May 1976).

gives a quick overview of the problems our optimism has generated. The apparent destruction of many fish species through overfishing is a classic illustration of the problems which arise when we confuse "improvements in the pump," as Aldo Leopold has called our technologies, with improvements in the well. Because we temporarily catch more fish when we get better at fishing, we are lured into thinking there *are* more fish.

The papers by Reddy and Galtung consider the relationship between India and the ocean— suggesting on the one hand the potential of the ocean to provide food to a hungry nation, and on the other one of the ways not to go about providing it.

And in case it seems to the reader that surely we have by now learned our lessons, there are also included here three brief pieces on krill. Before this energy-conscious decade had even opened, the biological economics of krill-catching were scathingly laid out in a widely popular book, *Population, Resources and Environment*. The authors, Paul and Anne Ehrlich, pointed out that whales had been ideally fitted by nature for krill-exploitation, and that in terms of net protein production it made most sense to let the whales catch the krill and then catch the whales. At that time, the Ehrlichs quoted Dr. Roger Payne of Rockefeller University to the effect that killing off the whales and harvesting krill was "like wiping out beef cattle in order to have the pleasure of eating grass-protein concentrate." If one considers the krill's largely arctic habitat and the overall energy inefficiency of long-distance fishing illustrated in the last chapter, one can only marvel at the wistful willfulness of humanity.

And should we learn in time to cultivate the sea for food—to become agriculturists/herdsmen of the oceans instead of hunter/gatherers—we will need to be attentive, much more attentive than we are at present, about the chemicals we charge it with, about the radioactivity we leak into it. The ocean is no more an unlimited sink than it has turned out to be an unlimited source.

And finally, some words, optimistic, harsh, questioning, troubled, about the Green Revolution, that breakthrough which promised not so long ago to end hunger, if not forever, then at least until we had brought population under control. The Green Revolution teaches us lessons not only about the incredible complexity of natural systems, but about the incredible complexity of the social systems which various groups of humans have built up to make use of them. The "backward peasant" is not so backward after all—only a man who has learned to hedge his bets under circumstances in which a losing throw means starvation.

The readings go full circle—from the incautious technological optimism of Norman Borlaug, the undoubted father of the Green Revolution, to the cautious optimism of Robert Rodale, whom Borlaug would view as among the worst of those "emotional environmentalists." The message perhaps is that while no one is all right, no one is all wrong either.

The final selection, one of my favorites in the volume, is by the noted ecologist Raymond Dasmann. It may be, in the real world the most optimistic paper of all. For in a time when the big solutions, like nuclear energy, seem terrifying but perhaps inevitable, he tells us that they are not only not inevitable, but that they don't even work. No matter how large our police forces, no matter how many rules we invoke, we cannot *make* people take care of the systems on which all our lives depend. The only people who can decide whether the last leopard lives or dies will be the people who live where the last leopard lives. *They* will preserve what is necessary for their ecosystem. "Bigness," Dasmann reminds us, "creates dependency. Economies of scale lead to sociologies of economic helplessness."

We have automated our agriculture and produced a "welfare problem." The best solutions, the only lasting solutions (as Barbara Ward's paper pointed out in chapter 2) are those which are small and patient and work with nature.

For what it all adds up to is that if we *fight* nature, we lose...in the end.

One final ecological story. Some time ago a method was developed of encapsulating a highly toxic pesticide (parathion) in a time-release capsule. No pesticide was released as long as it was in solution, as it was while being applied. Only when the capsule got onto the plant and dried off was the pesticide released. This was very good for the agricultural workers. Unfortunately for the bees the capsules turned out to be about the same size as pollen grains, so they adhered to foraging bees, who carried them back to the hives and promptly wiped them out. When a local specialist was contacted by the bee-owners, his memorable comment was that the bees were "trespassing" on the sprayed orchards.

Teaching a bee not to trespass surely presents a significant technological challenge. With any luck, we will meet that challenge before the bees are wiped out. But we had better hurry. Pesticide "accidents" have already caused a striking loss in bee colonies throughout the country, and especially in California. And bees—as those of us who remember our sex education will recall—are still required to fertilize everything from almond orchards to hybrid soybeans.

"We need to re-orient our minds, and remember three basic things about the soil, the land, the countryside. The first is the fact that it is our home, and that our mental and physical well-being is dependent upon its condition. The second is that it is our only source of food. Townsmen sometimes talk as though food came naturally from tins and freezers, and it needed only the profit motive to keep the supply flowing forever; farmers know better. And the third point is that we're stuck with this world for a long time, and can't possibly rely upon short-term expedients. We have to think in terms of permanently sustainable systems."[8]

[8]Schumacher, 1974.

CHAPTER 7

Epilogue: What Can I Hope For?

I had hoped to open this section with a series of pictures. The first was to be a newspaper ad for *Glamour* magazine showing a brisk young woman in a floppy man-tailored suit striding toward the camera. The opening line of copy was **"A young woman's first priority today is herself. Openly so."** *Glamour* was very discouraging about giving permission to have its ad reprinted. So we have not printed it here. The second picture was to be an ad for *Playboy*. Its headline was **"Today's young men are no longer committed to poverty."** It pictured a smug-looking young man seated at a table filled with edible delicacies. At about the level of his elbow the ad copy read **"He doesn't worry about the future because 'that's tomorrow, and it's not worth a cent today.' He's very much focused into today and what he can do for himself today. Tomorrow's for tomorrow."** We didn't get permission to run that ad either. What you see below is what we did get permission to run. We assume it speaks for itself.

Keeping Up

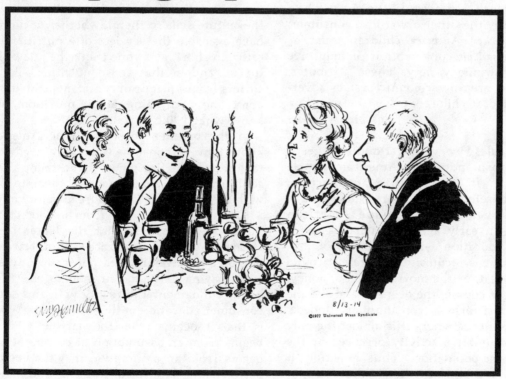

"Look, quit worrying—nothing's going to run out before we do."

Reprinted with permission from Universal Press Syndicate. Copyright 1977 by Universal Press Syndicate.

"We have met the enemy and he is us."
—Pogo

Consuming in the Year 2000

JOAN DYE GUSSOW

Homo sapiens trains his children for the roles they will fill as adults. This is as true of the Eskimo three-year-old who is encouraged to stick his little spear into a dead polar bear as it is of an American child of the same age who turns on TV to absorb commercials; the one will be a skilled hunter, the other a virtuoso consumer. In contemporary America children must be trained to *insatiable* consumption of impulsive choice and infinite variety. These attributes, once instilled, are converted into cash by advertising directed at children.

Jules Henry, 1965

As Jules Henry's bitter quote suggests, consumption is as American as apple pie. It seems quite appropriate, therefore, that there should be a growing movement to provide American children at an early age with what is called "consumer education"—usually a set of prescriptions for wise acquisition centered around getting the best, or the most, for one's money.

Eating is, of course, the original, and still the most universal form of consumption. (Indeed, there are countries where it is almost the only form of consumptive activity practiced by the majority of the population.) Thus, hopefully, it can be argued that a nutrition educator ought to be viewed as an expert in some kinds of consumption.

Unfortunately, nutrition educators have long tended to forget this fact, seeming to behave as if those they taught were ingesters merely of facts, and not of food. As Margaret Mead observed, "The educators have not differentiated food habits from any other type of habit. If children could be taught to write by the Palmer method... then they could be taught to eat foods which contained vitamins instead of foods that did not." Children, as it turns out, cannot be so taught. They, like everyone else, eat what the culture makes acceptable to them (or, in the case of contemporary America, what the culture sells to them), whether or not they have available the services of a nutrition educator. In short, everyone thinks he knows how to eat; and in that sense nutrition, like art, suffers from a plague of confident amateurs—"I don't know anything about nutrition, but I know what I like to eat."

In the broader sense, as well, Americans know how to consume, and they need to be taught only the fine points: to postpone signing contracts before they have read them; to check with the Better Business Bureau before buying a $300 living room set from a door-to-door salesman; to assume that the larger size is cheaper unless the unit price says otherwise; to buy bread by weight, and not by size, so as to avoid paying extra for air, and so on.

The fundamental difficulty with this sort of consumer education in the contemporary world is that it begins from too narrow a base. It begins from an assumption of consumption. It begins from an assumption that the choice is between one kind of dishwasher and another or, if you are a child, between one kind of plastic toy and another—when the real question ought to be whether you need any kind of dishwasher or plastic toy at all.

Early in 1973 Dr. John Knowles, president of the Rockefeller Foundation, spoke to the members of Washington, D.C.'s Urban Institute. He said that the world was coming close to the brink of a Malthusian disaster, with starvation and misery for millions. Dr. Knowles called for a new ethic of *austerity* for the United States as a world leader to help the world avoid disaster. There must be a new recognition, he went on to say, that world civilization is tightly interdependent, and that concern for conservation must replace the traditional concerns for production and growth. If Dr. Knowles is right, then real consumer education for the last quarter of the twentieth century ought to be education to teach people how not to consume at all unless absolutely necessary.

The inhabitants of the United States are the world's most diligent consumers. Less than 6 percent of the world's population, they manage to consume almost half of all the world's nonrenewable natural resources, about 35 percent of the world's total energy supply, and roughly a third of all the world's animal protein. The annual United States per capita consumption of cereal grains is almost twice that of Europe and close to four times that of the developing countries taken as a whole. In some places the disproportion is greater. Early in 1974 the per capita grain ration in Calcutta—for those who held ration cards—was cut from 4.6 to 4.4 pounds a week, an amount considerably less than the average American consumes (mostly in the form of milk, meat, and eggs) in a *day.*

Major Social Influence

Just as we consume more than our share of the world's material goods, we also consume the majority of the world's advertising. In 1973, the 210-million-odd people in the United States were exposed to some $23 billion worth of advertising—$115 worth per capita—while the 3-billion-plus people who make up the other 94 percent of the world's citizens, consumed only $12.5 billion dollars worth—that's about $4 apiece. Altogether we 6 percent of the world's people consumed 65 percent of the world's advertising.

That Americans are subjected to the majority of the world's advertising and consume a dis-proportionate share of the world's things are not unrelated facts, for the nation has achieved its dazzling level of consumption at least partly as a *result* of advertising. In a small and brilliant book, *People of Plenty,* first published some twenty years ago, historian David Potter pointed out that advertising in its flamboyant American manifestation began as a response to an astonishing level of abundance. "In a society of abundance," Potter wrote, "the productive capacity can supply new kinds of goods faster than society in the mass learns to crave these goods or to regard them as necessities. If this new productive capacity is to be used ... society must be adjusted to a new set of drives and values in which consumption is paramount."

The instrument of this consumption-adjustment was—and is—advertising. Advertising in America rapidly became an instrument of persuasion, the only institution we have had, Potter points out, for instilling new needs, for training people to act as consumers, for creating wants sufficient to exploit the country's productive capacity.

Potter saw advertising as being—like the school and the church—a major social influence; and he raises some unsettling questions about the effect on a society of having as one of its major instruments of social control an institution whose sole aim is to promote consumption. Leaving aside such moral questions, the point to be emphasized here is simply that the purpose of advertising at this time, in this country, is to stimulate wants and to instill needs, to promote consumption beyond need—i.e., overconsumption.

This is true whether the potential customer is a housewife who is being convinced that her private parts require deodorizing or a child who is being convinced that the last set of plastic people he acquired were nothing compared to the new improved version now available. Yet according to observers as astute as Dr. Knowles, the nation is coming into a time—is indeed in the midst of a time—when overconsumption (translated as waste) of any of the world's increasingly scarce resources is wrong.

Combatting Overconsumption

What can be done about the habits of over-consumption which advertising has encouraged and continues to encourage, now that the world is beginning to run short of many of the things it needs to survive? How can the next generation be helped to learn the real consumer wisdom for the coming decades—how *not* to consume, how to put the minimum burden on the planet earth?

Such questions are particularly poignant—and urgent—where food is concerned. Waste of anything, in a world of finite resources, is wrong—waste of food is obscene. On September 14, 1973, the *Wall Street Journal* published an article entitled "The Growing Threat of World Famine" in which the author, an agricultural development worker, showed that, if America and the other overdeveloped nations bid for the world's tightening supplies of food grains, they could drive prices high enough to make starvation inevitable for a number of hard-pressed developing countries. Recall that the $115 Americans invest per capita in advertising is somewhat more than the yearly per capita income of the world's 800 million poorest people.

The author of the article suggested a massive public service advertising campaign aimed at saving food, urging such voluntary steps as reduction in the size of restaurant portions, immediate commencement of planned diets on the part of potential dieters, and a reduction from two to one predinner drink—thus saving half of the grain used for alcohol. In September 1973, the need for action seemed urgent. Since then, despite a broadening awareness of the crisis and a near universal[1] agreement with the underlying premise of the projected campaign, there has been no organized public service effort to promote food conservation by any governmental body.

Margaret Mead once pointed out that it was difficult for overfed Americans to keep in mind that people elsewhere were starving because they were always having the experience of refusing food. It is also difficult to keep hunger in mind in an American supermarket or in front of an American television screen. Americans are encouraged to waste food—and to deal with it frivolously—at least in part by the very nature of the food products advertised and the appeals made on their behalf. Novelty, fun, sparkly colors and shapes, irresistible sweetness for children, and sexual or social triumph for adults are the characteristics to be sought in food, not repletion, true sociability, or survival.

So the first consumer education issue that needs addressing is absolutely fundamental, namely, what can be done about the cultural press toward consumption in a time of growing shortage. How shall we deal with an instrument of social control, advertising, which promotes self-indulgence, when we need to teach our children self-restraint? . . . If the world is to eat, our consumption of more than food must be restrained. It would be ironic, indeed, if our children's children had to live without spaghetti because in this energy-hungry generation it was decided we could not live without strip-mining the lands on which the nation grows its Durham wheat.

In some ecological circles these days, plans are going forward for the Post-Famine Society. Such resignation[2] ought not to be surprising. Warnings have been issued and ignored for a number of years. Paul Ehrlich exploded his *Population Bomb* in 1968; in 1967 the Paddocks told us there would be *Famine 1975*. There is. There is megafamine.

Obviously, things could be done to stave off widespread starvation. In the short term, the overfed nations could cut back on their own consumption to make available emergency food aid to the countries where famine is most imminent and most widespread. For the long term, of course, only population control and the development of a productive and sustainable agricultural capacity among the poorest farmers in the developing world can hope to stave off

[1]Federal officials, most notable among them Secretary of Agriculture Earl Butz, have been prominent exceptions.

[2]Or optimism—some would argue there will *be* no post-famine society at all.

disaster. As Robert McNamara of the World Bank has pointed out, the developed nations must funnel sufficient aid to the poor countries to enable them to begin to solve their own food and population problems, and the aid must be used (in some cases in near defiance of local leadership) to promote the kind of grass roots development that has been shown to be effective in reducing birth rates in developing countries where it has been tried. Population has begun to decline, historically, when death rates among children go down, when populations have hope that their own lives will be tolerable and their children's somewhat better, when social planning has provided some alternative to childbearing as the only form of old-age security.

A new study done for the Club of Rome by a German-American research team suggests that an investment reaching a level of $250 billion a year by the industrialized nations will be required if the developing nations are to become self-sufficient by the end of the century. The World Bank suggests the much more modest figure of $24 billion per annum by 1980 in order to keep the poorest countries from experiencing *negative* growth rates. Given the projected rates of growth of GNP, $24 billion would represent in 1980, .3 percent of the GNP of the developed aid-giving nations in that year. The United States' contribution to Official Development Assistance, however, has declined from 2.79 percent of the GNP in 1949 to less than one-third of 1 percent of the much larger 1970 GNP to a projected one-fifth of 1 percent by 1975.[3] Given such a penurious history at a time when our affluence was growing, it is doubtful that we shall be more generous when our own economic fortunes are on the decline. Tragically, we seem unable to use what economist Herman Daly has called "our scarce moral resources" to arrange a more equitable distribution of wealth—even within our own country.

Therefore, the *Food and People Dilemma*, in geographer Borgstrom's phrase, can only get worse. If these are realities, and each passing day makes their reality more inescapable, then we are obligated to prepare the coming generations to live *with honor* in the kind of world there will be for them to live in. And food being one of the three essentials for life (air and water being the others), some thought must be given to teaching diets suitable for the year 1990 and beyond.

But suppose—a dissenting voice replies—suppose the predictions prove wrong? Suppose a technological breakthrough once again discredits the neo-Malthusian prophets? Here, after all, is the voice of a United States Department of Agriculture economist speaking at Columbia University on the eve of the first World Food Conference. "We are very concerned about the world food situation . . . but in general there is well-founded hope. No, the world does not face a decisive battle between the forces of plenty and starvation. Yes, the neo-Malthusians are wrong."[4] Given such a countervailing optimism, how is it possible to propose a wholesale educational effort to change the diets of "the best fed people in the world"?

Diets for the Future

There are areas of life in which such a concern may be justified. Fortunately, diet is not one of them. In prescribing diets for the coming decades—even for the optimistic—it is easy to heed that ancient physicians' dictum *primum non nocere*—first do no harm. American diets are not, as it happens, the best in the world, if length of life and health in life are the criteria. The civilization of abundance has fallen far short of producing optimum health, producing instead an epidemic of obesity, heart disease, cancer, and other degenerative maladies. Despite an array of astonishing medical advances, life expectancy for those over twenty-one has increased hardly at all in decades.

[3]Compare the United States' projected .2 percent to Sweden's .7 percent of her GNP given as Official Development Assistance. In percent of its GNP given for ODA, the United States ranks fourteenth out of seventeen developed nations. Only Austria, Italy, and Switzerland give less.

[4]J.R. Barse, "World Hunger, Food and Farming," remarks at the Workshop on Hunger in the World, Earl Hall Center, Columbia University, New York, October 24, 1974, mimeo.

If one were to prescribe the dietary conduct which appears on the basis of present evidence to be most conducive to health, it would be very close to the diet which is most ecologically and morally responsible. The rules of such a diet are very simple. Eat only as many calories as are needed to attain and maintain normal weight; eat only nutritious foods—that is foods which contain significant amounts of protein, vitamins and/or minerals, and are not debased by excessive amounts of added fat or sugar; eat less fat, especially less animal fat; eat more fiber, especially that associated with whole grains and vegetables; and eat lower down on the food chain.

Eating only enough to maintain normal weight is perfectly consistent with a view of the world which says: Food is scarce—one ought to eat only what one needs and no more. In teaching children, it ought also to be made clear that to take a kind of Dorian Gray approach to gluttony—to maintain normal weight by eating food which is "calorie-free" because it is made with synthetic sweeteners and methylcellulose (which humans can't digest)—is obscene in a world where too many people can't get enough calories. Such foods consume energy without producing any.

Wasting food is equally wrong. It is not true, as earlier generations of children were taught, that cleaning up one's plate will help feed starving children elsewhere. Cleaning up one's plate will not do that. But putting onto the plate only as much as can be eaten, putting less on the table in the first place, and buying less to put on the table will both reduce the demand on the food supply and reduce the temptation to overeat. Waste of food (whether by eating too much of it or by throwing it away) implies that there is more of it than can be used. Tragically, because of maldistribution of money and resources, this is sometimes locally true; witness the recent wastage of calves. But in a world where food is increasingly recognized as a precious commodity, children ought to be taught, by deed as well as by word, that waste is wrong.

Choosing foods which are nutritious usually also means choosing foods which are minimally processed, since processing tends to destroy nutrients (requiring that such products have their vitamins "restored"). Unnecessary processing wastes not only nutrients, but energy and money as well. Consider the waste—nutritionally and energetically—in taking a nutritious cereal grain which contains all the nutrients for its own metabolism, stripping it of its vitamins and minerals, boiling and flattening it, toasting it, making some new nutrients and spraying them back on, dying it red, covering it with sugar and putting it—along with some red marshmallow bits—into a four-color printed box, calling it a breakfast cereal, distributing it all over the country, and selling it for $1.39 a pound. A country where such products are marketed to innocent children can hardly be expected to take food—or hunger—seriously.

Eating more "whole foods," as the British call them, means automatically that one will eat more fiber, since it is fiber that is removed in the processing of grains, and it is the lack of fiber that is now thought to be responsible for a host of civilization's ills, including that one for which generations of mothers prescribed "roughage." Fiber has also been displaced from the American diet as meat has come to occupy much of the space on the dinner plate once occupied by potatoes and other vegetables.

To eat more vegetables and less meat, more vegetable and less animal protein—in short, to move down on the food chain—goes happily with the prescription to eat less animal fat. It is not a question of recommending universal vegetarianism. If Dr. Butz is right that "we will always be a nation of meat eaters," it does not necessarily follow that we need be a nation of "beefaholics." Surely a country which has doubled its beef consumption in twenty years—to the apparent detriment of its health—can equally well halve its beef consumption without undue sacrifice.

In terms of the world food supply, the impact of living high on the cow has been widely discussed. The statistics are well known—it takes twenty-one pounds of plant protein to make one pound of beef protein—but according to the Livestock and Meat Board, one 10-oz. steak actually represents seventeen pounds of corn, five pounds of hay, and two pounds of protein supplement. Humans can live on plants, just as other animals can; indeed, most humans *do* live largely on plants. Since there is a loss of energy, as well as protein, with each step along the route from the primary energy source to the ultimate consumer, getting all, or even some, of our protein and energy from plants is more efficient than getting it from animals.

This thesis has been most eloquently put forward in recent years in a book entitled *Diet for a Small Planet.* The author of this small and influential volume has argued that the United States with its high consumption of "intensively" fed beef has become a kind of protein "sink" into which pour millions of tons of grains, legumes, fishmeal, and other foods which might otherwise be directly eaten by people. Since this conversion causes a large net reduction in the total food available, the more meat consumed the faster the world will run out of food. Through this is a grossly oversimplified statement of Ms. Lappé's thesis, the basic point is that grain-feeding of cattle—who are efficient converters of hay, grass, and other humanly inedible substances—is an inhumanely wasteful process in a world where men and women are competing for available stocks of grains.

The lessons then are simple. Eat less, waste less, eat less animal protein and animal fat, more vegetable proteins and other "whole foods." It is almost as simple to teach these lessons to our children. People eat, as was suggested earlier, what their culture makes it acceptable to them to eat. People eat what they like, but they also like what they eat. The next generations will eat as we eat, wastefully if we model wastefulness, frugally and responsibly if such is our lesson. There is no guarantee that such behavior will save the world. It is possible that nothing we can do will make any difference in the long run, given the proliferation of an atomic technology whose "peaceful" hazards are only now becoming fully evident. It is possible there will be no post-famine society at all. If there is, and if the neo-Malthusians are right, the way to eat well in the coming decades, the way to eat well while keeping in touch with one's own conscience, will be to learn to live happily lower down on the food chain—selecting foods for their nutrition as well as their taste, learning not to waste, learning not to overeat.

What is so astonishingly rewarding about these lessons in a time when so little gives cause for optimism is that they are wholly beneficial. For once it is not necessary to make a choice between the lesser of two evils. For even if the neo-Malthusians are wrong, children raised on diets designed for an austere world will be healthier than their parents, whatever kind of society they have to live in.

References

Borgstrom, G. *The Food and People Dilemma.* North Scituate, Mass.: Duxbury Press, 1973.

Butz, Earl L., "We Will Always be a Nation of Meat Eaters," address before the California Livestock Symposium, May 30, 1974. Quoted in CNI Weekly Report, June 13, 1974.

Committee on Food Habits. *Manual for the Study of Food Habits,* NAS-NRC Pub. 111. Washington, D.C.: U.S. Government Printing Office, 1945.

Daly, Herman, ed. *Toward a Steady State Economy.* San Francisco, Calif.: Freeman, 1973.

Ehrlich, Paul R. *Population Bomb.* New York, N.Y.: Sierra Club-Ballantine, 1968.

Henry, Jules. *Culture Against Man.* New York, N.Y.: Random House, 1965.

Lappé, F. M. *Diet for a Small Planet.* New York, N.Y.: Friends of the Earth-Ballantine, 1971.

McNamara, Robert, address to the Board of Governors of the World Bank, Washington D.C., September 30, 1974.

Mesarovic, M. and Pestel, E. *Mankind at the Turning Point.* New York, N.Y.: E. P. Dutton, 1974.

Paddock, W. and Paddock P. *Famine, 1975: America's Decision: Who Will Survive?* Boston, Mass.: Little, Brown, 1967.

Potter, D.M. *People of Plenty.* Chicago, Ill.: University of Chicago Press, 1954.

Revelle, Robert. "Food and Population," *Scientific American,* Vol. 231, September 1974, pp. 161-170.

Reprinted with permission from *Teachers College Record,* 76(4): 665-673 (May 1975).

Epilogue: What Can I Hope For?

"Indeed, I tremble for my country when I reflect that God is just."
—Thomas Jefferson, *Notes on the State of Virginia,* 1781-1785

"dear boss, i relay this information without any fear that humanity will take warning and reform."
—Don Marquis, *Archy and Mehitabel,* 1934

"I would feel more optimistic about a bright future for man if he spent less time proving that he can outwit Nature and more time tasting her sweetness and respecting her seniority."
—E. B. White, *Essays,* 1977

This chapter is probably unnecessary. Its existence may reflect an educator's unwillingness to end the lecture without a summing up, or the reluctance of a preacher to let the congregation depart without a call to repentance. Or, as I would urge, it may merely be that the optimist within will not let the book expire without hope.

The title of the volume, *The Feeding Web,* was suggested by my husband when all but this final chapter had been written. It says, in three well-chosen words, what I think all this is about. As I observed in the Prologue, our problem is that as living human organisms we are utterly dependent on complex foodstuffs for survival—and to make those complex foodstuffs we are utterly dependent upon the continued functioning of a feeding web—an as-yet-unfathomable set of biological interconnections maintaining the flows of energy and materials through living matter.

In one sense this book is circular—it begins and ends with limits to growth. But the limits it begins with tend to be physical, while the limits it ends with are biological. It is not the limited availability of *things* that is our most serious problem. It is the limited tolerance-to-disruption of processes. What will stop us in the end is not the fact that we cannot find more energy, fix more nitrogen, mine more potash, or impose more technological fixes; our problem is that in the process of doing so we are threatening to impair the very food-producing systems we are striving to "improve." In short, it's not that we *know* how much harm we are doing; it's that we don't.

Though we cannot at this moment predict how much further down this road we can go before we have irrevocably damaged those processes that sustain us; it is certain that the longer we simply keep moving on, the less room we will leave ourselves to maneuver. The message, therefore is: "Repent Now!...*or* the end of the world is at hand."

"Desist!" says the reader. "I am convinced. What I may hope for then is not that all this is untrue, not that everything will resolve itself if I simply ignore it. What then *can* I hope for—since you promised me optimism?" At least three things: 1) that it is not too late already; 2) that we are capable of change; and 3) that we can find out how to change in appropriate ways, in time.

Is the world salvageable? Or has our careless affluence so fouled our nest as to have already doomed future generations to starvation—or worse? It is always possible that we are, in biologist Paul Ehrlich's depressing but memorable phrase, "too far into the tube already"—in which case we will end up in the chronicles of life-on-earth as just one more failed species, albeit the one that did more damage than any other. Only time can provide a definitive reply to such an assertion.

But I would submit that the very same ignorance (of how the natural world *really* works) that argues against our heedless continuance, argues as well against hopeless pessimism. We cannot *know* whether it is too late unless we fully understand how Nature operates—and if we wait until then to take action, it may well *be* too late. It is the same kind of argument that one must ultimately use against *triage*. Certainly if we go on as we are, we will find ourselves, probably within the lifetimes of many now living, too far into the tube. But to assume that it is already too late on the basis of fragmentary evidence, is to counsel inaction; and to counsel inaction is to opt for the continuance of present trends, which will lead inevitably to the self-destruction of humanity—even if some human beings survive.

Hope is, in short, essential to our survival, as Eric Bentley recently pointed out. For "if the minimum commitment is to continuation, persistence, survival, the maximum commitment is to changing the world. Clearly if we don't believe the world can be changed, that is going to be a self-fulfilling prophecy and the world will not be changed. It is worth seeing if it can be changed by acting on the assumption that it can."[1]

Which brings us to the second thing we must hope for: that humans are capable of change—that we are capable of learning to *want* to save the world, even if there is a cost in terms of our own material comfort. Linda Stewart's essay which opens the book expresses confidence in humanity's ability to become more self-sacrificing—even if *she* could not stop smoking.

My students are less sanguine about our prospects for salvation. Sometime along in my course they always need a session on "hope." They are, by that time, well beyond the hope that they can simply deny the need for change. They believe we are in trouble, and they want me to tell them why they should hope that "selfish" humanity *can* or *will* reform.

And the tenor of what they say is this: "Here are we, people concerned with the food supply; yet we did not know until now that farmers were in trouble; we did not know of energy costs and topsoil losses and acid rain and of the frightening persistence of toxins in our food chain. What we have read and heard seems to us to be the truth, but that truth has not made us—even us—free. Even we yearn for 'convenience,' so how can others change? We know a hundred reasons not to buy those foolish and unhealthy foods. Still we do."

Children of the TV generation, they are stunned to recognize the depth of their own and their culture's conditioning. "Are all of us," they ask despairingly, "irrevocably ruined? Are we so permeated with 'pecuniary pseudo-truth' and so corrupted by 'monetization,' that we are as a people no longer capable of rational action—even rational action on behalf of our own survival?"

They are, in their anguish, their own best answer. Of course they—and we—can change; but what they fear is what others have feared before them, the socially noxious character of the citizens produced by a culture so dedicated to consumption.

The only reading I have included in this chapter is an essay written when "the food crisis" was on every front page. It raises some questions about the lessons our consumer society teaches its children about food. The same questions have been raised more broadly by economist Robert Heilbroner in a recent book, *Business Civilization in Decline*. A business civilization like ours, he points out, is based on the underlying assumption that social contentment will result when man is freed from material insufficiency. But we have neglected to take into account "the extraordinary subversive influence of the relentless effort to persuade people to change their lifeways, not out of any knowledge of, or deeply held convictions about the 'good life,' but merely to sell whatever article or service is being pandered."[2]

What will destroy a business civilization, he says, is at least partly the character of the citizens it produces and its tendency to "substitute impersonal pecuniary values for personal nonpecuniary

[1] Eric Bentley, "Despair and Hope." *The New York Times* (3 September 1977).

[2] Robert L. Heilbroner, *Business Civilization in Decline*, p. 113 (New York: W. W. Norton & Company, Inc., 1977).

ones"—what Jules Henry called the "monetization" of values. When a society substitutes things for relationships, it turns out that there are never enough *things* to create satisfaction. Thus the risk, if we continue our headlong ways, is not merely that the earth will be unable to tolerate the demands which our insatiableness induces us to make, but that, in the end, we will not be able to tolerate ourselves—or each other.

Yet if we have been made to be as we are, then clearly we can make ourselves different. And, as Leon Eisenberg has taken pains to point out,[3] how we think about ourselves will help to determine what we can become. "What we believe of man affects the behavior of men, for it determines what each expects of the other . . . Is [man] educable? Is he actuated only by self-interest? Is he a creature of such dark lusts that only submission to sovereign authority can save him from himself? . . . What we choose to believe about the nature of man has social consequences."

"Pessimism about man," he continues, "serves to maintain the *status quo*. It is a luxury for the affluent, a sop to the guilt of the politically inactive, a comfort to those who continue to enjoy the amenities of privilege . . . Man is his own chief product."

And even now, ceaselessly urged as we are to give in to ourselves, not all of us are *Playboys* or *Glamour* Girls, irrevocably committed to living for ourselves forever. If there is anything that makes humanity uniquely human, it is our capacity to escape our programming, to imagine the future and to take steps to change it. If we refuse to imagine it, or if, imagining it, we turn away to more immediately pleasurable activities, then it will be clear we have abandoned something of what makes us human, in which case we will surely deserve our fate as a species.

Thus, I find I must operate on the assumption that the truth, continually searched for, *will* make us free; and I do not find these readings depressing, or the prospects they imply gloomy. Yet in the face of my students' yearly despair, I have had to ask myself why I feel that way. The first year I taught the course that inspired this book, a student came up to me after one especially doom-filled class and said with some asperity, "I think you're completely wrong. *I* think things are getting better and better." I, of course, disagreed. Then she went on, "Anyway, if you believe all this, I don't see how you can go on living." My response was flippant, conditioned by what I sensed was her approaching pain. "You have to have a good sense of humor," I said.

You do, of course, but that is not the whole truth. My answer did not explain how I have traversed the anxiety associated with coming to accept the unsustainability of the American Way of Eating; or how I have come out the other end with optimism. How had I come to accept almost cheerfully the need for changes I wasn't certain we could make peacefully—if at all?

I believed for a time that my optimism arose from my having grown up before World War II, before "the Bomb," at a time when *everyone* knew the only wars America fought were "just," at a time when *everyone* knew things would get back to "normal." But though the seeds of my hopefulness were perhaps planted by the fact of my birth in a more hopeful time, they have been nourished by more contemporary events.

It is only in writing this book that I have come to understand the real reason why I am not depressed by the pile-up of evidence that "mastery-over-nature" has failed, that technological optimism is romantic, that the world as we know it will have to be differently organized if we are to succeed as a species. My present optimism arises out of a conviction that increasing numbers of ordinary citizens are viewing with horror the automated, effort-free future the official "optimists" predict for us. They are finding it considerably less tolerable in its implications for our freedoms, our health and our sanity, than what is billed as a somewhat "lower standard of living." "If we're so rich," they are asking "why ain't we happy?"

---

[3]Leon Eisenberg, "The Human Nature of Human Nature," *Science* (14 April 1972).

I grew up in an era when "progress" went in only one direction, toward those *Popular Mechanics'* cities of the future, dominated by exotic freeways, climate controlled buildings, and "streamlined" cars. I grew up in Los Angeles at a time when that "modernistic" vision had yet to impose itself on the city—when orange groves still covered much of the land, when towering eucalyptus trees made lushly romantic windbreaks, when from most of that once-barren coastal plain you could see the mountains every day. I have seen Los Angeles progress toward the future, and like increasing numbers of Californians (and other less exotic Americans) I have come to the conclusion that such a future will not work, for us or for the rest of the world.

In accepting a high technology vision of the future as inevitable, we have sacrificed community for "progress," meaning for possessions, nurture for conquest, contentment for envy. "All societies, optimally, must allow for both change and stability," Philip Slater has written. "Our society... has traditionally handled the problem by giving completely free rein to technological change and opposing the most formidable obstacles to social change." But since technological change *forces* social change, he points out, we end up leaving our social structures in the hands of a "whimsical deity.... Our relation to change is entirely passive. We poke our noses out the door each day and wonder breathlessly what new disruptions technology has in store for us. We talk of technology as the servant of man, but it is a servant that now dominates the household, too powerful to fire, upon whom everyone is helplessly dependent."[4]

And in this "progressive" world we have lost our connections to the real sources of life and community. Food—the getting, preparing, and consuming of which has been a major organizing force in human society through most of history—we have reduced to a triviality. How easy it is to forget that within the lifetimes of many still living, a majority of the American people were still directly involved with the natural cycles that control food production. The extent to which we have been "freed" from that dependence on the land has long been seen as one of the major indicators of our advancement toward an earthly Nirvana. Yet a remarkable recent book by farmer-poet Wendell Berry reminds us that in the "unsettling of America," in the detachment of us as a people from our land, may lie the root of much of our present social unrest.[5]

To paraphrase Thomas Huxley, what is the end to which this food system is the means? Is it optimal nutrition for the greatest number? Is it health and well-being? Is it, in Berry's phrase, "kindly use" of the earth's valuable resources? Is it maximization of the length of humanity's sojourn on this planet? Is it "right livelihood?" Is it *really* living the good life?

Our food supply is full of fun and devoid of joy. Devoid, like much of our lives, of meaning or of connections to other living things. "The American Indians might say we have forgotten our mother the earth," one observer has written. "Do not all we creatures—people, grasses, birds, trees—drink of her creation? The clang of the quarter in the food vending machine makes it difficult to see this as suckling the breast of Mother Earth... Other cultures prepare with sacred care the things they eat. Our 'ritual sanctification' consists of the multitude of processes and chemicals that transformed the milk of the earth into our food. Stouffer's Frozen Spinach Soufflé. Screaming Yellow Zonkers."[6] Food comes from the land. We have forgotten that. If we do not learn it again, we will die.

We have trivialized food. In retaliation our food supply has made us helpless. Millions of American men, women and children are largely dependent for their sustenance on food products which have recipes for use written neatly on their labels. ("Eat me," they read, like the currants on the small cake in Alice in Wonderland. And with even less foresight than Alice—we do.)

[4]Philip Slater, *The Pursuit of Loneliness*, p.44.

[5]Wendell Berry, *The Unsettling of America, Culture and Agriculture* (San Francisco: Sierra Club, 1977).

[6]Philip Snyder, "Taking In and Giving Out: Food for Thought," *Human Ecology Forum*, 3: 5-7 (Spring 1973).

We have a generation of college graduates who do not know what to do with fresh spinach or a head of broccoli; and we are well into a second generation of Minute Rice users, "cooks" for whom Minute Rice is just like mother used to make. We are dependent upon experts to tell us what is nutritious, experts to tell us what is safe, experts to give us instructions on food acquisition and use. Mothers used to count on their senses to tell them whether a food was fit for their families, Ross Hall reminds us,[7] and now that food technology has managed to separate palatability from both safety and nutrition, we have tried to turn the Food and Drug Administration into a surrogate mother who will assure us of the safety, or at any rate the harmlessness, of the food objects about which our senses can no longer reliably instruct us.[8]

We have thus become dependent upon specialists while, as Wendell Berry points out, we ourselves are "freed" to occupy ourselves with one or another specialized task at which we make money to pay the specialists who control the remainder of our lives. Increasingly, these specialists include "mental health experts" who help us deal with the intolerable anxiety our progress has produced. But our anxiety is appropriate, says Berry. It is a warning to us that something is wrong. What is wrong is that we are helpless.

Are we not, in fact, more helpless than any people before us, less able to fend for ourselves, more cut off from the sources of nourishment? What would we do if we could not get to a supermarket? Is not our panic when they threaten to deprive us of our saccharin a frightening signal of our dependence? Could anything be worse than such pitiful vulnerability? Is it not more intolerable to live in a state of such anxious dependence, wondering when the next technological miracle will demand another human concession, than it is to plunge in, examine the alternatives and work to make the future compatible with *human* life? I believe that increasing numbers of Americans are coming to such a conclusion.

But how are we to free ourselves from this dependence? How can we escape "the system"? Some people have begun to look for ways for all of us to escape. But it would be foolish to suggest that it is, at this moment, easy. It is not always even *possible* in the short run, especially for those whose very livelihood depends, at least in the short run, on the continued functioning of the present food system.

What does a farmer do when *not* to spray his orchard with a suspected carcinogen will make his pears cosmetically unacceptable and hence unmarketable—thus helping to drive that farmer out of agriculture? What does a responsible food company, or a responsible food company employee, do when *not* to produce a new unneeded product results not merely in reduced company profits, but in the disappearance of hundreds of jobs? Or, as a *Wall Street Journal* reporter put it to me once after I had made it clear that I found the idea of fortifying Coca Cola profoundly troubling, "What would you do if you were the president of Coca Cola and suddenly developed a social conscience?" My reply, after a long pause, was that I would probably fortify Coca Cola.

And though I find I am content to leave to our economists the difficult question of how we can stop overconsuming without precipitating a depression, the moral issue seems to me to be more difficult. Like Hardin's responsible citizen who—listening to appeals to reduce population growth— has no more children, thus helping to breed conscience out of existence, the orchardist who refused to spray, or the corporation executive who suddenly proposed withdrawal from a profitable food market on the grounds of conscience, would each surely be replaced by someone less morally constrained. So, in time, we could breed all responsibility out of the food business. Thus, it must be

---

[7]Ross Hall, *Food for Nought, The Decline of Nutrition* (New York: Harper & Row, 1974).

[8]For a brilliant discussion of television's contribution to the confusion of our sense systems, see Jerry Mander's "Four Arguments for the Elimination of Television," *Co-Evolution Quarterly*, 16: 38-52 (Winter 1977-78).

seen as a matter of no small privilege where food is concerned, to be able to speak and act in concert with your conscience.

But merely because personal change is presently difficult, painful, and sometimes unacceptably expensive to individuals, does not argue that such conversions cannot and will not take place. If, as I believe, personal morality and social responsibility are much more widely desired than may be obvious, individuals given the chance to act unselfishly will surely do so; they need only the existence of social and economic structures that reward instead of punish such behaviors.

And so we come to the final hope that reality permits: the hope that there are answers, that change will happen, and that it will happen in time. I have struggled for months over what this chapter ought to contain—since it was originally conceived as a parallel to the "hope" session I conduct for my students. (That session now comes at the end of the semester—students having become more tolerant of despair—and is usually called "Yes, but what can I do?")[9] Over time, I have included in the session various reading about ideas, people, or organizations which I thought might suggest directions or models for action to the students. Thus, in thinking about this chapter I have contemplated including everything from an *Appropriate Technology* article on "Restoring Esteem for Green Leafy Vegetables," to an essay on "Industrial and Post-Industrial Images on Man" which appeared recently in *The Ecologist*. In the end, I have included no readings at all, except—as I indicated earlier—one of my own.

The reasons for this are twofold: one practical, one philosophical. The practical reason is simply this. There has been a truly Malthusian growth in the numbers of groups seriously "into" alternative ways of organizing both what they take from and what they give back to the environment; so that any selection of readings about "food chain pioneers of the future" would be entirely arbitrary, based more on those I happened to have room for than on any judgement of their relative worthiness.

If you accept the fact that all of man's activities that affect the environment are ultimately related to food (and the underlying fact that all of man's activities *do* affect the environment), then the extent of the problem will be manifest. For example, as earlier sections in this volume were intended to emphasize, all individuals and groups concerned with alternative energy sources are working on food chain issues: *ergo*, the Center for Rural Affairs in Walthill, Nebraska has set up a Small Farm Energy Project designed to guide plains farmers to greater profits through energy independence.

The remarkable depth and extensiveness of what one might call the "alternatives network" first came to my attention several years ago when I became concerned with the issue of appropriate farm size and sent for a bibliography on U. S. land reform. With the bibliography came a two or three page list of *organizations* working on land-ownership issues. Until that time I had not imagined that there were more than a few dozen individuals so involved.

Since then I have learned about literally hundreds of organizations devoted in one way or another to searching out what will be the appropriate parts of an appropriate food system. They are engaged in everything from organizing farmer's markets in New York City to raising backyard rabbits in San Francisco. They are reading, and writing for, a multitude of alternative publications, not all of them as phenomenally successful as the "Good Housekeeping" of the alternatives movement, *Mother Earth News*, which is based down in Hendersonville, North Carolina. *Mother* refers to itself editorially as MOTHER, describes itself as "more than a magazine...a way of life," and puts heavy emphasis on "alternative lifestyles, ecology, working with nature, and doing more with less." It is "into"

[9]The title was stolen from a special issue of *The New Internationalist*, which came out several years ago and was devoted to brief descriptions of various groups all around the world "doing something" to combat indifference, pollution, waste, nuclear plants, hunger, selfishness, and other negative influences standing in the way of a new age.

homesteading. Were it not for this country's tendency toward faddism, it would be easy to be encouraged by the fact that in December of 1977 MOTHER had 2,154 *lifetime* subscribers (at $350 a throw) and that its expanding regular subscription list is widely considered one of the publishing phenomena of the decade.

MOTHER's success may be less encouraging in the light of the report in the summer 1977 issue of *The Co-Evolution Quarterly* that the most popular monograph ever produced by the Stanford Research Institute's Business Intelligence Program was entitled *Voluntary Simplicity*. This account of a growing movement among relatively affluent people to give up material excesses and to find a "new balance between inner and outer growth"[10] reported to the business community that people who didn't want to buy very much were members of the fastest growing "market." Skepticism is healthy: too many trends toward simplicity in this country have ended up as markets for pre-faded jeans.

But whether or not MOTHER's subscribers actually raise goats, build solar ovens, and forage for clams, or only want to stay in touch with those who do; and whether or not the readers of *Voluntary Simplicity* are "into" alternative life styles or are merely trying to find a way to make simplicity sell, it is impossible to spend any amount of time dipping into the alternative publications without being convinced that something authentic is going on out there.

In various parts of the country groups of gleaners now follow the harvesting machinery into the fields, salvaging formerly wasted but still usable food to be used to feed the hungry here and abroad. In Woods Hole, Massachusetts, and more recently in Prince Edward Island, the New Alchemists experiment with self-sufficient "Arks," structures whose windmills and passive solar systems are designed to make them energy independent, and whose greenhouses are intended to produce sale-able food in excess of the needs of their inhabitants. In a somewhat less rural setting, Washington D.C.'s Institute for Local Self-Reliance devotes itself to rooftop food growing and basement fish culture, and to economic analyses which deal with restoring the self-sufficiency and viability of neighborhood communities.

In my more metaphorical moments, I have seen the likely end point of all these scattered activities as being similar to what happens when you pour a packet of dry yeast into a mixture of honey and warm water. The yeast falls to the bottom and the water gets cloudy, and for ten minutes or so nothing appears to be happening. Then, if you don't stir the mix, puffy mounds of growing yeast pop up to the surface—and cover it. To anyone who attends to the signs, it is clear that the yeast, while hardly visible, is working.

Last year at my university in New York we had a conference to bring together local farmers who wished to farm in an ecologically responsible way and co-ops who were looking for local sources of good food. For two days the halls of the university were filled with bearded young men (and some who were not so young) in lumbermen's shirts and jeans, and with young women in jeans or long dresses, some of them nursing babies. Backpacks were piled up along the edges of the corridors, since it was a two-day conference and most of the participants were going to sleep on the floor of the Barnard Gym. It looked like the return of the 1960's except that there was no rock concert going on and everyone was there to learn and work. They were friendly, cooperative (when the workshops got off to a late start, they simply started without the conference organizer), committed, and hard working.

The following Monday, one of my faculty colleagues laughingly said to me, "I didn't know there were that many of those people left."

"They aren't 'those people'," I replied. "They're the generation after; and they're determined to make it work."

---

[10]Duane Elgin and Arnold Mitchell, "Voluntary Simplicity (3)," *The Co-Evolution Quarterly*, 14:4 (Summer 1977).

What is "it"? What are they working toward? Responsibility toward themselves, the land, the food it produces, the next generation. Alternative forms of social organization that will replace those business-society values that have not given us the happiness they promised. And there are a lot of "them," so many, in fact, that as I said earlier, I have not chosen to end this book with a little list because no "little" list would do.

As I also said earlier, there is a second reason for not including any specific "solutions" in this chapter, a philosophical reason. It has to do with what I believe to be the nature of the ultimate resolution of our population/food/resource *problematique*. The ultimate solution is to come to terms with the fact that there is no ultimate solution—and that "they" won't solve "it" for us.

We are in trouble partly because we have been seduced by the chimera of the ultimate material superlative. We have sought not the good life, but the best life through possession of the whitest wash, the strongest glue, the sweetest cereal, the fastest drain cleaner, the slowest catsup and the sexiest blue jeans. Yet we know from experience that each "best" will be followed by an even better best which "they" will provide for us. They will not make things better. We must. This is what the alternatives network is about.

There is not one person, or ten people, or a hundred or a thousand who know what to do in this nation, on this continent, on this globe. There are only local men and women working to find ways of living that will allow for the preservation—in their communities and regions—of those things which they have come to understand must be preserved for the sake of the long-range survival (and rehumanization) of the species.

How will we get there? *If* we get there it will surely be by a great variety of paths, each of them in its own way respectful of the earth and its systems. For if there is no single answer, there is at least a single criterion which can be applied in judging the reasonableness of particular "solutions": they must reflect both global awareness and local reality.

In the very first reading in this volume, Linda Stewart began with the observation that the reason we have so much difficulty in conceiving that the world might end is that it has never ended before. It was a while before I understood that her assumption is really untrue. The world has, of course, ended before. It ended for the Indians who built Mesa Verde, for the sophisticated builders who constructed Machu Picu, for the Mayans who piled up those huge and mysterious earth-mounded pyramids in the Yucatan jungle. And on other continents it ended for the Greeks, and before them for the Etruscans, and for the Egyptians—several times. For the world is only as large as any culture knows it is. The limits of the world are what one knows those limits to be; and if the worlds that have ended before were less than planetary in extent, their end was no less total for that. So the world has ended before, and men have worried before that the world *would* end, and sometimes they have been wrong, and sometimes they have been right.

The threatened end of the world then is not new. What *is* new is that to an extent never before known in the history of mankind, we are fully aware of the *real* boundaries of our world (if not of the real limits of its biological systems). We have even seen our globe, with its fragile crust of green, from space. Hence, we *must* cooperate. As Barbara Ward reminded us in Chapter 2, we must love one another, or we die. "The idea of brotherhood is not new. What is special to our times is that brotherhood has become the precondition for survival."[11]

What we know for a certainty now is that it will not do for anyone anywhere to destroy carelessly his ozone layer (whether with spray cans or nitrogen fertilizer) since it is our ozone layer too. Too much release of CO_2 (whether from careless destruction of forests in the underdeveloped countries or from heavy use of fossil fuels in the overdeveloped ones) will inundate indiscriminately the

[11]Eisenberg, *op. cit.*

coastlines of every continent—if the "greenhouse effect" produces melting of the polar icecaps. If waterways anywhere become dumping grounds for toxic wastes, it is mankind's oceans that will be defiled. So to focus on the local is not to urge a new kind of anarchy, a 1980's version of "doing your own thing," but a new kind of responsibility and self-restraint in which we, of all peoples, could be a voluntary model to the world.

And since we do not know what is ecologically optimal even on a small scale, we must encourage a multitude of experiments aimed at finding ways of living carefully on the planet. I am grateful to have discovered in the writing of an anthropologist the very useful term *relocalization* to encompass many of the changes that look most promising where the food supply is concerned. It is the very essence of relocalization that there is no single group, no single solution, no applicable universal that will work—except that we must all move toward a way of living more lightly on the earth. We must not keep looking for "the" way, but settle (perhaps even with some relief) for "a" way which seems to solve many different kinds of problems at once in a given locale.

Saving Massachusetts' farmland turns out not only to preserve open land as an amenity, and to sustain Massachusetts' farmers as a knowledge resource, but to decrease the dependence of Massachusetts' citizens on food "imported" at a high energy cost from elsewhere. Groups like the Center for Studies in Food Self-Sufficiency in Vermont are well-along in investigating the feasibility of a largely Vermont-based diet. Such alternatives seem extreme to many people, the food choices they offer so restricted as to be absurd and intolerable. But in a time when a snow storm or a truckers' strike can cut off all food from a city the size of Boston, such research is surely at least as potentially useful as that aimed at designing one more packaged cake mix.

It is part of the source of my optimism that ideas which once seemed merely wistful have given way first to serious consideration, then to dedicated investigation, and finally to trial. The idealistic notion that small children should not be sold sugar on television is moving, on the day I write this, from an increasingly tolerable idea to a matter of active consideration before the Federal Trade Commission. The "absurd" notion that city people might even grow some of their own food became less absurd with the publication of *The City People's Book of Raising Food*, and took on a mainstream cast when agricultural extension agents were assigned to cities to teach food growing to the urban poor. The late Dr. E. F. Schumacher milled his own wheat and baked his own bread because he believed that we all had to start somewhere.

It turns out to be very hard to end a book such as this, since to be open to change means that what seem like the right answers at the time one begins a chapter may be modified by events, or the changed perception events evoke, before one has brought it to completion. But just last week I came across what seemed to be the right conclusion—in both meanings of the word—for this chapter and for the book.

I was looking through an issue of *Family Health* and was stopped short by the headline: "If I Die Tomorrow, It Ain't Going to be My Fault!" The article, an interview with Dr. John Knowles of the Rockefeller Foundation, was largely about health, and about the steps Knowles personally was taking, and believed others should take, to stay healthy. Ultimately the discussion turned to Knowles' view of the world, a view, I will venture, similar to the one put forward in this book. The interviewer's last question was: "That's a very grim picture you paint, yet you call yourself an optimist."

I would like to let Knowles' final words stand for my own: "I'm practical about these things, but I think there is great hope in the world. There are substantial numbers of well-intentioned, well-educated people who are passionately committed to making things better in this country and around the world. They are working hard on these problems and making substantial gains. I gotta be an optimist. If I wasn't laughing, I'd be crying. I mean, why else would I be knocking myself out?"[12]

Joan Gussow
Congers, New York

February 28, 1978

[12]Carol Kahn, "If I Die Tomorrow, It Ain't Going to be My Fault!" *Family Health*, pp. 43-45 (February 1978).

Index